the manual of dental assisting

4e

Dental Assistants' Association of Australia Incorporated

Edited by Leah Vern Barnett, BA, DipEd, MEd

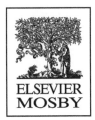

ELSEVIER
MOSBY

Sydney Edinburgh London New York Philadelphia St Louis Toronto

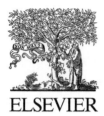

ELSEVIER

Mosby
is an imprint of Elsevier

Elsevier Australia
Tower 1, 475 Victoria Avenue, Chatswood, NSW 2067

This edition © 2005 Elsevier Australia
(a division of Reed International Books Australia Pty Ltd)
ACN 001 002 357

This book has been previously published as the *Dental Assistants' Manual*, NSW Dental Assistants' Association.

National Library of Australia Cataloguing-in-Publication Data

The manual of dental assisting.
4th ed.
Includes index.
ISBN 0 7295 3737 4.
1. Dentistry. I. Dental Assistants' Association of
Australia.
617.6

Publisher: Vaughn Curtis
Developmental Editor: Rhiain Hull
Edited, project-managed, proofread and indexed by Forsyth Publishing Services
Picture research and coordination by Lisa Petroff
Cover by Modern Art Production Group
Illustrators: Shelly Communications Pty Ltd and Joe Lucia Diagraphics
Internal design and typesetting by Grizzly Graphics
Printed and bound in Australia by Griffin Press

Contents

acknowledgments

The Dental Assistants' Association of Australia Inc (DAAA) was formed in 1939 under the name of the Nurses' Club. Its members worked voluntarily helping dentists with their war effort in keeping the armed services members' teeth in good condition, so they could go to fight in World War II.

The association became the professional voice for dental assistants and held training evenings throughout the following years. Specialist dentists were invited to give lectures on dental subjects and together with the Dental Assistants' Committee gave their time as voluntary workers.

In 1956, the first training course was commenced with 32 dental assistant students. With the assistance of the Australian Dental Association, the education standards were formed to comply with the professional ethics and goals of dentistry. Today, the educational activities of the association remain the focal point. The first dental assistants' manual was published in 1967.

This text has been developed as a comprehensive resource, replacing the third edition of that text; *Dental Assistant's Manual: An Australian text*. All chapters have been updated and modified to take into account the latest techniques, equipment and materials. All information in this text complies with Australian Standards.

It is a great pleasure to be associated with Elsevier Australia in the development of the fourth edition of *The Manual of Dental Assisting*. Thanks to Vaughn Curtis, Rhiain Hull, Helena Klijn and the publishing team at Elsevier Australia, and to the copyeditor, Jon Forsyth.

The Dental Assistants' Association of Australia Inc wishes to extend its deepest gratitude to the dentists and dental assistants who generously contributed their time and extensive expertise in the following areas:

Dr Ernie Altman — General and oral pathology
Preventive dentistry and oral health promotion
Communication
Dr Brian Vern-Barnett — Removable prosthodontics
Dental radiography
Dr Graham Thomas —   General and head and
neck anatomy
Dr Melissa Kah —   Fixed prosthodontics
Dr Kevin Todes —   Periodontics
Dr Angus Kingon — Oral surgery
Anaesthesia and sedation
Prof Anthony Martin — Endodontics
Mrs Dee MacPherson and
Dr Keith Powell —Orthodontics
Dr Sarah Raphael and Dr Kareen Mekertichian —
Paediatric Dentistry
Dr Emma Jay and Dr Roger Lindsay — Dentistry
for the aging
Dr Emma Jay — Patients with special needs
Dr Alex Forrest — Forensic odontology
Dr Tony Zahra — Implant dentistry
Dr Nectarios Andrews — Oncology patients
Linda Hunter and Barbara Hayes — Clinical and
office duties
Anne Fahey OAM— Occupational health and
safety

Editorial contributors
Kathy Vern-Barnett OAM
Leah Vern Barnett

Special mention must be made of the contribution of Kathy Vern-Barnett who co-ordinated this complex and time-consuming project over several years and who did so in a voluntary capacity.

Marie Wells CDAA
President
Dental Assistants' Association of Australia Inc

introduction
to Certificate III in Dental Assisting

Welcome to the fourth edition of *The Manual of Dental Assisting*.

This book is intended to be the teaching and learning text for the nationally accredited Dental Assistant Certificate III course. Job satisfaction comes from a job well done. The more underpinning knowledge you have, the better you can understand the processes and techniques that you work with every day.

The text will be a useful reference for dental assistants who are being trained on the job and for members of the dental health team who are responsible for providing supervision and training.

It will also be a useful reference for experienced dental assistants who wish to refresh some of their underlying knowledge and check that their day-to-day procedures comply with current legislation and standards.

Dental assistants wishing to further their studies, for example by completing a Certificate IV, after achieving a Certificate III in Dental Assisting will also find this a useful reference. Ongoing study will improve your interest level in your work, increase your chances of advancement, open new career paths to you and make you a more competent dental assistant.

We wish you all the best with your studies and with a fulfilling career in dental assisting.

How to use this book

Content

Each of the sections in this book focuses on an aspect of your work in the dental practice.

- Section 1 is a general introduction to dental assisting with information about the non-clinical aspects of your work.

- Section 2 focuses on human biology and will introduce you to the terms and concepts that are the underlying basis for all the clinical work that you do.

- Section 3 covers clinical dentistry and describes the day-to-day work undertaken in a dental practice.

- Section 4 focuses specifically on restorative dentistry, which will probably be the most frequent type of dentistry that you will assist with.

- Section 5 describes preventive dentistry techniques.

- Section 6 briefly outlines specialist areas of dentistry.

- Section 7 provides information and advice for those dental assistants seeking employment.

The Study Skills at the end of this section contains information that will help you to successfully complete your studies and/or training.

Glossary

Down the side of each page are brief definitions of new terms as they are introduced to the text. The terms that appear in this page-side glossary are highlighted in bold in the text the first time that they appear.

A more comprehensive glossary appears at the end of the book. Look to this glossary for more detailed and additional definitions. You might like to write some of these definitions onto the page-side glossaries as a reminder and aid to understanding if there are terms that you find difficult.

Procedures

Some frequently used procedures have been identified and placed in boxes through the text. You may wish to copy these procedures to a laminated sheet and keep them as a handy reminder in appropriate places throughout the practice/clinic.

Appendix

At the end of the text is an appendix where you will find lists of useful contacts for your local area. Duties and legislation relating to the tasks undertaken by the dental team vary from state to state and are regularly updated. It is not possible for this text to cover all variations for all states. You should consult the organisations listed in the appendix for the most up to date information for your location.

Study skills

Some general tips

Start each study session with an achievable goal in mind. Reading a long chapter and hoping to remember it all may not be a very efficient use of your time. Instead, work on a shorter section, take some notes, draw some pictures, test yourself. Revise what you did in your last session and plan what you will do in your next. Perhaps set yourself a little test to do when you next sit down to study.

People have different learning styles. Some people really need to see something written down before they can make sense of it. Others need a picture. Some people like to hear something explained. Other people benefit from using or making a working model or by colouring in anatomical drawings, for example.

Try to work out what your learning style is because by understanding how you learn best, you can improve your speed and depth of learning.

Do some mental 'warm-ups'. For example, try to jot down from memory the key points from your last lecture or tutorial, or what you were reading the day before.

Have a regular place of study. It doesn't need to be the only place you study but it should feel like it's your own working space and should set the mood for a productive study session. Try to have a good chair, good light and writing materials at hand.

Have regular breaks where you stretch, walk around, have a drink of water and assess how the study session is going. Do you need to change your goals for the session? Do you need to make a list of questions or problems to take to the next tutorial?

If you are having a real problem with a concept, it may be time to take a break, particularly if you are tired. Go back to the problem with a fresh outlook the next day.

Time management

It is important to try to set yourself a routine and stick to it. Studying can be difficult when you are tired or stressed but sometimes the discipline can actually make you feel better. Try to stick to a timetable of study for a few weeks and then take time out to consider whether it is working for you or if it needs 'tweaking'.

Find the optimal study time for you. Some people like to have an uninterrupted, extended block of time to work. Others prefer a series of shorter, more focused periods.

Before you can develop a plan, you need to think realistically about your regular time commitments. Make yourself a chart into which you can mark your usual week. Don't forget to mark in travel time, time for family and friends, exercise, work time, class time, shopping, cooking, cleaning, eating, washing and your other commitments.

Next make a list of all the study activities you need to do each week, such as:

- pre-reading to prepare for lectures and tutorials (the more you know about a topic before you go in, the better you will understand what happens in class and the more interesting you will find it);
- reviewing notes after the lecture;
- preparing assignments;
- writing assignments;
- preparing for exams; and
- general studying.

Plot the best time to do each of these activities. Do you have travel time that can be comfortably spent doing pre-reading? Do you work best early in the morning or in the evening? Schedule the hardest activities for your best hours.

Remember that plans are meant to suit you and you might need to readjust them after trying them for a few weeks. And there will be times when you need to be flexible; for example, when special events occur, or 'spur-of-the-moment' opportunities.

Often we fool ourselves into thinking that we need a long block of time available in which to work. Instead, look at ways you can split your workload into smaller tasks achievable in smaller timeframes.

For example, you could spend 15 minutes planning the week's work, spend 20 minutes reviewing notes, and a short period reading a small part of the textbook and taking notes. Try to see your study as a set of small, achievable tasks rather than a huge unfocussed mess of work.

Taking and using notes

One of the best things you can do is to take notes during lectures and tutorials and then review them as a part of your regular study program. It is best to go back to your notes within a day or two of a lecture or tutorial. There are many good reasons for doing this, for example:

- to be an active learner — learning something is not the same as flipping the top of your head open and pouring the information in; you have to be an active participant and build on what you already know, and reviewing your notes helps you to do this;

- to firm your understandings — if you don't look at your notes until the week before the exams, it is likely you will have forgotten everything and you will need to start all over again;

- to prepare for new learning in the week ahead; and

- to develop a set of good quality, clear notes in your own words that you can use to prepare for exams and assignments.

Reviewing your notes does not mean reading them over or writing them out neatly. It means:

- organising the information in the notes into logical groups and restating the information so that it is clear — remember, you will be going back to review these notes before the exam and they will need to be clear or you will not be able to make sense of them;

- locating new terms to remember;

- identifying areas where you need clarification or more information — if there are things you don't understand, make a note and then go to your textbook and your tutor to 'fill in the gaps'; and

- integrating additional information (from your experience, from previous learning, from books) into the notes.

When you are taking notes, don't try to write down everything that is said. Try to filter the important from the unimportant. If you have spent a little time before the lecture looking through your textbook for the topic of the lecture, you will know what is in there and you don't need to write that down again! What you are trying to have at the end of the lecture is a list of the main points and possibly some useful examples.

Don't try to copy everything down from overheads. What is on the overhead is more than likely in your textbook. If it's really important and not in the textbook, the lecturer will probably give you a photocopy. Instead, use the overhead to help you concentrate on what the lecturer is saying.

Use colour to highlight important points.

Tutorials and lectures

Tutorials and workshops are good opportunities to practise skills and communication, to clarify your own understandings and to get help if you need it. They also allow you to meet with people with common interests and experiences. It is important to take advantage of these opportunities by coming to these sessions with a positive attitude and prepared with questions for clarification.

Don't be afraid to ask questions. You might think you are the only person who doesn't understand something but it is likely that others are puzzled, too, and are wishing that someone else will put their hand up to ask for clarification.

Knowing what is important

This textbook is based on the skills and experiences of many dental assistants and dentists, learned over many years. There have been contributions made by experts in a wide range of areas. Reference has been made to government standards, education and training requirements and professional organisations. So, although you might not immediately be able to see the relevance of something, you can be confident that if the information were not relevant to you and your job, it would not be included!

Try to think about the way in which the information will be used. By thinking of ways in which it might be applied, you will also be able to determine the best way to learn it. For example, is it a practical skill? If so, you should be practising the skill, not just learning the procedure by heart.

Also remember that learning about something might be dependant on other knowledge. So, although the building blocks of information might not be useful in themselves, they might be crucial to understanding something really important later on.

Exams

Exams are hard if you try to learn a term's work in the two days before the exam. If you keep up with assignments, pay attention during classes and use good study techniques in between, the exam will not be a problem for you.

If possible, look at examples of past papers so you know what sorts of questions to expect.

Pace yourself. There is nothing worse than spending too much time on an answer you are having trouble with and then running out of time to answer the questions you know. Spend some time looking at all the questions before you begin writing. Sometimes a question later in the paper helps you remember answers to earlier questions. It also lets you know roughly how much time you should spend on each section and each answer in each section.

Mnemonics

Mnemonics are memory 'tricks' that you develop to help you remember facts. For example, 'MRS C SLENDER' is often used to remember body systems

Muscular
Respiratory
Skeletal

Circulatory/Cardio-Vascular

Skin
Lymphatic
Endocrine
Nervous
Digestive
Excretory
Reproductive

Another technique is to take a mental walk around your house or workplace, using your imagination to leave information in each room. When you need to remember the information, you take another mental walk to collect it.

There are many other techniques that people use and you might want to borrow a book about mnemonics from the library if you think they might be useful to you.

Memorising information

There will be some information that you will need to memorise. Information is always easier to remember when you understand it and can link it to things you already know. More importantly, though, you will need to be able to use the information that you memorise in practical ways.

Do not just try to remember lists of things without a framework. For example, there will be some anatomical terms that you need to remember and it will be easier to remember them if you try to build a picture of where the new terms fit into what you already know. Draw a diagram that includes the new terms. If there is already a picture in your textbook, try to draw it from another angle, or re-draw the picture and colour code the information in groups. Try to see how each part fits into the whole and see if there are any common letter patterns between terms. Then try to use the terms correctly by describing where they fit into the body or how they work.

With terminology, it is sometimes possible to see patterns in the words that can help you to remember the meaning of the word. Many examples of these are listed at the beginning of the glossary.

As another example, if a job has to be done in a particular order, try drawing a plan of your surgery and mapping the steps of the process onto your plan. This is particularly useful if you are a visual learner.

Try formatting information into a table of facts by grouping the information logically (for example, group anatomical terms according to the body system they belong to). By grouping the information into a table or grid, you might find that there are common features that can be learned — and this will reduce the amount that you have to learn. For example, if you know the common qualities of a virus, you don't have to remember all of the details of how individual viruses behave.

Remember that the more you know, the easier it is to learn additional information. This is because you have more of a framework to hang new learning on.

Test yourself

Don't just sit in front of your textbook trying to memorise chunks of information. Try to think of challenging ways to use your knowledge in different situations. For example, as you eat your breakfast, try to envisage and name the muscles that are being used as you chew, as you swallow and digest. As you clean your teeth, run through the names of the tooth surfaces. Think about the last time you visited the dentist and run through, in your mind, what happened and why.

Find a study buddy that you can role play with. Your buddy can ask you to pass instruments and you can pass pictures of the instrument that your buddy checks for correctness. Your buddy can ask you to chart for them. You will be able to think of many other activities to role play — 'the nervous patient', 'the angry patient', 'the patient with wandering hands', etc.

Make a set of cards with terms and definitions on separate cards. Shuffle the two sets and see if you can match the terms. Or play memory with a study buddy. Make a huge 'pin the tail on the donkey' style picture and pin the names of body parts onto the picture.

Write some test questions each week for your study buddy and have them do the same for you. Your questions should try to cover the main ideas from the week's topic and you might like to add one or two revision questions from previous weeks' work.

Motivate yourself

You might need to take the time to go through the benefits of completing the course. For example, your real goal might be to complete the Radiography Certificate, or to progress to Practice Manager in a few years' time. By re-focusing on the big goal you can feel better about the commitment you are making to this course.

Perhaps you can find someone who has completed the course successfully and can tell you about the ways in which it has assisted them at work. Perhaps you can talk to your study buddy and see if they can perk you up.

Also think about your general health. Are you getting enough sleep, exercise and good food? Is there another problem that may be carrying over into your study — for example, a work, finance or relationship problem? If so, you may need to get some external help from a counsellor. Perhaps you need to talk to your lecturer who may be able to give you some useful advice.

Spelling

Spelling is important in all your business correspondence, note taking, applications, etc. If you find spelling difficult you might try the following technique to learn specific words.

Look   Cover   Write   Check

- **Look** at the word. Are there any strange letter groups (e.g. the gh in rough)? Do you know other words with the same combination? Can you break the word into syllables and learn them separately? Underline letters you often have trouble with.
- **Cover** the word and try to see it in your mind.
- **Write** the word. Remember which letters you have trouble with. Try to get them right.
- **Check** to see if you are right. If you made a mistake, write the correct spelling underneath.

Repeat the whole process until you can spell the word correctly three times.

Section 1

Introduction to dental assisting

Dentistry is one of the major branches of the health sciences. Everyone in the community is likely to require dental services at some time in their life.

Scientific advances in the last century (for example, local anaesthetic, safe x-ray technology and antibiotics) mean that dental practitioners can offer their patients a high standard of care.

The addition of **para-medical** and **para-dental auxiliaries** to the dental team has placed greater emphasis on the role played by the dental assistant. This section is an introduction to dental assisting. It will introduce the roles of different members of the dental health team. Chapter 2 discusses ethics for dental assistants and the basics of legal responsibilities (jurisprudence). Chapter 3 provides an introduction to basic psychology for dental assistants and Chapter 4 discusses communication for dental assistants. Chapters 5 and 6 cover reception duties and account keeping and financial duties respectively.

An important note

Duties, qualifications, training and legislation relating to the tasks of the dental team vary from state to state and territory. Duties of dental assistants also vary according to particular practices/clinics and the requirements of the dentists with whom the assistants are working. Note also that legislation, national competency standards and training options are regularly reviewed.

It is not possible for this text to comprehensively cover all variations for all states and territories. The descriptions that follow are a general indication only. You should consult local organisations such as your state Australian Dental Association (ADA) and Dental Board for the most up to date information relevant to your location. A list of organisations that can provide you with assistance and information is provided in the appendix.

■ **para-medical and para-dental auxiliaries:** staff whose work supports medical or dental practitioners.

chapter one
the dental health team

Introduction

The dental health team in a dental practice or clinic typically consists of the dentist and the dental assistant. The team may also include a secretary/receptionist, practice manager, dental radiographer, dental hygienist, dental technician and dental prosthetist.

Dental therapists and specialist dentists (e.g. orthodontists) are also recognised as members of the dental team.

The team

The dentist

The dentist or clinician may work in general practice, in public health clinics, health fund clinics or specialist practice. The dentist is responsible for all clinical treatment in the oral cavity.

The education and training of a dentist involves a minimum of five years undergraduate study or four years following a degree in a related field; for example, a science degree. On graduation, all dentists have to apply for registration with their state/territory's dental board before they can treat patients.

Dentists with overseas qualifications have to undergo an extensive theory and practical examination to gain registration in Australia.

During their studies, dentists become proficient in patient care. This includes:

- recognising patients' needs relating to physical and emotional wellbeing;
- diagnosing and treating oral conditions;
- developing technical dexterity in restoring or replacing diseased teeth; and
- educating patients in the prevention of disease.

Specialist practice includes:

- oral surgery, which includes extraction of teeth, soft tissue surgery, bone surgery and fracture repair, and removal of pathology in the region of the mouth and face;
- orthodontics, which involves the correction of mal-positioned and crowded teeth;
- periodontics, which is the treatment of soft supporting tissues of the teeth and surgical procedures for dental implants;
- paedodontics, which is the practice of dentistry for children;
- endodontics, or root canal therapy, which involves the treatment of the roots of non-vital teeth and the pathology associated with teeth; and
- prosthodontics, which involves full and partial replacement of fractured or lost teeth or other parts of the facial anatomy.

These and other areas of specialist dentistry are discussed in detail in section six.

Dental assistants

Dental assistants, also known as DAs or chair-side assistants, prepare patients for oral examination and assist the dentist in providing treatment. The responsibilities of the dental assistant are outlined in more depth later in this module.

The minimum age for entry to dental assisting is 16 years or on completion of Year 10 schooling. The Higher School Certificate is preferred but not required. An acceptable level of skill in English and Mathematics is expected.

Practical/clinical training is received while working on the job.

National Competency Standards for dental assistants have been developed and endorsed by the

Australian National Training Authority. Students are assessed against this set of competencies and must demonstrate all of those competencies if they wish to obtain a:

- Certificate III in Dental Assisting HLT31802;
- Certificate IV in Dental Assisting (Dental Radiography) HLT40702;
- Certificate IV in Dental Assisting (Oral Health Education) HLT40602; or
- Certificate IV in Dental Assisting (Assisting during General Anaesthesia and Conscious Sedation) HLT40802.

There are courses available in all states and the ACT (but not the Northern Territory) that prepare dental assistants to achieve Dental Assistant Certificate III. Some teaching institutions also offer distance and online examination.

All these courses enable dental assistants to gain a better understanding of their function, to get a formal qualification and to improve their job satisfaction and pay. Students completing the Certificate III course are eligible, if they wish, to sit externally for the Dental Assistants' Association of Australia Inc (DAAA) National Registration examination.

Course providers include TAFE, private training companies, the Dental Assistant's Association (NSW) and the Australian Dental Association (SA and Qld).

Most states offer traineeships. Contact your state Industrial Relations Departments, state branches of the Australian Dental Association (ADA) or New Apprenticeship Centres for information.

Some states also offer pre-employment introductory courses and dental-specific infection control courses.

The DAAA conducts regular conferences and triennial conventions that coincide with the ADA congresses. In some states local professional organisations for dental assistants conduct occupational health and safety (OHS) training sessions and regular continuing education lectures.

Secretary/receptionist

Some practice/clinics employ staff whose only role is as secretary or receptionist. In other practice-clinics, these duties fall to the dental assistant.

Duties include making appointments, answering phones and greeting patients, surgery correspondence, report writing, filing, bookkeeping, account and record management and handling financial transactions.

Practice managers

Practice managers are usually employed in larger multi-dentist practices and are responsible for the smooth running of the practice. Their duties include human resources management, staff selection and supervision, rosters, financial management and developing practice protocols.

Training tends to be on the job. Senior qualified dental assistants progress into the position of practice manager. Some universities offer Practice Managers Certificate IV and diploma courses.

Dental radiographers

Dental assistants who have completed a Certificate III may choose to undertake further training and gain a Certificate IV in Dental **Radiography**. When licensed, they are able to carry out **intra-oral**, in some states, and **extra-oral** dental radiographic procedures. Dental assistants without licences must not take radiographs. Not all state legislation permits dental assistants to carry out radiographic procedures. Check with your state's legislation and training organisations for more information.

Dental hygienists

Dental hygienists are widely utilised in many countries and increasingly in Australia. The hygienist must work under the direct supervision of a dentist.

The dental hygienist is trained and legally qualified to perform procedures on the soft, supporting tissues of teeth (the periodontium). These may include:

- **prophylaxis** (removing calculus and stain);
- **root planing**;
- diagnostic radiography;
- fissure seals;
- impression taking;
- simple orthodontic procedures;
- application of topical fluorides; and
- educating patients in preventive measures.

Hygienists also record case histories, complete dental charts and complete other tasks largely related to preventive dental care. The role of the dental hygienist is to free the dentist to complete tasks that require the dentist's skills. Hygienists may also at times be called upon to assist at the chair-side.

There are a number of courses available for hygienists, ranging from an 18 month technical college course in South Australia to a three-year degree

radiography: creating images using x-rays . **intra-oral:** within the oral cavity (mouth). **extra-oral:** outside the oral cavity (mouth). **prophylaxis:** measures taken to prevent disease (e.g. removing calculus and plaque). **root planing:** smoothing of root surfaces during scaling before polishing the teeth.

course in oral health in Queensland (soon to be available in New South Wales).

Dental therapists

Dental therapists work under the supervision of a dentist within the Government School Dental Services. They are usually legally permitted to perform some types of fillings, fissure sealing and extractions of **deciduous teeth** and also scaling, radiography, fluoride applications and dental health education for young people between the ages of five and 18.

In Victoria, dental therapists can also work in private practice on patients who are up to the age of 25 years and the therapists can provide a range of services including:

- examination;
- diagnosis;
- restorations on permanent teeth; and
- impression taking.

Training is two years full-time, which leads to a Diploma of Dental or Oral Health Therapy, depending on which state is issuing the qualification.

Dental technicians

The dental technician fabricates dentures, crowns, inlays and bridges on prescription of the dentist. The technician has to complete a four-year diploma course in association with on-the-job training in a laboratory. Dental technicians are highly skilled craftspeople but are not qualified or trained to treat patients.

Dental prosthetists

In some states, on completion of a dental technology diploma, graduates may choose to continue for two years part-time to become dental prosthetists. This enables them to deal directly with patients to construct and fit dentures without a dentist's written prescription. Prosthetists must be licensed to practise by the Dental Technician's Board.

The role of the dental assistant

As a well-trained and educated dental assistant, you are a very important asset to a dental practice/clinic. You can assist the dentist to offer a health service of the highest quality.

The need for auxiliaries in dental practice has increased in recent years due to demands from the public for dental services. At the same time, dental equipment and techniques have become more sophisticated and, therefore, your duties as a dental assistant have become not only more complex and demanding but also more interesting and rewarding.

The duties of the dental assistant are covered in depth in other modules in this series. Duties vary according to individual employers and from state to state. However, in summary, you may be responsible for:

- surgery preparation;
- infection control procedures including equipment disinfection, cleaning and sterilisation of instruments;
- provision to the dentist of instruments and equipment;
- maintenance of instruments and equipment;
- chair-side assisting including preparation of filling materials;
- charting and recording of findings from oral examinations;
- processing, mounting and filing dental radiographs;
- clearing the patient's mouth of fluid and debris during treatment by using handheld suction and/or triplex syringe;
- pouring and trimming study models;
- constructing mouthguards;
- reception of and caring for patients;
- stock control and replenishment of supplies;
- making appointments, keeping records of treatments and sending reminders for re-examination and general office duties;
- preparing accounts and collecting payments;
- educating patients on proper oral care (following a Certificate IV Oral Health Education Course qualification); and
- practice administration and management (senior, promotional position).

It is important to remember that you have the first contact with the patient and are a representative of the dentist. The practice/clinic is judged by your manner and appearance. Consequently, you must endeavour to make the patients feel as relaxed as possible and to inspire confidence in them by being friendly and efficient.

deciduous teeth: teeth of the primary dentition that are shed naturally.

Responsibilities of the dentist and dental assistant

Responsibilities of the dentist and dental assistant are governed by a Code of Ethics and by the Dental Practice Acts in each state/territory. These are discussed in greater depth in Chapter 2.

Your responsibilities to the dentist

You should:

- give complete and loyal support to the practice/clinic;

- accept the dentist's method of work;

- contribute to the ethical standards of dentistry in dealing with patients, other dentists and the public;

- carry out duties and accept responsibilities in compliance with Occupational Health and Safety (OHS) Acts and regulations;

- treat the dentist with the respect that they would expect and do not criticise the dentist;

- hold in the strictest confidence all things heard or seen in the surgery;

- realise the scope and limitations of the dental assistant's duties and only perform those that are permitted;

- carefully follow instructions and work to the best of your ability;

- keep complete and accurate records to protect the employer in the event of **litigation** for malpractice (you may be called upon as a witness);

- always behave in a professional manner to reflect favourably on the dental team, the practice and the profession;

- realise that direction, supervision and criticism are occasionally necessary and accept these with grace;

- develop knowledge and skills by utilising recognised training schemes;

- maintain a positive attitude to working relationships with colleagues and not let personal problems affect professional activities; and

- air problems and grievances through accepted channels before they become major — try to work out minor difficulties quickly when they occur.

Your responsibilities to the patient

You should:

- perform all duties to the best of your ability and within the scope permissible;

- respect and accept the patient, recognising all cultural and social diversity;

- know that each individual's needs vary and learn to meet these needs; at the same time help the patients accept the situation they find themselves in;

- be tolerant of behaviour you may not understand and be pleasant and empathetic even though the patient may be irritable and demanding;

- at all times take due care in looking after the physical needs of the patient and alert the dentist of any signs of distress — the patient's safety is paramount; and

- hold in the strictest confidence any information regarding patients and/or their treatment — you should not repeat gossip you hear in the surgery.

The dentist's responsibilities to you

- The dentist is expected to provide employment for you and a fair day's pay for a fair day's work. The dentist must comply with the current *Industrial Relations Act* and no less than the minimum provisions of the **Award**.

- The dentist must provide a safe work environment for you, free from any perceived harm in compliance with Occupational Health and Safety Acts and regulations.

- The dentist must provide you with the necessary training and education to enable you to carry out allotted duties to the best of your ability.

- The dentist is expected to detail permissible duties that you may perform without direct supervision and should make sure that you properly understand these with regard to their limitations.

- The dentist should ensure that your presentation and behaviour are of suitable standard and in keeping with the dental practice.

- The dentist should show the same respect to you as the dentist demands from staff.

Copies of the Industrial Relations Act are available from your local trade union as well as from government publishers or on the internet. Copies of Occupational Health and Safety Acts can be obtained from your local OHS office. A list of offices is provided in Appendix 1.

■ **litigation:** legal action. ■ **Award:** conditions of employment laid down by industrial legislation.

Industrial obligations of employers and employees

Employment conditions are governed by the industrial relations legislation in each state of Australia. There is also a Federal Act, called the *Workplace Relations Act*. This covers employees who work under Federal Awards, or in the territories.

This Act is enacted by state and Federal Parliaments and its regulations are binding on all employers and employees. Other Acts and regulations cover OHS, holidays, long service leave and many other conditions.

The various Acts are revised regularly.

Industrial Awards

There are specific industrial Awards for most occupations. One such Award is the Dental Assistants and Secretaries (State) Award in New South Wales. Similar Awards exist in other states. The Award describes the minimum wages and work conditions under which dental assistants are employed. Each state's Award has differing negotiated pay rates. Also included are such provisions as hours of work, overtime, sick leave, allowances, classifications (levels) of education and responsibilities.

Under the Industrial Relations Act, employers are obliged to have a full copy of the relevant Award on the premises. It must be available for all employees to read.

The Industrial Relations Act also expects employers to maintain a wages and hours of work record. This can be either electronic (a computer printout) or a time and wages book. A pay slip must be provided to employees which details gross and net pay, how much tax is taken out, any overtime worked, superannuation paid, any sick days and leave taken. You can find more information about the wages book in Chapter 6.

Personal qualities of the dental assistant

Dental assisting is a vocation requiring a special type of person. The work is technical, complex and demanding. Dental assistants must be perceptive, intelligent and have a pleasing personality. They must be patient and understanding and show integrity, tact, diligence and good manual dexterity.

To perform the duties of a dental assistant you require the following qualities.

- Adaptability — you should be able to adapt to varying duties within the dental practice/clinic. You require a good memory, must be organised and mature, have good time-management skills and be able to accept responsibility.
- Impeccable appearance — clothing should be clean and professional in style.
- Strength of character — you should be ambitious, dependable, honest, kind, sympathetic, enthusiastic and sincere.
- Impeccable conduct — you should show no evidence of unsatisfactory conduct and should abide by appropriate social and professional etiquette.
- Cooperation — this is necessary to a very high degree and can best be achieved in a friendly, professional atmosphere. There is a great deal of satisfaction to be gained from being an integral part of a successful team.
- Conversational ability — you must be able to maintain friendly conversation without being intrusive. Patients often require confident reassurance before dental procedures.
- Dependability — dental assistants should always strive to be punctual and to carry out responsibilities carefully and thoroughly. Tasks delegated to you should always be completed.
- Initiative — this is displayed when you carry out duties without constant reminders. You should also strive to maintain and improve knowledge and capabilities in dentistry.
- Good health — this should be reflected in your behaviour and appearance.
- Honesty — the dentist must be able to have complete faith in your honesty, not only in regard to financial transactions within the practice but also in all other dealings with the dentist, staff members and patients.
- Personality — no matter how efficient you are, it is also important to be pleasant and friendly.
- Courtesy — this is of vital importance in the practice/clinic. Courtesy to all patients, employer, visitors and all other staff members is crucial to a pleasant working environment. Your manner should be smart and business-like while conveying calmness, sincerity, confidence and sympathy when required.

You should endeavour to maintain a positive self-image and self-esteem. Take pride in your knowledge, skills and ability. They contribute to every procedure and assist in the patient's needs being met.

7

Personal appearance of the dental assistant

Good personal hygiene is essential for all members of the dental health team. It is crucial not just for appearance but also for good infection control in the practice. (Chapter 14 discusses infection control in depth.)

A daily bath or shower and the use of a good deodorant are essential. Make-up should be used with discretion as should perfume, deodorant or after-shave. Patients may have allergic responses to these.

Special attention must be paid to your breath. Smoking leaves a lingering odour on the breath, so it is important to use a breath freshener if you smoke. It is inadvisable to smoke during working hours. Most establishments have 'no-smoking' policies in place. For the same reason, avoid eating highly seasoned foods, onions and garlic. It is unprofessional to chew gum during working hours and you must not drink alcohol during working hours.

Fingernails must be short and well manicured with no nail polish. Long nails easily puncture rubber and vinyl gloves. Hands should be well cared for and free from abrasions. A cream compatible with the hand washing solution should be applied in the morning before work and again after work, but not during the working day.

Hand washing should be carried out regularly and frequently, including:

■ before donning and after removing gloves;

■ before assisting at the chair-side;

■ before instrument preparation;

■ after touching soiled instruments and linen;

■ before touching the telephone and before returning to the chair-side;

■ when visibly dirty;

■ before leaving the surgery for lunch or tea/coffee breaks; and

■ before and after visits to the toilet.

Your uniform or other prescribed clothing should be clean and wrinkle free. It should be worn in the surgery only, not to and from work. A spare uniform should be kept in the surgery in case of accidents. Underwear must be changed daily. Hosiery should be kept in good repair.

Rings should not be worn in the dental surgery for two reasons. Firstly, if gold or silver come in contact with some metals and chemicals used in the surgery, claw settings may be destroyed and the remaining surfaces can be damaged. Rings can also put at risk the integrity of gloves by puncturing them. Additionally, correct hand washing cannot be carried out when wearing jewellery. Wedding bands may be worn on a small chain around the neck.

Small, non-dangling earrings can be worn, as can unobtrusive necklaces or chains that can be tucked inside the uniform.

As it is most important when preparing materials to adhere to correct mixing times, the wearing of a fob or nursing watch is useful for this purpose.

Good posture is also crucial for a good public image and personal health. Feet should be well cared for, and correctly fitting, closed shoes should be worn. Occupational health and safety regulations state that shoes should afford support and protection. As sharp instruments may be dropped, open-toed shoes or sandals are not safe. Shoes should be cleaned daily and kept in good repair. More information about posture can be found in Chapter 15.

Hair should be clean and kept tidy. If hair is long, it must be tied back and kept off the face. If a fringe is worn, this should be kept well trimmed to enable good vision.

Organisations representing the dental health team

The dental boards

The dental boards of the various Australian states and territories are statutory bodies (arms of government) that control the practice of dentistry through the medium of their individual dental legislation. The Acts define the practice of dentistry, the qualifications necessary for registration, the ethical standards required, the conditions under which a charge of professional misconduct may be laid, and the penalties which may be imposed. More information about dental boards, Dental Practice Acts and regulations can be found in Chapter 2.

The Australian Dental Association (ADA)

This is a voluntary association of dentists. It is made up of state branches, country divisions and study groups. Its role is to:

■ set and enforce the professional Code of Ethics for dentists;

■ look after the interest of members;

■ provide dental health education to the public (e.g. Dental Health Week);

■ organise post-graduate education, courses and congresses;

■ be the voice of the profession nationally;

■ arrange benefits for members;

■ provide for indemnity insurance for members; and

■ at its discretion, provide legal representation for members.

Dental Assistants' Association of Australia Inc

The national body, called the Dental Assistants' Association of Australia Inc (DAAA), is made up of state branches, affili-ates and individual members. Its role is to:

■ be the voice of dental assistants at national and state level;

■ set and enforce its professional Code of Ethics;

■ look after the interests of members;

■ conduct on-going education by organising seminars, workshops and conventions;

■ issue certificates and badges following a registration examination and register them; and

■ provide an internet website publicising its activities.

There also exist various state interest groups that promote educational programs for dental assistants.

Dental assistants are encouraged to belong to a professional organisation (either state or Federal). In states where there is no association, the Dental Assistants' Association of Australia Inc welcomes individual members.

Trade unions

Trade union organisations tend to concern themselves more with working conditions and remuneration than with ethics. You should be encouraged to join your trade union should you so desire but should not suffer any discrimination if you elect not to join.

The New South Wales DAA also looks after dental assistants industrially and is party to negotiations of the Award.

Unions represent dental assistants in settling workplace conflict and give support to members in resolving pay and other disputes. Conflicts can arise from time to time and union representatives may even call for industrial action, but this is very unlikely.

Other organisations

Other organisations that represent members of the dental team are:

■ the Dental Therapists' Association;

■ the Dental Hygienists' Association;

■ the Dental Technicians' Association; and

■ the Dental Prosthetists' Association.

All these organisations have their own codes of ethics and their own aims and objectives.

Summary

As a dental assistant, you are a very important member of the team that provides dental care. Dental assistants today are more highly trained and required to accept more responsibility than their predecessors. A well-trained and qualified dental assistant acquires many skills that create career opportunities both within and outside of dentistry.

chapter two
ethics and jurisprudence

Introduction

Ethics are:

- a set of moral principles and values;
- a discipline dealing with what is 'good' and what is 'bad', with moral responsibility and obligation; and
- a particular system of rules applying to a duty or 'calling'; that is, professional morals, customs and manners.

It is the last of these definitions that is most applicable to the dental assistant.

The moral principles, customs and manners to which the dental assisting profession adheres are laid down in a Code of Ethics. This set of rules lays down minimum standards of behaviour required to maintain and improve the status of dental assisting within the dental profession and the community. In the health care professions (dental assisting included), the main feature of codes such as these is an emphasis on the welfare of the patient.

Although it is a voluntary code, the standards are set by professional colleagues (in this case the Dental Assistants' Association of Australia Inc). All dental assistants should act by this minimum code.

The code lays down a more stringent system of behaviour than is provided by law. Something might be unethical but not illegal. However, anything that is illegal is definitely unethical.

Dental jurisprudence is the law applied to the practice of dentistry. It consists of three parts. These are:

❶ the provisions of the state/territory Dental Practice Acts;

❷ common law, which has evolved through the ages; and

❸ the 'laws' of the profession; that is, dental ethics.

These three units are not separate and distinct. They merge into each other. However, as a general rule common law is a matter for the courts, the dental Acts are the concern of the dental boards and ethics are the prerogative of the Australian Dental Association and its state branches.

Laws relating to dentistry are discussed later in this chapter.

The dental assistants' Code of Ethics

This code was developed by and for members of the Dental Assistants' Association of Australia Inc (DAAA) and, with the exception of item one, applies equally well to all dental assistants, whether they are members of the association or not.

The dental assistant should:

❶ foster the aims of the association and maintain association standards;

❷ maintain honesty, loyalty and diplomacy in all contacts with the profession and society;

❸ give to the employer the cooperation and show the initiative and efficiency needed to serve all patients capably and efficiently;

❹ work in a collaborative manner with all health care professionals and others involved with providing care, respecting their particular contribution within the care team;

❺ work cooperatively with patients and their families, recognising their involvement in the planning and delivery of care;

❻ respond to the patient's need for care and comfort, exercising courtesy, kindness and consideration irrespective of origin, religious and culture beliefs, or the nature of their health problems;

❼ not advise any treatment for patients which requires the professional expertise of a dentist, at the same time acknowledge any limitations in knowledge and competence and decline any duties or responsibilities unless qualified and able to perform them in a safe and skilled manner;

❽ keep in confidence all professional details of dental colleagues, individual patients and the dental profession in general;

❾ refrain from criticising the employer's treatment of patients or any previous dental treatment and the dental profession in general;

❿ contribute to and maintain a safe and effective care environment for patients and colleagues;

⓫ maintain and increase professional knowledge and competence by taking advantage of every educational opportunity available; and

⓬ assist professional colleagues to develop their professional competence and assist others in the care team.

In summary, your ethical duty to the patient is to:

- be competent in work and to keep abreast of the progress of dental science applicable to the work situation;

- understand the patient as a human being and not merely as a case;

- bring to bear the full resources of training and not to exceed the legal range of duties; and

- observe the rules of professional confidentiality and secrecy — a patient in a dentist's rooms retains the right of privacy (you should not gossip about patients).

Additionally, employers, solicitors, insurance companies and similar bodies are often anxious to obtain information about the condition and progress of a patient, especially when it relates to road accident or workers compensation cases. This information must never be disclosed without the consent of the patient.

Dental Acts

Each state in Australia has its own Act and regulations that define the practice of dentistry in that state. All dentists are legally required to understand their obligations under those Acts. State Acts are administered by a dental board. You can get a copy of the Act for your state or territory from government publishers or from the dental board website.

Under the terms of the dental Acts only a dentist or a licensed dental auxiliary may practise dentistry. The dental assistant is not licensed.

Dentistry is defined to include the giving of any dental treatment, attention or advice to any person or the examination of the natural or artificial teeth for any purpose. That means that, if in your role as a dental assistant you carry out any of these, you are breaking the law. You and your employer are both liable to prosecution by or on behalf of a dental board.

The legal position of a dental assistant employed in four-handed dentistry can be clarified as follows.

- Not more than one person can practise dentistry on a patient at any time. That means, when a dentist is attending to a patient, it is legal for you to carry out procedures such as cheek and lip retraction or aspirating fluids from the mouth.

- A dentist cannot practise dentistry on more than one patient at the one time. Unless a dentist is working at the chair-side, it is illegal for you to undertake any intra-oral service for the patient.

The Medical Protection Society does not indemnify a dentist in cases arising out of illegal practice by a member of staff. The DAAA cannot defend any dental assistant who carries out any illegal procedure.

State dental boards

Dental boards administer state Dental Practice Acts. Although they differ slightly from state to state, a typical board may consist of members made up of:

- registered dentists elected by the dental profession;

- a dentist, appointed by the Health Minister, and who is an officer of the Department of Health or an employee of a public health organisation;

- a registered dentist appointed by the minister involved in tertiary education; for example, the dean of a Faculty of Dentistry;

- a registered dentist appointed by the minister's own choosing;

- a dental auxiliary (therapist or hygienist) appointed by the minister;

- a legal practitioner appointed by the minister; and

- two consumer representatives appointed by the minister.

The board is headed by a president (usually a dentist) and administered by a registrar. The board is an arm of government and its duties include:

- administering the Dental Practice Acts that define the practice of dentistry;

- advising the Health Minister on matters relating to the registration of dentists, dental auxiliaries, and standards of dental practice;

- enforcing standards and regulations;

- providing for the accreditation and recognition of qualifications entitling a person to registration as a dentist or dental auxiliary;

- inquiring into competence of a dentist or dental auxiliary;

- overseeing the requirement for registration of competence as a dentist or dental auxiliary by requiring proof at the time of registration of continuing education having been undertaken;

- publishing and distributing information covering the Act and regulations to dentists, dental auxiliaries, consumers and other interested persons; and

- providing a channel for patient grievances to be heard.

The board may also have a sub-committee known as the Dental Care Assessment Committee. This committee decides (among other things) on penalties to be imposed for misconduct; for example, prosecuting those who practise dentistry illegally.

There is also a tribunal, which hears disputes between patient and dentist or dentist and dentist or any other party involved with a registered dentist. A tribunal is like a court of law.

State and Federal Acts

The *National Privacy Act 2000*

The National Government Privacy legislation was amended in 2000 to include the private sector. This Act sets the standard for the way in which organisations, including health care providers such as dentists, collect, use and disclose information about individuals. This standard is contained in 10 National Privacy Principles that govern the collection of (patients') personal information. There are penalties imposed for anyone contravening these principles.

Health information in an individual's dental records must be considered to be highly confidential and all members of the dental team must undertake to keep those patient details confidential.

Patients must be given information about their rights under the privacy provision and be asked for permission to give health information to another person; for example, when referring to a specialist.

Some practices/clinics provide new patients with a statement setting out the policy of that practice/clinic.

Patients may have access to their own records through the *Freedom of Information Act*.

Child protection legislation

All people looking after children and young people have a responsibility to provide a safe environment for them. All states have some form of child protection Act, although their names and content differ. You should obtain copies of local legislation and ensure that you meet all obligations under the Act.

Additionally, in some states there is legislation requiring the compulsory reporting of suspected child maltreatment, child abuse or neglect. If you have concerns that a child may have been maltreated in this way, you should report your concerns to the dentist who should then take appropriate action.

Occupational Health and Safety Acts

Each state and territory in Australia has an Act and regulations that aim to protect the safety and welfare of people at work.

For example, in New South Wales, the WorkCover Authority administers this Act. It lays down general requirements that must be met at the workplace by both employers and employees. WorkCover oversees workers compensation and rehabilitation following injury. WorkCover inspectors are available to advise and inspect premises and to impose fines for breaches of the Act.

One of the major changes in the 2000 Act is that employers are now obliged to consult their employees on all occupational health and safety (OHS) issues. All workplaces employing 15 or more people must have a committee made up of representatives of employees and management. In smaller establishments a responsible person is appointed to ensure that the workplace complies with the provisions of the Act and regulations.

Provisions in other states are similar and there is a move towards national standardisation. See the appendix for a list of OHS organisations in your state or territory to get the most up to date information for your location.

Consumer Acts

All states and territories have an Act that protects consumers. The dentist is responsible to the patient for the quality of service and treatment. If dissatisfied, the patient can complain to the Department of Fair Trading, or similarly named department depending on the state or territory. Staff can be sued for malpractice under Common Law.

Radiation Control Act 1990

This Act regulates the ownership and licences of x-ray equipment and people operating such equipment. It lays down rules for the protection of patients and operators from radioactive substances and sets fees for licences.

Dental assistants who continue their studies with a Certificate IV in Radiography must also apply for a license upon successful completion of their course. Most states in Australia provide training for, and license, dental radiographers. The exceptions are Victoria and Tasmania.

The *Therapeutic Goods Act 1989*

This Act defines and registers all dangerous and hazardous substances and equipment. It regulates the use and distribution of drugs and all chemical substances and establishes drug schedules.

Common law in dentistry

Duty to the patient

The dentist's duty to patients has, over the years, been defined by judges of the Supreme Courts. The law presupposes that the prudent practitioner will observe forethought, judgment, skill and care in all actions. The standard of skill and care that the law demands from a dental practitioner is that which might reasonably be expected from the average practitioner of the class to which the dentist belongs.

The duty of a dentist to a patient is a personal duty that applies irrespective of the circumstances under which the dentist is practising. Whether the dentist is a principle or a partner, an assistant or an employee, this duty to the patient remains and the dentist is liable for all his or her actions. This is called **vicarious liability** (see below).

Similarly, you are required to exercise skill and care and should also be responsible for all your actions.

Cases have been reported where a patient has been injured by a spilt solution or a sharp instrument dropped by the dental assistant. In such cases, if legal action is taken, it is likely against the dentist. However, you may also be sued under Common Law.

There is a time limit placed upon people being able to sue for negligence or assault. The limits vary from state to state and territory (usually referred to as statutes of limitation). Under certain circumstances the courts may extend the time limit during which legal proceedings may be brought.

Vicarious liability

According to the master and servant relationship in employment, the employer is deemed to be responsible for the negligent act of an employee if committed in the course of work.

Under the New South Wales State Law — *Employers' Liability, Indemnification of Employer Act 1982* — the employer cannot recover costs from the employee.

There is no protection against serious or wilful misconduct.

Negligence

There are a number of legal definitions of negligence. Despite the increasing use of the term 'negligence' by the public and the media, a dentist is usually only liable when the standard of treatment offered falls below the standard of a reasonably competent practitioner in the field, so much so that the dentist's conduct is inexcusable. In this circumstance the dentist's professional association has the discretion not to support or offer legal assistance. If negligence is proven the dentist may be deregistered for a specific term, or if serious enough, for life.

Negligence is a term used in regard to a failure to discharge a public or private duty. Since a duty can only be assessed in the light of all relevant circumstances, so must negligence be assessed. Accidents do happen in dental surgeries and often these accidents are due to lack of care rather than lack of skill.

Assault

Assault can be defined as a wilful act without consent.

From time to time dental boards receive complaints from members of the public alleging that an assault

■ **vicarious liability**: the employer is responsible for any negligent act of an employee if committed in the course of work.

has occurred in the dentist's room. Such complaints are infrequent but they do occur in sufficient numbers to illustrate the need for care and vigilance.

The most common complaint received is that the dentist had acted without consent or had gone beyond the limit of the consent given as, for example, a child who attends a dentist to have a tooth filled and returns home with several teeth missing.

However, there have also been rare instances where the wrong tooth has been removed. In cases such as these, the dentist who has operated must accept the final responsibility.

Complaints have also been received from parents who claim that excessive physical measures have been used to control their child. Finally, there is the rare occasion when indecent assault is alleged.

There may be occasions when a dental assistant may be called upon as a witness to give evidence in court for the dentist. For this and other reasons it is essential that you are always present when the dentist is treating a patient.

Informed consent

Everyone has the right of freedom from interference with their person and this right forbids a dentist (or anyone else), as a general rule, from doing anything that involves physically touching a patient without the patient's consent.

When patients enter the dentist's surgery they consent to the touching that is necessary for a dental examination. The patient need not manifest agreement to this touching, as their presence in the dental chair implies permission for the dentist and the dental assistant to touch them. However:

- consent to carry out treatment must still be obtained; and
- touching in excess of that necessary for the examination or treatment may constitute assault.

Before embarking upon treatment, a dentist must obtain informed consent. Normally this is obtained from the patient but there are certain groups who are unable to give consent. These include children, adolescents who are supported by their families, and some adults with intellectual disabilities. For consent to be valid, the patient or the person acting on the patient's behalf must realise what the dentist has in mind and understand the consequences of the treatment they are consenting to. Appropriate explanations must be given and the individual concerned must be capable of assessing the facts and making a logical decision.

Before giving consent to proceed with treatment the patient is entitled to be fully informed of:

- the type of treatment;
- the alternatives (if there are any);
- the number of appointments required;
- the cost of the treatment;
- the prognosis; and
- any side effects or complications.

Some dentists delegate the duty of obtaining consent to the dental assistant, and some have designed a consent form that authorises the dentist to undertake all necessary treatment. However, the use of such forms has been questioned by some legal authorities who have pointed out that the basic requirements for informed consent still apply. In any litigation the dentist may be required to prove that the patient understood the information given at the time of signing the consent form. An example of an extraction consent form is shown in Figure 2.1.

The dangers of proceeding with treatment without consent are:

- that the dentist may not be paid for services undertaken; and
- the dentist could face a charge of assault.

All matters relating to patient management (i.e. consent for treatment) must be relayed directly to the dentist and kept with the patient's record.

Contracts

A contract is an agreement between two or more parties whereby obligations are created that may be enforced by law. These may be written or verbal.

In the course of your duties, you may enter into a number of contracts for or on behalf of your employer. Opinions vary as to which of such duties a dentist should delegate but these may include making appointments, issuing instructions to a dental laboratory, ordering stock, obtaining informed consent and quoting fees.

A dental appointment is a contract between the dentist and the patient. Patients contract to present themselves at the dentist's rooms at a specified time and the dentist contracts to provide the patient with a professional service at the time that has been specified. The contract may be varied by mutual consent but in the absence of such consent, if either party fails to fulfil the contract they could be held liable.

The control of the appointment book is one of your most important and challenging duties, particularly with regard to requests for emergency service.

Extraction Consent Form

About the proposed treatment

An extraction involves removing one or more teeth. Depending on their condition, this may require cutting the tooth or gums or removing bone. If any unexpected difficulties occur during treatment, I may send you to an oral surgeon, a dentist who specialises in extracting teeth and performing other surgical procedures.

Benefits and alternatives

The proposed treatment will help to relieve your symptoms and may also enable you to proceed with further proposed treatment. There is no reasonable alternative treatment that will relieve your symptoms.

Common risks

Although they are rare, you should be aware of the following risks:

1. Bleeding, swelling, discomfort and infection: Following treatment you may experience bleeding, pain, swelling and discomfort for several days, which may be treated with pain relieving medication. You may possibly also experience an infection following treatment, which would be treated with antibiotics.

2. Reaction to anaesthesia and/or sedation: You will receive a local anaesthetic and possibly a sedative (tranquilliser) to keep you comfortable during treatment. In rare instances patients have an allergic reaction to the anaesthetic, which may require emergency medical attention, or find that it reduces their ability to control swallowing, which increases the chance of swallowing foreign objects during treatment. Sedatives may temporarily make you drowsy or reduce your coordination.

3. Stiff or sore jaw joint: Holding your mouth open during treatment may temporarily leave your jaw feeling stiff and sore and may make it difficult for you to open your mouth wide for several days afterwards. Treatment may also leave the corners of your mouth red or cracked for several days.

4. Dry socket: The blood clot that forms in the empty tooth socket may disintegrate or become dislodged, for example, as a result of smoking or drinking through a straw. This painful condition, called dry socket, lasts a week or more and is treated by placing a medicated dressing in the tooth socket to aid healing.

5. Damage to adjacent teeth: In some cases, the instruments used in extracting a tooth can chip or damage adjacent teeth, which could require further treatment to restore their appearance.

6. Opening into sinuses: With upper posterior teeth, the roots sometimes extend up beyond the surrounding bone into the sinuses, the natural cavities in the bone behind your cheeks. Removing these teeth may temporarily leave a small opening into the sinuses. Antibiotics and additional treatment may be needed to prevent a sinus infection and help this opening to close.

7. Bone fracture: Depending on the location of the tooth or teeth to be extracted, treatment may cause a fracture in the surrounding bone. In rare instances the tooth or teeth to be extracted may be fused to the surrounding bone. Both situations may require further treatment.

8. Tooth fragments: Depending on the condition and position of the tooth or teeth to be extracted, tooth fragments may be left in the extraction site following treatment. Generally, this causes no problems, but on rare occasions tooth fragments become infected and must be removed.

9. Changes to nerve sensations: The nerves that control sensations in your teeth, gums, tongue, lips and chin run through your jaw. Depending on the tooth or teeth to be extracted (particularly lower teeth or third molars), in rare instances it may be impossible to avoid touching, moving, stretching, bruising, cutting or severing a nerve. This could change the normal sensations in any of these areas, causing itching, tingling or burning (called paresthesia) or the loss of all sensation (called anaesthesia). These changes could last from several weeks to several months or in some cases, indefinitely.

Consequences of not performing treatment

This course of treatment will help to relieve your symptoms. If no treatment were performed, you would continue to experience symptoms, which could include pain and/or infection, deterioration of the bone surrounding your teeth, changes to your bite, discomfort in your jaw joint and possibly the premature loss of these and other teeth.

Additional information:

Every reasonable effort will be made to ensure that your condition is treated properly, although it is not possible to guarantee perfect results. By signing below, you acknowledge that you have received adequate information about the proposed treatment, that you understand this information and that all of your questions have been answered fully.

___I give my consent for the proposed treatment as described above.

___I refuse to give my consent for the proposed treatment as described above. I have been informed of the potential consequences of my decision to refuse treatment.

_____	_____	_____
Patient's signature/Date	Dentist's signature/Date	Witness's signature/Date

Figure 2.1 Extraction consent form

Such requests must be assessed and dealt with without undue effect on the schedule planned for subsequent patients. You will find more information about appointment scheduling in Chapter 5.

Another type of contract is the contract between the dentist and a **dental laboratory**. In dealing with a dental laboratory, the laws relating to contractors and sub-contractors apply. Under such laws the sub-contractor is entitled to precise specifications and a reasonable time in which to complete the work.

The instruction sheet that is forwarded to the dental laboratory with details of the requirements, including denture design, is a contract in writing. If you prepare it, it should be rechecked and signed by the dentist before despatch.

When a fee is quoted to a patient it should be in specific terms, full details of the quotation should be given to the patient in writing and should be recorded for future reference. There is a misapprehension that only written contracts are binding. This is not correct. Although it is harder to prove, a verbal contract can be upheld in the courts. If you are authorised to quote fees and/or obtain consent to treat, good communication between you, the patient and the dentist is vital.

There are occasions when a dentist and patient agree upon the work to be done but neither discuss nor arrive at the fee to be charged. In this situation, the law implies an obligation to pay on the part of the one receiving the service. It is also implied that the fee charged by the dentist will be reasonable, that the work will be completed within a reasonable time, that the dentist will conform to customary standards, that the patient will follow instructions, and so on.

Records

All matters relating to patient management should be kept with the patient's records. This includes updated medical histories, medical and laboratory prescriptions or instructions, correspondence and any other information about, by or for the patient with the exception of business or financial documentation. More information about patient records can be found in Chapters 5, 6 and 17.

Changes should be made to records by crossing out the incorrect entry and by adding a dated correction and initialling the card. Entries should never be erased or deleted in any way. A new card should not be made to replace an incorrect card.

Taxation records

The *Income Tax Assessment Act 1936* requires that every taxpayer keep sufficient records to enable assessable income and allowable deductions to be ascertained. These records must be kept for at least seven years from the date of the transactions to which the records relate.

The patient's card serves as a record of treatment rendered to that individual and of the financial return derived from that treatment. The Trustees of a Professional Indemnity Fund require that each member shall at all times keep adequate, faithful and detailed records of the professional services carried out for each patient and that such records shall be written legibly in ink. Any changes and amendments should be initialled by the dentist.

Practising dentists have different ideas with regard to record keeping. Some make a point of personally writing up the patient's card. Others use an electronic system of record keeping.

Whichever method is used, the dentist should have readily available, and for each patient, a detailed record of the advice that has been tendered, the consent that has been given, the fees that have been quoted and the treatment that has been carried out.

Ownership of records

Radiographs taken as an aid to diagnosis are a part of the clinical records of a case and remain the property of the dentist. They should be filed and preserved with the patient's other records. The patient pays a fee for the dentist's opinion of the x-ray picture and not for the film itself.

Patients' requests for their radiographs should generally be politely refused. However, there are instances where a patient who is moving out of the district requests the recent radiographs, perhaps to avoid further radiation exposure or expense. This is not an unreasonable request. It is preferable to send the radiographs directly to the patient's future dentist.

If there is a likelihood of the patient being referred for specialist treatment it is preferable to take a double x-ray film. One radiograph produced can be kept by the dentist as a permanent record and the other can be provided to the specialist. Radiographs can also be photocopied but good results cannot be guaranteed. Digital radiographs can be emailed.

Patients may have access to their own records through the *Freedom of Information Act 1982*.

dental laboratory: manufacturer of dental prostheses, for example, dentures.
radiographs: often but incorrectly called x-rays.

Supply of dentures

In addition to the other legal obligations to the patient, a dentist who contracts to make a denture agrees to provide that patient with an article that is reasonably satisfactory for the purpose for which it is intended, provided always that the patient is reasonably cooperative.

A contract to supply a denture is not a contract for work or labour done but a contract for a sale of goods. Since the denture has a value in excess of $20, a verbal contract is not binding and under such circumstances the patient can withdraw from the contract at any time, and the dentist has little or no redress. Dentists can protect themselves against this risk by requesting a contract in writing or a small deposit, usually about one-third of the final fee, for which a receipt is issued. However, cases of withdrawal are so rare that few dentists consider this precaution to be necessary.

In any sale of goods, the moment arrives when the goods change hands. In denture construction this is when the patient leaves the surgery with the new dentures in the mouth. Even though the account may not be paid, the dentures thereafter belong to the patient. The dentist can use accepted procedures to collect the fee, but cannot deprive the patient of the dentures, nor can they be returned without the consent of both parties.

If a dentist undertakes to repair a denture, then there is an implied obligation to return the denture to the patient in a condition as near as possible to its former state. Consequently, before accepting a denture for repair, the dentist should confirm that the patient had been wearing the denture and that it was considered to be satisfactory. Otherwise the dentist may have to remake the dentures if the patient maintains that they are now ruined, and the dentist is in no position to refute the charge.

Professional indemnity

Despite all skill and care, sometimes treatments fail, complications arise and accidents occur and these may involve the patient in pain, suffering and expense. Under such circumstances some patients seek compensation.

The number of dental defence cases that are heard in court are increasing but statistics indicate that a large proportion of dentists and dental assistants will never be involved in such cases. Nevertheless, the possibility is always there and practitioners should carry insurance cover that indemnifies the dentist and staff against legal actions arising out of the practice. No matter how fully a dentist is insured, the involvement in a legal action never pays even if it is successfully defended in court. No compensation is paid for the time lost in defending the case, or for the weeks of anxiety or for the adverse publicity that is received.

The assistant is often the first to learn that the patient is considering legal action and the assistant's handling of the situation may be crucial to the future of the case. The essential criterion is to be a good and sympathetic listener and to make detailed notes of the conversation that has occurred. It is the responsibility of the dentist and the insurers to attempt to reach an equitable solution.

Summary

Your career as a dentist's assistant must be seen within the context of your personal and professional ethics and your legal responsibilities. It is crucial that you know and understand your ethical and legal obligations and apply them in all aspects of your work.

chapter three
psychology for dental assistants

Introduction

Psychology is the scientific study of behaviour. Behaviour is a term used to include a variety of activities — thinking, seeing, hearing, speaking, reading, learning and reacting. We usually think of it as the observable actions people make as responses to different situations. Psychologists are interested in all forms of behaviour exhibited by human beings and animals.

To practise psychology as a profession requires extensive training at university. The intention of this chapter is not to encourage untrained people to practise psychology. However, a great deal of human behaviour is irrational and carried out for reasons that the individuals themselves do not understand and you will see examples of this in your work. Some competence in understanding human behaviour and some skill in dealing with people are essential.

A principle of behaviour is a general rule that explains the behaviour of the majority of people. As a result of psychological research, many principles of behaviour have been discovered. This chapter will deal with several principles of behaviour and show how these principles may be applied in the dental surgery for the purpose of:

- understanding behaviour;
- improving methods of patient management; and
- developing an efficient and productive dental practice.

Personality and traits

Personality

It is important to remember that each individual's personality is unique and is closely related to the way that person usually behaves.

In the dental surgery, there are usually at least three people involved; the dentist, the patient and the dental assistant. Each of these people has a unique personality. This determines their behaviour and, in particular, the way they relate to the personalities of others. Because of this, it is important to understand some of the personality characteristics that are commonly exhibited in dental surgeries. It is also important to understand some of the ways in which behaviour may be affected by personality characteristics and problems.

Learning social behaviour

Psychologists believe that personality characteristics may be learned through life experiences. Some people may learn to be outgoing and friendly in relationships with others while other people learn to be shy and dependent. There are three processes responsible for most learned social behaviour in human beings:

❶ operant conditioning;
❷ modelling; and
❸ classical conditioning.

Operant conditioning

Operant conditioning is a form of learning that occurs when reward or punishment shape behaviour.

Smiling and encouraging statements, such as, 'that's good', are rewards that are frequently used to shape children's behaviour. When a child behaves well in the dental surgery, a smile, a statement (e.g. 'you sat very still, Susie — that was good') or even a little gift (e.g. a new toothbrush with the child's name engraved on it with the dental drill) may all reinforce this good behaviour and encourage the child to behave well in the future.

It is most important that reinforcers follow closely in time to the behaviour to be reinforced. Where there is too long a delay, rewards and punishments become less effective in producing desired changes in behaviour.

Modelling

Modelling is a form of learning that is very important in human learning. A person watches or hears someone else say or do something, then attempts to imitate it. Children may develop negative attitudes to dental treatment simply by hearing their parents or friends describing painful dental experiences. These children may then present in the dental surgery with a high degree of anxiety even though they themselves have never had unpleasant dental treatment.

Cultural, racial, social and family influences are all important in shaping personality and behaviour. For example, some cultural groups are not as time-conscious as we are in Western culture and may arrive late for appointments without being aware that we regard this as impolite and annoying. In order to deal effectively with patients it is necessary to understand these sources of variation and to

remain uncritical and accepting of 'strange' behaviours, remembering that our behaviour may appear equally strange to others.

Classical conditioning

This is a learning process in which a person's behaviour is influenced by the experiences they have. It is obvious that the kind of experiences a patient has had in the past with dentists plays an important part in forming the patient's present feelings. If for example, the individual has suffered a painful dental treatment in the past, the patient will probably feel very anxious about another treatment.

Other kinds of experiences can also contribute to the way the patient feels about a visit to the dentist. For example, unpleasant or painful experiences with a doctor or painful experiences that friends or relatives have had with a dentist will also play a part.

Self-concept

As we grow and learn, we develop a self-concept. This self-concept changes as a child grows older, as a result of experiences and of the opinions that other people hold about the child and communicate to the child.

The concepts that people hold about themselves may differ from the concepts that another person holds about them. The way in which people believe other people see them is another important factor in understanding their personalities.

For example, in Figure 3.1, Mary is a dental patient who is anxious about dental treatment but who is

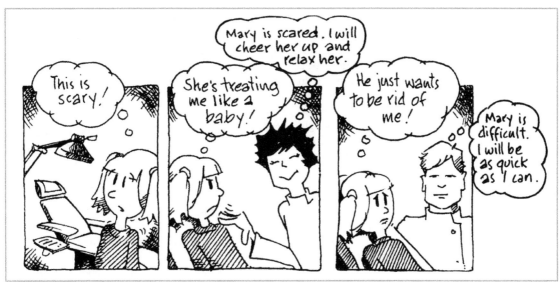

Figure 3.1 Our perceptions of ourselves differ from other people's perceptions of us

able to hold herself in control so that she doesn't cause 'a scene'. She sees the dental assistant as being flippant and insensitive. She believes that the dental assistant thinks of her as dull and un-interesting because she is too worried to listen to what is being said. She believes that the dentist is being abrupt and negative and sees her as a bad patient and a nuisance because she is so upset. Because she thinks that the dental assistant and the dentist think of her in this negative way she becomes even more anxious.

The only way of developing objective and correct concepts of oneself and others is to communicate about them. You should discuss your impressions of a patient with the dentist, particularly where the patient's behaviour indicates to you that the patient is disturbed or unhappy in the dental surgery.

Also remember that the patient's self-concept is strongly related to the body-concept. Patients who are told that they have bad oral hygiene may become anxious or angry because their self-concepts as attractive people have been threatened.

Anxiety

Anxiety is a physiological and psychological response to a threatening situation. The threat may be physical (e.g. a painful dental operation) or it may be psychological (e.g. lack of confidence about being able to cope with pain).

Where the threat is observable, the emotional state is termed 'fear'. Anxiety is the term used when the person is not quite sure why they are afraid. For example, a dental patient who doesn't know what is going to happen next in the treatment may become anxious.

When a person is anxious, a number of physio-logical changes are experienced including increased heart rate, increased blood pressure, increased muscle tension and palmar sweating. Changes in emotional expression, particularly crying, out-bursts of anger or nervous laughter may also occur. The person may also experience changes in thought processes. For example, the patient may have problems remembering instructions or inform-ation presented in the dental surgery.

It is important to know enough about a person to have some understanding of his or her feelings. This involves going beyond the spoken words of the patient. There are many patients who are very anxious about the dental treatment but steadfastly claim that they are not frightened. A good working principle is that no patient attends a dental surgery without experiencing some degree of anxiety.

Many dentists and assistants find it difficult at times to understand how a patient can be so afraid of treatment that is so painless and so harmless. You need to understand that what seems trivial to you might have great significance for the patient.

Defence mechanisms

There are a number of ways of thinking or behav-ing that help to reduce anxiety. These are called defence mechanisms because they serve to defend the person against anxiety and help to cope with problems. Defence mechanisms are highly effective methods of coping with anxiety and everybody uses them at times. However, to the non-anxious observer, they may sometimes give rise to state-ments or actions that appear odd, irrational or unrealistic.

In dealing with a patient who appears to be anxious or frustrated you should be accepting and uncritical. Encourage the patient to express their feelings openly so that the treatment program can be tailored to suit the patient's psychological needs, as well as dental needs.

Most people do learn to cope with their anxiety without special help. However, sometimes they learn inappropriate strategies for coping with anxiety. For example, avoiding the dentist is a highly effective way of relieving dental anxiety on a short-term basis, however, it may lead to more serious consequences later on, such as dental disease or greater treatment needs.

Some typical defence mechanisms are the following.

- Repression — upsetting or dangerous thoughts are pushed down into the unconscious mind. They may, however, return to conscious aware-ness in moments of extreme stress (e.g. where a usually docile, gentle person suddenly lashes out at the dentist).

- Projection — a person blames someone else quite unjustly for his or her own faults or undesirable behaviour. For example, a patient might say, 'My dentist is unhelpful and not at all interested in me', while it is the patient who is uncooper-ative and disinterested in the dental treatment.

- Rationalisation — people make excuses for their undesirable behaviour. For example, 'I can't help it if my teeth decay because I've got naturally chalky teeth', when the truth is that their teeth are covered in plaque due to poor oral care.

- Displacement — emotions are discharged onto 'safe' sources rather than onto the original cause. For example, the dentist might become angry with the dental assistant rather than with the patient who caused the bad temper.

- Substitution — a desired but frustrated goal is replaced by a less desirable but more easily obtained one. For example, a patient frightened of root canal therapy may choose the less desirable option of having the tooth removed.

- Denial — a person denies their actions or feelings. An example is when a very tense, pale, shaking patient states that they are feeling perfectly alright and that the treatment didn't hurt a bit.

- Regression — in this case, the person acts childishly or reverts to a more primitive way of behaving. This defence is frequently used by children of about five years of age who might revert to crying or bedwetting as a way of coping with anxiety.

- Affiliation — this is when the person seeks out others who share the same perceptions or values. Dental assistants may find that active involvement in organisations of their peers is an effective method of reducing anxieties related to work problems.

The dental team sometimes 'teaches' patients undesirable strategies for managing dental anxiety. An example of this is making false promises. It is a mistake to tell a patient that a particular treatment will not hurt when this guarantee cannot be made. When the procedure *does* hurt the patient, the patient is forced to conclude either that the dentist or dental assistant is insensitive or a liar. The patient may then feel unable to manage or control anxiety in future dental situations.

True, realistic information given before the event is an important way of producing the best coping behaviour. In the dental surgery it is important to give patients information that will allow them to have realistic expectations about the treatment, particularly about the length of time it will take, the degree of pain it is likely to cause and what is happening during the dental operation. The patient knows what to expect before, during and after treatment and will not be unnecessarily worried by unfamiliar sensations.

Incidental factors that have an impact on anxiety

The reception area

The waiting room should be planned with the well-being of the patients in mind. It should be relaxing and contain magazines that are varied, in good condition and up to date. In this way, the patients may feel that their needs are considered by the dentist and staff. It is not just that the surroundings are more pleasant to be in, in these circumstances — concern for the patient as a person is implied. Without being able to specifically pinpoint the reason, the patient may feel a 'personal touch' in the reception area. Lack of facilities (for example, old and untidy magazines) may be regarded by an anxious patient as an indication of lack of consideration.

People sometimes feel angry about the reception areas of some doctors and dentists. A lot of this anger may stem from the underlying feeling that if doctors and dentists permit an unattractive reception area, they do not really care about their patients.

The importance of the individual

If the patient has been to the dentist before, or has made an appointment, they will appreciate the courtesy of you addressing them by name. Although it may not be apparent, patients may feel rather put out if you cannot remember who they are.

In a situation where a person is anxious it is important for them to feel that those providing the treatment know who they are, for it can make the patient feel reassured that you and the dentist are aware of their particular treatment needs. This has an effect on the patient's confidence in the dentist and the treatment.

Delayed appointments

If the patient is punctual for the appointment, and for some reason there will be a delay before the dentist is about to see them, the patient should be told of this delay and the expected waiting time. The patient may choose to go away and come back later or may prefer to settle down to read. But if the delay is not explained, the patient may become increasingly tense as time passes. The patient might begin to imagine what is going on in the surgery, and to build up a false picture of what may be going to happen to them. This results in the dentist's work with this patient being made more difficult when the patient finally arrives in the surgery for treatment.

Some patients feel a sudden increase in anxiety as they leave the reception area to enter the surgery. The main part of the work of reassurance will fall to the dentist in this situation.

Behaviour shaping

Sometimes it is useful to be able to shape the patient's behaviour by using techniques that relieve the patient's anxiety and assist them to be co-operative. Dentistry tends to place the patient in a passive role rather than allow active participation in the treatment. It is important, therefore, that you do what you can to acknowledge the patient's needs and to help the patient to feel actively involved.

You should be as relaxed and as natural as is possible. It is a common error to treat the patient formally, coldly and in a strictly business-like fashion. These ways of behaving can be interpreted by the patient in a way that makes them feel even more passive than necessary and increases feelings of helplessness.

A behaviour-shaping technique that is especially effective in managing anxious patients is the 'tell – show – do' method. In this procedure, you or the dentist explains the work that is going to be done, using language that the patient can understand. Sometimes it is too difficult to describe the whole procedure. In this case, the description should be undertaken in steps.

Before commencing the procedure, you or the dentist demonstrates the procedures to show the patient exactly what is going to be done. The procedure is then carried out in exactly the way described.

Dental assistants will come to learn that they have to adapt in many ways to differences between patients. The kinds of information that can be sensibly communicated to adults will be different from the kind of information that can be communicated to children. Additionally, some adults learn quicker than others and may resent being told the same thing over and over again, while others may welcome this repetition. All of this draws attention to the important need for you to get to know as much as possible about the individual peculiarities of each patient so that each patient can be dealt with as an individual.

While extremely fearful patients may require the professional assistance of a clinical psychologist to desensitise their anxiety, good results can be ob-

tained for most patients using two simple techniques that do not require special training for their use. These are contact desensitisation and modelling.

Contact desensitisation

One of the special problems of dental anxiety is that patients often fear dental procedures, not because they are frightening in themselves but because the sensations they produce are cues that they are likely to experience pain. To reduce this anxiety it is necessary to desensitise the patient to these special sensations.

The contact desensitisation method is based on simulation of these dental sensations.

Contact desensitisation for fear of drilling

The sensation of drilling is mainly one of vibration transmitted through bone. This can be simulated by an electric toothbrush or any vibrating instrument (e.g. an electric shaver). A patient who is afraid of the drill is instructed to work through the following steps, repeating each step until no anxiety is experienced. If at any step in the process the patient feels anxious, they must not progress to the next step until this anxiety is alleviated.

- Step 1 — holding the vibrating instrument in the hands, feeling the sensation of vibration and thinking, 'This is like the sensation of drilling'.

- Step 2 — holding the instrument against the cheek so that the vibration is felt through the cheekbones and mandible, although cushioned by the soft tissue of the cheek, and thinking, 'This is like the sensation of drilling'.

- Step 3 — holding the instrument against the mouth with the mouth closed so that the vibration is felt through the upper and lower incisors, although cushioned by the lips, and thinking, 'This is like the sensation of drilling'.

- Step 4 — using the electric toothbrush to clean the teeth, thinking that the sensation of the bristles vibrating against the teeth is like the sensation of drilling, or using a cotton bud held against the electric shaver (or other instrument) with a rubber band, manipulating the cotton bud around the surfaces of the teeth while thinking, 'This is like the sensation of drilling'.

- Step 5 — reversing the electric toothbrush so that the plastic is against the teeth and using this to produce a drumming against the tooth surfaces while thinking, 'This is like the sensation of drilling'. Or using the same procedure as in step 4 but with a teaspoon strapped to the shaver instead of a cotton bud, stimulating the tooth surfaces while thinking, 'This is like the sensation of drilling'.

This technique significantly reduces fear of drilling in most patients by familiarising them with the vibration of drilling. In fact, because most dental drilling involves less vibration than that experienced during step 5 of these exercises, some patients say it is not as bad as the exercises themselves.

Some patients report that because they are familiar with the vibration sensation, it no longer seems as painful as it did previously to have teeth drilled or polished.

Contact desensitisation for fear of injections

A similar simple technique may help patients who are afraid of having injections. The sensation of a local injection consists of a sharp pin-prick felt as the needle is inserted, followed by pressure as the fluid is injected into the tissues. These sensations can be simulated using a long straight sewing pin in the following way.

- Step 1 — to simulate the sensation of having an injection in the palm of the hand, the pin is first held in a vertical position against the skin of the palm until a pin-prick sensation is felt, although at no time does the pin puncture the skin.

- Step 2 — maintaining this pin-prick sensation, the pin is then held horizontally with the shaft lying across the palm. Pressure is applied to the tissues lying beneath the shaft of the pin. The patient is instructed to repeat this procedure a number of times while thinking how similar it feels to the sensation of having an injection in the hand. When the patient can do this without feeling too anxious about it, the patient may then go on to practise simulating sensations of having injections in parts of the body where local injections are usually administered; the back of the hand inner elbow, upper arm and gums.

- Step 3 — to desensitise the gums the patient should use a small mirror to see what he or she is doing. Strong wooden toothpicks or inter-dental stimulators may be used instead of metal pins if there is any danger that the patient may slip and prick himself or herself. It may be necessary for some patients to repeat the procedure with another person holding the toothpick in order to more realistically simulate

the real local anaesthetic injection situation. This technique effectively reduces anxiety and many patients report that injections seem less painful after completing the simulated practice.

A small number of patients fear the sensation of numbness involved in local anaesthesia. This fear may be reduced by providing the patients with a small amount of topical anaesthetic paste to take home and apply daily to lips, gums and tongue until they becomes less anxious.

Modelling

Modelling is the form of learning by imitation that was described previously. It may be used to help patients to cope with their anxiety about dental treatment. While it may be used with adult patients, it is particularly useful with paedodontic patients (children) because it helps to establish socially acceptable ways of behaving in the dental surgery.

The anxious child (or adult) is booked in to attend the surgery at the same time as one (or preferably more than one) non-anxious, friendly, 'good' patient. The anxious patient accompanies the non-anxious patient into the surgery where the anxious patient watches the dental treatment. It is important to ensure that the treatment being demonstrated to the anxious patient is simple and straight-forward, unlikely to be painful or to produce bleeding. A good example is restoration of a small cavity (with local anaesthesia) followed by a prophylaxis.

The anxious patient, while permitted freedom of movement to observe the model patient, should be ignored. Attention, smiles and praise for good behaviour should be directed to the model patient so that the impression of the dental surgery as a comfortable, happy and rewarding place is communicated.

While this technique can be used with groups of children, it is best to have no more than two anxious children per group or the technique may backfire and anxious behaviour will be modelled. If using a group technique, it is preferable for the dentist and staff to concentrate on introducing sensations; for example, the feeling of a rubber polishing cup against a fingernail, the taste of prophylaxis paste, the sensation of topical anaesthetic on the lip.

Children also enjoy learning how the dental equipment works; which buttons fill the cup with water, how the apparatus can suck water out of the cup, what the air and water sprays do and, most importantly, how the chair goes up and down.

When a child exhibits dental anxiety, it is highly likely that the parent also suffers from dental anxiety. In this case, the parent would be the model from whom the child has acquired the anxious behaviour. Some dentists permit the parent to stay in the surgery with the child while the child is being treated. In the situation where the mother is anxious, to keep the parent in the surgery serves to keep an anxiety model before the child. To avoid this complication, it is preferable to see the child alone without the anxious parent.

Often 'bad' behaviour in the dental surgery may result from ignorance rather than from anxiety. It is a good idea to check that children understand the surgery 'rules' for good behaviour; for example, always sit still during dental treatment, do not move your tongue suddenly, do not try to touch the instruments in your mouth, do not grab the dentist's arm, and so forth.

Providing the child with a means of communication during dental treatment may be of assistance in controlling behaviour. For example, it may be worthwhile to tell the child, 'If you want to tell us something, wiggle your fingers like this, then as soon as possible the dentist will stop and see what you want'. This provides the child with some control over the situation and may relieve anxiety considerably.

Pain

Pain, and particularly the infliction of pain, can be a very difficult problem for the dental team to cope with. Pain can occur before treatment (e.g. a toothache), during treatment (e.g. exposure of sensitive **dentine**) or after treatment (e.g. post-surgical pain). However, the cause of pain is not always clear.

Pain is a highly individual experience. Pain can occur where no tissue damage is evident or where previously damaged tissues have completely healed. Pain of this type is referred to as psychogenic pain. It is as real to the patient as pain for which a **somatic** basis can be found (somatogenic pain).

The experience and the expression of pain may be influenced by a number of factors.

- Pain threshold — people vary in their sensitivity to pain. Some people experience drilling of dentine as severely painful while others do not classify this sensation as painful in any way. Fear can cause increased sensitivity to pain.

- Pain tolerance — people also differ in the amount of pain that they are able to tolerate. Some are unable to tolerate a twinge while others can bear severe degrees of pain without complaint.

- Age — although a reduction in pulp canal size within a tooth (a response to the ageing of dentine) can reduce sensitivity, older people (60 plus) appear to be less able to tolerate pain than younger people. Previous experience can also make older patients more anxious.

- Sex — women report experiencing greater levels of pain than do men undergoing similar experiences. It is possible that this results from social pressures that encourage men to 'be brave'.

- Personality — people who are anxious or depressed are more sensitive to pain than people who are not. Anxiety is the most common reaction to **acute** pain conditions while depression frequently occurs in patients who have suffered chronic pain (pain lasting six months or more). Extroverted people are more fluent in pain expression than shy or introverted people.

- Culture — some racial and cultural groups encourage a stoic attitude to pain while others do not. A great deal of misunderstanding can occur where staff and patients have different cultural backgrounds.

Any method that assists the patient to control anxiety will have the effect of reducing the patient's sensitivity to pain and helping them to cope better with the pain experienced. Perhaps the simplest method is to provide the patient with clear, concise, logical explanations of treatment procedures and effects. This provides realistic expectations concerning treatment with an understanding of the likely duration and severity of the pain experience. Expectation of pain can sometimes be worse than the pain itself.

Providing the patient with a means of control (e.g. a method of signalling to let the dentist know when the pain is becoming intolerable) can reduce anxiety related to feelings of helplessness and vulnerability. Special psychological techniques such as hypnosis are also highly effective in pain control.

Chronic pain is different from acute pain and is not easily controlled. Most chronic pain presenting in dental surgeries results from disorders of the temporo-mandibular joint and associated musculature. (See Chapter 8 for information about this joint.) It may be that patients experiencing this kind of chronic pain will require professional assistance to learn to cope with it.

■ **dentine:** the main mineralised substance of the tooth that surrounds the dental pulp and is covered by enamel on the crown and cementum on the root. ■ **somatic:** of the body. ■ **acute:** of sudden onset. Having a short and relatively severe course. ■ **chronic:** long, continued, not acute.

Attitudes to health

People's attitudes to dental health and dental treatment are also important. A patient may have a dental condition requiring treatment but they may not believe they need treatment. A number of other factors can influence a patient's decision to seek dental care, particularly preventive dental care.

- Perceived susceptibility — patients must believe that they are susceptible to dental diseases. Unless they hold this belief, they will not seek preventive treatment. Some people believe, 'This won't happen to me' and are less likely to seek treatment.

- Perceived seriousness — in the days when dental caries could lead to septicaemia and ultimately to death, the disease was clearly more serious than it is today. How serious individuals believe dental disease to be depends upon how they weigh the consequences of dental disease against other factors; for example, inconvenience, getting time off to attend the dentist, adverse effects on appearance, etc.

- Perceived benefits — some patients believe that dental disease is unavoidable; for example, as a result of a **hereditary** tendency to poor teeth. These patients often do not believe that dental treatment is very beneficial.

- Perceived salience — decisions about seeking dental treatment will also be based on how important (or salient) dental needs are in comparison with other needs. The most important factor here is financial. As a rule, people seek dental treatment when they feel that they can afford it. Patients have differing views on the benefits and costs of the recommended treatment and whether the benefits will outweigh the costs.

- Fear of dental treatment — it is generally accepted that fear can be a major factor in reducing dental visits by some people.

- Demographic factors — age, sex and socio-economic status are important. Dental treatment is more frequently sought during teenage years and decreases over time. Women utilise dental services more than men. Higher socio-economic groups (i.e. people with higher levels of income and education) make greater use of dental services than lower socio-economic groups.

- Service factors — easy access to dental treatment is also important. Dental insurance is another factor. Patients receiving treatment through public institutions may have waiting list problems. Dental health insurance has some effect on increasing dental utilisation.

Summary

Many different factors influence a patient's behaviour in the surgery. Understanding these factors can help you to make a better assessment of the patient's needs. This in turn will improve relations between the patient and the dental staff and lead to better outcomes for all.

An understanding of a patient's behaviour can also help you to provide them with appropriate oral health education.

■ **hereditary**: having the characteristics passed on from parents to children before birth.

chapter four
communication

Introduction

Dental assisting is a helping profession. In such a role, it is important to communicate effectively. Good communication is important in the achievement of a number of goals including:

■ the development of a mutually trusting, co-operative relationship with each patient (this is sometimes referred to as rapport) — patients who have good rapport with the dental health team are more likely to stay with the team and refer other people to the surgery, to accept treatment recommendations, to pay for those treatments on time and to be punctual for appointments;

■ effective transmission of information;

■ understanding of the patient's special needs and problems; and

■ efficient, effective and non-confrontational working relations with the dentist and other staff members.

Why do we communicate?

We communicate to reduce the uncertainties in our environment and to satisfy some essential basic needs.

Practical needs

Practical needs for communication encompass everyday transactions that require the sending and receiving both of factual information and of attitudes, feelings and emotions. Dental assistants may be involved in:

■ gaining knowledge and passing exams;

■ obtaining employment or convincing a selection committee that they are the best person for a position or a place in a graduate program;

■ interacting with other health professionals who may well be more experienced, knowledgeable or trained in a different field (e.g. dental therapists, practice managers, dentists, dental technicians, dental prosthetists); and

■ selecting, motivating and training staff.

Physical needs

Some interactive communication is essential for both physical and psychological health. Levels of need for social contact vary between individuals but some social contact is essential for wellbeing. Health professionals who are poor communicators risk feeling undervalued, misunderstood, professionally isolated or professionally unfulfilled.

Good communication at work will help to:

■ build and maintain rewarding and effective dentist–patient relationships; and

■ reduce professional stress and tension and prevent 'burnout'.

Ego needs

Communication is necessary for us to develop and clarify our own beliefs and attitudes. We decide on who we are based on how others react to us. Our sense of identity, self-worth, self-image or self-esteem partly derive from the quality and quantity of our interactions with others.

Social needs

This is the need to establish and maintain meaningful and rewarding relationships for inclusion, control and affection.

Inclusion

Inclusion is the sense of having some individual and group relationships, either formal (family, marriage, religious denomination) or informal (sporting team, study group, group of friends, professional organisation, practice team).

Control

Control is the need to have a sense of influence, control or power over our immediate personal environment. It includes the need to influence others, which may be demonstrated in a positive caring way, or in a negative destructive form, such as a complaint, nagging or hostility.

The dental situation can become impersonal with patients feeling physically powerless (lack of control), de-personalised and excluded from the group dynamics of the dental team. Effective use of interpersonal communication skills can make patients feel a sense of inclusion, while appropriate explanation and presentation of options will ensure that they perceive an appropriate share of control.

Affection

This is the need to care for others and know that others care for us. This includes love, friendship and approval.

The process of communication

Communication is dynamic. Communicators simultaneously send and receive verbal and nonverbal messages.

The more that the communicators have in common, the easier it is to interpret and understand the messages passing between them.

Some of the most common communication problems are the following.

- For communication to be successful, the receiver must be listening. Frequently speakers neglect to ensure that they have the listener's attention before they start.

- The language chosen by the speaker may not clearly convey the idea. In communicating with patients it is best to use simple, non-technical terms. However, it is also important to avoid 'talking down' to the patient.

- Communication is an exchange of ideas within the context of the attitudes and emotions of the people involved. Often we focus on the information content of the message but neglect the emotion and attitudes that accompany the message. These are often transmitted via body language. Body language is discussed in more depth later in the chapter.

- If the medium is rejected by the listener, it is highly likely that the message will also be rejected. For example, a patient who is terrified of dental surgeries may find it extremely difficult to concentrate on anything said to them while they are in the surgery. In rejecting the medium of the surgery, the patient is also unable to accept the messages conveyed there.

- The receipt of a message is dependent upon the listener's ability to receive it. Not all information is registered. Which parts of the message we attend to depends upon our attitudes, existing beliefs, interests and so on. For example, a patient who has undergone oral surgery may be in a mild state of shock and be unable to attend fully to instructions regarding post-operative care. A sensible precaution would be to provide such instructions in writing for the patient to read at home.

- The fact that a listener can repeat the message is no guarantee that the message is understood. Understanding depends upon the ability to decode the message to understand the idea intended by the speaker.

- The fact that a listener understands the message is no guarantee that the message is accepted. The listener can hold attitudes or beliefs in relation to the information transmitted that prevent the message from being persuasive.

In all communication it is necessary that the speaker receive feedback from the listener to assess whether the message has been received correctly. Dental assistants frequently neglect this important step in establishing whether patients have heard and understood post-operative instructions.

Communication barriers

There are psychological and physical barriers that can cause the 'noise' that leads to breakdowns in communication.

Psychological barriers can include fear, anger, jealousy, irritation, distraction, tension, lack of empathy, resentment, arrogance, embarrassment, defensiveness, preoccupation, intolerance, prejudice, low self-esteem, frustration, shyness and boredom.

Physical barriers can include offensive smells, intellectual disability, language difficulty, lack of knowledge, educational deficit, speech or hearing impediment, depressing overcrowded surroundings, uncomfortable temperatures, distracting or unpleasant sounds, hunger, fatigue and illness.

Physical barriers can often be minimised or removed by developing strategies to deal with them. Psychological barriers require behavioural changes to enable effective communication.

Breakdowns in communication

Physical noise

This concept describes identifiable physical or environmental barriers to communication. Physical 'noise' includes:

- distracting or excessive sound levels (traffic, argument, radio, dental equipment);
- offensive smells (personal, foodstuffs, cosmetics, antiseptics, dental materials);
- uncomfortable temperatures (excessive heat or cold);
- depressing, unattractive surroundings (overcrowding, dampness);
- hunger and fatigue;
- physical illness or pain;
- hearing, intellectual or visual impairment; or
- language difficulty.

Some of these physical barriers can often be anticipated and eliminated by choosing appropriate timing and surroundings, arranging for interpreters, etc. Recognising that all communication does occur in an environment, permits the option of establishing the most favourable circumstances for communicating.

Psychological noise

It is the psychological elements present in all communicators that are the most difficult to overcome. Psychological barriers often trigger powerful, negative and usually involuntary non-verbal signals or impede active listening. These barriers can and do affect communication between dentist and patient. Both patient and dentist can be the cause of the problem. Psychological 'noise' includes:

- anticipation of pain (whether correctly or incorrectly perceived);
- fear;
- anxiety or apprehension (for example, 'The worst is going to happen!'; 'How much will it cost?');
- preoccupation (for example, 'Has the parking meter expired?'; 'Will the appointment be over by a certain time?');
- emotions or attitudes such as prejudice, intolerance, defensiveness, irritation, distraction, tension, embarrassment, lack of empathy, confusion, hostility, anger, jealousy, arrogance, resentment and apathy.

Overcoming barriers to communication

Some techniques will assist in overcoming the effects of negative emotions.

Self-disclosure

Assess your own characteristics, attitudes and behaviours. Identify those that you consider destructive or unhelpful and attempt to avoid them. Try to avoid important communication transactions until you have had time to assess your emotions and bring them under control. Make others aware of your concerns.

Empathy

This is best described as trying to feel the other person's emotions. It is not the same as sympathy for someone's problems. Rather it is an attempt to share their feelings. It requires an assessment of the other's perceptions and feelings; that is, the responses or attitudes produced in them by those perceptions. Developing empathy can be demanding on the dental team but the reward is more relaxed and cooperative patients and reduced environmental stress.

Openness

Many of the identified psychological barriers will be eliminated by a frank, open and informative dental team providing explanation and introduction to the surgery and its procedures.

Perceptual screening

This barrier to communication is produced by the communicator's social and cultural experiences, gender roles, self-concepts and occupational roles. To lower your own perceptual screens and open the way to more effective communication try to:

- Gather all the facts — it is a common error to be unduly influenced by the obvious, loudest, most repetitious messages.

- Evaluate first impressions — perceptual screening results in stereotyping of others on first impressions. Holding on to negative first impressions can develop into a permanent and negative self-fulfilling prophecy.

Focus on the positive — it is easier and probably more newsworthy or exciting (and it makes a better story!) to highlight another person's negative qualities. Better communication requires an effort to identify and give prominence to favourable behaviour and attitudes.

Don't assume that others share your opinions, motives, attitudes and values. An educated guess based on all the available facts is better than an assumption. Testing and validating your opinion by asking questions of the other person is preferable but only if you employ active listening when the answers are given.

Listening

Between 60 per cent and 80 per cent of our waking hours are devoted to some form of communication. This communicating time is subdivided as follows.

- 53 per cent is listening (21 per cent of which is actual face-to-face listening).

- 16 per cent is talking.

- 17 per cent is reading.

- 14 per cent is writing.

The significance of listening is immediately obvious. However, listening is an acquired skill that must be practised in order to become effective. Of all the barriers to effective interpersonal communication, poor listening is the most significant.

Listening is an active psychological process, not simply the process of hearing. Listening requires a disciplined, active effort on the part of the communicator. Not all listeners receive the same message.

An effective listening process involves:

- hearing (the physical act);

- attending (concentrating on the message) — attention increases with the perceived importance of the message;

- understanding; and

- remembering, based on the amount of repetition and on the intensity of the relationship.

Assess your own listening habits so you can develop strategies to improve listening skills.

Attending skills

Good attention is necessary for good communication. Paying careful attention demonstrates to the patient that you respect them and that you are interested in what they have to say.

Postural position (including gesticulation and facial expression)

Good postural position includes:

- having your body face the other person;

- having hands either on your lap or loosely clasped or occasionally being used to gesticulate what is being communicated verbally;

- being responsive facially (spontaneous smiling or nodding of the head in agreement or understanding and frowning when not understanding); and

- an erect but not rigid body, and occasionally leaning toward the person.

Poor postural position includes:

- sitting with the body, and head not facing the other person;

- slouching;

- sitting in a very fixed, rigid position without moving;

- being restless or fidgety;

- being preoccupied with hands, papers, fingernails;

- making no gestures at all with hands;

- constant movement and thrashing of hands and arms;

- no facial expression (poker-faced); and

- too much (inappropriate) smiling, frowning or nodding of the head.

Eye contact

Good eye contact includes:

- looking at the person while they are talking to you or vice versa; and
- maintaining eye contact by means of spontaneous glances which express interest and desire to listen and respond.

Poor eye contact includes:

- never looking at the person;
- staring at them; and
- looking away from them as soon as they look at you.

However, be aware that some cultures find eye contact offensive and this should be respected.

Some habits of poor listening

Pseudo-listening

This involves pretending to listen by giving the impression of being interested and attentive, while actually thinking about something totally unrelated to what is being said because the message or the person delivering it is considered unimportant.

Stage hogging

This is practiced by persons who are only interested in hearing themselves talk. These people are good at making speeches but can also be annoying because other people do not have an opportunity for inclusion.

Selective listening

This involves filtering messages so that only those aspects that interest the listener are received.

Filling in the gaps

This is a common habit where the listener assumes to know what the other person is going to say or has heard the message before. This behaviour leads not only to incomplete messages but also to distorted messages.

Assimilation to prior input

This involves a selective and distorting form of listening that mutilates the message to ensure its consistency with what the receiver has heard in the past.

Defensive listening

This can be a common problem when clinicians are faced with apparent criticism from patients. Innocent comments or justifiable enquiries are interpreted as personal attacks. It is often a tactic used by people with low self-esteem to project their own insecurities onto others. If one feels criticised, it is more productive to seek precise information, listen with an open mind to the criticism and, where possible, agree with the speaker (e.g. agree with the truth or a principle). These non-defensive responses will permit constructive dialogue leading to a resolution.

Ambushing

These people listen very carefully to your argument, waiting for a particular statement or phrase that can be used to attack what you are saying. Habitual ambushers will create defensive listening habits in others.

Rehearsing a response

This is similar to ambushing and is a common error in which all listening ability is suspended while the person runs through the 'best response'; often a putdown to something that has been said.

Ineffective listening

When the listener gives an opinion, criticises or gives information, these responses have the effect of pulling the patient up, inhibiting or redirecting their line of thought. These responses communicate the message that the patient has no right to complain or, if they do complain, won't receive a truly sympathetic hearing.

Active listening

One of the most important skills in communication is learning to become a good listener. In active listening the listener 'bounces back' or paraphrases what the speaker has said. It is a skill that requires carefully attending to patients and the ability to put yourself in their shoes and see things from their points of view.

In its simplest form, paraphrasing is a simple re-statement of a word or a phrase. More usually, the objective of paraphrasing is to say back to the patient the essence of what they have just said. To do this you reveal the meaning that their comment has for you so that they can check whether it matches the meaning they intended to convey.

Paraphrases serve three purposes.

❶ They convey to the patient that you are trying to understand what is being said.

❷ They crystallise a patient's comment by making it more concise, thus helping give direction to the interaction.

❸ They provide a check on the accuracy of your perception.

Paraphrasing is not an attempt to mind-read but it is an aid to accuracy and additional clarification. If your paraphrase is successful, it will often be rewarded with a 'yes' or 'right' and the patient will continue to talk in more depth about the issue at hand.

Good paraphrasing involves restating the patient's basic message in similar, but usually fewer, words. If you are not sure whether you have got it right, it is useful to preface your paraphrase with a phrase such as:

- 'Are you saying...'; or

- 'It seems to me that you're...'

Suggested guidelines for good paraphrasing are:

- listen for the basic message;

- restate a concise and simple summary of their basic message; and

- observe a cue or ask for a response that confirms (or otherwise) the accuracy and helpfulness of the paraphrase.

Poor paraphrasing includes:

- introducing your analysis, interpretation, or value judgment of the patient's message;

- responding to a minor part of the message rather than the main theme; and

- using inappropriate words or phrases (e.g. jargon).

Exploratory responses

A second method that facilitates communication is exploratory responding. An exploratory response is a way of responding that encourages the person to continue talking and at the same time provides the speaker with freedom to talk about concerns. The listener could simply say, 'Tell me more about that,' or 'Why do you feel that was?' It can also be done by just saying 'Oh?' and looking interested.

The important thing is that the speaker is encouraged to continue talking without being directed towards the listener's line of thought.

In summary, good listening includes:

- maintaining your full and undivided attention;

- listening to all that is being said;

- listening to the whole person (their words, feelings and behaviour), sensing their total message; and

- directing whatever you say to what the person has said.

Poor listening includes:

- allowing yourself to be distracted by other noises, or the view behind the patient;

- forming judgments about the person before they complete their message;

- formulating a response to the person's message before they finish; and

- jumping from topic to topic.

Communicating without words

Non-verbal communication, or body language, is an important part of all communication. The messages transmitted in the non-verbal medium often carry information about feelings, attitudes and emotions.

In the dental surgery, because the mouth is immobilised for long periods, the communication process may depend heavily on body language. Sometimes, the nature of dental treatment and the structure of the dental surgery may mean that some body language rules must be modified or broken. Since each body language signal has a specific meaning that we all recognise, it is important to understand how body language operates in the special environment of the dental surgery.

Attention and sensitivity to the non-verbal messages communicated by patients and by the dental team will improve the overall effectiveness of communication. Remember, the non-verbal component of a message is very powerful. Matching non-verbal signals will enhance a verbal message. Non-verbal signals that do not match the verbal message will undermine that message. This can often be seen in patients who say that everything is fine but whose body movements contradict their words.

Distance

The physical distance chosen by two people having a conversation depends upon factors such as the intimacy of the relationship, age, sex and racial background, as well as upon circumstances of the physical environment. As a rule, close proximity (distances of less than a metre) is tolerated only in intimate relationships and tends to produce a rise in anxiety or tension when it occurs in other interactions.

Dental treatment may necessitate distances of as little as 200 mm between the people involved and often the patient may have two other people within their personal 'territory'. This produces an increase in discomfort. Better communication is achieved at distances of a metre or greater. It is advisable to use this more acceptable distance for conversation and to use the closer distances only during treatment.

Posture

When communicating, people usually adopt postures that are similar in the degree of relaxation, the amount and direction of leaning and the placement of limbs. Dissimilar postures usually indicate that there are different circumstances in the inter-actions; for example, that one of the people has higher status than the other.

Supine postures (lying or reclining) lower than the other person, are usually only adopted in intimate relationships. Patients, lying in a dental chair, can feel very threatened in this position.

Tension in hands, feet or shoulders may indicate anxiety.

Body contact

Body contact is bound by strict 'rules' in every culture. Generally, contact in any area other than hands and arms is regarded as a gesture of intimacy or as a threat. Contact with the oral area is understood by the patient to be necessary for dental treatment. Other contacts, for example, wiping instruments on the patient's bib, should be avoided.

Facial expression

Facial expression is a complex form of non-verbal communication involving movement of the eyes, eyebrows and the mouth. We are capable of inter-preting very small muscle movements.

During dental treatment, the patient's use of facial expression is curtailed because the mouth is immobilised. For this reason, the patient may rely upon eyes and eyebrows to communicate or may make use of body movements and muscle tension to express feelings such as anxiety or stress.

Eye movement

Eye movement is another complex and fast-moving medium of non-verbal communication. There are three basic rules of eye movement.

❶ We look in the direction of our interest.

❷ We look less at people in close proximity.

❸ We use eye movement to provide feedback cues in speech (e.g. to tell each other when it is our turn to speak).

Sometimes patients stare at the dentist or dental assistant during treatment and may make them feel quite uncomfortable because it contravenes the rule of looking less at people in close proximity. Patients may do this because you are talking (a speech feedback cue to show the patient is listening), or because they are worried about what is happening or because looking at the ceiling is boring (both reasons indicating looking in the direction of interest). Placing an interesting picture on the surgery ceiling or talking less compulsively can help to prevent this problem.

Conflict resolution

Effective communication often breaks down due to the way people make sense of verbal, written or non-verbal messages that they receive. Poor listen-ing is often a source of conflict as it can result in messages being incorrectly decoded.

As well as ineffective communication, conflict can stem from:

■ different attitudes, values and beliefs; and

■ conflicting needs.

Attitudes, values and beliefs

The lifelong influences on an individual combine to form their perception of the world. A clash of world views is often a source of conflict. Some of these influences are family, media, climate, gender, culture, books, era, friends, education and economy. When two people have different world views they can have different expectations of appropriate behaviour.

Needs

Maslow's psychological theory of 'hierarchy of needs' (1970) provides a useful framework for examining how conflicting needs are often a source of conflict. He argues that we all have the following needs in common.

- Physical needs — job security and a reasonable income are needed to meet the physical needs of food, shelter and clothing. If these are threatened, then conflict can occur.

- Safety needs — any threat to safety can be a source of conflict. Some of these threats at work could include unsafe working conditions or verbal or physical aggression.

- Self-esteem — work can be an important source of self-esteem. Meeting self-esteem needs can be threatened by feeling unappreciated, having work performance criticised or devalued, feeling excluded from decision-making or being ostracised.

- Self-actualisation — being hampered from achieving full potential is another source of conflict. This can happen when opportunities for advancement are threatened or requests for further training are denied.

Ways of dealing with conflict

Some ways in which people deal with conflict are:
- avoiding it, ignoring it or pretending it isn't there;
- competing and trying to always get their own way;
- giving in to others even when it means that one person is making an uncomfortable compromise;
- working out ways where there will be mutual compromise by all parties; or
- collaborating to find a solution that meets as many needs as possible.

Obviously, some of these methods are better than others and no one method will work for all people for all situations. Sometimes there are times when it is possible to ignore a conflict. At other times, to ignore the conflict simply escalates it.

Dealing with difficult people can be unpleasant but sometimes thinking about dealing with a conflict is worse than actually dealing with it. The key to conflict resolution is to find the right method for the issue at hand.

Assessing the conflict to determine the best way to go forward

- Try to clarify your own position and role. For example, does it only seem bad because of some other reason (for example, you are unwell or tired or have an unrelated personal relationship problem that is causing stress)?

- Try to judge just how important the issue really is. Is it more important than your job or your relationships with others?

- Decide whether you are just trying to get your own way.

- Try to identify multiple actions you can take to resolve the conflict and list the pros and cons of each (perhaps with the help of a sympathetic friend).

Wait a short time to see if the situation resolves itself (but set a deadline for when you want the improvement to occur so you know if you will need to take action). When trying to resolve a conflict:

- Try to keep the process private by moving away from other people.

- Use all your best communication skills including active listening, attending and exploratory responses.

- Let go of trying to get what you want. You might get what you want, at the other person's expense and then the other person gets back at you later.

- Try to agree on what the best outcome would be before you work out a way of reaching that outcome.

- Make it clear on what points you agree and disagree.

- Do not interrupt.

- Ask questions to clarify the other person's motives. What does the other person think the conflict is about? Perhaps you are arguing about two different things.

- Don't blame the other person for everything that is wrong. You are part of the problem, too.

- State your own assumptions about the issue so the other person knows your thoughts but focus on the conflict, not on the person you are in conflict with.

- Don't be shy about asking for what you want and working to get it.

- Thank the other person for taking the time to try to find a solution with you.

- Do whatever you can to stay calm, including keeping your voice low, taking deep breaths etc.

- Keep your eye on the 'big' picture. Your job and your relationship with other staff is more important than the conflict.

- Try to establish a list of actions that everyone in the conflict can take part in.

- Be very careful not to take offence or retaliate.

- Establish whether a mediator is needed.

- When you think you have a good solution, try it for a week or so and make a date to go back and assess whether it is working or not.

Conflict with patients

Prompt resolution of complaints or misunderstandings is a crucial facet of communication between the dental health team and the patient. It is important to use good communication skills to ensure that the patient's complaints are resolved.

It may well be necessary to have the dentist solve the issue, in which case it is possible to tell the patient that the dentist will call them at a particular time. Ensure that this does happen.

Summary

Learning any communication skill is difficult at first but improvement quickly follows with practice and can extend your function and effectiveness in the dental practice. Remember the following points:

- Communication is a shared responsibility.
- Communication is irreversible.
- Verbal communication is conscious and voluntary.
- Non-verbal communication can be involuntary or voluntary. It is very powerful and very difficult to fake or disguise.
- What we do when communicating conveys far more meaning than the spoken words.
- Words do not have meaning. People have meaning.
- Silence is a powerful form of communication.
- Listen to the major points and the supporting arguments.
- Share the communication responsibility.
- Clarify and seek feedback by asking questions.
- Listen with an open mind and with empathy.

Good communication is crucial to an efficient and effective practice and improves relationships between dental staff and the patient.

Reference

Maslow, G. (1970) *Motivation and personality* (2nd edn). Harper & Row, San Francisco.

chapter five
reception duties

Introduction

Some surgeries have secretary–receptionists or secretary–bookkeepers. The duties of these staff members are outlined in Chapter 1. However, in many surgeries, reception, secretarial work and bookkeeping fall to the dental assistant. For this reason, it is important for you to have an understanding of these duties.

This chapter covers the duties of the dental assistant as a secretary–receptionist.

These duties generally include:
- arranging appointments;
- reception of patients and visitors;
- answering the telephone;
- writing correspondence; and
- sending recall notices.

Account keeping and financial duties are discussed in the next chapter.

A note about computer systems

There is a range of different computer systems that are available on the market and can be used in the dental surgery. Some are generic systems (not specifically designed for dentistry). For example, some practice/clinics have generic bookkeeping systems to handle all account information.

There are also software packages designed specifically for dental practice/clinics. Each year, there are more on the market and the existing packages are updated. If a computer package or packages are used in your workplace, you will need specific training to use those systems. This training can sometimes be organised through the package supplier.

If electronic systems are used, regular backups should be made of all information that is stored electronically and these backup copies should be kept away from the premises.

The appointment book

The focal point of a dental practice/clinic is the appointment book. The efficiency of your practice/clinic depends primarily on your skill in booking appointments correctly. A sample appointment book page is shown in Figure 5.1.

To ensure that the maximum number of patients receive satisfactory treatment in one day it is necessary to plan how appointments will be booked. There is an optimum number of people who can be seen profitably in a given number of hours. In this case, profitably means both financially profitable and achieving completed work for the patient.

The type and amount of work to be done is different in each practice/clinic. The dentist sets policy in this regard and should be consulted. Booking should ensure that:
- the maximum number of patients is treated within a day;
- patients are seen on time;
- time is used economically so that each patient's needs are attended to;
- the appointments are well balanced so appointments are not hurried, and stress and tension are minimised;
- a variety of treatments is scheduled for maximum efficiency;
- the maximum number of working hours in the day is not exceeded;
- essential rest breaks (e.g. lunch time) are adhered to; and
- periods of wasted (non-productive) time are avoided.

Thursday 11 January	Treatment	Friday 12 January	Treatment	Saturday 13 January	Treatment
8:00 Johnnie Brown	C/U	8:00		8:00	
8:15 Sarah Brown	C/U	8:15		8:15	
8:30 Mrs I Jacobs	Prep	8:30		8:30	
8:45	Imps Crown	8:45		8:45	
9:00		9:00		9:00	
9:15		9:15		9:15	
9:30 Mr S Jones	Dent	9:30		9:30	
9:45		9:45		9:45	
10:00 Tom Sharp	Comp fill	10:00		10:00	
10:15		10:15		10:15	
10:30 Mrs C Daniel	Try in F/-	10:30		10:30	
10:45		10:45		10:45	
11:00 M H Dang	RCT	11:00		11:00	
11:15		11:15		11:15	
11:30		11:30		11:30	
11:45 Bob Allen	T/A	11:45		11:45	
12:00 Anna Taylor	S4C	12:00		12:00	
12:15		12:15		12:15	
12:30 Mr H Trapovski	C/U N/P	12:30		12:30	
12:45 ph. 9750 8906		12:45		12:45	
1:00		1:00		1:00	
1:15		1:15		1:15	
1:30 LUNCH		1:30		1:30	
1:45		1:45		1:45	
2:00 Rotary meeting		2:00		2:00	
2:15		2:15		2:15	
2:30 Mrs O Dumper	MOD Amal	2:30		2:30	
2:45		2:45		2:45	
3:00		3:00		3:00	
3:15 Robin Smith	EXO 14	3:15			
3:30		3:30		**Standby Patients**	
3:45 Jodie Smith	(E)	3:45			
4:00 Rowan Green	fill	4:00		Bob Allen C/U 1/2 hour	
4:15		4:15		9647 5401	
4:30 Yvonne Foley	(E) N/P	4:30			
4:45 Mother Anne	5 years	4:45		Book in February Recalls	
5:00 Bonny Foley	Fill	5:00			
5:15		5:15			
5:30		5:30		**Notes**	
5:45		5:45			
6:00		6:00		Call Technician for	
6:15		6:15		Mrs Jacobs Crown	
6:30		6:30		next week	
6:45		6:45			
7:00		7:00			
7:15		7:15		**Hours Worked**	
7:30		7:30		**No. of Patients**	
7:45		7:45		**Days Off**	

Figure 5.1 Sample appointment book page

The biggest challenge is striking a balance between under- and over-crowding of the daily list. With practice, you should be able to manage the appointment book so that the dentist is comfortably busy, the patients are content with their appointments and you can carry out your duties efficiently.

There are various types of appointment books. The most common one is a hardcover diary-style book in which appointments can be made as far as necessary in advance. There is also a loose-leaf appointment book that shows an entire week's work when open. Many practice/clinics use computer appointment scheduling and you will need training in the specific system used if that is the case.

It is usually best if only one person makes the appointments. If more than one person will be making the appointments, a method must be used to identify who made the appointment so any confusion or error can be quickly resolved. If using an appointment book, use a soft (2B) pencil to make appointments, not ink.

It is useful to have a list of patients who can attend at short notice should cancellations occur.

Appointment arrangement

New appointments are usually made by telephone. The patient states why he or she is ringing (for example, for a check-up, a lost filling, a toothache, a new denture). Knowing this information is crucial to arranging the appointment. It may be a waste of time to reserve a full appointment, for example, and then find that there is no work to be done.

A card may be sent for confirmation of the day, date and hour. Many patients need to be reminded of their appointment. Most practice/clinics call the patient a day or two before the appointment to confirm the appointment and as a reminder.

A patient who is continuing treatment makes the next appointment at the desk before leaving the surgery. The patient's name is entered in the appointment book or computer immediately, with the nature of the treatment in the adjacent column. The patient is given an appointment card with the date and time of the appointment.

Scheduling appointments

It is useful to know what treatment is planned and the duration of the treatment so that scheduling may be carried out logically.

Long appointments are more productive than short ones. If there is a free period in the day, suggest this time to the patient. Try to steer the patients away from the busiest times and towards free periods.

Patients with multiple appointments should have a complete list of appointments appended to their treatment card and preferably their next appointment should be noted alongside their current time. This allows accurate rescheduling if an appointment is broken or cancelled.

Any difficult work is usually best scheduled in the morning while the dentist and patient are fresh. Prosthetic appointments may be scheduled more suitably for the early afternoon. Remember to consult with the dental technician about the length of time to complete prosthetic work to ensure that each stage of work is completed well before the patient's arrival. Selecting shades of denture teeth and similar work is best done in the middle of the day.

Young children (aged nine years and under) are more tolerant before 10.30 am. Children are better patients early in the day than they are after school. Where there are a number of children in a family, parents may prefer to bring them in together or on the same day as their own appointment. This may save them many visits.

Routine multiple appointments should be made only in the special circumstances indicated by the particular course of treatment that has been predetermined, e.g. root canal therapy, crown and bridge, elderly patients with disabilities or patients who travel long distances. Note should be taken of how many days are required for laboratory work between appointments. If possible, make serial appointments on the same day of the week and at the same time. This makes them easier to remember.

Staying on time with appointments is important. Patients resent being kept waiting, especially when it is a perpetual problem with the practice/clinic.

New patients

It is advisable to ask new patients to come a few minutes early to allow them to fill in the medical/dental history form. (Medical/dental history forms are discussed in depth later in this chapter.) Some practice/clinics send medical/dental histories that can be filled in at home. However, all forms should be checked for completeness when they are returned.

It is also common for surgeries to send out information packs to new patients containing a map, information about the availability of parking, office hours, emergency numbers, payment policies and information about the services offered by the dentist.

Blocking out the appointment book

The appointment book should be prepared many months in advance, with entries made to indicate:

- the number of dentists and hygienists working and the number of rooms in use;
- times when the surgery is closed;
- holidays, public holidays and away days (conference attendance for example);
- meeting times;
- lunch hours;
- continuing education lectures; and
- times scheduled for last minute or emergency appointments.

Computer systems used in some dental surgeries allow easy entry of this kind of information.

Note should also be made of school or public holidays when the surgery is open but schools and businesses are not. It can be useful to save these days for patients who cannot attend during usual office hours. (Be careful when making appointments during school holidays as families often go away and forget their appointments.)

Appointments are usually booked in units of time (either of 15 minute or 30 minute duration). The dentist should be able to tell you approximately what length of time to set aside for each treatment.

Entries should include:

- the name of the patient;
- contact phone numbers (home and business hours);
- treatment type and appointment length; and
- any special information that may be relevant to the appointment. For example, if the patient

requires premedication or needs to complete a medical history, this can be noted in the appointment book.

If the patient is at the reception desk, an appointment card can be completed and handed to the patient once the appointment has been made, containing the same details as those written in the appointment book. If the appointment is being made over the phone, the information should be verbally confirmed. Impress upon patients the importance of keeping appointments.

A certain period may be kept each day for emergency appointments. Learn to distinguish between true urgency and panic on the part of the patient.

Patients who drop in without an appointment can disrupt the entire schedule. They should be reminded that if they make an appointment a time can be reserved so they do not have to wait. It is important you understand the dentist's policy on patients who walk in from the street without an appointment. Some dentists will see patients if they are previous patients of the surgery, some will insist that an appointment be made, some will see new patients who walk in, others will not. Make sure you know the dentist's view before the situation arises, so that patients can be turned away politely if necessary.

Broken appointments

If a patient does not arrive for an appointment, try to telephone them in the first 10 minutes of the time booked for their appointment. It is quite important to let them know politely that they have broken an appointment. Failure to do this may allow the patient to believe that they were not missed (for example, that you were so busy that it took you five hours to get around to reporting the broken appointment).

Be tactful. For example, 'According to our appointment schedule, we had a $3/4$ hour appointment reserved for you at 1.45'. It is always possible that you may have made an error and recorded the appointment for Tuesday, for example, but recorded it for Monday in the book. Alternatively, the patient may have cancelled and the appointment was not erased. It is wise to note cancelled and broken appointments on the treatment card (showing the time and date) for future reference and action as necessary.

Some patients find it difficult to remember appointments. A telephone call can be made two hours before the appointment to remind them.

Charging for broken appointments

It must be understood that a patient may occasionally forget or run late for an appointment. However, some patients regularly do not arrive for their appointments and don't seem to care. A suitable method for these patients is to insist on them leaving a deposit for their next appointment. If they keep the appointment, the deposit forms part of the fee to be paid. If they break the appointment the deposit is forfeited.

Some practices have a sign stating that broken appointments will be charged for. Unfortunately, this may be ignored by some patients. It is doubtful that this is enforceable in law.

Buffer times

Some surgeries like to have a 'buffer period' scheduled each day. This might be a 15 minute period at the end of the morning session and again at the end of the afternoon session. These periods are never filled more than 24 hours in advance and are used, for example, for emergencies, relief of pain, patients who walk in off the street, or for last minute adjustments. Sometimes they simply allow 'breathing space' when the surgery is running behind schedule.

The telephone

Most practice/clinics establish protocols for the handling of incoming telephone calls. All staff members must follow these protocols.

The telephone should be answered as promptly as possible. Do not forget to remove your gloves and wash hands before picking up the phone.

Be cheerful, courteous and tactful. Pleasantness can be transmitted by the tone of voice more than by what is said. Listeners can hear in your voice whether you are smiling, or if you are anxious, angry or tired. Your voice should be calm, low and well modulated, friendly and interested and the enunciation should be clear and slow.

In a single dentist practice, the telephone can be answered with, 'Dr Smith's surgery' and then your name as the person speaking. When there are two or more dentists in the practice the appropriate title of the surgery should be established with the dentist/dentists.

If the patient or some other caller does not give a name immediately, ask who is speaking and continue the conversation only when you have taken note of the name. Use the person's name occasionally from then on and always at the end of the conversation, e.g. 'Good-bye Mr Smith. We'll see you on the 25th'.

Next, ask the reason for requesting an appointment, the degree of urgency and whether it is a genuine emergency; that is, whether there is toothache, fracture of a denture, etc. With this information an appointment can be made. If the caller is in pain or a denture is fractured, arrange the appointment for the same day.

Ask if the speaker has been to the surgery before. If so, you should have a record card for the patient. If the patient is new, ask for initials and have the name spelt correctly. Also, make sure you ask for the patient's address and telephone numbers (work and home).

If for any reason it is impossible to make an appointment for a patient, try to explain why but never refuse to see a patient without referring the matter to the dentist. If in doubt, ask the advice of the dentist before finishing the conversation with the patient. It is better to ask the dentist's opinion on an appointment before 'overbooking' or alienating a patient who could be fitted in with some re-arrangement of the schedule.

Personal calls should not be taken during working hours. If they are unavoidable, they should be brief.

Avoid coughing or sneezing near the handset. Do not quote fees over the telephone. Fees vary according to the exact treatment and can only be quoted in the surgery after an examination has taken place.

If an irate patient telephones to complain about an account or appointment it is best to tell them that you will investigate and call them back. Once the complaint is investigated and clarified with the dentist, the patient should be called back. Usually they will have cooled off by the time of the second call and a more useful discussion can be held.

Placing patients on hold

Never place anyone on hold without first asking their permission. A patient should not be kept on hold for more than a minute (which will seem much longer than that to the person on hold). If a long delay is likely, it is wiser to take the patient's number and arrange a time to call them back.

If the telephone system has a recording that plays while the patient is on hold, effort should be made to ensure that the quality of the recording is good

and the content is appropriate. Many patients object to having to listen to loud or static-filled music while they wait.

Messages for the dentist

A pad and pen should be kept next to the phone to note calls that must be returned and for messages that must be brought to the dentist's attention. These messages should be brought promptly to the dentist's attention. If appropriate, also hand the patient's records to the dentist when passing on the message.

Effort must be made to ensure that all the information recorded is accurate. Ensure that you have the correct name, time and date written down. Some surgeries have a specially printed 'phone log' and record *every call* that comes in to the surgery.

Some callers will insist that they will only speak to the dentist. If this is the case it is appropriate to say, 'Dr Smith is with a patient now. Is there something I can help you with or would you like me to take a message?'

Some dentists have a regular 'call back' time each day when they can call patients with queries or complaints. If this is the case, it is appropriate to tell the caller that the dentist will return the call at that time.

Some dentists like to set rules for whom they wish to speak to immediately (for example, family members or suppliers) and whom they wish to call back. Make sure you know the dentist's preferences. Bear in mind that interrupting a treatment has implications for infection control. Protocols should be in place to prevent the possible transmission of infection from the surgery to the reception area and telephone.

Voicemail and answering machines

All surgeries should have a recorded message for patients who ring out of hours. Think carefully about any message that you leave. Most messages would contain:

- the name of the surgery or dentist;
- office hours;
- an invitation for the patient to leave a message or call back during office hours; and
- a phone number in case of emergencies.

The message bank should be checked as soon as the office opens each day or after any period that the machine has been turned on.

Receiving patients and visitors

The physical environment

The physical surroundings of the reception area and surgery should be warm and inviting. Furniture, carpets and curtains should be clean and free from wear and tear. All areas should be dust free and an attempt should be made to keep reading materials (magazines, for example) up to date and tidy. Fresh or dried flowers, provided they are free from dust and do not look shabby, can make the reception area much more welcoming. Dental educational pamphlets and posters add colour and interest for waiting patients. In practice/clinics where families with young children are seen, a children's toy corner creates a welcoming atmosphere.

If furnishing or furniture needs repair, this should be brought to the dentist's attention.

Many people, not only patients, may visit the surgery (dental company representatives for example). These people must also be received promptly and courteously. The dentist should instruct the receptionist on appropriate times for visitors to call.

Greeting the patient

Reception of the patient at the door, in the hall or the reception area follows the same general principles as answering the telephone but here you have the advantage of seeing the patient and making some assessment of their mood and personality.

It is also the first time the patient sees you and they will often make an assessment of the quality of the practice from this first impression. A ready, natural smile should always be given to a patient when coming and going. This is vital with children.

Patients should be greeted by name and a smile as soon as they arrive. If the patient is new, introduce yourself. Use the patient's correct title (Mrs, Mr, Dr, etc.) unless they tell you their first name, and mark on the card the patient's preferred form of address. Collect necessary information from patients who are new to the practice/clinic and give them any necessary forms to complete; for example, the medical/dental history.

It is important to know how patient's names are spelt and pronounced. If it is a difficult name, write it on the treatment chart with phonetic spelling, e.g. 'Meyn' pronounced Mine'.

It is important to learn children's nicknames, sports, and hobbies and to mention these when greeting or seating them in the surgery. Make a note on their card to prompt your memory. Also note if their parents' surnames are different. Some more suggestions for working with children are in Chapter 35.

Patients become frustrated if their presence in the reception room is not acknowledged very soon after their arrival. They do not know whether to sit down or try to announce their arrival in some way. After the patient has been greeted correctly and is seated, inform them if there is to be a short wait. If a long wait is anticipated, 20 minutes or longer, inform the patient the dentist is delayed with an involved case but will see them as soon as possible. You can usually judge the waiting time by the type of treatment the dentist is giving. Offer a drink or suggest re-appointing if the patient is in a hurry and can't wait. Inform the dentist of the patient's arrival by a recognised signal, e.g. marking off the patient's name on the day sheet.

Recording patient details

It is usually the receptionist's role to obtain personal details and record them on the patient's card. These details will include name, contact information, etc. Refer to Chapter 18 for more information.

Medical/dental histories

Why histories are taken

There are many conditions of patients' general health that will influence their dental treatment. Even a seemingly healthy young adult may have a medical condition or be utilising a medication that could have an impact on any proposed form of treatment.

A few examples that illustrate this point are:

- Allergy — for example, to red food dyes (disclosing solution) or to latex (operator gloves, dental dam, etc).
- Asthma — the patient may need to bring a **bronchodilator** to each visit. There is a possibility of oral candidiasis (thrush) from use of preventive corticosteroid medications.
- Diabetes — there is a possible risk of **hypoglycaemia** and a possible effect on status.

bronchodilator: a drug used by asthmatics to relax air passages to the lungs and make breathing easier.
hypoglycaemia: a medical condition where the patient has too little blood sugar.

There is also an increased risk of wound infection or delayed healing and **hyperglycaemia** with the resulting acetone breath and high blood sugar. (See Chapter 22 for information on medical emergencies in the surgery.)

- Heart murmur — history of heart murmur may indicate a need for antibiotic cover before invasive treatment such as deep **subgingival scaling**. It is essential to distinguish this type of murmur from 'innocent' murmurs in healthy patients. Consultation with the patient's cardiologist may be required.

- **Epilepsy** — epileptic conditions are usually very well managed with medication and sufferers can function normally within the community. There may be some dental effects such as gingival enlargement from medication or fractured teeth due to previous trauma. Clinicians should be aware of the nature of a seizure in the unlikely event that one does occur.

- Medication — there is a possible risk of drug interaction.

- Pregnancy — there is a possibility of hormonally influenced gingival enlargement. Diagnostic radiography may be restricted or postponed. (This is not necessary if proper radiographic procedures are followed but many patients prefer to delay radiography until after the birth of the baby.) Use of drugs should be avoided wherever possible.

A sample medical/dental history form is shown in Figure 5.2 (overleaf).

Ethical, legal and privacy issues

Any information obtained during medical history taking, whether from a colleague or from a patient, remains strictly private and confidential. It may not be disclosed to other parties, including members of the patient's immediate family. Exchange of this information is permitted between bona fide health professionals involved in the patient's care, if the patient's permission is sought and given. This information may not be used to discriminate against the person, either in provision of treatment, in employment or in any other manner.

At all times, the patient has to be reassured that confidentiality is guaranteed.

Additionally, the history only becomes legally acceptable if the patient has fully understood its purpose and the exact nature of the questions.

Uses of medical histories

Medical histories are essential for the provision of comprehensive holistic health care, treatment planning and the patient's protection and safety.

Medical histories are essential for the protection of patients and good infection control. Standard precautions should always be adopted for every patient but transmission-based precautions may be required in specific instances, such as when patients have CJD (Creutzfeldt-Jacob Disease) or antibiotic resistant tuberculosis.

The medical history also aids the diagnosis of many periodontal and oral mucosal lesions, some of which may be drug induced. Other conditions such as **xerostomia** require an understanding of the patient's medication and medical condition.

It is, of course, essential to avoid any drug to which the patient has a history of **allergy** and the medical history form should alert you of that. It is also essential to avoid interactions between the patient's medications and dentally prescribed drugs such as local anaesthetic solutions or antibiotics. For example, some antibiotics **potentiate** the effects of some anticoagulants and may inactivate oral contraceptive medication.

Some invasive procedures require prior prophylactic antibiotic cover. An example is if the patient has a history of heart valve disease or prosthetic valve replacement. There may also be a necessity to modify existing medication such as systemic corticosteroids and anti-coagulant medication before extractions.

Scheduling and length of appointments may need to be modified to accommodate the patient's abilities, or the need for meals and medications at certain times.

Filing patient records

For safekeeping and accessibility it is essential that all patient records and other relevant information is filed in a systematic manner. Filing should be done at regular intervals to avoid unnecessary accumulation and to maintain easy access to cards when needed.

Several different filing methods are used. Remember, if your place of work uses electronic systems, you will need to be trained in the specific systems used. Don't forget that regular backups should be made of all information that is stored electronically and these backup copies should be kept away from the premises.

hyperglycaemia: a medical condition where the patient has too much sugar in the blood. ■ **subgingival scaling:** scraping away of subgingival calculus. ■ **epilepsy:** a medical disorder that can result in loss of consciousness and convulsions or 'fits'. ■ **xerostomia:** dry mouth caused by reduction or complete lack of saliva. ■ **allergy:** hypersensitivity to a substance. ■ **potentiate:** increase the effectiveness of a drug.

Pearl E. White, BDSc, LDS
Dental Surgeon
1 Sea Street
Port Macquarie 2444

ph: 02 9222222
fax: 02 9333333
e-mail: pewhite@midcoast.com.ua

PATIENT INFORMATION

Welcome to our DENTAL PRACTICE. We appreciate the opportunity to provide dental services for you. To assist us in helping you, please complete the following form. The information provided on this form is important to your dental health. If there have been any changes in your health, please tell us. If you have any questions, don't hesitate to ask. All information supplied will be held in the strictest confidence.

Patient name: _____ Date of birth: _____ Age: _____
Home address: _____ Post code: _____
Postal address (if different): _____ Post code: _____
Home telephone: _____ Mobile: _____ Bus. phone: _____
Employer/Occupation: _____ Next of kin: name & phone: _____
Dental Health Insurance Fund: _____ Name of your general practitioner: _____ Tele. number: _____
Date of last visit to medical doctor: _____ Name of previous dentist: _____ Date of last visit to dentist: _____

DENTAL HEALTH HISTORY

Please tick any that apply:	Yes	No	Please tick any that apply:	Yes	No
Are you apprehensive about dental treatment?			Do you gag easily?		
Have you had any problems with previous treatment?			Do you wear dentures?		
Do you have difficulty in chewing your food?			Do you have difficulty in chewing your food?		
Do your gums bleed easily?			Have you noticed slow healing sores in or about your mouth?		
Do your gums bleed easily when you floss?			Do you take fluoride supplements?		
Do your gums feel swollen or tender?			Are you unhappy with the appearance of your teeth?		
Do you chew gum or smoke a pipe?			Do you want complete dental care?		
Does your jaw make a noise that bothers you or others?			Do you clench or grind your jaws frequently?		
Do your jaws ever feel tired?			Does your jaw get stuck so that you can't open it freely?		
Does it hurt when you chew or open wide to take a bite?			Does it hurt when you chew or open wide to take a bite?		
Are you unable to open your mouth as far as you want?			Do you have earaches or pain in front of your ears?		
Do you avoid brushing any part of your mouth because of pain?			Do you have any jaw symptoms or headaches upon waking in the morning?		
Do you feel twinges or pain when your teeth come into contact with:			Do you take medications or pills for pain or discomfort (pain relievers, muscle relaxants, antidepressants)?		
• Hot foods or liquids?			How often do you brush? _____		
• Cold foods or liquids?			How often do you floss? _____		
• Sour or sweet foods or liquids?					

MEDICAL HEALTH HISTORY

Do you have, or have you had any of the following?	Yes	No	Please give details
Heart condition such as chest pain, heart murmur, heart valve problems, rheumatic fever, high or low blood pressure, heart valve or bypass surgery			
Blood problems such as bruising easily, frequent nose bleeds, blood diseases (like anaemia), have you ever required a blood transfusion			
Allergies such as asthma, hay fever, skin rashes, sinus problems			
An adverse reaction to anaesthetics, antibiotics or other medication, to latex rubber, or any other substance			
Bone or joint problems such as arthritis, back or neck pain, joint replacement			
Intestinal problems such as constipation/diarrhoea, ulcers, sudden weight loss or gain			
Frequent or severe headaches			
Fainting spells, seizures or epilepsy			
Kidney or bladder problems			
Thyroid problems			
Diabetes class I or class II			
Tuberculosis or other respiratory disease			
Persistent cough or swollen glands			
Hepatitis or other liver trouble			
History of head injury or other accident			
Infectious childhood diseases such as chickenpox, measles, glandular fever, cold sores			
Do you wear contact lenses?			
Do you drink alcohol?			How much?
Do you smoke?			How many?

Please list any medications (including non-prescription and supplements) that you are taking: _____

Is there anything you would like to discuss confidentially in private with the dentist? _____
Thank you for completing this form. Please notify us of any changes in your health at each visit.
Completed by: self/parent/guardian   Signed: _____   Date: _____
Dentist's signature: _____

Figure 5.2 Medical/dental history form

Alphabetical

This is the most common filing method. Patient files are sorted in alphabetical order by surname. If more than one patient has the surname, the initials of the first names are sorted alphabetically.

Chronological

Here, files are sorted according to the order in which they need to be done. For example, recall notices are sometimes filed in the order they need to be sent out.

Numerical

Each file is given a number. This system is rarely used in dental practice.

Subject

Information is filed by subject matter. This is useful, for example, for business files, professional journals, tax information.

General headings

Patient records are usually filed under three headings.

❶ The 'Current' file contains cards of patients currently being treated. When a recall appointment has been confirmed, the patient's card is usually placed into this file for easy access.

❷ The 'Account' file contains the cards of patients whose treatments have been completed for the time being but who have money owing.

❸ The 'Completed' file contains cards of patients whose treatment has been completed for the time being and all fees are paid.

Remember, these three systems need to be checked and sorted regularly. This could be something done during quiet periods in the practice/clinic.

Recalls

Preventive dentistry is based around the periodic recall of patients for examination, prophylactic treatment and bitewing x-ray examinations. That is, the patient receives a card in the mail, an email or a phone call that reminds them that they are due for a check-up. All patients should be told this recall service is available. Only those patients who consent to be notified should be recalled.

Advantages of a recall system for the patient are:

■ that regular examination and treatment keeps the mouth as healthy as possible — it does not uncover more disease, rather it discovers any disease at the earliest stage when treatment will be simplest, cheapest and most beneficial;

■ protection from a major breakdown of dental health;

■ checking of previous treatment and home care; and

■ maintaining goodwill and confidence in the dental team.

Advantages of a recall system for the dentist are:

■ the dentist's job of keeping the patient's mouth healthy is simplified;

■ emergency calls are minimised;

■ a steady flow of patients and treatment is maintained; and

■ there is opportunity of maintaining good rapport with the patient.

A simple method for recall is to book each patient for recall when current dental work is completed. At the last appointment, check with the patient whether a recall is desired, and if so, what day and time is suitable. This is entered into the appointment book. An appointment card with details can be given to the patient. On a printed form which folds into an envelope, the patient's name and address is written and, on the other side, the day and time. This is then stored with the recalls to be sent for that month. Make a note on the patient's card that this has been done. The advantage of this system is that there will be opportunity to change the day and or time closer to the appointed day if necessary.

Alternatively, where envelopes are used for filing all patients' records, a small recall card for each patient can be kept along with all other records until the current work is completed. Then the card is placed in a special 'come up' recall file. From this file, patients are recalled at an appropriate time and the fact is noted on their recall cards stating the method of recall used and whether contact has been made and an appointment allotted. When the patient returns, the card is taken from the recall file and placed in the envelope, whether the patient comes in response to the recall or not.

In some practices/clinics a telephone call is the only system used for recall. Lists are kept of patients to be recalled and these lists are consulted daily. With this system there is sometimes a tendency to put off calling patients if the appointment book is booked heavily in advance.

Computerised recall systems are used in some practices/clinics and if this is the case in your practice, you will need training in the specific system used.

Letter writing

Business letters use clear, direct language to convey the message. A large proportion of business letters concern a limited number of subjects (overdue accounts, treatment outstanding, referring a patient, replies to treatment queries, and so forth). A series of sample letters can, with simple variation, handle most these and save a lot of time.

The content should be clear and specific. For example, rather than suggesting 'as soon as possible', 'in the near future', or 'about this amount', give the exact time, date and amount of money. Technical words should be avoided where possible.

The letter should be neat, well set out, with good grammar and no spelling or typing errors. Good letters result from careful planning. Copies should be kept of *all* letters. Computers keep the filing and use of these letters simple and efficient. Clean paper, careful presentation of content and a thoughtful letter create a good impression.

The divisions of a business letter (as seen in Figure 5.3) are:

- letterhead — usually on pre-printed office stationery;
- date;
- name and address of the person the letter is being sent to;
- the salutation — Dear Sir/Madam/Ms Smith etc;
- the body of the letter (i.e. the subject matter);
- the complimentary close — Yours faithfully, Yours sincerely;
- the writer's signature;
- the writer's identification — printed below the signature;
- the reference — the initials of the typist.

Letter styles

Although there are different letter writing styles, the fully blocked letter is recommended for dental practices. Every line begins at the left-hand margin. This is the most common type of business letter because it is neat and easy to type. An example is provided in Figure 5.3.

Courtesy letters

Some employers like to send courtesy letters to patients, recognising significant events in their lives or thanking the patient. Instances where a courtesy letter might be appropriate include:

- thanking the patient for referring a new patient;
- a thank-you for prompt payment of obligations;
- a bereavement; or
- congratulations on a new baby, graduation, an engagement or marriage.

Summary

Dental practices can be one-dentist practices or large practices with many dentists and many support staff. Regardless of their size, there are office and reception tasks that must be completed to maintain the efficient running of the practice.

In a small practice, you and your colleagues should devise a system of handling the work efficiently; for example, allocating duties to the same section of each day or doing necessary office work during appointments when you will not be required to assist at the chair-side.

In a large practice/clinic, appropriate duties should be divided between the dental assistant(s), receptionist and dental office staff. Throughout the day, as the opportunity arises and according to the most pressing needs, radiographs should be processed and filed, autoclave water levels checked, dental cabinet contents tidied and replenished, reserve supplies checked, the following day's charts arranged, and all office records, filing, correspondence and the recall system kept up to date. All non-essentials should be kept out of sight, and treatment cards and other records should be filed promptly to avoid loss and confusion arising from their accumulation.

Pearl E. White
Dental Surgeon
BDSc, LDS

I Sea Street
Port Macquarie NSW 2444
ph: 02 9222222
fax: 02 9333333

18 November, 2004
(2–5 blank lines)

Ms Jill Smith
Manager
The Pharmacy
99 Main Street
Port Macquarie NSW 2444
(2 blank lines)

Dear Ms Smith
(1 blank line)
This letter uses a fully blocked open punctuated format, the most popular modern business letter layout.
(1 blank line)
Note that the date is written out in full, and the name, title organisation and address of the person receiving the letter are all included above the salutation. Your contact details are included in the pre-printed letterhead. You can also create and save a letterhead template on your computer.
(1 blank line)
Paragraphs are indicated by a blank line rather than indenting, and the only punctuation used is in this section, the body of the letter.
(1 blank line)
Yours sincerely,

(3-5 blank lines)
(the dentist signs)

Pearl E. White
per *(if you sign on the dentist's behalf)*

ref: FJ

Figure 5.3 Fully blocked business letter

chapter six
account keeping and financial duties

Introduction

Dental assistants are often required to:

- produce the accounts to patients;
- convey estimates and arrangements for payments;
- handle banking of money received;
- render accounts and issue receipts; and
- disburse cash from the petty cash.

The dental assistant's duties vary with each practice/ clinic and you should be trained in the systems used at your practice/clinic.

Some dentists engage firms of accountants to do some of the accounting work. However, this does not excuse you from careful account keeping because the accountant will need complete and accurate records.

Duties connected with accounts are:

- the recording of treatment and charges following each completed stage of treatment;
- the rendering of accounts at intervals, usually the end of the month (as postage is now a heavy expense, many dentists have adopted the practice of handing the account to the patient at the completion of treatment, or at agreed intervals should the treatment extend over a long period of time);
- recording of receipts (credits) on the account;
- the following up of unpaid accounts; and
- transferring cards to the proper section of the card filing system (e.g. from 'Accounts' to 'Completed').

Fees for service

The efficiency of any venture is based on the ratio of productive time to non-productive time. *Productive time* is the time spent with the patient for which a

fee is charged. *Non-productive time* is that time spent with a patient for which no fee is charged (e.g. a denture adjustment). Non-utilised time comprises time not used between patients, appointments that are incorrectly timed, and appointments that are cancelled or broken. This time must be kept to a minimum.

The dentist should give the estimated cost of treatment to the patient after the initial examination, when the treatment plan is completed. The patient can judge if the treatment is affordable or if a payment schedule will be needed. Some choose to pay a set amount at regular intervals and their chart should be marked accordingly (e.g. 'budget account'). Each month, a reminder is sent of the total amount and how much payment is expected at this time.

Some patients may find treatment beyond their financial means and, in these cases alternative treatment plans should be discussed with the dentist.

Patients' accounts

In most practices, each patient has a clinical card with financial records attached. An example of a financial record is included in Figure 6.1.

Mr George Smith 15 Arrow Street Glen Iris VIC 3146		Debit	Credit	Balance
31.3.03	To services	$170		
8.4.03	By cash		$20	
				$150

Figure 6.1 Patient financial record
Note: Great care should be taken with the accuracy of all entries.

Many dentists request that accounts be paid on the day of treatment and many offer EFTPOS facilities to patients for this reason. EFTPOS stands for Electronic Funds Transfer Point Of Sale and includes all payments that are done electronically using credit or debit cards. Each EFTPOS machine and each practice will have its own routines for processing these transactions. There are also manuals that come with the machines and most organisations that provide the machines will also provide training. You will need to ensure that you receive the appropriate training for your practice.

Patients should be told before their first visit, usually during the first telephone contact, that this is practice policy. You will need to have some change available for those patients who pay in cash.

Some practices send accounts on the completion of treatment. Many larger surgeries utilise alphabetical cycle billing. The A's are posted on the 3rd of the month, B's on the 4th, C's on the 5th and so on. Such a procedure spreads the office load of sending out accounts in one batch.

Most surgeries have pre-printed account forms, called tax invoices, as shown in Figure 6.2.

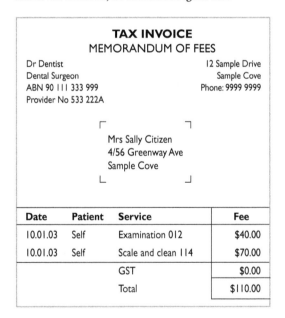

Figure 6.2 Tax invoice
Note: Most tax invoices will also include item numbers for medical benefit funds.

These pre-printed forms include Australian Dental Association item numbers that describe treatments undertaken. All medical benefit funds recognise these item numbers.

Some dentists have account forms with the commonly used numbers and their descriptions listed at the bottom of the account form. Some also have a cut-off or tear-off section to be used as a receipt.

Partial-payment plans or budget accounts

These plans allow the patient to make small, partial payments on a regular basis until the account is cleared. They are usually discussed by the dentist and patient at the same time as the treatment plan. The dentist may suggest a plan but you will possibly be left to work out the details with the patient at the end of the treatment.

You will need to work out:

- the total amount due;
- an interest fee, if there is one;
- the number of payments;
- the date of the payments; and
- the amount of each payment.

A copy of the payment schedule should be kept by the practice and another copy given to the patient.

Receipts

When a patient pays an account, a receipt must be issued. A proper receipt book or computer generated receipt should be used and a carbon or electronic copy kept of each receipt. An example of a manual receipt is shown in Figure 6.3.

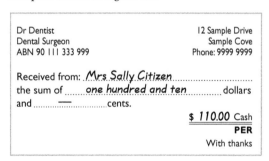

Figure 6.3 Manual receipt

Issue receipts and enter them on the patient's card together with the receipt number. Always mark the duplicate receipt to indicate that it has been marked off on the patient's card.

Most surgeries now have pre-printed receipt books into which the details can be added. Other practices use computerised accounts. Considerable variations occur between practices and you must familiarise yourself with the system used in your practice.

All receipts should:

- be numbered consecutively and be dated;
- show the patient's initials, surname and address for identification, as there could be more than one patient with that name;

- show how the payment was made; for example, by cash or cheque (if a cheque, then the cheque number should be recorded); and
- have the signature of the person writing the receipt.

All patients should be issued with a receipt regardless of the method of payment.

If your practice uses a computerised system it is crucial that the information you enter is correct. It will be used to calculate practice records as well as daily, monthly and yearly account information. Your practice will also have a routine for backing-up data at the end of every day to ensure that spare copies of records are kept outside the office in case the computer fails or is damaged by fire, theft, etc.

Veterans' Affairs and medical benefits

If your patient's dental work is paid for by Veterans' Affairs you may need to complete the paperwork and have the form signed by the patient and the dentist. Whether you fill in the form or the patient fills it in depends on the policy of your practice.

In most cases, patients with medical benefit cover will deal with the paperwork themselves and you are only required to provide the correct item numbers on the receipt you give them after payment. However, some practices have electronic funding for health funds. If this is the case for your practice you will need to ensure that you receive the correct training for the particular program.

Professional courtesy discounts

Some dentists offer discounts to colleagues, family members and friends, to patients paying 'up-front', etc. The dentist will tell you if this is the case and you will need to make a note on the patient's card stating the type and amount of discount.

Collection of overdue payments

As noted earlier, most dentists now ask patients to pay at the end of every treatment. In some cases, though, patients are issued with accounts and inevitably some have money owing on their accounts. At regular intervals, statements should be sent to patients who have not paid their accounts. A statement that follows an original account is an 'Account Rendered'. This term means 'An account has been sent previously'.

Although unpaid accounts should be followed up to ensure that payment is completed, you need to be familiar with the routines used in your practice. A patient who is upset or offended by collection methods is less likely to pay their bills!

Some patients will take the statement with them after the treatment, or a statement is sent in the post. This statement will have the due date written on it (usually 30 days after the date of treatment).

If the account is still unpaid after 60 days (from the date of treatment), a second statement is sent as a reminder with some polite but firm collection information (for example, the terms of the payment of the statement, or perhaps an offer to organise a payment or part-payment schedule). Alternatively, a telephone call might remind the patient of the overdue statement.

If the account is still unpaid after a further four weeks a stronger note is sent, usually advising that if payment is not made within ten days the account will be sent to a collection agency.

After that time, the account is sent to a collection agency.

Note that this is just a suggestion and you should find out the policy of your practice.

Bad debts

If a patient is unable to be located, or after accounts have been outstanding for some time and it appears that the patient has little intention of settling the debt, the account may be given to a debt collector, if that is the wish of the dentist. This increases the chances of being paid but it also incurs service and legal fees.

Wherever possible, fees should be stated before treatment starts and, if necessary, an acceptable payment plan agreed on. Often financial problems arise because treatment is continued without any attention to helping the patient accept their responsibilities regarding payment.

Many practices now adopt a 'pay at the end of each treatment' policy. This saves time, ensures a regular income stream to the practice and saves writing and sending invoices. It also reduces bad debts.

Handling of remittances received

Cheques

A cheque is a written promise to pay a sum of money to a designated person or persons. It is not money received until it has been cleared by the bank on which it is drawn. There are two types of cheques commonly used: cash cheques and not negotiable cheques.

Cash cheque

This is a cheque marked 'Pay Cash'. This form of cheque is not desirable in dental practice since the cheque can be cashed if stolen. It is generally only used to draw wages and in that instance, the bank must be authorised by the drawer to honour the cheque. The person collecting the money must also provide appropriate identification.

This type of cheque can be taken by any person to the drawer's bank and, provided the drawer has credit in the account to meet the sum of the cheque, the bank will honour the cheque and pay cash to the person presenting such a cheque.

Not negotiable or crossed cheque

This is a cheque crossed by two straight lines and marked 'not negotiable' between the lines. Such a cheque cannot be cashed but must be paid into the bank account of the person or business named on the cheque. The sum of money represented by this cheque will only be credited to that account when that cheque has been cleared through the account of the drawer. Such a cheque is desirable since no-one else can draw on it, and if it is lost the drawer can cancel the cheque by notifying the bank. A new cheque can then be issued. Both the dentist and the patient are protected.

Examine in detail cheques received from patients, keeping the following in mind:

- Is the date recent? A cheque is 'stale' after 12 months. Post-dated cheques cannot be negoti-ated. A cheque only becomes legal tender at the entered date.

- Do the words and figures agree?

- Is it signed by the drawer?

- Ask the patient to print their name and address on the back of the cheque.

- Some cheques require more than one signatory; for example, many associations (such as the DAAA) choose to have two signatures for each cheque.

- Cross the cheque immediately, if it is not already crossed.

- Check that the payee is made out correctly.

Dishonoured cheques

Sometimes the patient's cheque is returned to the dentist by the bank for various reasons, some of which are:

- the cheque has been post-dated;

- the patient does not have sufficient funds in their account for the bank to pay the cheque;

- there has been an alteration that should have been initialled by the patient; or

- the figures or words differ (a cheque such as this should be paid in for the lower amount and the patient sent an account, with explanatory letter, requesting the additional payment; for example, if the words on the cheque say 'One hundred and twenty dollars' but the number says '$100', the cheque is paid in for $100 dollars and an account sent for the outstanding amount).

It is essential that the person accepting the cheque carefully reads the writing on the cheque to avoid the cheque being dishonoured by the bank due to discrepancies. Most of the problems described above can be avoided.

If a cheque is returned because of insufficient funds, you should advise the patient at once. The cheque should be retained until satisfactory arrange-ments have been made to pay it. Dishonoured cheques carry a dishonour fee and the patient should also pay this fee.

Some states levy stamp duty on monies received. Ascertain the correct procedure and note it in the front of your receipt book for ready reference.

Money orders

A patient may not be able to go to the dentist's rooms to pay or may not have a cheque or credit account. Money in the form of notes and coins should not be sent through the post. The patient will, there-fore, send a money order. This is organised through a post office.

You should write on the top of the money order the name and address of the sender. Money orders must be signed by the dentist as having been received. They may be cashed at the post office or paid in through the bank.

Books and records

Good records are obligatory by law. The *Income Tax Act 1936* requires that everyone carrying on a business keep sufficient records (in the English language) of their income and expenditure to enable their assessable income and allowable deductions to be readily ascertained. These records must be kept for a period of at least seven years after the completion of the transactions.

The following books and records are required.

1. Receipt book.
2. Cash received book or cash inwards book.
3. Bank deposit book.
4. Cheque book.
5. Cash outward book or analysis book.
6. Petty cash book.
7. Bank statement.
8. Bank reconciliation.
9. BAS statements (see separate heading below).
10. PAYG payment summary.
11. Time and wages books.
12. Patients' record cards, study models, radiographs and photos.
13. Account form.

The office accountant should always be consulted in setting up the recording system. Records are factual and if kept properly can aid in costing, budgeting and establishing fees. This enables the dentist to see where adjustments must be made.

Australian Business Number (ABN)

This is the identifier for your employer's dealings with the Australian Taxation Office (ATO). It should be provided on all financial documents (statements, receipts, and so forth).

Business Activity Statement (BAS)

A Business Activity Statement (BAS) is a form you use to account for GST (Goods and Services Tax) and some other taxes. GST is added on to cosmetic dentistry fees. Usually 10 per cent is added to the fee, depending on the practice. Computerised practices can use item number 999 for the GST component of a bill. GST is added to any merchandise sold; for example, toothbrushes. Who calculates GST and invoices the patients depends on the practice.

Business Activity Statements are lodged monthly or quarterly according to the preference of the business. The BAS covers withholding tax from employees, the GST you have charged patients and the GST you have paid on supplies and other taxes that may apply to individual practices. Quarterly, the surgery pays tax on its gross income.

In some practices an accountant will complete the BAS or it will be done by the dentist or practice manager. In most practices the dental assistant does not deal with the BAS. However, you will need to refer to your practice manual or the accountant to find out how records are kept for your practice and if you are required to do the recording.

Cash inwards book

All receipts are entered in the cash inwards book. Entries are totalled and balanced against cash and cheques before banking. Banking should be completed frequently; daily if possible. An example of a cash inwards book is shown in Figure 6.4.

Dr Bite Family Dental Care Balance as per Cash Journal			Income (cash inwards) $112,667.88			March 2003 c/f February 2003	
Date	Name	Rec #	Total Amount	Dental Services	Misc T'brush	GST rec'd	Total Banked
01.03.03	Mrs A. Sudin	87315	$745.00	745.00			
01.03.03	Mr G. Bridge	87316	$272.00	272.00			
02.03.03	Mrs V. Zandin	87317	$469.00	469.00			
02.03.03	C.J. Dean	87318	$1013.00	1013.00			
03.03.03	D. Vandezee	87319	$988.00	988.00			
03.03.03	Mr G. Catlin	87320	$6.05		6.05	0.55	3493.05
04.03.03	J.I. Senz	87321	$2173.00	2173.00			
04.03.03	A. Bell	87322	$2182.00	2182.00			
05.03.03	K. Weiner	87323	$1030.00	1030.00			5385.00
08.03.03	C. Kahlin	87324	$428.00	428.00			
09.03.03	Z. Chen	87325	$2402.00	2402.00			
10.03.03	L. Yeung	87326	$895.00	895.00			
11.03.03	K. Araki	87327	$121.00	121.00			
12.03.03	P. Williams	87326	$4026.00	4026.00			7872.00
15.03.03	I. Miller	87329	$789.00	789.00			
16.03.03	T. Vladimir	87330	$1701.00	1701.00			
16.03.03	J. McKay	87331	$992.00	992.00			
17.03.03	A. Best	87332	$521.00	521.00			
18.03.03	D. McRobie	87333	$700.00	700.00			
19.03.03	D. Mehan	87334	$897.50	897.50			5600.50
22.03.03	B. Chalkley	87335	$210.00	210.00			
23.03.03	D.P. Green	87336	$615.00	615.00			
23.03.03	T. Haydn	87338	$412.00	412.00			1237.00
29.03.03	W.D. Flynn	87339	$487.00	487.00			
30.03.03	K. Louden	87340	$948.00	948.00			1425.00
31.03.03	E. Khan	87341	$1299.00	1299.00			1299.00
			$26,321.00	26,315.55	6.05	0.55	$26,321.55

Figure 6.4 Cash inwards book

Cash outwards book or analysis book

This is where the details of cheque butts are recorded and an analysis made of the expenses of the practice. It is usually written up by the accountant and requires accurate and complete entering of all payments. An example is in Figure 6.5.

It is suggested that columns be provided for each of the expenses that are allowable deductions for income tax purposes, and these include drawings of the dentist, wages, anaesthetics, stock, laboratory fees, plant, repair, car, gas and power, laundry, travel, subscriptions, insurance, stationery, rates and taxes, rent, donations, postage and telephone, refunds, staff refreshments, leasehold improvements and GST.

Bank deposit book

Most banks now only accept deposit slips that are correctly computer coded with the dentist's account number. Single deposit forms should be avoided. If used, they should be immediately stuck into your deposit book in chronological order.

Carbon copy deposit books should be used. Enter the amount of cash and details of each cheque separately, showing drawer, bank and amount. Balance this against the cash inwards book before paying in at the bank. The bank teller will stamp and sign the deposit slip or deposit book. An example of a bank deposit book page is shown in Figure 6.6 on the next page.

Dr Bite Family Dental Care			Expenses				March 2003
Date	**Drawer/Details**	**Chq. No.**	**Amount**	**Personal**	**Wages**	**Electricity/ Gas**	**Rent**
01-Mar-03	Rainwater Supplies	139	$18.00				
01-Mar-03	Cash	140	$1,412.00		$1,412.00		
01-Mar-03	Cash	141	$ 49.25				
04-Mar-03	Doalson P/L– Surgery Rent (April)	142	$3,426.00				$3,426.00
07-Mar-03	Dental Express	143	$1,541.00				
07-Mar-03	Smith's Pharmacy	144	$27.00				
07-Mar-03	Horsley Dental	145	$724.35				
08-Mar-03	Cash	146	$1,327.00		$1,327.00		
08-Mar-03	Cash	147	$42.95				
08-Mar-03	Telstra	148	$112.00				
12-Mar-03	Cash	149	$200.00	$200.00			
14-Mar-03	Coastal Power	150	$87.00			$87.00	
15-Mar-03	Cash	151	$1,426.00		$1,426.00		
15-Mar-03	Cash	152	$54.85				
22-Mar-03	Waterfront Services – home	153	$49.25	$49.25			
22-Mar-03	Cash	154	$1,460.00		$1,460.00		
23-Mar-03	Cash	155	$47.00				
24-Mar-03	Medfin – Equip Lease May	156	$213.00				
27-Mar-03	J. G. Smith Autoclave Services	157	$149.00				
28-Mar-03	M. D. Sweepaway – Cleaner (April)	158	$230.00				
28-Mar-03	Cash	159	$1,237.00		$1,237.00		
28-Mar-03	Cash	160	$34.75				
28-Mar-03	Woolworths	161	$218.25	$218.25			
28-Mar-03	Visa Cards	162	$1,739.65	$246.00		$10.85	
28-Mar-03	Dental Design – Electrosonic cleaner	163	$2,374.00				
28-Mar-03	Port Laboratories	164	$1,380.00				
28-Mar-03	P. Woods – Refund Overpayments A/c	165	$25.00				
28-Mar-03	Dishonoured cheque		$10.00				
28-Mar-03	Bank Fees		$12.00				
	March Total		**$19,626.30**	**$713.50**	**$6,862.00**	**$97.85**	**$3,426.00**

Figure 6.5 Cash outwards book

Note: This figure is continued on the next page.

(continued)

Dr Bite Family Dental Care				Expenses				March 2003
Supplies	Equipment	Repairs	Petty Cash	Phone	Surgery Cleaning	Misc	Bank Fees	GST
$18.00								$1.60
			$49.25					$3.90
								$311.45
$1,541.00								$128.41
$27.00								$1.80
$724.35								$65.85
			$42.95					$3.20
			$112.00					$4.28
			$54.85					$4.47
			$47.00					$3.56
	$213.00							$19.36
		$149.00						$13.54
				$230.00				$20.90
								$2.80
								$8.93
$1482.80								$134.80
$2,374.00								$215.81
$1,380.00						$25.00 Refund		$97.35
							$10.00	
							$12.00	
$5,173.15	$2,587.00	$149.00	$228.80	$112.00	$230.00	$25.00	$22.00	$1,042.01

Figure 6.5 Cash outwards

THE BANK •
ABN 99 222 222 222

Please fill in the following particulars of cheques

DEPOSIT

Date 02 / 03 / 03

Drawer	Bank	Branch	Amount	
1. Mr John Smith	The Other Bank	Sample Cove	100	00
2.				
3.				
4.				
5.				

Teller		Paid in by/ Signature	*Ms Reception*	Teller Use		Notes	500	00
				$100	$10	Coins	10	00
						Merchant		
No.Chqs		Account Identification No: 005 8234333 333333		$50	$5	Cheques	100	00
		Account Name: Dr Dentist Branch: SAMPLE COVE		$20	$	TOTAL	610	00

Figure 6.6 Bank deposit book

Cheque book

It is most important that every cheque be entered accurately and completed with all details. See the example in Figure 6.7. As well as entering details on the cheque itself, details should also be added to the cheque butt. The butt should show the date, payee, purpose of the cheque, particulars and amount. The face should be entered and crossed 'not negotiable'. Should you wish to draw a cheque for cash, then at the top left-hand corner write 'Please pay cash' and have this instruction signed by the authorised signatory(ies).

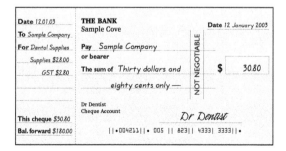

Figure 6.7 Cheque book

Petty cash book

As its name implies, the petty cash book records petty cash; those small amounts used to purchase small items (such as stationery, tea, milk, pencils) but may also be planned to include larger items (such as laundry, papers and stamps). These items are small and do not justify the writing of a cheque, or it may be more convenient to pay by cash. The best system for accounting for petty cash is called the 'impress system'. See the example in Figure 6.8.

A suitable amount is selected as the impress amount — say $50.00. A cheque is drawn for this amount and the money kept in a separate petty cash box. Each item purchased is entered in the petty cash book and when the amount runs low (monthly or quarterly) a cheque is drawn to reimburse the amount spent.

Bank statement

This is a copy of the dentist's account with the bank. The deposit book and cheque book are reconciled with this bank statement at regular intervals.

On the bank statement you may find some entries that do not tally with corresponding entries in the deposit book and cheque book; for example, the bank charges (a fee for keeping the account) and also interest on any overdraft. By agreement, regular payments such as a housing loan may be automatically paid without a special cheque being written out. Some companies and the Department of Veterans' Affairs prefer to pay dividends or fees directly into the bank. These will obviously appear on the statement without a corresponding receipt or cheque butt. Some dental suppliers also offer direct debit. These appear as separate entries on the statement, as seen in Figure 6.9 (overleaf).

Bank reconciliation

The monthly bank statement is balanced against the cheque book and deposit book to ensure that all debits and credits have been recorded correctly. Enter any special debits or credits in your analysis book and, if necessary, onto the patient's card and receipt book.

Bank reconciliation statement

The effective credit position at any given time may be obtained by adding any deposits not yet credited to the bank statement and then subtracting any outstanding cheques. See Figure 6.10 for an example.

Payment of sundry accounts

Accounts payable by the dentist will include:

- dental supply house accounts;
- rents;
- cleaning;
- electricity and gas;
- insurance;
- registration and association fees; and
- conference, continuing education and training expenses.

Date	Item	Amount	Postage	Morning Teas	Materials, medications	Laundry	Magazines, papers	Stationery	Sundry	GST
June 1	Postage Stamps	18.00	18.00							1.63
	City Laundry	15.00				15.00				1.36
	Newsagency									
	Newspaper	1.20					1.20			.10
	Milk	1.60		1.60						
June 3	Chemist, Aspirin	3.50			3.50					.58
	Chemist, Band-aids	2.95			2.95					
June 6	Door key cut	12.00							12.00	1.09
	Ball Points	2.75						2.75		.25
June 9	Coffee	5.40	5.40							.49
	Milk	1.60		1.60						
	Flowers	18.00							18.00	1.63
	Totals	$82.00	$18.00	$8.60	$6.45	$15.00	$1.20	$2.75	$30.00	$7.13

Reimbursed by cheque No. 437 for $82.00	$ 82.00
In cash box	$ 18.00
Total	$100.00

Figure 6.8 Petty cash book

STATEMENT

Page 1 of 1

Statement begins	1 July 2003
Statement ends	31 July 2003
Closing Balance	$560.50 Cr

THE BANK •
ABN 99 222 222 222
Enquiries: 13 1111

Dr Dentist
12 Sample Drive
Sample Cove

Cheque Account A/C No. 05 8234 33333
Name: Dr Dentist
Branch: Sample Cove BSB 05 8234

Date	Transaction Details	Debit	Credit	Balance
01 July 03	Opening balance			100.00Cr
01 July 03	Merchant fees	30.00		70.00Cr
10 July 03	Deposit cash		500.00	570.00Cr
13 July 03	Withdrawal cheque 00457	10.00		560.00Cr
20 July 03	Credit interest		0.50	560.50Cr

Figure 6.9 Bank statement

Routine for payment of accounts

■ Keep all invoices and statements received in a loose file until, say, the 21st of each month. (Note: telephone, gas and electricity accounts may have to be paid at particular times.)

■ Check the details of invoices and statements and initial if they appear correct.

■ Write out a cheque for each account, ensuring that you deduct the cash discount where applicable and cross cheques not negotiable.

■ Place the statement with the completed cheque for the dentist to sign.

■ Attach signed cheques to invoices or statements (which will be returned) and post in sealed envelopes.

■ When receipts are received, file receipt statements and invoices in numerical sequence of cheque numbers. Most companies do not issue receipts except on request so you will need to request one if your auditor insists on receipts. If this is the case, follow up accounts where receipts aren't received within one month.

It is prudent to make a copy of the account before sending it off with the cheque.

Payment by cheque

When preparing cheques for signature by the dentist, care should be exercised to ensure that:

■ the payee is named correctly and the date is correct;

■ the words and figures agree;

■ fraudulent alteration is not possible;

■ the cheque is crossed;

■ the butt corresponds with the cheque; and

■ attention is drawn to any alterations so that they may be initialled.

Dental supply house accounts

Delivery docket

When goods are delivered they should always be accompanied by a list of the goods enclosed. This is called a delivery docket. The goods should be checked against this list and, if correct, the list signed and placed on the file.

Dr Bite Family Dental Care			Expenses for March
BANK RECONCILIATION MARCH			
Balance as per Bank Statement			$115,584.13
Less O/S Deposits	0		
Add Unpresented Cheques	163	$2,374.00	
	164	$1,380.00	
	165	$25.00	
		$3,779.00	$3,779.00
Balance as per Cash Book			**$119,363.13**
Cash Book Bal c/f – Feb			$112,667.88
Add Deposits Mar			$26,321.55
Less Expenses Mar			$19,626.30
Balance as per Cash Book			**$119,363.13**

Figure 6.10 Bank reconciliation statement

Invoice

Either at the same time or subsequently, the supplier will forward a list identical to the delivery docket but added to this will be the itemised cost of the goods. Some suppliers routinely combine the delivery docket with the invoice, issuing only one price list at the time of delivery of the goods. Place this in the file. See Figure 6.11 for an example.

Statement

At the end of the month the supplier will forward a statement of account listing the invoice numbers and a total price for the goods supplied. This should be checked against the delivery docket and invoices. Alternatively, many suppliers now routinely request payment against invoices to save the additional cost of statement postage. Delivery dockets can be discarded after checking to see that they correspond with the invoices.

Sample Company ABN 99 333 333 444
Unit 3, 33 Test Drive, Sample Ville
Enquiries: 9333 4444 Fax order: 9333 4422
Email: samplecompany@anything.com.au

TAX INVOICE

Invoice No: **1189923**
Date: 10.01.03
Our ref: 2345

Deliver to:	Invoice to:		
Dr Dentist	Dr Dentist	Order Date: 05.01.03	
12 Sample Drive	12 Sample Drive	Order No: 123	
Sample Cove 2999	Sample Cove 2999	Rep: 100	
		Customer No: S4367	
		Despatch Date: 06.01.03	

NETT TERMS	7 days
Over 90 days	
Over 60 days	
Over 30 days	$300.00

Code	Description	Unit	Ordered	Shipped	Back Order	Unit Price	Discount	Amount	GST
55555A	Alginate fast	1	2	2	0	10.00	0.00	20.00	2.00
678989	Yellowstone	1	1	0	1	80.00	0.00	0.00	0.00
						Freight/Handling		8.00	0.80
						Subtotal		28.00	
						GST		2.80	
						TOTAL		30.80	

REMITTANCE SLIP

Detach this stub and return with payment to:
Sample Company
PO Box 33
Sampleville
ABN 99 333 333 444

Invoice No: 1189923
Date: 10.01.03
Our Ref: 2345

Figure 6.11 Supplier tax invoice

Check that:

- any discount has been allowed;
- any amount shown as 'account rendered' is correct;
- that there is an invoice for each entry on the statement;
- that payments made during the month have been included and deducted; and
- that goods returned have been credited on the statement.

Also note any undelivered items on back order.

Stock control

Stock ordering

When ordering supplies, a stock book will aid in efficient and economical purchasing. The stock book should show details of the name, make and size of the item to be ordered. It should also show the amount kept in stock, when to re-order (when stock is at minimum required level), where to re-order and problems of delivery; for example, if the supplier obtains the required item from interstate or overseas.

The shelf life on dental materials should be shown in the stock book as it is important to have supplies that are fresh and uncontaminated. The **quantity rate** buying prices should also be shown.

If you are required to handle all the ordering of stock for the practice, it is most practical to set up a loose-leaf indexed book. It should be divided into four sections — surgery, laboratory, office and miscellaneous and each section should show the above details, as shown in Figure 6.12.

In some practices the dental assistant is only required to handle the ordering of stock for the surgery. Similarly, the secretary–receptionist will be responsible for office and miscellaneous stock. The dental technician will be responsible for laboratory requirements. In each case the employee stock book should show details of who is responsible for particular stock ordering.

Stock ordering is often computerised. Orders can usually be placed by phone, through the dental representative, over the internet or by fax.

Stock storage

An orderly storage system is necessary for dental supplies to help eliminate frustrations and un-expected shortages. Shelves, no more than 200 to 300 mm deep, permit supplies to be ordered neatly, within the line of vision and arranged in the order in which they are used; for example, filling materials — alloy, composite resin, cavity lining, etc.

- The shelves should be labelled to make it easy to check supplies quickly.
- The inner door of the supply cupboard could be used for pasting a surgery stock book sheet.
- Small items, such as burs, can be stored conveniently in shallow boxes, with divisions to keep the burs in order if necessary.
- Items that are not carried in large stocks can often be suitably stored on narrow shelves attached to the doors of the cupboard.
- When a new stock item arrives it should be dated and placed behind the other materials so that the older product will be used first. Failure to do this could mean that some stock could be retained for years, becoming unsuitable for use or even dangerous.
- Some impression materials have a particularly short shelf life.
- Antibiotics and x-ray films are usually labelled with their effective life and are probably best stored in a refrigerator.

Item	Brand Size	Amount in stock	When to order	Company	Quantity to reorder	Price	Date ordered	Back order/ due date	Date received	Notes
Alloy	250g	500g			60g BTs					
Analgesic	2.2mL	2 boxes			10 boxes					10% off on bulk orders
Cotton rolls	1000/box	2 boxes			Carton					
Needles, disposable	100/box	4 boxes			12 boxes					Imported (so allow longer delivery time
X-ray film	50/box	1 box			6 boxes					Short shelf life
All orders should be written into a duplicate order book, the original given to the dental representative or marked 'phoned' and the duplicate checked against the delivery docket or invoice.										

Figure 6.12 Surgery stock book

■ **quantity rate:** some companies offer a discount if you buy in bulk.

- Remember to always check the manufacturer's instructions for storage of any stock items you receive.

Wages and salaries

When you accept a job you enter into an agreement with the employer. This may be verbal or in writing. It covers work conditions and rates of pay. These conditions are laid down by industrial Awards. Under the agreement or contract of employment, both the employer and employee have certain responsibilities. These are discussed in Chapters 1 and 2.

Income tax deductions from wages and salaries

It is compulsory for tax to be deducted from every employee's wage or salary where they are in excess of the exempted minimum. This is called PAYG or Pay As You Go taxation.

In each case, it is necessary to calculate the amount of tax to be deducted. This is done by taking the gross wages and deducting the amount of tax as shown on the Schedule of Deductions provided by the Australian Taxation Office (ATO). This form is obtainable from newsagents. Care must be taken to obtain a declaration from each employee as to dependants, if an employee has any, and to calculate the tax according to the appropriate column in the schedule.

When the PAYG Payment Summary system is used, after calculating the wages due to the employee, the tax payable from all employees is totalled each month and a cheque forwarded to the ATO. At the end of the financial year, a PAYG Payment Summary is issued to each employee and a reconciliation done.

It is important that, if an employee leaves before the end of the financial year, a PAYG Payment Summary is issued at the termination of employment. Stationery and very clear instructions are provided by the ATO.

Superannuation

All employers in Australia are required by the Superannuation Guarantee legislation to make contributions to a complying superannuation fund for most employees. The amount contributed by employers is 9 per cent of an employee's salary (as of July 2002), generally based on ordinary time earnings. Under Federal Government Superannuation Guarantee legislation, contributions must be paid for employees who earn $450 or more in a calendar month. Contributions do not have to be made for employees who: earn less than $450 per month; are aged 70 or over; or are under age 18 and working 30 hours or less per week. Superannuation Guarantee amounts must be paid to a super fund.

Employers are required to make superannuation contributions on behalf of their eligible employees at least quarterly, as per Table 6.1.

Quarter	Due date
September	28 October
December	28 January
March	28 April
June	28 July

Table 6.1 Quarterly superannuation contribution dates

Within 30 days of having made the final contribution for each quarter, the employer must supply a written report to the employee with the following information:

- employer's name;
- employee's name;
- the total amount of superannuation guarantee contribution made;
- the name of the superannuation fund/RSA;
- the employee's account or membership number if known.

The employer must keep a record of when, what and how they reported the information to their employees.

Calculation of superannuation

The superannuation contribution is calculated as a percentage of the basic gross wage. The contribution does not include allowances, overtime or bonuses. For example:

Basic wage			Overtime		
hours	rate	amount	hours	rate	amount
40	10	400	3	20	60
Allowance		**Bonus**	**Gross**	**Tax**	**Net**
10		200	670	200	470

Superannuation for the example above would be $9\% \times \$400.00 = \$36.00$

Tax file numbers

When you start a new job, and at the same time as you fill in the form for the ATO where you declare the number of your dependents, you will need to complete a Tax File Number declaration form. If you do not submit one of these forms to the ATO your wages will be calculated with the highest level of tax payable.

Time book

By law, it is obligatory for each employee to record the hours of work in a time book, which is subject to inspection by the Department of Industrial Relations and Employment, and the relevant union. This is to ensure that the employee is being paid accurately for the hours worked and the conditions of the Award are being observed. The employer is responsible for ensuring that the entries in the book are made daily.

Wages book

Once again, the law requires that a wages book be maintained to keep on record the wages paid and tax deductions made for each employee. Holiday and sick pay records, annual holidays, sick leave, leave without pay and compassionate leave for each employee must also be recorded. See the example in Figure 6.13.

Many practices now use computerised systems.

Employees should check the details in the wages book or computer printout and sign at the time of payment of wages.

Wages and tax deductions

The following is the procedure necessary for payment of wages.

- Calculate the hours of attendance, including the overtime as a separate item, on a time sheet or in the wages book.
- Consult your employer as to the gross wage payable. It may be the normal Award rate or a margin above the Award rate. The pay rate is usually agreed to at the time of employment.
- Calculate overtime (refer to the Award for rates payable). Enter normal wage plus overtime, deduct time off without pay, and superannuation, thus arriving at the total wage. Determine the tax payable by reference to current tax deduction scales.

- Enter tax in the wages book and calculate the net wage in the appropriate columns.
- Draw an open cheque for the net wages and obtain cash of the required denominations at the bank. (The employer must apply to the bank for approval to present a wages cheque.)
- The pay envelope should show full details, either on the envelope or on an enclosed slip, as seen in Figure 6.14.
- If you have trouble calculating wages, you can contact your state association or union for assistance. This is especially the case if you have a disagreement about your wage with your dentist.

At the end of the financial year:

- give employees their portion of the PAYG Payment Summary;
- send to the ATO the appropriate portions of the reconciliation and duplicates of the PAYG Payment Summary and PAYG Payment Summary Statement; and
- send to the ATO any dependent declarations.

Summary

Efficient and careful account keeping is crucial. Establishing good systems for maintaining accounts can improve the productivity of your practice and considerably reduce staff stress. Everyone in the practice who has a role in account keeping should have a good understanding of the systems in place (make sure they are written up in the practice's procedures manual).

Many of the tasks described in this chapter are now computerised. Staff members should have thorough training to allow them to operate computer systems effectively.

ZIONS

WEEKLY TIME, PAY

EMPLOYER'S NAME & ABN .... ADDRESS ....

EMPLOYEE'S NAME Nicola Spencer ADDRESS 12/35 Mooney St, Avalon 2107 AGE/DATE OF BIRTH (IF UNDER 21) 15/2

APPLICABLE AWARD/~~AGREEMENT~~ Dental Assistant & Secretaries (state) Award CLASSIFICATION/DESIGNATION OF EMPLOYEE Dental Assistant

WEEK ENDING	1st DAY 10th Mon				2nd DAY 11th Tues				3rd DAY 12th Wed				4th DAY 13th Thurs				5th DAY 14th Fri				6th DAY				7th DAY			
	STARTED	STOPPED	HOURS WORKED ORD.	HOURS WORKED OVER-TIME	STARTED	STOPPED	HOURS WORKED ORD.	HOURS WORKED OVER-TIME	STARTED	STOPPED	HOURS WORKED ORD.	HOURS WORKED OVER-TIME	STARTED	STOPPED	HOURS WORKED ORD.	HOURS WORKED OVER-TIME	STARTED	STOPPED	HOURS WORKED ORD.	HOURS WORKED OVER-TIME	STARTED	STOPPED	HOURS WORKED ORD.	HOURS WORKED OVER-TIME	STARTED	STOPPED	HOURS WORKED ORD.	HOURS WORKED OVER-TIME
14.2.03	8 am	6 pm	9	–	9 am	7.30 pm	7	@1½ 1½	8 am	12 pm	4	–	12 pm	9 pm	6	3	8 am	6 pm	9	–								

© ZIONS SYSTEMS – No. 500

TOTALS

SYSTEMS

AND WAGES BOOK

SHEET No. 24

TERMS OF EMPLOYMENT ☐ FULL TIME ☐ PART TIME ☐ PERMANENT ☐ TEMPORARY ☐ CASUAL

EMPLOYMENT COMMENCEMENT DATE 20/01/2001

EMPLOYMENT TERMINATION DATE ....../....../......

The Regular Daily Breaks for meals, etc. for the employee (except where specially otherwise mentioned) are:-
From 12pm To 1pm
no break Wed, Thurs

RATE OF WAGES

DATE	AMOUNT	PER
2003	$450–	40hrs

ORDINARY TOTAL			OVERTIME TOTAL			ALLOWANCES		GROSS WAGES	DEDUCTIONS					NET WAGES PAID	EMPLOYER SUPER. CONTRIB.	EMPLOYEE'S SIGNATURE (For Fines, Record & Receipt of Pay)
HOURS	RATE	AMOUNT	HOURS	RATE Time + ½ hr	AMOUNT	uniform laundering	meals after 7pm		TAX				TOTAL			
35½	11.25	450 00	4½	14.06	49 20	6 75	19 –	524 95	120 30				120 30	404 65	40 50	

Figure 6.13 Time and wages book

Pay Slip (Sample Only)

Employer's name: Dr Sample
Employer's address: 23 Sample Drive, Sample Ville
Employee's surname: SMITH   Given names: Mary Sue
Date of payment: 12 April 2003   Period of payment: 1 April 03 to 8 April 03
Form of employment: Full time ✓   Part time ☐   Casual ☐

No. of ordinary hours	40	Rate	18	Total	$720.00
Overtime hours	02	Rate	32	Total	$64.00
Allowances		Rate		Total	
Bonus					
				TOTAL	$784.00

Superannuation for which quarter Jan to March 03   Member Number   999999999
Paid to which fund   Health Super

Gross $784.00
Tax $200.00
Net $584.00

Figure 6.14 Pay slip

Section 2

Human biology

To be a competent and efficient dental assistant, you need a thorough understanding of the knowledge that underpins the tasks that you perform daily. You need to understand how the body works, and in particular the functions and structures of the head and neck.

The topics covered in this section are:

- body systems (including cells, tissue and organs);
- **anatomy** and **physiology** of the head and neck;
- oral and dental anatomy, dental **embryology**;
- microbiology;
- general **pathology**;
- oral pathology; and
- dental **pharmacology**.

■ **anatomy**: the study of the structure of living things. Therefore, human anatomy is the study of the individual parts, organs and tissues that form the human body. ■ **physiology**: the study of the functions of the individual parts, organs and tissues that form the human body. That is, it is a study of how these parts work together – how the body works. ■ **embryology**: the study of the development of human embryos, from conception to birth. ■ **pathology**: the scientific study of the nature and causes of disease. ■ **pharmacology**: the study of drugs and their action.

chapter seven
body systems

Introduction

It is important for you to be familiar with general anatomy and physiology. Knowledge of anatomy will help you to be more efficient at chair-side assisting during complicated procedures. It will also allow you to better understand the problems faced by general dentists, endodontists, periodontists, oral surgeons, orthodontists and prosthodontists. (See Section 6 for information about these specialist areas of dentistry.)

The organisation of the body

Organisation is a vital feature of body structure. Every cell, tissue, organ and system consists of smaller parts arranged in a precise way. If this organisation fails the result is disease.

The body is made up of:

- **CELLS**
  which are grouped or organised into
- **TISSUES**
  which are organised, according to their function, into
- **ORGANS**
  and these are organised into
- **SYSTEMS**
  arranged to carry out complex functions.

Survival is the body's most important business. Survival depends on the body maintaining a state of **equilibrium** in spite of changes in the environment or level of activity. This is called **homeostasis**. It depends on the exchange of materials between the body's environment and its cells (for example, metabolising food and integrating the body's many

activities). Ultimately, body functions depend upon the functioning of individual cells.

Body function alters over the years. Infancy and old age are the least effective times as the body is involved in maturing or ageing processes.

Cells

The cell is the basic building block of the body. It is the smallest unit in an animal or plant that can function independently. There are many different kinds of cells but they reproduce in the same way.

Each cell is a tiny mass of **protoplasm** surrounded by a thin cell wall (membrane). Each cell is made up of a **nucleus** and **cytoplasm**, as can be seen in Figure 7.1.

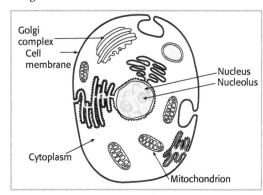

Figure 7.1 Structure of a cell

The nucleus has its own nuclear membrane. Inside that membrane is chromatin, a substance that contains **DNA**, **RNA** and various proteins.

This nucleus is surrounded by cytoplasm. Cytoplasm consists of all the chemical compounds in the cell that are not the nucleus; for example, the cytoplasm also contains **organelles**.

Cells can change nutrients into energy. They can grow and reproduce. As they grow, differentiation takes place. That is, groups of specialised cells begin to form. Each group is different in structure from others and is adapted to provide one or more specific functions. For example, blood cells have different functions from cells in the kidneys or the brain.

Tissues, organs and body systems

Tissues

Millions of cells together make **tissue**. Tissues combine in different proportions to form structures such as bones, nerves, muscles, blood vessels and body **organs**.

■ Nerve tissue receives and transmits messages around the body.

■ Epithelial tissue covers the body (i.e. the skin). It also lines, as mucous membrane, the internal cavities (e.g. mouth, intestines, etc). It is often referred to as the common integument. It also makes glandular tissue.

■ Connective tissue supports and connects other tissue. It may consist of **collagen**, elastic and reticular fibres, fatty tissue, blood, lymph, cartilage, bone marrow or bone.

Organs

Organs are made up of tissues that perform a specific function. For example, the kidneys, the heart and the liver are all examples of organs.

Organs are parts of body systems. These body systems keep the body functioning. Examples of body systems are the respiratory system, which includes the lungs, or the circulatory system, which includes the heart.

None of the body systems can work without the other systems. Also, each organ may carry out several functions so it may be part of more than one system. For example, the pancreas produces enzymes for the digestive system and insulin as part of the endocrine system.

Body systems

These are:
■ the bony or skeletal system;
■ the muscular system;
■ the digestive system;
■ the circulatory or cardiovascular system;
■ the respiratory system;
■ the nervous system;
■ the excretory system;
■ the lymphatic system;
■ the endocrine glands;
■ the reproductive system; and
■ the integumentary (skin) system.

This chapter gives brief overviews of the functions of each system. The following chapter contains more information about these systems as they relate to head and neck anatomy.

The bony (or skeletal) system

Functions of the skeletal system

The skeletal system:

■ supports the body and acts as its basic framework;

■ allows for the attachment of muscles;

■ protects vital organs (for example, the skull protects the brain, the spinal chord is encased in the spinal column and the ribcage protects the lungs and the heart); and

■ forms blood cells in the bone marrow (haematopoiesis).

Components of the skeletal system

There are 206 bones in the body. The skeletal system also includes cartilage, joints, and bone marrow.

The two parts of the skeleton are:

❶ The axial skeleton, which consists of the skull, the vertebral column, the sternum and the thorax (or rib cage). It holds the body erect and protects most of the body's vital organs.

❷ The appendicular skeleton, which is comprised of the limbs and is further subdivided into the upper and lower extremities.

Composition of bone

Bone, or osseous tissue, is a very hard substance consisting of a matrix of connective tissue (collagen) impregnated with organic salts (calcium hydroxy-apatite). That is, the matrix is **calcified** and that is what makes the bone rigid. These salts make up about two-thirds of the mass of the bone tissue.

The other third is made up of **organic matter** such as collagen, blood vessels, nerves, cartilage and other cellular material.

Structure of bone

Bones vary in size and shape and are often quite complex in structure. Figure 7.2 shows a cross section of a long bone and the different parts of the bone.

A typical bone has:

- Cortical (compact) bone — this is the outside layer of bone. It is very dense and, as a result, very hard. The exterior surface of bone is covered by the periosteum. It is tough and has many blood vessels but is very sensitive and easy to damage.

- Cancellous (spongy) bone — this is the inner part of the bone. It has a lattice (or honeycomb) appearance.

- The medullary cavity — at the centre of the long bone is a cavity or canal called the medullary cavity. The medullary cavity is lined with endosteum. (If the content of the cavity is rich in blood tissues then it is called red marrow. Many of the cells found in the blood stream develop and mature in the medullary cavities of the long bones. If the marrow has fewer blood elements and is richer in yellow fatty tissue it is called yellow marrow.)

Some bones are formed from a sheet of membrane, others from cartilage. The **articulating** (joint) **parts** of some long bones are covered by cartilage.

Types of bones

- Long bones (arms, legs, fingers, toes).

- Short bones (wrist and ankles).

- Flat bones (skull, ribs, pelvis).

- Irregular bones (vertebrae, sacrum, mandible).

Markings on bones

Bones have many 'landmarks' in the form of openings, depressions or projections.

A depression and opening can be a:

- fossa (a hollow or depression);

- sinus (cavity within bone);

- foramen (hole into or through bone); for example, mental foramen; or

- meatus (tube shaped opening); for example, external meatus or ear hole.

A projection can be a:

- condyle (a rounded projection entering into a joint), such as the condylar head of the mandible;

- head (a rounded projection beyond a narrow neck-like portion);

- crest (a bony ridge) to which muscles are attached, such as the mylo-hyoid ridge of the mandible;

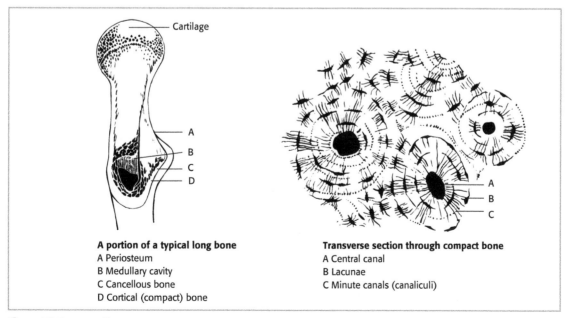

A portion of a typical long bone
A Periosteum
B Medullary cavity
C Cancellous bone
D Cortical (compact) bone

Transverse section through compact bone
A Central canal
B Lacunae
C Minute canals (canaliculi)

Figure 7.2 Structure of bone

■ **organic matter:** matter made of living things (cells, for example). ■ **articulating parts:** the parts that allow movement.

■ tuberosity (a large, rounded projection) such as the maxillary tuberosity; or

■ tubercle (a small, rough projection), such as the genial tubercles of the mandible.

Cartilage

Cartilage is a strong elastic tissue found, for example, in the flexible tip of the nose. It is sometimes called gristle. Articular cartilage covers and protects the joint surfaces of the bones.

Joints

Joints are the places where bones come together. The terminology and various classifications of joints are quite confusing. The simplest way to remember is to divide them into two main structural types, which are:

❶ Diarthrotic (or diarthrosis) joints — these types of joint have a small space or joint cavity between the **articulating surfaces** of the two bones forming the joint. The **bearing surface** is covered with cartilage and the joint cavity is lined with **synovial membrane**. Diarthrotic joints are freely or slightly movable joints (ball and socket or hinge) and the bones forming them are locked together by ligaments and muscles.

❷ Synarthrotic (or synarthrosis) joints — these types of joint do not have a cavity. The bones are united by fibrous cartilage. They are fixed joints (for example, the bones forming the skull).

The two joints of most relevance in dentistry are the temporo-mandibular joints (TMJ). These joints are diarthrotic joints that are involved in movement that relate the mandible (the lower jaw) to the temporal bone at the base of the skull every time we swallow, talk or move our jaw.

The muscular system

Functions of the muscular system

The muscular system:

■ allows movement of the external body parts from place to place (arms legs, head, jaw);

■ allows movement of internal body parts to allow breathing, swallowing, beating of the heart, movement of body fluids, **peristalsis**; and

■ regulates blood flow and body temperature.

Components of the muscular system

The three types of muscle tissue are:

❶ Skeletal muscle — this muscle is also called striated muscle because there are light and dark stripes (or striations) in the muscles fibres. The cells in this muscle tissue are extremely long and **distensible**. These muscles attach to the skeleton to make voluntary movement (like walking or chewing) possible.

❷ Visceral muscle —this muscle is also called smooth or non-striated muscle. These cells are shorter, have no striations and are less **contractile**. Smooth muscle is responsible for less active movements. It forms the muscle wall of organs such as blood vessels, the stomach and the intestines. It contracts more slowly and less vigorously than striated muscle. These muscles are responsible for involuntary movements such as transporting food in the alimentary canal.

❸ Cardiac muscle — specialised muscle for the heart only. This muscle is striated *and* involuntary.

These types of muscle are shown in Figure 7.3.

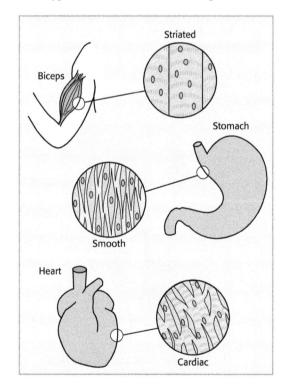

Figure 7.3 Types of muscle

The main specialty of muscle tissue is its 'irritability'. That is, muscle is responsive to stimulation, which causes it to contract. The strength of contraction of any muscle will depend upon the number of individual fibres stimulated to contract; the greater the number, the stronger the contraction. However, each muscle fibre contracts to its maximum capacity when stimulated. It is an 'all or nothing' response.

Voluntary muscle fibres are much longer than involuntary muscle fibres and there is a tremendous variation in the size of muscles, from the tiny slip that erects individual hairs to the gluteal muscle of the buttocks.

Altogether there are about 30 muscles in the facial region. Most of these are involved in the making of facial expressions. In dentistry, the muscles of significance are those responsible for the movements of the **mandible** during eating, talking and swallowing.

The digestive system

Functions of the digestive system

The digestive system:

- prepares food for digestion in a form that can be used by the body cells;
- absorbs food;
- absorbs nutrients; and
- eliminates solid waste.

Components of the digestive system

The digestive system is made up of:

- the mouth, including teeth, the tongue and salivary glands;
- the oesophagus (or food pipe);
- the stomach;
- the small intestines (or small bowel);
- the large intestines (or large bowel);
- the rectum and anus; and
- associated organs, such as the liver and gall bladder.

Digestion

Digestion is the process of breaking foods into a form that can be used by the body cells.

- Food is chewed, mixed with saliva and swallowed using the masticatory apparatus (the first part of the digestive system).

- The food goes down the **oesophagus** and into the **abdomen** where it enters the stomach. Food stays in the stomach for a few hours while the stomach **enzymes** begin the first stage of digestion.

- After leaving the stomach, the partially digested food enters the small intestine where digestion is completed. The small intestine makes its own enzymes to do this but also receives some help from the pancreas.

- Anything that could not be digested is of no use to the body and passes into the large intestine. The large intestine absorbs water from the waste food elements and carries waste to the rectum, which then carries the waste to the external orifice, the anus.

- Food that is digested passes through the wall of the small intestine into capillaries where the blood carries it to the liver. The liver distributes food to the parts of the body requiring it.

The circulatory system

Functions of the circulatory system

The circulatory system:

- collects nutrients (from foods) from the digestive system for delivery to cells;
- collects oxygen from the respiratory system for delivery to cells;
- collects wastes (produced during the metabolism of foods) from cells and delivers them to excretory organs; for example, carbon dioxide is given off via the lungs and nitrates and phosphates are given off via the kidneys in urine;
- assists in the metabolism of cells;
- assists in the maintenance of fluid volumes;
- assists in the maintenance of **pH**;
- assists in the control of body temperature;
- produces and distributes antibodies as a defence against pathogens;
- enables blood coagulation (clotting); and
- assists in tissue repair.

Unfortunately malignancies (cancers) can be spread by the circulatory system.

■ **mandible:** the lower jaw. ■ **oesophagus:** long tube, which passes through the neck (behind the trachea) and chest (behind the heart and lungs) and into the abdomen. ■ **abdomen:** the part of the body that contains the stomach, intestines and other organs. The abdomen is immediately below the chest but is separated from it by a sheet of muscle called the diaphragm. ■ **enzymes:** proteins produced by cells and which start biochemical reactions. ■ **pH:** hydrogen ion concentration. Neutral pH is 6.8 to 7.0. Anything lower is increasingly acid. Anything above is increasingly alkaline.

67

Components of the circulatory system

The circulatory system consists of the heart, blood vessels and blood. There are two major circulatory subsystems, which are:

■ pulmonary circulation, in which blood flows from the heart, through the lungs where it collects oxygen and flows back to the heart; and

■ systemic circulation, in which the oxygenated blood flows to all the other parts of the body.

The circulatory system is sometimes called the cardio-vascular system (see Figure 7.4).

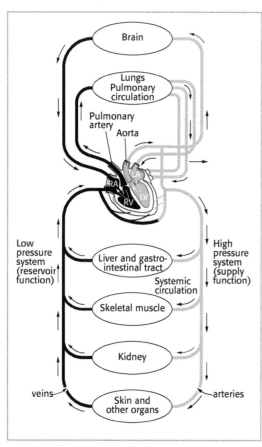

Figure 7.4 Circulatory system

The heart

The heart is a muscular organ, normally about the size of a man's fist. It is the centre of the circulatory system and acts as a pump to circulate blood through the body. The heart pumps about 6800 litres of blood a day, even when the body is at rest. It is controlled by the cardiac centre of the brain. This centre is influenced by changes in blood pressure, oxygen and carbon dioxide levels in the blood.

The heart contracts and beats approximately 70 times per minute but this varies from person to person, and also varies within a person under differ-ent circumstances. The rate of the muscle contraction (or beat) can be felt as a wave of contraction along the arteries and is referred to as the arterial pulse. The pulse is usually felt on the inside of the wrist (radial pulse) or on the neck (carotid pulse).

The heart is divided into right and left sides, as shown in Figure 7.5. Each side is then subdivided; that is, there are four chambers in the heart. The top cham-bers on each side are called atria. The bottom chambers are called ventricles. The atria are the chambers that receive the blood and the ventricles are the pumping chambers that push blood to other parts of the body.

The right side of the heart circulates the blood through the lungs. The left side forces blood through the body. There is no direct connection between the two sides of the heart. The divider between the right and left side is a strong muscular wall called the septum. Reflux (back flow) of blood is prevented by a system of valves, so the flow of blood can only go in one direction.

The heart supplies blood to itself via the coronary arteries. Blockages of these at any point by a blood clot or other kind of **embolus** causes a coronary occlusion or myocardial infarct, which can result in the death of an area of cardiac muscle supplied by that coronary artery. This is commonly known as a heart attack.

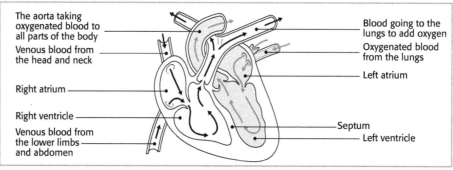

Figure 7.5 The heart

■ **embolus:** may be a blood clot, bacterial or an air bubble that blocks a blood vessel. It may be carried to other parts of the body (e.g. the brain) by blood vessels.

Circulation

Blood circulates continually through the body through the network of arteries, veins and capillaries. The blood is forced around the body by the pumping action of the heart.

- The heart drives deoxygenated blood through the lungs and when the oxygen supply has been renewed, the blood is returned to the heart and pumped out to other parts of the body.

- Blood is carried away from the heart by the arteries and returned to the heart through the veins. (There is one exception to this rule: the pulmonary artery, which carries deoxygenated blood to the lungs, and the pulmonary vein, which returns the oxygenated blood from the lungs to the heart.)

- Before entering the tissues, the arteries divide into smaller vessels called arterioles, which then divide into minute vessels called capillaries. Blood passes through the tissue in the capillaries, which are drained by venules that combine to form veins, and is then returned to the heart via the superior and inferior vena cava.

Blood vessels

The blood vessels are a network of 'pipes' that carry blood to and from the tissues. Blood is carried away from the heart by the arteries and returned to the heart through the veins. As noted before, the exceptions to this rule are the pulmonary artery, which carries deoxygenated blood to the lungs, and the pulmonary vein, which returns the oxygenated blood from the lungs to the heart.

Arteries

Arteries carry oxygenated blood away from the heart through the body. The arteries have thick walls to cope with the pressure of blood pushed with considerable force by the contraction of the left ventricle. The outer wall of an artery is a loose fibrous sheath. Inside this is a thick, elastic muscular layer that gives the artery its strength. The inner lining is made of a smooth layer of cells that allow the blood to flow smoothly.

The blood pressure measured within the arteries results from the force of contraction of the heart as it pumps blood through the circulatory system. If an artery is cut, blood spurts out rhythmically because of the beat of the heart.

The largest artery is the aorta, which splits into numerous smaller arteries to supply the organs, the head, the neck and the limbs. The arteries become progressively smaller, finally becoming arterioles. These arterioles supply the capillary beds in the various structures.

Veins

Veins carry deoxygenated blood back to the heart. Veins are similar in structure to arteries but the muscular wall is not as strong and the central channel, or lumen, is much bigger than an artery of the corresponding size. If a vein is cut, the blood flows steadily.

When they leave the capillaries, the small veins are called venules. These progressively increase in size to carry larger volumes of blood. The largest veins are the inferior and superior vena cava which enter from above and below, respectively, the right atrium of the heart.

The longer veins have a system of valves in them to stop the back flow of blood due to gravity; for example, in the arms and legs. The failure of these valves causes varicose veins.

Capillaries

Capillaries are the tiniest of the blood vessels. Each one consists of a very thin layer of tissue rolled into a tube and surrounded by an equally thin membrane. Capillaries have to be thin enough to allow substances (such as nutrients, oxygen and waste products, for example) to pass in and out of the blood. In addition to this function, the capillaries in the skin have a special role of regulating body temperature. For example, when constricted they prevent the loss of body heat, when dilated they assist in cooling the body.

Being thin walled, capillaries damage easily and those near the skin are most at risk. If the skin is cut or scratched or receives a blow, the capillaries release their blood. The result is a haematoma (bruise).

Neuro-vascular bundles

Neuro-vascular bundles are groups of nerves, arteries, veins and lymph vessels which usually pass through naturally occurring holes in bone, called foramina; for example, the mental foramen in the mandible. The arteries in these bundles have relatively strong walls but the veins are larger and thinner walled than veins in normal tissue. Dramatic bleeding can occur if they are punctured.

Blood

Blood is connective tissue. It is 55 per cent fluid (plasma) and 45 per cent cellular (solids known as blood **corpuscles**). The solids are red blood cells,

■ **corpuscles:** a cell in the blood or the lymph.

several types of white cells and platelets and these are suspended in the plasma.

Plasma is 90 per cent water. The remaining 10 per cent is made up of serum electrolytes (salts), **plasma proteins**, gases, hormones, vitamins, minerals, antibodies, foods and wastes.

One of the main functions of the blood is to transport nutrients to the tissues of the body. There, the cells use the nutrients to build new cells or to convert to energy for carrying out body processes. The second important function is defence against foreign bodies such as micro-organisms. The red and white blood cells undertake these two functions.

Red blood cells (or erythrocytes) act as transporters. They carry oxygen to the tissues and transport carbon dioxide back to the lungs for us to breath out. They are able to do this because they contain millions of molecules of a substance called haemoglobin. Red cells are produced in the red marrow.

White blood cells (or leucocytes) are involved in the body's defence against disease. White corpuscles are much bigger than red corpuscles and are capable of moving with a 'creeping' motion. White blood cells are mostly made in the spleen although some are also made in the red marrow. They are classified into five main groups. These are:

❶ neutrophils, which engulf germs and thereby fight disease;

❷ eosinophils, the number of which increases with allergic conditions;

❸ lymphocytes, which are important in giving the body its natural immunity to disease — they produce antibodies to attack infected cells/disease;

❹ monocytes, which dispose of dead and dying cells and other debris; and

❺ basophils, which are involved with inflammatory and allergic reactions — they contain large amounts of **histamine** and also **heparin**, which help to maintain a balance between clotting and anti-clotting processes.

Platelets are the tiniest cells in the body. One millilitre of blood contains about 250 million platelets. Platelets initiate blood clotting when an injury to a blood vessel occurs. The platelets stick to the wall of the blood vessel and to each other so that a plug is formed that stops the bleeding. Clotting normally starts within five minutes of injury to a blood vessel occurring.

Blood groups

There are four major classifications of blood in humans. There are various classifications but the most common one is represented as: O, A, B, AB.

A person's blood can also be RH– (negative) or RH+ (positive). These groupings are important when blood transfusions are required. The blood types have to match otherwise the body will reject them.

The universal donor is O (RH)+, the universal recipient is AB.

The respiratory system

Functions of the respiratory system

The respiratory system:

- oxygenates venous blood;
- removes waste carbon dioxide; and
- removes some water waste.

Components of the respiratory system

Structures involved are:

- the upper respiratory tract (the nose, pharynx, mouth, epiglottis, larynx and trachea);
- the bronchi (one bronchus on each side of the chest) and bronchioles;
- the lungs (right and left); and
- the diaphragm.

These can be seen in Figure 7.6.

Lung tissue is very elastic. Contraction of the respiratory muscles causes the thoracic (chest) volume to expand and this sucks air into the lungs. Air, rich in oxygen, enters the body through the nose, passes the pharynx and then the larynx. The air reaches the **epiglottis**, passes between the vocal chords, into the trachea (windpipe), via the bronchi then into the lungs.

Because the blood in the lungs has a low oxygen/carbon dioxide concentration relative to the inspired (inhaled) air, oxygen is taken up by the blood and carbon dioxide passes out of the blood.

The respiratory muscles relax, thoracic volume decreases and air is expired (exhaled).

70

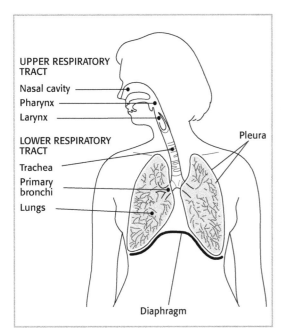

Figure 7.6 The respiratory system

The rate of respiration is under the control of the respiratory centre of the brain. Although we can control it to some extent, there is an overriding reflex control initiated by the rises and falls of oxygen and carbon dioxide levels in the blood.

The nose

The nose is divided into the external, visible portion and the nasal cavity. Air enters through the nares (nostrils). The nose filters air, warms and moistens it, screens for irritants, senses smells and is important in the formation of sounds in speech (phonation).

The nose is lined by **ciliated mucous membrane** which, with the aid of mucous secretions, helps trap any foreign matter. Four pairs of sinuses open into the nasal cavity. Of these, the maxillary sinuses have the greatest relevance to dentistry.

The pharynx

This is the space at the back of nasal and oral cavities through which air passes to and from the larynx. The pharynx is a tube-like structure about 12 cm long reaching from the base of the skull to the oesophagus. It is comprised of muscle and lined with mucous membrane. It is divisible into three parts. These are:

❶ the nasopharynx, which is located behind the nose and above the soft palate;

❷ the oropharynx, which goes from the soft palate to the epiglottis (this is the part of the pharynx that you can see when you open your mouth); and

❸ the laryngopharynx, which goes from the epiglottis to the larynx below.

There are five openings into the pharynx, which are:

❶ the **Eustachian tubes**;

❷ the posterior nares (the back opening of the nasal cavity);

❸ the oral cavity;

❹ the larynx; and

❺ the oesophagus.

The pharynx acts as a passageway for the respiratory and digestive tracts. Additionally, changes in its musculature affect various speech patterns. The pharynx is commonly called the throat.

The larynx

The larynx, or voice box, consists largely of laryngeal cartilages and muscles. These muscles play an important part in breathing, speech and **deglutition**.

The functions of the larynx are:

▪ to protect the airway against ingestion of foodstuffs or liquids during swallowing.; and

▪ voice production.

The protection of the airway is achieved by a network of nerves, the pharyngeal plexus. Its activity is controlled in the lower brain stem, which brings together information from both the respiratory and the swallowing centres high in the brain.

The trachea

This is a rigid pipe passing through the neck to the bronchi in the lungs. The trachea ensures free flow of air to the lungs. It is a tube about 115 mm long, reaching from the larynx to the bronchi in the thoracic cavity. It is comprised of smooth muscle that incorporates C-shaped rings of cartilage that keep the opening in shape. You can feel this part of the trachea quite easily with your fingers through the skin at the base of your neck.

The trachea is also lined by ciliated mucous membrane like the nose, to filter any bugs or dust that are pushed into the oesophagus (during swallowing) from entering into the bronchi.

▪ **epiglottis:** a leaf-shaped flap at the entrance to the larynx. It assists in closing the airway when food is swallowed. It prevents food from 'going down the wrong way'. ▪ **ciliated mucous membrane:** a moist lining that secretes mucous and that is covered in tiny hairs (ciliated). ▪ **Eustachian tube:** a tube that connects the middle ear to the back of the throat. The tube allows air pressure on both sides of the ear drum to equalise. ▪ **deglutition** swallowing.

The bronchi

The bronchial tree distributes air within the lungs. The bronchi commence at the inferior end of the trachea where it divides into two primary bronchi (bronchus is the singular). The right main bronchus is larger and more vertical than the left, hence any inhaled foreign body is more likely to lodge in the right main bronchiole. The structure of the bronchi is similar to that of the trachea, except that the cartilaginous rings become complete (O-shaped) when they enter the lungs.

The right and left main bronchus divide into secondary bronchi, then into **bronchioles**, then terminal bronchioles and finally into alveolar ducts.

The lungs

The lungs are large cone-shaped organs that are divided into lobes. The left lung has two lobes because the heart cavity encroaches more on the left side than the right, and the right has three lobes. The lungs themselves are made up of a dense latticework of tubes. The bronchioles terminate in air sacks called alveoli.

A second system of tubes is formed by the pulmonary arteries, which enter the lungs alongside the right and left bronchi. They also branch into smaller vessels that run alongside the bronchioles and become capillaries at the alveolar sacs. This is where the gaseous exchange takes place.

The diaphragm

The diaphragm is a sheet of muscle and fibrous tissue that forms a complete wall between the chest and the abdomen. It lies horizontally across the body. Looking from the front, the diaphragm appears as a dome, attached by muscular strings to the inside of the lower six ribs. The muscular fibres of the diaphragm contract when we breathe in and flatten the dome, drawing the highest central part into the abdomen. This increases the volume of the lungs and draws air into them.

The nervous system

Functions of the nervous system

The nervous system:

■ controls movements and regulates body functions such as breathing;

■ receives stimuli such as pain, pleasure, touch, taste, heat and cold, sight and sound;

■ transmits such information to the brain; and

■ assists in the development of language, thought and memory and the maintenance of homeostasis.

Components of the nervous system

At the centre of the nervous system are the brain and the spinal cord, which ultimately control all the nervous tissue in the other parts of the body.

The nervous system is divided into two major systems, which are:

❶ the central nervous system (CNS), made up of the brain and spinal cord; and

❷ the peripheral nervous system (PNS), made up of cranial nerves, spinal nerves, autonomic nerves and ganglia.

The central nervous system (CNS)

The central nervous system (brain and spinal cord) is the control centre for the movement and actions of the entire body. Messages from outlying receptors and sensors arrive at the CNS where they are interpreted. The CNS then sends out reaction impulses.

The peripheral nervous system (PNS)

The peripheral nervous system (cranial nerves, spinal nerves, autonomic nerves and ganglia) is divided into two further parts. These are:

❶ the afferent system, which carries messages from the sensors to the CNS for processing; and

❷ the efferent system, which carries the commands of the CNS to the muscles and organs.

■ **bronchioles:** smaller branches of the bronchi which carry air to all parts of the lungs.

Somatic and autonomic systems

There is a further division of the nervous system. That is:

- the somatic nervous system involving reflexes, movement and conscious actions; and
- the autonomic nervous system, which regulates body function, controls sphincters, cardiac and respiratory rates, glandular secretions and other unconscious actions.

Nerve cells

Nerve cells, like all other cells of the body, have a nucleus and fluid cytoplasm enclosed by cell membrane. Nerve cells are called neurones. A number of fine root-like fibres, called dendrites, project from the cell body. These carry impulses to the cell body. There can be up to 200 dendrites in each neurone. A picture of a nerve cell can be seen in Figure 7.7.

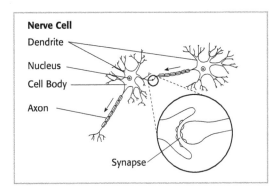

Figure 7.7 A nerve cell

Also projecting from the cell is a single long fibre called the axon, which carries messages from the cell body. At its far end, the axon divides into a number of branches, each ending in a number of tiny knobs. Each of these knobs is in close proximity to, but not actually touching, a dendrite of another neurone. This gap is called a synapse. Messages are transmitted across the synapse by chemicals called nerve transmitter substances.

The brain

The brain is a giant computer that receives information, analyses it and produces necessary impulses to cope with a given situation. It is the storehouse of all kinds of reflexes, has centres controlling speech, and all body functions, emotions, etc. It has the function of memory and is the seat of thought.

The nerves that give the brain its information are the sensory nerves responsible for touch, taste,

smell, pain, sight, heat and kinaesthetics (movement); in other words, all sensation.

The nerves that carry out the commands are the motor nerves. Their activity results in muscle contraction or glandular secretion.

The spinal cord

The spinal cord is a roughly cylindrical column of nerve tissues about 40 cm long that runs inside the spine from the brain to the lower back. It acts as a two-way conduction system between the brain and the peripheral nervous system.

The excretory system

Functions of the excretory system

The excretory system removes waste products from the body.

Components of the excretory system

The excretory system depend on various organs and glands for waste removal. The major ones are:

- the large bowel and rectum for the end products of digestion;
- the lungs for the removal of waste gases;
- the gall bladder, which stores the bile produced by the liver for the emulsification of fats;
- the sweat glands of the skin for the removal of water, thus regulating temperature; and
- the urinary system for the removal of liquid waste from the body.

The urinary system

The urinary system consists of:

- two kidneys;
- two ureters;
- one bladder; and
- one urethra.

The function of this system is to filter out the waste product of protein, which is nitrogen. This leaves the blood stream in the form of urea, is filtered by the kidneys and excreted in the form of urine via the ureters to the urinary bladder. Here it is stored until it is excreted from the body via the urethra.

Urine is made up of nitrogenous waste, electrolytes (salts), toxins and toxic substances, pigments, and hormones, all in water. Urine is normally sterile when excreted. A breakdown in any part of this system could very quickly lead to symptoms of poisoning, usually referred to as uraemia.

Many antibiotics are excreted by the urinary system.

The lymphatic system

Functions of the lymphatic system

The lymphatic system:

- drains fluids from the tissues back to the veins (it is a supplementary tissue drainage system);
- assists the veins in the transportation of nutrients and waste products to and from capillaries and cells;
- defends against disease; and
- conserves plasma proteins.

The lymphatic system may also be responsible for the spread of malignancies (cancers).

Components of the lymphatic system

The lymphatic system is made up of lymph fluid, vessels, lymph nodes (containing white cells called lymphocytes), thymus gland, tonsils and spleen (see Figure 7.8).

Lymphatic vessels

Lymphatic vessels are similar to veins but have thinner walls and many more valves. Fluid is forced along lymphatic vessels by muscle contraction. Small vessels collect to form larger vessels, which in turn form one vessel and this drains into the venous system. Vessels drain tissue fluid back to the veins.

Lymph fluid

Lymph fluid is similar to blood plasma, except that there are not as many proteins in it. The function of the lymphatic system is to return fluid and protein that has 'leaked' into tissue spaces from the vascular system, back to the blood.

Lymph nodes

Lymph nodes occur in the 'chains' of lymphatic vessels. Nodes filter out bacteria and foreign matter and foreign organisms/infection are destroyed. A swollen gland is an enlarged lymph node. The most usual cause is bacterial or viral infection. Cancer can **metastasise** (spread) along lymph vessels to the nodes.

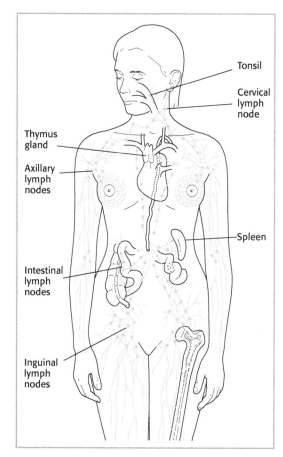

Figure 7.8 The lymphatic system

The spleen

The spleen is situated under the diaphragm on the left side of the abdominal cavity (just above the pancreas). It is rich with lymphatic tissue. Its functions are to:

- act as a blood reservoir (stores about 380 mls of blood);
- manufacture some white cells (haematopoiesis);
- break up old or damaged red cells (iron and globin are returned to the liver and bone marrow); and
- remove micro-organisms (infection).

metastasise: transfer disease from a primary lesion to a secondary site via blood vessels or lymph channels.

The thymus gland

The thymus gland is a structure (small in adults, large in children) situated in the base of the neck. It plays a very important part in the production of the antibodies necessary in overcoming infection. It plays a vital role in controlling the T and B lymphocyte cells which are called 'immune cells'.

Tonsils and adenoids

Tonsils and adenoids are masses of lymphatic tissue at the back of the nose and throat. They form a protective circle of lymphatic tissue.

The endocrine system

Functions of the endocrine system

The endocrine system:
- controls many of the body's functions (for example, growth); and
- helps to maintain homeostasis.

Components of the endocrine system

The pituitary gland, the thyroid gland, the parathyroid glands, the adrenal glands, the pancreas and the gonads are **ductless glands** and help to keep parts of the body working harmoniously. The hormones secreted into the blood stream relay messages to organs and stimulate them to carry out processes such as growth and reproduction.

The pituitary gland

The pituitary gland is the 'master' gland of the body. It is a little more than a centimetre in diameter, located on the under surface of the brain. It is connected to the **hypothalamus** by a stalk of nerve tissue and works closely with this area of the brain. It produces hormones that control growth, the activity of the thyroid gland, the development of the reproductive organs, secretions from the ovaries and testes, the stimulation of the mammary glands to provide milk, blood pressure, the performance of smooth muscles, the re-absorption of water in the kidneys and the functioning of the adrenal cortex (which becomes active during times of stress).

The thyroid gland

The thyroid gland is made up of two lobes located on either side of the trachea. It secretes iodine-based hormones that regulate physical and mental growth, oxidation, heart rate, blood pressure, temperature, glucose absorption and the utilisation of glucose. It also has a role in controlling the calcium metabolism.

The parathyroid glands

The parathyroid glands are located next to the thyroid. Their secretions control the use of calcium in bone growth, muscle tone and nervous activity.

The adrenal glands

The adrenal glands are located above the kidneys and produce hydrocortisone. This regulates the metabolism and the balance between salt and water levels. During emergencies they also secrete adrenalin (epinephrine), which increases the heart rate and stimulates the liver and the nervous system.

The pancreas

Although this gland has a duct, there are islands of tissue that secrete directly into the blood stream. They produce insulin, which plays a very important part in maintaining normal blood sugar levels. Sugar diabetes may result when the levels of insulin in the blood are relatively low or not functioning efficiently.

The gonads

The ovaries (in females) control ovulation and hence fertility, by means of hormones (oestrogen and progesterone). The ovaries are influenced by the pituitary gland. The testes (in males) control spermatogenesis. They produce testosterone, which controls the growth of body hair, body size and the deepening voice in maturing boys.

The reproductive system

Functions of the reproductive system

The function of the reproductive system is the production of new life.

ductless glands: because secretions go directly into the blood stream, endocrine glands are referred to as ductless glands.

hypothalamus: an area at the base of the brain which controls many of the body's automatic and hormone-related activities.

Components of the reproductive system

In men, the reproductive system includes the penis and testes and in woman the ovaries, fallopian tubes, uterus and vagina.

The structure and operation of the reproductive system do not fall within the scope of this text.

The integumentary system

Functions of the integumentary system

The integumentary system:
- protects the body; and
- regulates body temperature.

Components of the integumentary system

The integumentary system consists of the skin, hair, sebaceous glands, sweat and nails. It is usually referred to as the common integument.

This body system keeps bacteria from entering the body, excretes liquids and salts and absorbs rays from the sun to produce vitamin D. The skin also has nerve endings that send messages to the brain to register touch.

The structure and operation of the integumentary system do not fall within the scope of this text. However, there are some conditions that affect the integumentary system that can have dental implications; for example, ectodermal dysplasia (refer to Chapter 35).

Summary

An understanding of body systems is crucial to an understanding of head and neck anatomy, which is covered in the next chapter. Anatomy is also important to the understanding of microbiology and the processes of infection.

chapter eight
anatomy and physiology of the head and neck

Introduction

Just as knowledge of anatomy of the body is a basis for understanding your work, so is an understanding of anatomy of the head and neck; the anatomy of most relevance to dentistry. This knowledge underpins knowledge of dental anatomy, which is crucial to your work. Knowledge of head and neck anatomy is also helpful when assisting with radiographic procedures, including the mounting, labelling and identifying of radiographs.

Before we look at this anatomy it is necessary to explain some of the terms we will be using to describe body parts. An understanding of these terms will assist communication between you and the dentist and is especially helpful in radiography, clinical photography and orthodontics.

Descriptive terms used in anatomy

A summary of terms

Midline	an imaginary line that divides the body into equal left and right halves
Superior	above
Inferior	below
Posterior	towards the back
Anterior	towards the front
Medial/mesial	towards the midline
Lateral	towards the sides away from the midline
Proximal	near, adjoining
Distal	away from the midline

Proximal, mesial and distal have particular meanings when describing tooth surfaces and these are discussed in Chapter 9.

Body planes

Body planes are imaginary lines that divide the body into sections. They can be thought of as pairs of opposite directions (like up and down).

The horizontal plane divides the body into upper (superior) and lower (inferior) parts.

The coronal plane is an imaginary line that divides the body into front (anterior) and back (posterior) parts.

The sagittal plane is at right angles to the frontal plane, so it divides the body into left and right parts. When this plane divides the body into equal left and right parts, it is called the midline. See Figures 8.1 and 8.2.

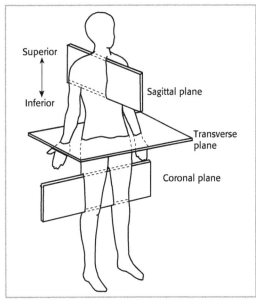

Figure 8.1 Body planes

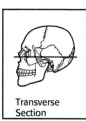

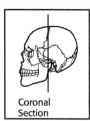

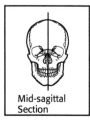

Figure 8.2 Body planes

The coronal and sagittal planes are named after the best-known sutures of the skull, as shown in Figure 8.3.

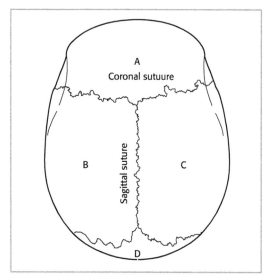

Figure 8.3 Sutures of the skull

Planes used in dentistry

Some important planes in dentistry are:

■ The Frankfort plane — a horizontal plane running from the lower border of the orbit (eye socket) to the opening of the ear.

■ The Alar-Tragal line — from the **ala** of the nose to a point near the opening of the ear. This is often used as an exterior indicator of the occlusal plane.

■ The occlusal plane — the plane passing through the tips of the **cusps** of the upper posterior teeth and the incisal edges of the upper anterior teeth.

■ The curve of Spee (see Figure 8.4) — also known as the smile line. This is the anatomic curvature of the occlusal **alignment** of teeth, beginning at the tip of the lower canine, following the buccal cusps of the natural premolars and molars and continuing to the anterior border of the ramus. (See Chapter 9 for a description of types of teeth.)

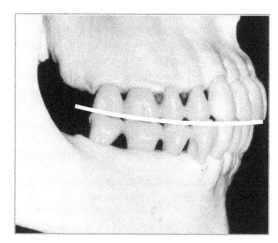

Figure 8.4 The curve of Spee

The skull

The skull consists of the brain case and the facial skeleton. It protects the brain and the organs of special sense (hearing, sight, taste and smell). It also provides the mount for the teeth.

The skull is made up of a large number of bones but only seven of them are freely movable. The sutures uniting the non-movable joints of the skull form very serrated edges, like the teeth of a saw.

The movable bones are the:

■ mandible (lower jaw); and

■ six tiny ossicles (three each side) that convey sound waves from the eardrum to the nerve centres in the middle ear.

The bones of the skull can be divided into two groups; the bones of the cranium and the bones of the face. (There are also the six auditory ossicles mentioned above.) See Figures 8.5 to 8.8.

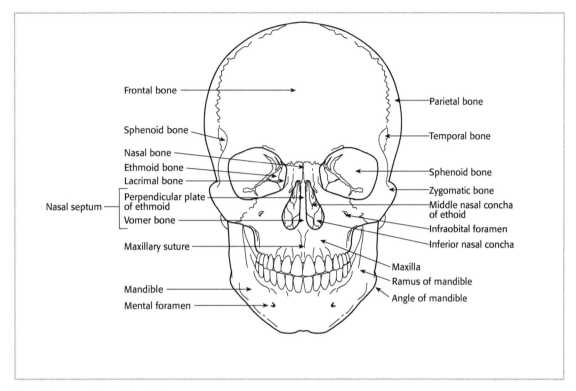

Figure 8.5 Frontal view of the skull

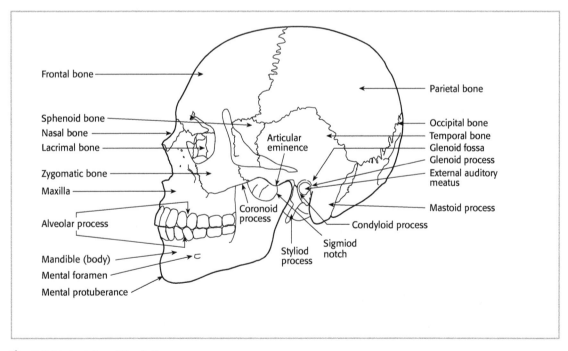

Figure 8.6 Lateral view of the skull

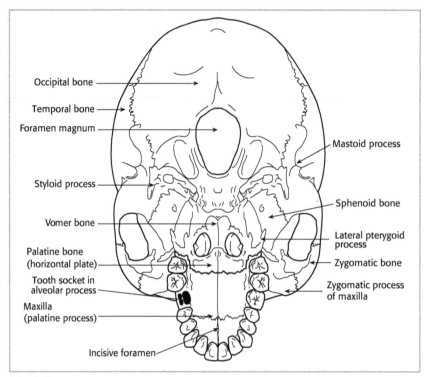

Figure 8.7 Base of the skull

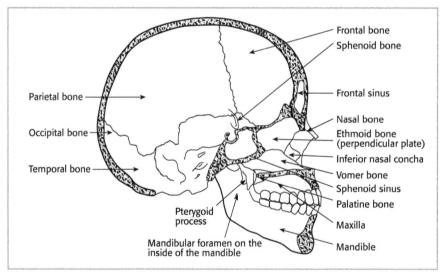

Figure 8.8 Mid-sagittal view of the skull

Bones of the cranium and the face

Bones of the cranium

These are the:

■ frontal bones (2), which form the forehead, part of the cranium and most of the top of the eye sockets;

■ parietal bones(2) — these two bones form most

of the top part of the skull and join along the top at what is called the sagittal suture;

■ occipital bone, which forms the back of the cranium;

■ temporal bones (2), which form the sides and the base of the cranium around the ears;

■ sphenoid bones (2), which form the back of the eye sockets and join to the temporal bones; and

■ ethmoid bones (2), which form part of the back of the eye socket, part of the floor of the cranium and some of the nasal cavity wall.

Bones of the face

These are the:

- mandible, which is the lower jaw (this will be discussed in greater depth later);

- maxilla (2), which make up most of the upper jaw and are fused together at the midline (the maxilla, plural is maxillae, will also be discussed in detail later);

- nasal bones (2), which form the bridge of the nose;

- palatine (2), which form the posterior part of the hard palate and the floor of the nose, and join at the maxilla at the front;

- zygomatic bones(2) which form the cheek bones and some of the wall and the floor of the eye socket;

- lacrimal bones (2), which are small bones that make up part of the inner wall of the eye socket;

- vomer, the base of the nasal septum; and

- inferior conchae (2), which are small projections from the wall of the ethmoid bone into the nasal cavity.

The hyoid bone

This bone is not joined to any other bone. It is suspended between the lower jaw and the larynx and is a support for the tongue.

The mandible and maxilla

The mandible and maxilla are the bones of most importance in dentistry so it is worth looking at these in detail, which we do in the following pages.

The mandible

This bone is the lower jaw and is the largest and strongest bone of the face. It consists of a body and two broad rami (singular is ramus) projecting up from the posterior ends of the body.

The body is horseshoe shaped. Its upper border contains the teeth and the lower border is rounded and broad, as can be seen in Figure 8.9.

The mandible forms initially as two bones, but it hardens into one bone in early childhood. The join at the midline is called the symphysis and there is a slightly protruding triangular area there known as the mental protuberance. At each corner at the base of the triangle is a raised area called the

mental **tubercle** which, together with muscles and covering skin, we call the chin.

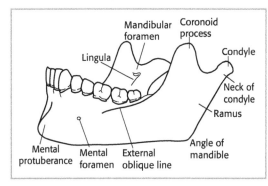

Figure 8.9 The mandible

Mental foramen

A **foramen** is a hole in or through bone. The mental foramen is a small opening lying between the roots of the first and second premolars (also known as bicuspids) on the outer aspect (the facial side) of the mandible. This foramen opens upward and backward. An injection into this region is made to produce mental nerve analgesia (mental block).

Oblique ridge

This is a thick, prominent ridge on the facial surface of the mandible, which passes upwards and becomes the anterior border of the ramus.

Coronoid and condylar process and the sigmoid notch

A process is a part of the bone that grows on or sticks out of the bone.

- The coronoid process is the anterior (front) portion of the ramus. It rises from a point immediately behind the third molar.

- The posterior portion of the ramus is the condylar process, usually called the condyle. This is made up of a large portion called the head and a narrower portion, directly underneath, known as the neck.

The dip in between the coronoid process and the condyle is called the sigmoid notch.

Angle of the mandible

The ramus is roughly rectangular and the angle of the mandible is where the body of the mandible and the ramus meet.

■ **tubercle:** a small prominence or projection.
■ **foramen:** a naturally occurring hole in bone through which pass blood and lymph vessels and nerves.

Mylohyoid ridge

This is on the inside of the body of the mandible. It starts behind the third molar and runs down and forward towards the base. The mylohyoid muscle is attached to this ridge and forms part of the muscular floor of the mouth.

Mandibular foramen and lingula

This is an opening on the inner aspect of the ramus. It opens to a canal that runs through the body of the mandible and divides between the bicuspids/premolars. One part continues as the incisive canal running forward beneath the incisor teeth and the other canal, the mental canal, passes to the mental foramen. This canal system carries the inferior dental nerve and the blood vessels supplying the lower teeth.

The lingula is a small projection of bone that partly covers the mandibular foramen.

Other foramina of the mandible

There are additional accessory foramina:

■ on the inner surface of the mandible;
■ a midline foramen at the symphysis; and
■ others related to the premolar and molar teeth.

Although chiefly for bone nutrition, they may also transmit nerve fibres, some of which supply the teeth.

The maxillae

The upper jaw consists mainly of two maxillary bones, one on each side of the midline, which are fused to each other. See Figure 8.10a. The other parts of the upper jaw are the palatine bones.

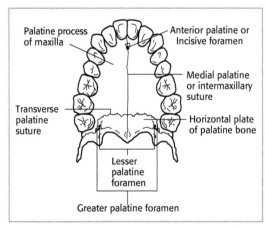

Figure 8.10a The maxillae

(The forerunners of the two maxillary bones fuse together about six weeks after conception. If they do not do this, a condition known as cleft palate results.)

The maxillae are fixed to the base of the skull and form the basic shape of the face above the lips and below the eyes. They also form the base of the nose, the cheekbones and the roof of the mouth, and give bony support to the teeth of the upper jaw.

Each maxilla contains a maxillary air sinus and has four processes that project from the central body of the maxilla to join with other bones of the skull. These processes are the:

■ nasal;
■ zygomatic;
■ palatine; and
■ alveolar processes.

Maxillary air sinus (antrum)

This is a large hollow, air-filled cavity in the body of the maxilla. Its walls are thin and it opens into the nose. The floor of the sinus is in close proximity to the roots of the upper posterior teeth and the floor may be damaged during difficult extractions of the roots of these teeth. Figure 8.10b contains a side-on view of the maxillae.

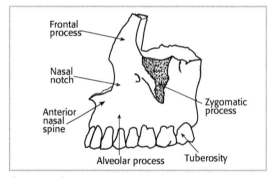

Figure 8.10b Side-on view of the maxillae

Foramina of the maxilla

Each maxilla has four foramina that carry the nerves and blood vessels that are needed to keep the surrounding tissue alive. As these holes are in fairly constant positions, it is possible to find and anaesthetise the nerves that pass through them.

The foramina are:

■ the anterior palatine foramen — there is only one of these, half in each maxilla, situated just **lingual** to the central incisors in the midline;
■ the greater, or posterior, palatine foramen, which are situated on the palate just lingual to the last molar (there is one in each maxilla);

■ the posterior superior **alveolar** foramen, which is on the cheek side just above the last molar in each maxilla; and

■ the infra-orbital foramen, just below the eye socket on the anterior side of the maxilla.

The alveolar process

The **alveolar process** (sometimes called the **alveolar ridge** or alveolar bone) is that part of bone that supports the teeth.

The outlines of the roots of the teeth are very clearly seen on its surface. The alveolar process is particularly thickened over the bicuspids/premolars root to form what is called the cuspid eminence. The alveolar process finishes behind the third molar at the tuberosity, which is a bony swelling.

Both the maxillae and the mandible have an alveolar process, the function of which is to retain the teeth. This process distributes the stresses of mastication (chewing) to the basal bone. It atrophies (that is, the bone is gradually reabsorbed) when the teeth are lost or removed.

This is important to note. The teeth are not set in bone-like pegs in concrete. Bone is living tissue with cells that live and die. Bones continually change shape and size by a process called re-modelling. In this process, some cells (osteoblasts) lay down new bone on one surface and at the same time other cells (osteoclasts) reabsorb bone on another surface.

The temporo-mandibular joint

The name of this joint comes from the two bones that are the basis of its formation — the temporal bone (at the base of the skull) and the mandible.

As can be seen in Figure 8.11, the temporo-mandibular joint is made up of:

■ the **mandibular fossa** of the temporal bone, behind the **articular eminence**; this is at the base of the skull;

■ the condyle of the mandible;

■ a joint capsule and ligaments that attach the mandible to the cranium completely surrounds the joint — it is attached to the condyle and the temporal bone;

■ the muscles of mastication that hold the mandible in position;

■ articulating surfaces of fibro-cartilage;

■ a synovial membrane producing a sticky lubricating fluid (like the white of an egg) called synovial fluid;

■ synovial cavities (upper and lower joint cavities), which are spaces between the surfaces of the fossa and the condyle and the cavities are filled with synovial fluid; and

■ a disc of fibro-cartilage lying between the upper and lower cavities.

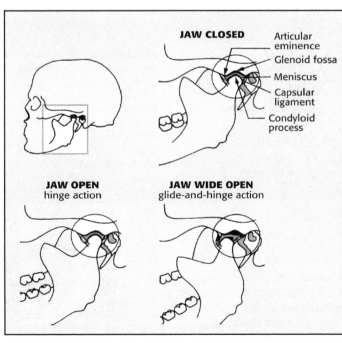

Figure 8.11 Movement of the temporo-mandibular joint

■ **mandibular fossa:** a fossa is a hollow or groove in a bone. The mandibular fossa is a hollow in the mandibular bone.
■ **articular eminences:** the articular tubercle of the zygomatic process of the temporal bone, forming the anterior boundary of the mandibular fossa.

Movements of the temporo-mandibular joint

As the mandible opens, the **condyles** rotate in the fossae of the temporo-mandibular joints, as shown in Figure 8.11. As the jaw continues to open, the condyles slide downwards and forwards onto the eminences. Insufficient support during extractions, or a blow on the mandible, can cause the condyle to slip over the eminence and out of the socket. This is called 'dislocation'.

The oral cavity

This is the space bounded:

■ interiorly by the lips;

■ laterally by the cheeks;

■ above by the hard and soft palate;

■ below by the floor of the mouth and the tongue; and

■ behind by the entrance to the pharynx.

See Figure 8.12 for a diagram of the oral cavity.

When the teeth are brought together and occlude, the space between the teeth and the lips is called the vestibule of the mouth.

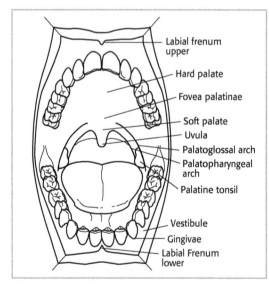

Labial frenum upper
Hard palate
Fovea palatinae
Soft palate
Uvula
Palatoglossal arch
Palatopharyngeal arch
Palatine tonsil
Vestibule
Gingivae
Labial Frenum lower

Figure 8.12 The oral cavity

The cheeks

The cheeks (buccinator muscles) are protected on the outside by the skin and on the inside by mucosa. At the entry to the mouth, the two coverings meet at a transitional area of thin red **epithelium**, which gives the lips their external character and outline form.

The hard and soft palates

These form the roof of the mouth. The anterior two-thirds are the hard palate and the posterior third is the soft palate.

The hard palate is formed by the palatal processes of the maxillae and the horizontal plates of the palatine bones. It is covered by a very tough epithelium, which has a median line (a raphe) ending just behind the upper central incisors in a small oval-shaped swelling or papilla. The anterior part of the palatal surface is roughened by folds of tissue known as rugae.

The soft palate is a movable fold suspended from the posterior border of the hard palate. It extends backwards and downwards between the nasal and oral parts of the pharynx. A small conical process called the uvula hands form the middle of its posterior border.

The soft palate plays an important part in swallowing, blowing and speech and aids in closing the mouth off from the nasal cavity.

The muscles contained in the soft palate pull it upwards and backwards between the nasal and oral parts of the pharynx where it meets a rounded ridge on the pharyngeal wall. Two folds of mucous membrane containing muscles run downwards from each side of the palate and between these two folds are the tonsils.

The floor of the mouth

This is largely formed by the anterior two-thirds of the tongue and the remainder by the reflection of the mucous membrane from under the tongue to the gingiva. In the midline, under the tongue is the lingual **frenum** and on each side, a ridge called the sublingual fold containing many openings of the sublingual gland.

Beneath the mucous membrane and the tongue is a sheet of muscle called the mylohyoid muscle. It forms the floor of the mouth proper and it is attached to the mylohyoid ridge of the mandible, as can be seen in Figure 8.13.

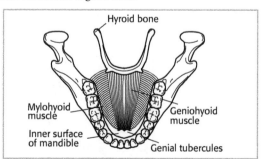

Hyroid bone
Mylohyoid muscle
Geniohyoid muscle
Inner surface of mandible
Genial tubercules

Figure 8.13 The floor of the mouth

The oral mucosa

The integument

Both the skin and the mucosa form part of the integument, which is the outer layer or membrane covering or lining any tissue or organ. The prime role of the integument is to protect the individual. An intact integument is the primary defence mechanism against successful invasion by micro-organisms.

Skin is the protective epithelial covering of the body. It has:

■ an outer layer called the epidermis — the surface layer of the epidermis consists of dead cells whose cytoplasm has been totally replaced by a protein known as keratin; and

■ an inner layer known as the dermis — the dermis contains structures such as hair follicles, sweat glands and sebaceous glands.

The vermilion is a transitional area of specialised non-keratinised epithelium separating the skin of the lips from the oral lining mucosa.

Oral mucosa

Oral mucosa lines the inside of the oral cavity proper and the **vestibules**. It is a moist mucous membrane that contains elastic tissue, minor salivary glands and mucous glands, but lacks hair follicles, sweat glands and sebaceous glands. The epithelium of the oral mucosa is variably **keratinising**.

Lining mucosa

The lining mucosa covers the soft palate, the inside of the cheeks and lips, the underside of the tongue and the floor of the mouth. It is non-keratinising and overlies loose connective tissue that contains elastic fibres. As a result, these tissues are relatively loose and movable, and blood vessels are readily distinguishable within them.

Masticatory mucosa

Those areas of the oral cavity that are directly subjected to the forces of mastication consist of dense connective tissue that does not contain elastic tissue, and is covered by keratinised epithelium. These areas include the upper surface of the tongue, the hard palate and the gingiva. This mucosa is firmly attached to the bone so it cannot move around like the lining mucosa.

Special characteristics of the gingiva

The gingiva is known as 'the gums'. The gingiva is the soft tissue surrounding the teeth as seen in Figure 8.14. It is subdivided into:

■ the attached gingiva; and

■ the free or marginal gingiva, which includes the triangular segments (interdental papillae) that fill the spaces between adjoining teeth.

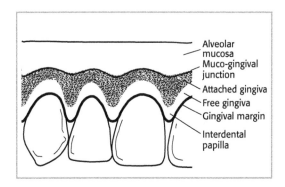

Figure 8.14 Periodontal structures

Healthy gingiva is a light coral pink colour in Anglo-Celtic and Caucasian persons. African Americans, Australian Aborigines, Mediterranean people, Asians, Africans and many South American people exhibit a wide and variable range of physiological gingival pigmentation ranging from yellowish to brown, purple or black.

A narrow crevice or gutter exists between the gingiva and the tooth surfaces.

In healthy individuals this gingival sulcus may range in depth from 0.5 mm to a maximum of 3 mm in health. The facial and lingual surfaces of the free gingiva may exhibit a free gingival groove, which corresponds with the base of the sulcus.

Both the oral lining mucosa and the free gingiva are smooth.

The attached gingiva may exhibit a pebbled, orange-peel-like appearance, known as stippling. This occurs in some 40 per cent of the population. Stippling is not regarded as an essential criterion for healthy gingiva.

■ **vestibules:** that part of the mouth between the cheeks and lips and the alveolar ridge.

■ **keratinising:** able to produce keratin, which is a fibrous protein that is the basis of hair and nails. Keratinised epithelium has a tough, protective layer.

The muco-gingival junction

Where the attached gingiva joins the oral lining mucosa, there is a line between:

■ the dense, tightly attached gingiva, in which there are no obvious blood vessels; and

■ the more delicate, red, smooth and movable lining mucosa in which blood vessels are easily seen.

This line is the muco-gingival junction.

Frena of the oral cavity

The inner surfaces of the lips and the cheeks are attached to their corresponding neighbouring gingiva by folds of mucous membrane known as frena (singular — frenum). Thus one can describe mandibular or maxillary labial or buccal frena.

The ventral surface of the tongue is attached to the floor of the mouth by the lingual frenum. If this frenum is abnormally thick and fibrous, it may interfere with speech and swallowing, a condition known as ankyloglossia, or as 'tongue tie'.

Blood supply to the head and mouth

The main blood supply to the head (and therefore to the teeth) is via an artery called the common carotid artery. It arises as a large vessel from the aorta, in the chest, and passes upwards to the neck.

At about the level of the thyroid cartilage (Adam's apple in men), and a little to the side, the common carotid divides into two branches, which are:

❶ the internal carotid, which enters the skull and supplies blood to the brain; and

❷ the external carotid, which passes upwards and gives off nine branches to the mandible and the maxillae.

The external carotid passes along the posterior border of the ramus and gives off a branch to the tongue (the lingual artery) and another important branch called the inferior alveolar artery.

This artery enters the mandibular foramen and then runs forward inside the mandibular canal, supplying the lower teeth as it goes.

It terminates at the mental foramen where it runs to the anterior teeth and across the chin and the lips.

As the external carotid continues up in the head region, it terminates as a large branch called the maxillary artery. This runs into the maxilla (upper jaw). This has several smaller branches that are interconnected: the posterior superior alveolar branch, the infra-orbital branch and the greater palatine branch.

Blood leaves the tissues and enters the veins. These correspond fairly closely to the passage of the arteries, though there are some variations from person to person. Finally, blood from the head is returned to the heart via the large jugular vein in the neck into the superior vena cava. See Figure 8.15 for a diagram of the blood supply to the face and mouth.

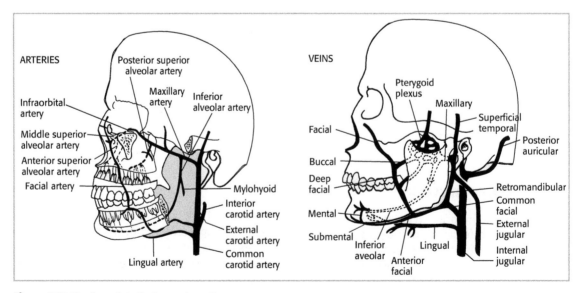

Figure 8.15 Blood supply to the face and mouth

The masticatory apparatus

The masticatory apparatus is the first part of the digestive system. It consists of:

- the bony skeleton of the head;
- the oral cavity (the space enclosed by the lips and cheeks) that contains the mucosa, the hard and soft palate, the tongue and the teeth and their supporting periodontal tissues;
- the muscles that move the mandible;
- the nerves that control movement, taste and smell; and
- the glands that produce saliva.

The main functions of the masticatory apparatus are:

- incision and mastication (the process by which food is broken up and mixed with saliva);
- deglutition (swallowing);
- speech (in association with the larynx); and
- appearance (which changes dramatically if the shape and conformation of teeth varies).

The muscles of mastication

There are four pairs of muscles that, acting together or separately, are largely responsible for the movements of the mandible.

The masseter muscle is attached to the mandible in the region of the ramus and passes upwards to the zygomatic arch. It raises the mandible and helps force the teeth together (occlude).

The temporalis muscle is a fan-shaped muscle joined to the side of the skull at one end and to the coronoid process of the mandible at the other. It also helps to raise the mandible and close the mouth.

The lateral pterygoid muscle is attached to the neck of the condoyle of the mandible at one end and runs forward towards the back of the maxilla to the sphenoid bone. It pulls cartilage forwards as the mouth opens. It also protrudes the mandible (moves it forward). Acting independently, this muscle is also responsible for lateral (side to side) movement.

The medial pterygoid muscle runs downwards from the sphenoid bone and joins onto the mandible on the inside of the ramus opposite to the masseter. It helps raise the mandible and close the mouth.

Other muscles involved in mastication

A number of other muscles also play a part in mastication.

Principal of these is the buccinator muscle. The buccinator muscle is the cheek muscle. It forces food across the teeth during chewing movements. It also plays a major role in the sucking process.

The tongue

The muscles of the tongue

The tongue is a complex muscular organ composed of muscles that are integrated and woven into a highly specialised organ with numerous functions, including assisting chewing and swallowing, tasting and speech.

There are two groups of muscles controlling the tongue:

❶ *extrinsic muscles*, which tether the tongue to the head; and

❷ *intrinsic muscles*, which control the tongue's ability to shorten and lengthen (longitudinal movement), widen and become thin (transverse movement) and lengthen and flatten (vertical movement).

The major muscles of the tongue are the:

- genioglossus muscle, which depresses and protrudes the tongue;
- hypoglossus muscle, which pulls the tongue back and down;
- styloglossus muscle, which retracts the tongue; and
- palatoglossus muscle, which lifts the base of the tongue and presses it against the soft palate while also depressing the soft palate towards the tongue.

The tongue's covering

The oral **mucosa** covering the dorsum (top surface) of the tongue is highly specialised to assist with taste, speech, **mastication** and deglutition, as can be seen in Figure 8.16 (overleaf).

There are epithelial elevations, or projections, on the tongue. The most numerous are the filiform papillae, which cover the anterior two-thirds of the tongue. These are the hundreds of pointed projections that roughen the surface of the tongue and

mucosa: moist epithelium and connective tissue. A moist lining that secretes mucous.

mastication: chewing.

enable it to grip and move food around the mouth during chewing. They have a fine core of connective tissue within them.

Interspersed among the filiform papillae are larger, red, dome-shaped elevations called fungiform papillae. These contain taste buds.

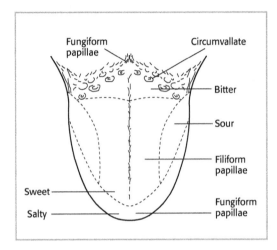

Figure 8.16 The tongue's covering

There is a v-shaped line that separates the anterior two-thirds of the tongue from the posterior third. Just in front of this line and parallel to it are eight to twelve circumvallate papillae. These are much larger than the other papillae and are round, dome-shaped structures that sit in troughs. They contain large numbers of taste buds, which also line the walls of the troughs surrounding them.

Along the lateral border of the posterior part of the tongue are several narrow parallel folds of mucous membrane called foliate papillae. These also contain taste buds. Taste buds in small numbers also occur in the mucosa of the soft palate and the pharynx.

The ventral (underside) of the tongue is covered by mucosa similar to the floor of the mouth to which it joins.

Other muscles of the head and neck

These are:

- the palatopharyngeus muscle at the back of the mouth, which helps to close off the nasopharynx;
- the sternocleidomastoid muscle, a muscle on the side of the neck;
- the trapezius muscle, which finishes in the back but starts on the outside of the occipital bone in the head;

- orbicularis oris muscle, which closes the lips and makes them pucker (it aids with speech and eating by keeping the lips closed);
- the mentalis muscle that pushes up the bottom lip;
- the zygomatic major muscle, which pulls the corners of the mouth upwards and backwards; and
- the muscles of the floor of the mouth — the mylohyoid, digastric, stylohyoid and geniohyoid muscles.

Saliva

Saliva is a watery secretion consisting of mucus and **serous** fluid. The body produces one and a half, or more, litres daily. It is colourless, tasteless and mildly alkaline. The sight, taste or smell of food cause the flow of saliva principally from the three main pairs of salivary glands, which can be seen in Figure 8.17.

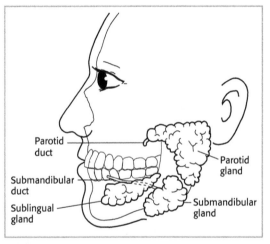

Figure 8.17 The salivary glands

Saliva:

- lubricates the mouth and food and makes swallowing easier;
- acts as a cleaning agent;
- aids in digestion as enzymes it contains act on food and make it more acceptable for use by the body;
- contains minerals and other chemicals to maintain a chemical balance in the mouth; and
- acts as a buffer against tooth decay.

The main salivary glands are the:

- parotid glands, situated on the side of the face just in front of and slightly below the ear opening, and close to the ramus — the saliva from these glands flows into the mouth via the parotid ducts (which opens at a small papilla on the mucous membrane of the cheek, opposite the upper second molar);

■ submandibular glands, which are medial to the body of the mandible — the submandibular duct carries the saliva forward and onto the floor of the mouth through the sublingual papillary under the tongue; and

■ sublingual glands, which are the smallest of the three — they are situated beneath the mucous membrane of the floor of the mouth and in contact with the inner surface of the mandible close to the symphysis. They have many ducts (8–18) that open on the sublingual fold close to the submandibular duct opening.

There are other small, minor salivary glands present in the lips, cheeks, tongue and roof of the mouth.

Nerves of the face, teeth and periodontium

The nerves of most significance to dentistry are the ones that supply the mouth and the face. These can be seen in Figure 8.18.

These nerves are:

■ the facial (seventh cranial) nerve, which supplies the muscles of facial expression (damage to this nerve may result in some facial paralysis); and

■ the trigeminal (fifth cranial) nerve, which has three branches (the ophthalmic nerve, the maxillary nerve and the mandibular nerve).

The proprioceptive system

As well as the usual sensory receptors mentioned here, there are also deeper receptors (situated in the muscles, joints and ligaments) that are stimulated by the contractions of the muscles and the movements of the joints. This proprioceptive system plays an important part in the control and regulation of body movements and posture.

This system is involved in the control of the path of closure of the mandible and the rest position of the mandible.

The branches of the trigeminal (fifth cranial) nerve

The ophthalmic nerve

This supplies branches to the eyeball and the lachrymal glands.

The maxillary nerve

This sensory nerve passes forward in the floor of the orbit and divides into four main branches.

❶ The infra-orbital nerve enters the infra-orbital grooves and passes out through the infra-orbital foramen just under the eye socket.

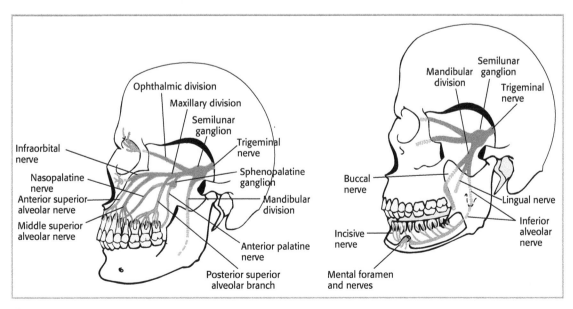

Figure 8.18 Nerves of the mandible and maxillae

❷ The posterior superior alveolar nerve supplies the roots of the maxillary second and third molars as well as some of the roots of the maxillary first molar.

❸ The middle superior alveolar nerve supplies the maxillary first and second premolars, some of the roots of the maxillary first molar as well as the maxillary sinus.

❹ The anterior superior alveolar nerve supplies the maxillary central, incisors, lateral and bicuspid/premolar teeth, their periodontal membrane and gingiva.

These nerves stay within the bone (except the branches to the gingiva). However, the maxillary bones around the teeth are porous enough to allow local anaesthesia to soak through from the surface of the bone to the nerves supplying the pulp of the teeth.

The mandibular nerve

The mandibular nerve passes downwards and forwards from the cranial cavity and divides into three branches significant in dentistry.

The inferior dental nerve enters the mandibular foramen on the medial surface of the mandible and passes along the mandibular canal where it supplies branches to the lower teeth. A branch passes out of the bone through the mental foramen to supply the lower lip. The bone of the mandible is not porous (except in the young or near the front of the mouth) so local anaesthetic must be deposited at the mandibular foramen, deep in the tissues, in order to obtain effective analgesia. This is called a mandibular block injection.

The lingual nerve runs downwards and forwards against the inner surface of the mandible and is sometimes seen during the removal of an unerupted wisdom tooth. It supplies the anterior two-thirds of the tongue, the floor of the mouth and the lingual side of the mandibular gingiva and mucosa. It is anaesthetised in association with a mandibular block injection.

The buccal nerve runs down the outside of the mandible and supplies the posterior part of the buccal surface of the gingiva and the cheeks in this region. It may require a separate injection when the mandibular block is used.

Summary

You have now covered the main elements of anatomy and physiology of the head and neck. Just as knowledge about the body systems is necessary to understand how our body functions, it is crucial to be familiar with the structures and function of the head and neck so as to move on to the next chapter, which covers the structures inside the oral cavity.

You have also become familiar with many descriptive anatomical terms used to describe body parts. Knowledge of these will assist communication between you and the dentist and is especially helpful in radiography, clinical photography and orthodontics.

To be a competent and efficient dental assistant, you need a thorough understanding and knowledge that underpins the tasks that you perform daily. With this, you will become more efficient at chair-side assisting during complicated dental procedures.

chapter nine
dental anatomy

Introduction

Dental anatomy involves the study of the teeth, the way they function and the structures that support them, including the jaws, muscles, glands and mucous membranes. A masticatory system cannot function properly unless all of these component parts are healthy and complete.

Consequently, you are required to have a working knowledge of the size, shape, location and number of teeth to:

- be able to chart correctly during the examination of the patient's mouth;
- understand the use of various instruments required for dental treatment;
- assist with radiography; and
- permit an appraisal, when making an appointment, of the patient's complaints and queries.

This chapter provides a more detailed description of the teeth and their associated structures.

Dentition

Deciduous and permanent dentition

Human beings (with some exceptions) have two sets of teeth in their lifetimes. The first set (known as deciduous or temporary dentition or 'milk teeth') are childhood teeth. These teeth are shed and replaced by more permanent teeth. Deciduous teeth are space maintainers for these permanent teeth. For this reason, it is important that they are cared for and remain in good condition and **caries** free until they exfoliate naturally.

The second set, known as permanent dentition, are the adult teeth.

- The deciduous dentition is composed of four incisors, two cuspids (also called canines) and four molars in each jaw — 20 teeth in all. Note, there are no deciduous bicuspids/premolars.

- The permanent dentition is composed of four incisors, two cuspids/canines, four bicuspids/premolars and, usually, six molars in each jaw — 32 teeth in all.

- Mixed dentition occurs during the time in which children lose their deciduous teeth and permanent teeth appear. An example is when the first (or six year old) molars have erupted.

Arrangement of the teeth

The teeth are arranged in two arches, an upper (or maxillary) arch and a lower (or mandibular) arch. The teeth in upper and lower jaws correspond (match) in number and type. This means that in any quarter (or quadrant) of the mouth, the pattern and arrangement of teeth is the same.

The maxillary arch is usually larger than the mandibular arch. The incisors and canines/cuspids of the maxillary arch normally project over the top of the mandibular incisors and bicuspid/premolars. This allows the cusps of the molars and bicuspid/premolars to match with the cusps of the opposing tooth (or between the cusps of two teeth).

This intercuspal relationship, as well as the muscles of the face and tongue, prevent the teeth from moving labially or lingually when the teeth are in occlusion (closed).

Mesial and distal contact between the teeth prevents their movement medially and distally.

The arrangement of the deciduous and permanent dentition can be seen in Figure 9.1.

■ **caries:** the process by which cavities are formed in teeth by gradual destruction of enamel and dentine.

■ **crown:** the part of the tooth that is covered with enamel (the part of the tooth usually visible in the mouth).

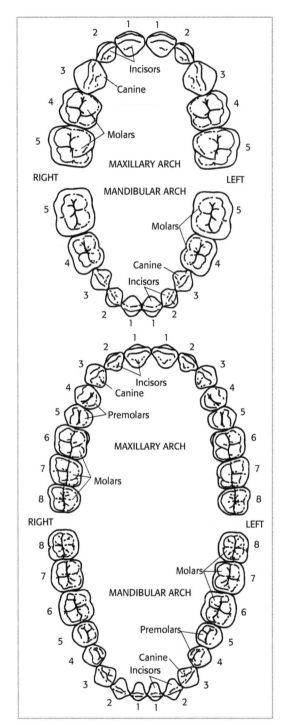

Figure 9.1 Arrangement of deciduous and permanent dentition

Teeth

Surfaces of the teeth

Surfaces are named for the direction in which they face in the arch of the teeth. The **crowns** of all teeth have five surfaces as shown in Figure 9.2.

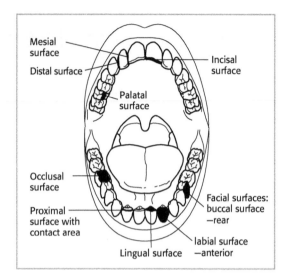

Figure 9.2 Names given to the surfaces of the crowns of the teeth

Teeth have the following surfaces:

- labial — the surface nearest the lips (La);
- lingual — the surface of mandibular teeth nearest the tongue (Li);
- palatal — the surfaces of maxillary teeth nearest the palate (P);
- mesial — the surface nearest the midline (M);
- distal — the surface furthest from the midline (D); and
- incisal — the cutting or biting edge (I).

Molars also have occlusal surfaces — the grinding surface with cusps (O).

The abbreviations shown in brackets are used in the charting of teeth to save time when describing tooth surfaces.

A proximal surface of a tooth is the surface adjacent to another tooth. The area between the teeth is called the inter-proximal space.

Characteristics of permanent teeth

Names of the teeth

The names of the teeth, to the right and left in each jaw, starting from the midline, are central incisor, lateral incisor, canine (also called cuspid), first bicuspid (also called premolar), second bicuspid/premolar, first molar, second molar and third molar (commonly known as the wisdom tooth). These teeth are shown in Figure 9.3.

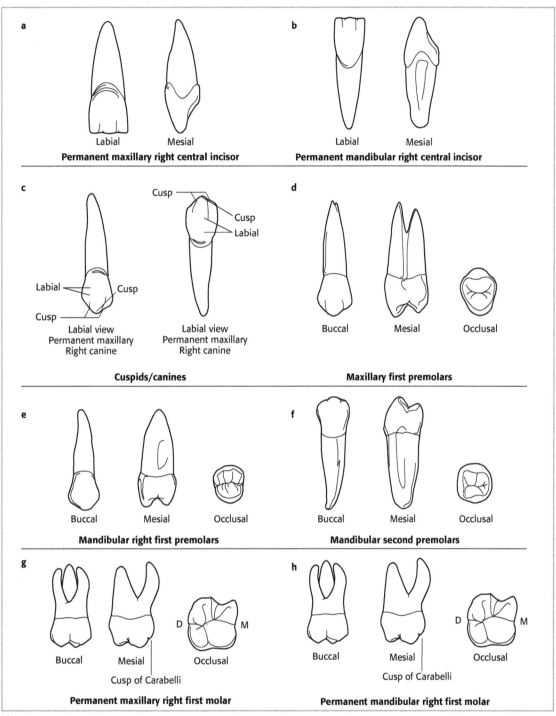

Figure 9.3 Views of teeth

Incisors

Incisors are at the front of the mouth and have one root. They have sharp edges for cutting food.

The maxillary centrals are larger than laterals. The distal angle is rounded.

Mandibular incisors are smaller but are more similar

to each other than the maxillary incisors. The lateral is slightly larger than the central and the distal angle of the central is not rounded.

Canines

Canines (or cuspids) have fairly sharp, pointy cusps. These are suitable for cutting and tearing food.

Cuspids/canines have a single, long root and are usually the most stable teeth in the mouth.

Maxillary cuspids/canines are larger than those in the mandible. The point of the cusp is nearer the mesial than the distal; one-third from the mesial, two-thirds from the distal.

First bicuspid/premolar (permanent premolar)

Bicuspids/premolars have points for grabbing and tearing food and also a broader surface for chewing. The maxillary first bicuspid/premolar usually has two cusps and two roots (which may be wholly or partly fused).

The mandibular first bicuspid/premolar has two cusps, with the lingual cusp poorly developed, and usually one root.

Second bicuspid/premolar (permanent premolar)

The maxillary second bicuspid/premolar is very similar in cusp to the first bicuspid/premolar but usually only has one root.

The mandibular second bicuspid/premolar has cusps much better developed than the first bicuspid/premolar. It may have two lingual cusps. It usually has one root.

First permanent molars (six year old molar)

Molars have broad surfaces that grind the more solid foods. They also usually have two roots in the lower jaw and three in the upper jaw. The third molars (also known as the wisdom teeth) in the lower jaw can have a varying number of roots.

The maxillary first permanent molar has four cusps (sometimes a fifth small cusp on the mesio-lingual, called Carabelli's Cusp). The mandibular first permanent molar has five cusps (three buccal and two lingual).

Second permanent molar (twelve year old molar)

The maxillary second permanent molar has four cusps and three roots.

The mandibular second permanent molars have four cusps. They also usually have two roots in the lower jaw.

Permanent third molars (wisdom teeth)

These vary greatly in number of cusps and roots.

Gross anatomy of the tooth

The following terms refer to parts of the teeth indicated in Figure 9.4.

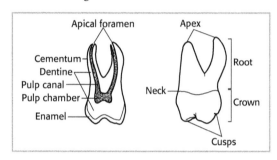

Figure 9.4 Gross anatomy of the tooth

- Crown — the portion of the tooth that is covered in enamel. This is the part of the tooth that can normally be seen in the mouth.

- Root — the portion of the tooth that is fixed within the walls of the alveolar bone.

- Neck — the portion of the tooth that forms the junction of the crown and the root.

- Cusp — a point or pronounced elevation on the crown of the tooth, usually on the biting (occlusal) surface. Teeth with more than one cusp (bicuspids/premolars and molars) have grooves on their biting surfaces that are formed by the depression between the cusps. These are called pits and fissures and when these are imperfectly formed, micro-organisms and food debris can collect there and cause decay.

- Apex — the end of the root of the tooth.

- Apical foramen — the opening of the pulp canal at the apex of the tooth.

- Pulp chamber — the cavity in the crown of the tooth that is normally filled by the dental pulp.

- Root canal — the pulp extends from the pulp chamber through one or more canals in the root to become continuous with the outside tissues through the apical foramen.

Microscopic anatomy of the tooth

The tooth consists of enamel, cementum, dentine and pulp tissue, as shown in Figure 9.5.

Enamel

Enamel is the hardest tissue of the body, composed of 96 per cent inorganic calcium hydroxyapatite supported by a small amount of inorganic material.

This forms the outer layer of the crown. It is formed of calcified rods that are held together with a **matrix** substance similar to the rods themselves. These rods run from the surface of the tooth to the outer layer of the dentine. Where the rods meet the dentine is called the dentino-enamel junction. If a tooth fractures, it is likely to do it along the length of these rods.

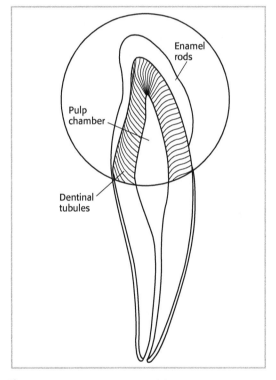

Figure 9.5 Microscopic anatomy of the tooth

Enamel is **non-vital** and like hair and nails can be cut without pain. It is completely formed before the **eruption** of the teeth but is capable of taking up some substances (like fluoride, for example).

Cementum

Cementum is a bone-like substance that covers the dentine in the roots of the tooth with a very thin layer that extends from the cemento-enamel junction to the root apex. A thin network of fibres (the **periodontal ligament**) holds the tooth in the socket in the alveolar process. These fibres are attached to the cementum at one end and the alveolar bone at the other, forming a sling that allows the tooth some movement.

The total amount of cementum slowly increases throughout life. Therefore, cementum is a vital tissue like dentine. It contains 45–50 per cent inorganic material.

Cementum is yellow in colour; darker than enamel but lighter than dentine.

Dentine

This is the vital, mineralised tissue that makes up the bulk of the tooth. It is covered with enamel at the crown and with cementum at the root. It forms before the tooth erupts (primary dentine) and continues to form at a slower rate throughout the life of the tooth (secondary dentine). Where a tooth has been damaged (for example by caries or attrition), new dentine may be laid down at a faster rate at the site of the damage. This is sometimes called reparative dentine.

Dentine is harder than bone but not as hard as enamel because it contains less inorganic material (67 per cent). The inorganic material is composed of calcium hydroxyapatite crystals randomly arranged in a collagen fibre organic matrix. The crystals are similar to the ones found in bone and cementum but are much smaller than the apatite crystals of enamel.

Dentine is elastic. That is, it can be deformed slightly and will return to its original shape.

The dentine is formed of tubules (dentinal tubules) that run from the outer junction with the enamel and dentine or the cementum and dentine (see Figure 9.5).

Each tubule contains minute processes of connective tissue cells (odontoblasts) that line the pulp cavity.

The health of these fibres and their associated cells in the pulp is crucial. If they are damaged, the first step towards the tooth becoming non-vital has occurred and there is a risk that the tooth may eventually be lost. For example, the odontoblasts and their fibres can be damaged permanently by:

- heat generated in cavity preparation if carried out without adequate cooling;

- excessive dehydration; or

- harmful chemical reaction on the dentine.

Pulp

The pulp occupies the pulp chamber and the root canals of the teeth. It has two functions:

matrix: a framework — basic material that binds together to form a mass or bulk. **non-vital:** not alive. **eruption:** the movement of the tooth through the gum surface, into its working position in the mouth. **periodontal ligament:** the ligament surrounding the root of the tooth and acting as a sling attaching the root to the alveolar bone (also called periodontal membrane).

❶ to form, repair and nourish the dentine; and

❷ to act as a sensory organ within the teeth. Decay processes, chemical or mechanical irritants or temperature changes can all cause pain.

The pulp contains all the components of normal tissue; blood vessels, lymph drainage and connective tissues as well as nerve fibres and odontoblasts.

Cavity preparation can be, and often is, painful. This is due to the cutting of the dentine but does not necessarily indicate nearness to the pulp of the teeth.

As we get older, the number of blood vessels in the pulp decreases and the amount of connective tissue increases. As the dentine grows, the pulp reduces in size.

The periodontal ligament

Teeth are held and supported in the jaw by their roots via the periodontal ligament as shown in Figure 9.6.

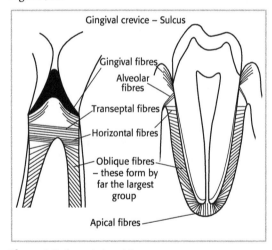

Figure 9.6 The periodontal ligament

That part of the jaws that surrounds the roots of the teeth and forms their sockets is the alveolar bone. The outer surface of the alveolar bone is denser than the inner bulk of bone and there is a continuous thin layer of compact bone lining the walls of the teeth sockets. This is called the lamina dura.

The periodontal ligament joins the roots of the teeth to this bone lining the socket walls. It is thin but very dense and tough tissue. Blood vessels and nerve fibres are interspersed between the tissue bundles.

Functions of the periodontal ligament

The functions of the periodontal ligament are:

■ Formative — the ligament contains cells that are continually replacing worn out fibres and remodelling the bone and cementum throughout the life of the tooth. They do this in response to stimuli that act on the teeth. This function of the ligament enables teeth to be moved in the jaw during orthodontic treatment.

■ Supportive — the ligament attaches and supports the teeth in the jaws in the correct relationship to each other and to adjacent tissues, and cushions the teeth against stresses caused by mastication and when they occlude.

■ Sensory — the nerve supply of the ligament is both sensory (to do with feeling and pain) and proprioceptive (to do with sense of location). So the ligament protects the tooth against excessive biting force by responding with pain. Sensory information localises the teeth in space to ensure correct positioning of the teeth and jaws when chewing.

■ Nutritive — the blood vessels and lymphatics supply essential nutrients to the ligament, bone and cementum and remove waste products.

Gingiva

The alveolar bone is covered in tissue called periosteum that blends with the mucous membrane of the mouth to form the muco-periosteum. This covering joins with a specialised part of the oral mucous membrane that surrounds and attaches to the necks of the teeth and acts as a seal.

This covering is called the gingival tissue. In Caucasian people, this soft tissue should be coral pink in colour, possibly with an orange peel or stippled appearance, and should be firmly bound down to the underlying bone. The colour may vary, with some pigmentation, depending on skin colour. It should have a streamlined relationship to the teeth, terminating with a knife-edge join immediately below the contact points of the teeth.

You should refer to Chapters 8 and 31 for more information about gingiva and the periodontium.

Dental embryology

Dental embryology is the study of the development of the teeth and other oral structures of a baby from the beginning of pregnancy through to the birth of the baby.

Development of the teeth in utero

The teeth start to form from the sixth to the eighth week of embryonic life with the development in each jaw of ten tooth buds (or tooth germs). These grow to form the ten deciduous teeth in each jaw.

About week 17, a second outgrowth from each tooth bud forms the permanent teeth. The tooth buds for the permanent molars form separately behind the deciduous molars. The permanent teeth develop below and lingual to the deciduous teeth. Therefore, there is a possibility of damage to the permanent tooth germs if the deciduous teeth are extracted prematurely.

At birth, babies normally have about 44 teeth at different stages of development. Enamel is developing on all the deciduous teeth and may be starting on the permanent teeth.

Tooth formation continues as the jaws grow throughout childhood and is not completed until after the third molars erupt at the age of 17–21 years.

Development of the enamel, cementum, dentine and bone

Mineralisation occurs from the fourth month in utero and continues at least until the child is 12 years old. The enamel forms from epithelial cells called ameloblasts. The outline of the tooth hardens as calcium (and some other mineral salts) is deposited.

The enamel is built in layers starting from the crown of the tooth and working down. If the tooth has more than one cusp, the enamel forms over each cusp and then these join to cover the occlusal surface of the tooth. (A fissure is an area where there is incomplete joining of the enamel and a pit is where the enamel overlaps, leaving a deep groove too small to clean with a toothbrush.)

The dentine, cementum and pulp develop from connective tissues called the dental papilla. The crown of each tooth grows before the root. After the tooth appears in the mouth, root formation continues for approximately two years. The alveolar bone and the periodontal ligament also develop from connective tissues at the same time as the dentine, cementum and pulp. See Table 9.1 for more information.

Stage	Description	Appearance
Thickening	Begins in week six of embryonic development; involves thickening of the embryonic oral epithelium to form the U-shaped dental lamina; thickening then occurs at twenty points (ten in the dental lamina of each arch)	area of thickening / dental lamina / epithelium / microscopic view
Bud	Twenty thickenings enlarge into bud-like clumps of tissue which appear to stretch out from the oral epithelium as they grow	tooth bud / (arrows show direction of future growth) / microscopic view
Cap	A dent develops as the deepest part becomes concave (pushed in) to form a cap	cap shaped epithelial in growth / microscopic view
Bell	Outline of the future tooth is determined by the way in which the cells grow; enamel production begins	dental papilla / dental sac
Eruption	Cycle finishes when root formation is complete (usually up to two years after eruption)	enamel organ / enamel / dentine / pulp

Table 9.1 Dental embryology – development of the tooth bud

■ **mineralisation:** the addition of minerals such as calcium to the body, which hardens certain tissues such as teeth and bone.

Eruption times of teeth

Teeth do not erupt into the mouth until well after the crown is completely formed (from 12 months to several years after the commencement of mineralisation). The approximate eruption dates are provided in Figure 9.7.

Exfoliation of teeth

When the deciduous teeth fall out, this is called exfoliation.

First, the root of the deciduous tooth is resorbed and eventually the crown falls out because it has no support from the root. The deciduous tooth is helped on its way by pressure from the permanent tooth. The crown of the deciduous tooth maintains a space for the permanent tooth when it erupts. More information can be found in Figures 9.7 and 9.8, and in Table 9.2.

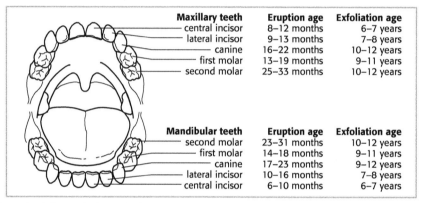

Maxillary teeth	Eruption age	Exfoliation age
central incisor	8–12 months	6–7 years
lateral incisor	9–13 months	7–8 years
canine	16–22 months	10–12 years
first molar	13–19 months	9–11 years
second molar	25–33 months	10–12 years

Mandibular teeth	Eruption age	Exfoliation age
second molar	23–31 months	10–12 years
first molar	14–18 months	9–11 years
canine	17–23 months	9–12 years
lateral incisor	10–16 months	7–8 years
central incisor	6–10 months	6–7 years

Figure 9.7 Eruption and exfoliation of primary dentition

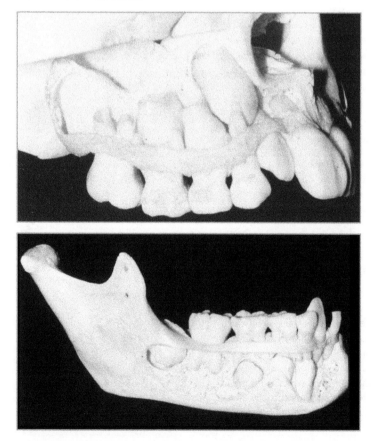

Figure 9.8 Examples of mixed dentition with primary teeth shed and permanent teeth erupting

Maxillary		Mandibular	
Central incisor	7–8 years	Central incisor	6–7 years
Lateral incisor	8–9 years	Lateral incisor	7–8 years
Cuspid	11–12 years	Cuspid	9–10 years
First bicuspid/premolar	10–11 years	First bicuspid/premolar	10–12 years
Second bicuspid/premolar	12–13 years	Second bicuspid/premolar	11–12 years
First molar	17–21 years	First molar	17–21 years
Second molar		Second molar	
Third molar		Third molar	

Table 9.2 Eruption of permanent dentition

Abnormalities of the teeth

Some common abnormalities are:

- congenitally missing teeth (anodontia), of which the lateral incisors, third molar and sometimes the second bicuspids/premolars are the most common;
- supernumerary (extra) teeth;
- microdontia, which are misshaped teeth; for example, peg-shaped incisors;
- hypoplasia, which are pits due to deficient formation of enamel;
- hypocalcification, which is abnormal softness and irregularity of surfaces; and
- extra cusps and abnormal tooth shapes.

These abnormalities can be caused by a range of factors including:

- genetics — problems can be caused by chromosome abnormalities; and
- environment — problems can be caused by the use of drugs by the mother, by illness, infection or radiation exposure.

There are also abnormalities that occur in the eruption of the teeth. For example, some babies are born with teeth (natal teeth) and others have teeth erupt in the month after birth (neonatal teeth).

In some cases a tooth will not erupt at all (an impacted tooth) or will become fused to the alveolar bone and only partially erupt (ankylosis).

Other conditions that you might see in the surgery that are not tooth related include cleft or hair lip, cleft palate and ankyloglossia. A cleft lip is the result of failure of the maxillary and medial nasal processes to fuse. A cleft palate occurs when the palatal shelves do not fuse with the primary palate. Ankyloglossia is also called 'tongue-tie' and occurs when the usually short lingual frenum is connected all the way to the tip of the tongue.

Some of these conditions are also described in Chapter 35.

Charting teeth

There are many styles of charts used in dentistry but the anatomical and the diagrammatic charts are the most common. Some examples can be seen in Figures 9.9 and 9.10.

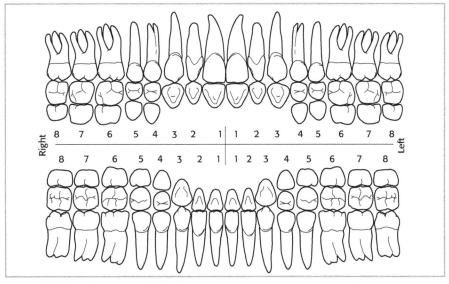

Figure 9.9 An anatomical chart (permanent dentition)

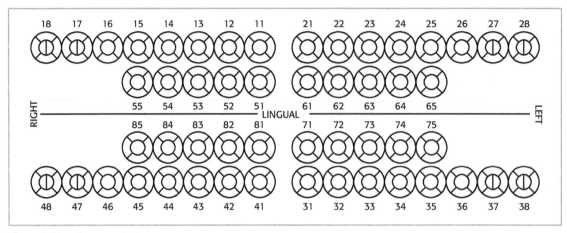

Figure 9.10 A diagrammatic chart

Anatomical charts, as the name implies, represent the actual tooth shape. They may be a little harder to use than diagrammatic charts, but they make it possible to record the various features of each tooth very precisely.

Some specialist practices may use specially designed charts, such as periodontal charts. Most charts contain both permanent and deciduous dentition.

The term 'charting' refers to the recording of the condition of teeth on the dental chart. Charting is a form of shorthand in which numbers are given to teeth to identify them and symbols are used to record their status (e.g. cavities). This is intended to make writing notes simpler than writing the full names of teeth.

There are two systems of notation that use shorthand forms to describe teeth:

❶ International (FDI — Federation Dentaire International) Notation; and

❷ Palmer's Notation.

These forms of notation can be used on both anatomical and diagrammatic charts. They are explained in more detail below and in Chapter 18.

International Notation

This system was developed by the International Dental Federation (IDF) from the older Palmer's Notation (see below). International Notation is easier for computer held records than Palmer's Notation as it uses only numbers to identify each tooth.

Each tooth is designated by two numbers. The first refers to the quadrant and indicates whether the tooth is permanent or deciduous. The second number refers to the position of the tooth in the quadrant.

The quadrants for the permanent teeth are numbered clockwise from 1 to 4, from the patient's upper right:

■ maxillary right quadrant = 1;

■ maxillary left quadrant = 2;

■ mandibular left quadrant = 3; and

■ mandibular right quadrant = 4.

The teeth in each quadrant are numbered 1 to 8 for the permanent teeth.

Maxillary right	Maxillary left
18 17 16 15 14 13 12 11	21 22 23 24 25 26 27 28
48 47 46 45 44 43 42 41	31 32 33 34 35 36 37 38
Mandibular right	**Mandibular left**

The quadrants for the deciduous teeth are also numbered clockwise, but range from 5 to 8 from the patient's upper right (as for permanent teeth):

■ upper right deciduous quadrant = 5;

■ upper left deciduous quadrant = 6;

■ lower left deciduous quadrant = 7; and

■ lower right deciduous quadrant = 8.

Maxillary right	Maxillary left
55 54 53 52 51	61 62 63 64 65
85 84 83 82 81	71 72 73 74 75
Mandibular right	**Mandibular left**

As an example, the upper right first permanent molar is 16 (pronounced 'one six') and the lower left deciduous molar is 75 ('seven five').

Palmer's Notation

In this charting system the dental arches are divided into a left and a right quadrant with a cross. Each of the permanent teeth is identified by the numbers 1 to 8 where 1 is the central incisor and 8 is the third molar. In Palmer's Notation the position of the tooth is defined by a right angle enclosing the number of the tooth.

For example, the upper right 3, or canine is represented as: $\underline{3}\,|$

The lower left 7, or second molar is represented as: $|\overline{7}$

For deciduous teeth, Palmer's Notation uses capital letters instead of numbers. These are:

- A for central incisor;
- B for lateral incisor;
- C for canine (cuspid);
- D for first molar; and
- E for 2nd molar.

Again the position of the teeth is defined by a right angle, this time enclosing the capital letter.

For example, upper left A or central incisor is represented as: $|\underline{A}$

Summary

The anatomy of teeth, the way they function and their supporting structures is complex. The better your knowledge of them, the more effective you will be in your work and the better you will understand the procedures being carried out by the dentist.

You will also be able, if requested by the dentist, to give better explanations to patients who require more information about their conditions and the procedures that they require.

chapter ten
microbiology

Introduction

Micro-organisms are living things that are so small they can only be seen with a microscope. 'Micro' means microscopically small and 'bio' means living organism. These organisms are found almost everywhere; in the soil, the air, in water, on vegetation, on the skin and mucous membranes, on our clothing, and so on. Microbiology is the study of these micro-organisms.

For hundreds of years it has been recognised that disease can be communicated (transmitted) from one person to another. Our knowledge of how this occurs is constantly increasing, aided by the development of research tools such as the electron microscope and the 3D laser microscopes and computers, as well as more advanced experimental techniques such as the findings in genetics. Two world wars, the increase in world travel, organ transplantation and the rise of dreadful viral infections such as HIV have dramatically stimulated research into disease control.

Most types of micro-organisms are quite harmless. In fact, some types of micro-organisms are essential to the body's efficient functioning. But some micro-organisms are capable of causing disease. These micro-organisms are called pathogens. The pathogens of most concern in the dental surgery are:

- viruses;
- bacteria; and
- fungi.

These pathogens are discussed on the following pages.

Viruses

Viruses are the smallest of the micro-organisms. Most can only be seen with the aid of an electron microscope. Viruses vary in shape and size. They look like rods, spheres or, if attached to other virus particles, like blocks.

Viruses can cause disease and death. Typical diseases caused by viruses are influenza (flu), mumps, measles, chicken pox, hepatitis (all types), HIV/AIDS, polio myelitis, herpes simplex (types 1 and 2) and warts. Some of the more exotic virus-caused diseases (like dengue fever, Ross River fever and encephalitis) are not yet very common in Australia but occurrences are increasing all the time.

Viruses are sometimes described according to the symptoms they produce. However, this is not very satisfactory as they can cause more than one disease depending on which organ they attack.

Viruses are responsible for many forms of infection. In some viruses, such as smallpox, chicken pox, measles and German measles, the virus particles get into the blood stream and are spread throughout the body. Other viruses produce more localised infections. The virus of hepatitis, for example, produces a disease primarily of the liver while the viruses of the common cold and influenza generally affect the upper respiratory tract.

Viruses can only reproduce within a host cell. Viruses invade a cell, replicate there (make copies of themselves) and these new copies then invade other cells. Viral reproduction within a cell does not necessarily cause the cell's death. However, in some cases (as in HIV) it does.

Unlike bacteria, viruses are not susceptible to (not killed by) antibiotics. They are also resistant to heat and chemicals. Viruses are also capable of **mutation**. This is why it is necessary to have a new flu vaccination each year as each flu season brings a different kind of virus.

No effective cure has yet been found for viruses.

Drugs such as Acyclovir, Zovirax, Retrovir and Interferon are used either alone or in combination and are effective in some instances. Some diseases caused by them are now preventable with vaccination but the most important preventive measure in the dental surgery is avoiding cross-contamination.

Virus-based dental diseases

Oral herpes

'Cold sores' are the most common virally caused lesion to occur around the oral cavity and affect some 20–30 per cent of the population. The intraoral lesions are painful ulcers affecting the keratinised mucosa, e.g. gingival and palatal masticatory mucosa.

Many initial infections with the herpes type 1 virus are painless. In some cases Primary Herpetic Gingivostomatitis is accompanied by fever, lymphadenopathy (swollen glands), dsyphagia (difficulty in swallowing), excessive salivation and multiple painful ulcers affecting the gingiva, cheeks, lips and tongue.

There is an increasing incidence of herpes type 2 oral lesions due to changes in sexual practices and, regrettably, subsequent to child abuse.

Active herpes lesions are highly infectious and can result in very painful herpetic paronychia (infected nail beds) and debilitating herpetic **kerato-conjunctivitis**.

Herpes zoster (shingles)

This very painful condition is due to reactivation of the herpes type 3 (chickenpox) virus in later life. The **trigeminal nerve** may be affected in 10–15 per cent of patients. The closely grouped ulcers occur unilaterally, are arranged in lines, and have been described as a 'belt of roses from hell' because of the excruciating pain. Patients can develop painful tongue lesions and the pain may mimic toothache.

Measles

This common childhood disease is highly infectious and is spread by droplet infection from the upper respiratory tract. Measles is accompanied by rash and high fever but before these are evident the oral mucosa becomes erythematous (reddened). Just before onset of systemic symptoms, small lesions called Koplik's spots occur in the mouth, commonly opposite the molar teeth. These bluish-white spots have a red halo and do not persist beyond 24 hours.

HIV/AIDS

Common oral manifestations in these conditions are severe oral candidiasis, hairy leukoplakia, Kaposi's sarcoma and ANUG (acute necrotising ulcerative gingivitis). See Chapter 12 for information on some of these diseases.

Bacteria and some of their characteristics

Bacteria are larger than viruses and can be seen using an ordinary microscope. They are minute, single-cell organisms of various shapes and sizes. Some are in the form of spheres, some are rods and some are spirals. Some are capable of independent movement.

Bacteria are the micro-organisms responsible for the large majority of diseases and so they probably concern us most in the dental surgery.

Spore formation

When environmental conditions are unfavourable, some bacteria (e.g. bacilli) are capable of going into a 'resting state'. This is known as spore formation; a kind of hibernation. **Metabolic activity** within the organism is reduced to a minimum and the organism becomes resistant to adverse conditions. That is, the bacteria remain alive in the spore form but they are inactive.

When conditions become favourable again, the spore resumes its original form. At this stage it produces exotoxins (poisons) that are capable of being very **virulent**. Spore-forming bacteria can cause diseases such as tetanus and food poisoning (salmonella).

Spores can survive heat and dryness and even disinfectant and radiation. Spores can only be destroyed by very high heat sterilisation.

Capsules

Some species of bacteria can form a slimy coating or capsule. This is a form of 'armour plating' that is very difficult to destroy and can resist attack from the body's defence mechanisms.

■ **kerato-conjunctivitis:** inflammation of the cornea and the conjunctiva of the eye. ■ **trigeminal nerve:** one of a pair of cranial nerves that supply movement and sensation to the jaw, face and nasal cavity. ■ **metabolic activity:** chemical interactions that provide the energy and nutrients needed to keep the organism alive. ■ **virulent:** extremely poisonous, infectious or damaging to organisms.

Motility (mobility)

Numerous bacteria are capable of independent movement. In some cases this is accomplished by long thread-like **processes** (flagella) or the corkscrew-like shape of spirochaetes.

Reproduction

Bacteria usually multiply by simple binary fission. That is, the cells split in two and then each of those cells splits again, etc. There is no **mitosis** as is seen with tissue cells.

Cell aggregates

When bacterial cells divide, the daughter cells may part company or remain attached to each other by their cell membranes. Aggregates formed in this way are very characteristic of bacterial species, particularly with cocci.

Oxygen requirements

Bacteria may be divided into three groups according to their oxygen requirements:

❶ obligate anaerobes, which cannot exist in the presence of free oxygen;

❷ obligate aerobes, which must have free oxygen to survive; and

❸ facultative anaerobes, which can adapt to the presence of free oxygen.

Cocci

These are small and roughly spherical (round). The cocci tend to produce localised infections in which pus is formed. They can be divided into:

- diplococci, which occur in pairs and cause disease such as pneumonia (caused by pneumococcus);

- streptococci, which appear in chains like strings of beads and cause diseases such as tonsillitis, scarlet fever and rheumatic fever;

- staphylococci, which grow in clusters like bunches of grapes and cause diseases such as skin infections, boils and carbuncles; and

- tetracocci, which occur in groups of four and cause diseases such as dental and pulmonary abscesses.

Bacilli

These bacteria have the shape of cylindrical rods. They may have rounded or pointed ends or be irregular in outline. The length and breadth of the rods can vary and some possess one or more flagellae (thin hair-like processes) attached to the outer wall. They have the ability to form spores. They can be **motile** or non-motile and cause diseases such as diphtheria, tuberculosis (TB), food poisoning and tetanus (spores).

Vibrio

These bacteria are cylindrical and curved on themselves (comma shaped). They are motile and cause illnesses such as diarrhoea, septicaemia and cholera.

Spirilla

These are elongated with a series of twists or curves, like a corkscrew. They are motile and cause illnesses such as human systemic disease, gastric attacks in children and can lead to abortions.

Spirochaete

These bacteria are long, thin and spirally coiled. They are capable of flexing and twisting movements. They are motile and often produce diseases of a severe and disfiguring nature such as syphilis and ANUG (acute necrotising ulcerative gingivitis).

Table 10.1 provides a summary of types of bacteria.

Fungi

These are plants that lack chlorophyll, such as yeasts and moulds. They reproduce by means of spores and may or may not be **pathogenic**.

Yeasts occur naturally in grapes and other fruits and are an essential ingredient in bread and beer brewing. They can cause diseases such as thrush (also known as candida albicans or monilia), ringworm and athlete's foot (tinea).

Moulds appear in 'woolly' patches that are made up of fine **filamentous** cells. A collection of mould can often be seen with the naked eye; for example, on stale bread. The antibiotic penicillin has been developed from bread mould.

Other groups of micro-organisms

Actinomyces

These are made up of long, branching, filamentous cells. They are non-motile and cause a condition called actinomycosis.

process: a part that grows on or sticks out of an organism. ■ **mitosis:** the way a cell divides into two daughter cells which both have the same number of chromosomes as the original cell. ■ **motile:** capable of independent movement. ■ **pathogenic:** capable of initiating infection. ■ **filamentous:** long strands of cells joined end to end.

Name	Description	Example of disease	Shape
Coccus (plural cocci)	Small, roughly spherical (round). Sub-divided into the following types of bacteria:		
Diplococci	Occur in pairs.	Pneumococcus – causes pneumonia.	
Streptococci	Appear in chains, like strings of beads.	Tonsillitis, scarlet fever, rheumatic fever.	
Staphylococci	Grow in clusters, like bunches of grapes.	Skin infections, boils and carbuncles.	
Tetracocci	Occur in groups of four.	Dental and pulmonary abscesses.	
Bacillus (plural – bacilli)	Cylindrical rods. May have rounded or pointed ends or be irregular in outline. Have the ability to form spores. Can be motile or non-motile.	Diphtheria, tuberculosis (TB), tetanus (spores).	
Vibrio	Cylindrical. Curved on itself (comma shaped). Motile.	Diarrhoea, septicaemia, cholera.	
Spirillum (plural – spirilla)	Elongated with a series of twists or curves, like a corkscrew. Motile.	Human systemic disease, abortion, gastric attacks in children.	
Spirochaete	Long, thin, spirally coiled. Capable of flexing and twisting movements. Motile.	Syphilis, ANUG (acute necrotising, ulcerative gingivitis).	

Table 10.1 A summary of bacteria types

Protozoa

Protozoa is a simple cell with a true nucleus. These are microscopic animals and include amoeba and malarial parasites. Protozoa cannot survive outside of the blood of a host so must be transmitted via **vector transmission**. They can cause diseases such as giardia lambia, trichomonas and malaria.

Rickettsiae

Rickettsiae are bacteria-like organisms, larger than viruses but smaller than bacteria. They are thought to belong to the vegetable kingdom. They may cause diseases such as typhus, trench fever and scrub fever and are transmitted to humans by the bite of an infected insect.

Helminths (also known as worms)

Helminths are multicellular organisms. There are round, tape, and hook helminths among other forms, and can be transferred from animals to humans.

Algae

Algae are green plants and include the blue-green algae polluting our waterways, as well as seaweed.

Prions

Prions are protein particles that contain no nucleic acid, do not trigger an immune response and are not destroyed by extreme heat or cold. Prions cause diseases such as Bovine Spongiform Encephalitis (BSE; Mad Cow Disease) and Creutzfeldt-Jakob Disease (CJD).

'Good' and 'bad' micro-organisms

Good micro-organisms

The great majority of micro-organisms that can live in humans are parasites. That is, they usually only reproduce on the surface or in the tissues of another form of life (which is called the host).

■ **vector transmission:** a vector transmits disease-causing micro-organisms from infected individuals to other persons. For example, a mosquito or a tick can carry infected blood from one animal to another. This is called vector transmission.

Remember that most micro-organisms do not cause disease. In fact, many are crucial to our wellbeing. For example, micro-organisms are involved in:

■ Soil replenishment — all living things die, decompose and return to the earth. This would not be possible without microbial action.

■ Garbage disposal and sewerage purification — this depends largely on bacterial action for breaking down waste matter.

■ Industrial production — bacteria are used in the production of foods (cheese, wine, beer, etc). Some drugs, particularly antibiotics, depend on bacteria for their production.

■ Physiological processes — without bacteria in the bowel we would be unable to synthesise or absorb many of the things the body requires.

Some good micro-organisms are nevertheless capable of producing disease if they are able to invade the tissues and subsequently multiply. Members of this group are known as facultative (or opportunistic) pathogens.

The presence of high levels of the bacterium Capnocytophaga, a facultatively anaerobic **gram-negative** rod-like organism, is associated with *a lower level of periodontal disease*. In this context it is a good bacterium, although how it produces its beneficial effect is not known.

Bad micro-organisms — pathogens

Micro-organisms that *do* cause disease are called pathogens. They invade the tissues and release toxins (poisons). This produces local signs of **infection** such as pain, **oedema**, redness and the formation of pus. In severe infections the organisms can invade the lymphatics (leading to 'swollen glands') and blood stream, which leads to widespread dissemination of the organisms.

During the process of invasion, some of the micro-organisms become damaged and ruptured and, as a result, toxins, known as **endotoxins**, are released into the tissues. These endotoxins are responsible for many of the symptoms accompanying infection, such as fever, headache, raised pulse and nausea.

Endotoxins are usually passively released from damaged micro-organisms. However, a few species of micro-organism can actively secret toxins known as exotoxins and these possess powerful and devastating properties. For example, the exotoxins produced by the tetanus bacillus can result in paralysis of the nervous system, and death.

Reproduction of micro-organisms

Cell division

Like all living things, micro-organisms reproduce to perpetuate their species. They are asexual and all equally capable of reproduction. Under suitable conditions, this reproduction occurs as soon as the organism has grown to full size.

Micro-organisms reproduce by division. Each new division is capable of further division.

In the presence of abundant foodstuffs, some micro-organisms may divide in this way every 20 to 30 minutes, whilst other micro-organisms require several days to reproduce.

Spore formation and germination

Those bacilli that can form spores usually only do so when the environmental conditions do not favour the growth of the micro-organism, or in the absence of an adequate food supply. In these instances the micro-organism will form spores that lie dormant until the environmental conditions improve.

Not only can spores remain in a state of 'suspended animation' more or less indefinitely but they can also survive treatments that readily destroy the bacilli from which they came.

When the spores are once again provided with foodstuffs and a suitable environment, they will germinate and reproduce as bacilli again. Re-emergence enhances their toxicity.

Causes of infection

The ways in which micro-organisms are transmitted, and ways of preventing transmission, are covered in considerable depth in Chapter 14. Causes, symptoms and treatment of infection are discussed in Chapters 11, 12 and 13.

For the purposes of this section, it is enough to say that when a body becomes infected with micro-organisms, the number of organisms that start the process by getting into the tissues is very small. If the organisms do not multiply they will produce no symptoms even though they may manage to stay alive. It is only the multiplication of the micro-organisms in the tissues that causes clinical signs and symptoms of infection. The more micro-organisms there are, the more likely they are to cause disease.

There is an exception to this. Some micro-organisms cause toxins to be produced in food. Before the food is eaten, the micro-organisms produce these toxins and it is the toxins that cause the symptoms, not the micro-organisms themselves.

Resistance to infection

The human body possesses some protective mechanisms that enable us to stay free of disease — to resist the disease.

Surface defences

The intact skin and mucosal surfaces act as an effective barrier against micro-organisms. Chemicals in and on the skin can also destroy many of the micro-organisms that come in contact with it. Mucous membranes act in a similar fashion and secretions such as tears, nasal mucous, gingival fluids and saliva are all able to rapidly destroy the micro-organisms that reach these surfaces.

Inner defences

There are two types of inner defences; phagocytosis and bacteriolysis. Phagocytosis is the process of large cells throughout the body engulfing and destroying foreign particles, including micro-organisms. This is very rapid and effective.

Bacteriolysis is the process of substances in the body rupturing the wall of the micro-organism, resulting in its destruction. When this happens, endotoxins are released and these are responsible for many of the symptoms of infection.

We get sick when these mechanisms fail. This allows the micro-organisms to multiply in our tissues, producing symptoms of infection. For example, a child with a cold may develop a middle ear infection. The healthier you are, the better chance your body has of resisting disease.

Reduced resistance can be caused by tiredness or fatigue, depression, injury, and poor living conditions or food. People using immuno-suppression therapy (which stops transplants from being rejected), undergoing chemotherapy or with diseases such as HIV are less capable of resisting other diseases. Elderly people are also more susceptible to disease.

Recovery from infection

It might seem that we recover from infection because the micro-organism is not capable of multiplying and staying alive in the patient, but this is not the case. In fact, in some infections, such as scarlet fever, diphtheria and typhoid, the micro-organisms can persist in the throat or intestines for many months after the patient has recovered. These micro-organisms are still capable of infecting other people. The person carrying them is called a 'carrier'.

The patient recovers because of a change in their body that makes them no longer susceptible to the disease. This change is the development of antibodies, which can stay in the body for many years.

Antibodies can act in several ways. They can:

- combine with and neutralise chemical substances on the surface of the micro-organism that protect the micro-organism against phagocytosis and bacteriolysis;
- neutralise bacterial toxins; and
- prevent the spread of micro-organisms.

If the cells that form antibodies can be stimulated to produce antibodies before a person comes into contact with the micro-organism, that person might escape infection. This is the process of **immunisation** where killed organisms (vaccines), such as influenza, and inactivated toxins, such as anti-tetanus toxoid, are injected into the circulation. The body then produces antibodies without the signs and symptoms of disease.

Culturing micro-organisms

When it is suspected that micro-organisms are causing disease, or when we need to determine the source of micro-organisms, we need to be able to identify the organism responsible. This is easier if the micro-organism can be reproduced away from the disease process. This is called 'making a culture'.

The micro-organisms must be provided with the same environmental conditions and foodstuffs they would have if growing in the body. They are placed in a **culture medium** and in an environment that encourages their reproduction.

Once the type of micro-organism responsible for a disease is identified it is possible to begin treatment with the correct antibiotic or drug, or to try to find the source of the micro-organism so further infection can be prevented.

■ **immunisation:** the process of rendering a person resistant to specific diseases or poisons, so protecting them against those diseases.
■ **culture medium:** nutrient substance used to grow biological material under controlled conditions.

Microbiological testing for the colony density of the mutants streptococci and lactobacilli can identify high caries risk patients, including those parents whose saliva may infect infants, resulting in 'nursing' or 'bottle' caries.

Summary

Equipment and instruments used in dentistry, hands and the mouth are all breeding grounds for micro-organisms. In order to make informed decisions about infection control techniques you must understand how micro-organisms grow and reproduce.

chapter eleven
pathology

Introduction

Pathology is the use of scientific methods to study the nature and causes of **disease**. A knowledge of pathology is essential for the accurate diagnosis and treatment of disease.

Methods of study include:

- physical examination; for example, 'check ups';
- biochemistry; for example, blood tests, urine tests, saliva tests;
- microbiology;
- radiology and nuclear medicine (branches of medicine in which x-rays and radioactive materials are used to diagnose and treat disease);
- ultrasound (a method of medical imaging that uses high-frequency sound waves for medical examination);
- scanning (imaging techniques used to obtain images of internal organs);
- **endoscopy**;
- **histology**; and
- **autopsy** (usually not for dental pathology).

Signs and symptoms of disease

Signs are objective. They may not always be obvious to the patient, but they can be described and measured by the doctor, for example:

- elevated blood pressure;
- abnormal test results;
- elevated temperature;
- altered pulse rate; or
- dental cavities.

Symptoms are subjective and are described by the patient, for example:

- pain;
- nausea;
- breathlessness;
- itching; or
- bad taste in the mouth.

In some cases (e.g. external bleeding), the sign and the symptom are the same. If the sign that the doctor observes and records is also obvious to the patient, then it is also a symptom.

Classification of diseases

Diseases may be classified as follows.

- Hereditary
  In this case disease is transmitted from parent to offspring via genetic factors. Examples of conditions which have a hereditary background are colour blindness, **haemophilia** and **anodontia**.

- Congenital
  Here the disease is acquired before birth but it is not due to hereditary factors. It may result from infection, e.g. syphilis transmitted from an infected parent, or it may be due to abnormal development.

- Traumatic
  This is disease produced as a result of mechanical injury such as a blow or cut. Examples are fractured bones, fractured teeth, lacerated soft tissue and bruised tissue.

- Caused by physical agents
  Agents such as heat, cold and excessive exposure to x-rays or electricity may cause tissue damage.

disease: any abnormality in the structure or function in any part of the body. The term 'lesion' is used to describe any area of tissue whose structure or function has been damaged or altered by disease or trauma. ■ **endoscopy:** insertion of a tube into the body for diagnosis. ■ **histology:** study of microscopic structures. ■ **autopsy:** examination of a dead body to determine the cause of death. ■ **haemophilia:** a condition in which the blood clots more slowly than normally. ■ **anodontia:** the absence of all or some of the teeth because they never formed.

109

■ Caused by chemical agents

Acids, alkalis and poisonous drugs may all damage tissues and cause disease.

■ Infectious

This may be caused by bacteria or by viruses. Infection plays a major role in the causation of common dental diseases such as dental caries, periodontal disease and **abscesses**.

■ Nutritional

Lack of vitamins in the diet can result in disease. Dental caries is caused by bacterial metabolism of sugars in the diet. The most common nutritional disease in Australian society is obesity. Bulimia and anorexia are diseases of nutrition, in addition to having a psychological component.

■ Endocrine imbalance

The normal growth and function of the body is dependent on a correct balance of the hormone secretions from the ductless glands of the body.

■ Allergic

Tissues may become sensitive to certain substances. As a result of this they may react excessively or even violently to a second contact with a similar substance at a later time.

■ Caused by blood dyscrasias

These are a group of diseases involving the blood cells and the blood forming tissues. Some examples are the **anaemias** (which may result from a deficiency in the number of red cells in the blood or a deficiency in the amount of haemoglobin in each cell), **leucopoenia** and the **leukaemias**.

■ Of unknown cause

The cause of many diseases is unknown or only partly understood. Also, one factor may tend to predispose towards another, for example nutritional deficiencies may lead to blood dyscrasias.

■ Psychological

Up to 20 per cent of the population may at some time suffer from conditions such as depression or bipolar disorder.

■ Combination of causes

Some diseases have more than one cause, e.g. bulimia is a disease caused by both psychological and nutritional factors. Dental caries is an infectious disease (caused by micro-organisms) but has an essential nutritional component.

Inflammation

The basic response of tissues to any form of injury or disease is to mount an inflammatory response. Inflammation is not a disease. It is the healing response to injury, and involves changes occurring in tissue. The purpose of this inflammatory response is to:

■ rapidly destroy or remove the cause of injury;

■ limit and localise the extent of the injury; and

■ repair and replace the damaged tissues.

The signs and symptoms of inflammation are:

■ redness;

■ heat;

■ swelling;

■ pain; and

■ loss of function.

The first change to occur in the tissue is an increase in the blood supply to the injured part. This is brought about by the opening (dilatation) of blood vessels in the area, which results in redness and heat.

Fluid escapes from the dilated blood vessels into the tissue, which results in swelling and pain due to pressure on the nerve endings.

Inflammation may be classified as either **acute inflammation** or **chronic inflammation**.

Acute inflammation

Acute inflammation is the body's sudden rapid response to an injury, usually with intense and obvious signs and symptoms. It may take a number of different courses. It may progress to:

■ Resolution — minor injuries or illnesses such as the common cold respond to inflammation by complete healing without the formation of any scar tissues. The tissues that were inflamed return to their previous healthy state.

■ Repair — as the inflammatory reaction develops, white blood cells (leucocytes) pass out from the dilated blood vessels into the surrounding tissue. They engulf and destroy bacteria, tissue debris, foreign bodies and other irritants.

■ Scar tissue — in the cleaning up process, new blood vessels and connective tissues (granulation tissue) grow into the area to replace the destroyed tissue. As this granulation tissue matures, it becomes more fibrous and less vascular, and is then known as scar tissue.

■ Suppuration — when bacterial infection is severe, large numbers of white blood cells may die in their attempt to destroy the bacteria. The result is the formation of a creamy liquid called pus. This pus consists of the accumulated bodies of the dead white cells, dead and dying tissue cells of the infected part, and both dead and living bacteria.

The accumulation of this pus in a solid tissue or organ results in an abscess (e.g. dental abscess). However, should the pus break out of this walled-off area and spread widely in the surrounding soft connective tissue, cellulitis results and a brownish-red swelling of the tissues underneath the skin may occur.

When localised inflammation occurs in bone it is called osteitis. Osteitis is an inflammation and not an infection. If the inflammatory reaction involves bacterial infection of all the bone elements (bone, bone marrow and the periosteum) then the condition is known as osteomyelitis.

■ Chronic phase — if the host defences are compromised, or the injury persists, chronic inflammation may develop.

Necrosis and gangrene

When tissue is severely damaged, the reaction may go beyond the stage of inflammation and progress to the death of the tissue. This is called necrosis. It results most frequently from the blood supply to the part being cut off by trauma such as crush injury, or the pressure of an inflammatory **exudate**.

If the necrotic or dead tissue undergoes **putrefaction**, the process is called gangrene. Gangrene usually occurs in the peripheral parts of the body furthest removed from the major blood vessels. Toes and fingers are common sites for gangrene. A good example in dentistry is gangrene of the tooth pulp.

Chronic inflammation

This is a longstanding form of incomplete, continually delayed or frustrated healing. Some of the usual signs and symptoms of inflammation may be less severe than in acute inflammation. Others, such as pain and limitation of movement, may be very severe.

Chronic inflammation results when the body tries to repair the diseased part. Some repair takes place, but does not go on to complete resolution. White blood cells (called lymphocytes and plasma cells) collect in large numbers. These white cells are part of the body's defence mechanism. The injured part continues to be inflamed for an extended period of time, and features of partial healing exist side by side with inflammatory changes.

Chronic inflammation may 'flare up' periodically to become acute; for example, the chronic dental abscess. This condition 'flares up' periodically to produce the acute stage with a tense red swelling on the mucosa over the apex of the affected tooth. The swelling comes to a head and discharges pus into the mouth through a sinus. After discharge it may go back to a chronic phase until another acute reaction builds up.

Ulceration

An ulcer is a crater-like, open sore on skin or mucous membrane in which the full thickness of surface covering (epithelium) has been destroyed, leaving the deeper parts of the tissue exposed, as can be seen in Figure 11.1. The base of the ulcer consists of inflamed, unprotected connective tissues which contain exposed nerve endings, which is why ulcers are so painful.

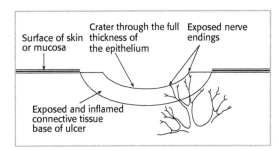

Figure 11.1 Diagrammatic representation of an ulcer

Ulcers occur in the mouth from a number of causes.

■ Trauma — hard foods, jagged or sharp meat or fish bones, sharp clasps on partial dentures, ill-fitting dentures and incorrect tooth brushing may all cause trauma and result in ulceration of the oral mucosa.

■ Infection — bacteria and viruses may cause ulceration in the mouth; for example, herpetic ulceration.

■ Chemical agents — some chemicals introduced into the mouth may cause ulceration of the oral mucosa; for example, strong acids such as etching liquids, trichloracetic acid, or aspirin applied directly to the mucosa in an attempt to relieve toothache.

■ Allergy — some ulcers of the mouth may be due to allergic factors.

■ **exudate:** fluid rich in plasma proteins, cell materials and debris, usually present when there is inflammation.
■ **putrefaction:** the decomposition of organic matter under the influence of micro-organisms and resulting in foul smelling discharge.

Some recurrent ulceration is of unknown origin.

Other less common causes of oral ulceration include nutritional deficiencies, hormone imbalance, **blood dyscrasias** and neoplasia (malignancy).

Tumours (neoplasms)

Normal tissue grows by multiplication of its cells to a definite pattern. The cells multiply by division, each cell dividing into two, and each daughter cell dividing into two more and so on. The cells that are produced are always of the same type and are histologically normal.

For some reason, cells in a part of the body may multiply abnormally and the result is the formation of a tumour or neoplasm (new growth). Therefore, a tumour is an increase in tissue size due to abnormal cell development. It serves no useful purpose and will not regress. That is, the tumour will not disappear or go away, and the word 'tumour' implies growth.

Benign tumours

A tumour may be **benign**, in which case it is walled off from surrounding tissue. Benign tumours are relatively harmless. They only cause trouble to their host because of their size and interference to function.

Benign tumours:

- are slow growing;

- are made up of excessive numbers of well organised cells of normal type for the tissue concerned, although they may be located in an organ or tissue where they are not normally found;

- are localised, well defined and usually contained within a fibrous capsule;

- are not locally invasive, but are walled off from surrounding tissues;

- do not metastasise (spread) to other parts of the body;

- are unlikely to recur when removed; and

- are only dangerous or potentially fatal due to their size if located in or near vital organs.

Examples of benign tumours are:

- papilloma, a tumour of epithelial tissue that may occur on the oral mucosa;

- fibroma, a tumour of connective tissue that may occur on the oral mucosa; and

- epulis, a benign tumour growing on the gingiva.

See Figure 11.2 for a diagrammatic representation of a benign tumour.

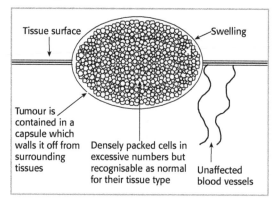

Figure 11.2 Diagrammatic representation of benign tumour

Malignant tumours

Malignant tumours are collectively referred to by the public as 'cancer' and are potentially fatal if not diagnosed and treated early.

In malignant tumours, the tumour is not walled off from the surrounding tissue but spreads into these tissues so that it cannot be completely removed from them, as shown in Figure 11.3. It may continue to grow. Pieces may break away from the tumour and travel by the blood stream and lymph channels (or some other pathway) to other parts of the body to cause secondary tumours called metastases.

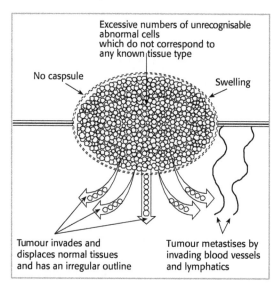

Figure 11.3 Diagrammatic representation of malignant tumour

Malignant tumours:

- grow rapidly;

- have an excessive number of disorganised, unrecognisable abnormal cells;

- infiltrate, invade and destroy surrounding tissues;
- are not well defined due to local invasion;
- metastasise (produce secondary growths) to other parts of the body by invading blood vessels and lymphatics; and
- have a tendency to recur after treatment.

They are divided into two main groups. These are:

❶ carcinoma, arising from epithelial tissue such as skin or mucous membrane. These are the most common malignant tumours occurring in the mouth. They affect mainly older age groups; and

❷ sarcoma, arising from connective tissues such as bone. These are comparatively rare in the mouth and affect chiefly the younger age groups.

Cancers of the mouth account for about four per cent of all cancer occurring in the human body. While they are not a death sentence, all malignant tumours are potentially fatal. Oral malignancies are very closely associated with smoking and with alcohol consumption.

Some types of lesions

Cysts

A cyst is a pathological cavity in tissue, filled with fluid, and contained in a fibrous sac which is usually lined by epithelium (see Figure 11.4). Cysts can occur in either soft tissues or in bone.

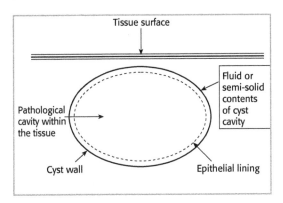

Figure 11.4 Diagrammatic representation of a cyst

Cysts can cause pain if they press on nerve endings or become infected. They can also grow quite painlessly to a very large size. If this occurs in bone, the bony destruction can result in a spontaneous pathological fracture.

The most common type of cyst occurring in the mouth is the radicular or dental cyst.

Other cysts that may be seen are dentigerous cysts. Here the tooth is un-erupted and the crown of the tooth is in the cyst. For example, the eruption cyst is a form of dentigerous cyst and is seen in the mouths of children as a bluish soft tissue swelling over the crown of a tooth that is about to erupt.

Atrophy

Tissue may respond to lack of use by atrophying. This is when there is a reduction in the size of cells and the bulk of the tissue in response to the reduced functional demands.

When a splint is removed from a limb after treatment for a fracture, the limb is smaller as the muscles have atrophied due to lack of use. This condition is reversible with exercise and physiotherapy.

Hyperplasia

When tissue is chronically irritated it may respond by multiplication of the cells, which enlarges the tissue. This is called hyperplasia. An example is the overgrowth of tissue seen in the mouth due to an ill-fitting denture. This hyperplastic tissue frequently becomes ulcerated from being rubbed by the ill-fitting dentures.

Other tissue enlargement

Hypertrophy

Hypertrophy involves an increase in the size of a tissue or organ. However, in this case it is an increase in tissue in response to increased demands of function. It is brought about by an increase in the size of the individual tissue cells (not an increase in the number of cells, as in hyperplasia). An example of this is the enlarged muscles of a bodybuilding enthusiast.

Summary

Although you are not required to diagnose disease in your work, a knowledge of general pathology allows a better understanding of dental pathology and the diseases you are likely to encounter in your work.

chapter twelve
oral pathology

Introduction

Oral medicine is the speciality of dentistry concerned with the diagnosis and therapeutic treatment of oral disease. It is not concerned with the surgical treatment of oral disease, which is the responsibility of oral surgery, although there is some overlap between these two areas. Oral pathology is the basis for both because it provides the knowledge of the causes and effects of disease. This knowledge is essential for correct diagnosis and effective treatment of disease.

Oral disease can be divided into:

■ disease primarily associated with the mouth; and

■ oral manifestations of systemic disease (that is, when an illness somewhere else in the body causes a disease in the mouth.)

This text cannot cover all of the wide range of oral diseases. Instead it will discuss briefly the more commonly occurring oral diseases. Caries and periodontal disease are discussed in depth in Chapter 27. The treatment of these diseases is also discussed in Chapters 27 and 31.

Drugs most frequently prescribed in the treatment of these diseases are discussed in Chapter 13.

Plaque and calculus

Plaque

Bacterial dental plaque is an organised colony of micro-organisms, i.e. bacteria, contained within an organic matrix and adhering to the tooth surface. Plaque is not soluble in water. The matrix is a sticky extracellular complex sugar produced by the bacteria during their metabolism.

Bacteria initially colonise the enamel surface by adhering to a clear layer of **pellicle**. This pellicle forms on a perfectly clean tooth surface within 12 hours, but does not by itself play any part in the disease process.

Although pellicle is a salivary glycoprotein, and although food debris may accumulate on plaque, plaque is not saliva and it is not food.

Calculus

Calculus is bacterial dental plaque that has become mineralised (calcified).

Supragingival plaque is found above the gingival margin. It can start to calcify within 2–3 days of being formed, the necessary minerals being derived from the saliva. For this reason, deposits are heavier on the lingual surfaces of the lower anterior teeth and the buccal surfaces of the maxillary first molars. These areas are located in close proximity to the openings of the ducts of the major salivary glands. Supragingival calculus is initially creamy yellow in colour, but can become heavily stained by tea, coffee and particularly by smoking. It is relatively easy to identify and remove.

Subgingival calculus adheres very tenaciously to tooth surfaces, and particularly to the cementum within periodontal pockets. Its minerals are derived from the gingival fluid and blood, making it dark brown to black in colour.

The surface of calculus is always covered by a layer of fresh, bacteriologically active plaque bacteria that perpetuate chronic periodontal inflammation. Meticulous calculus removal is an essential measure in the arrest and management of periodontal disease.

Dental caries

Dental caries is a chronic infectious disease affecting the calcified (mineralised) tissues of the teeth: the enamel, dentine and cementum. It occurs when micro-organisms in bacterial dental plaque metabolise sugars, resulting in the production of acid.

Over a period of time, this results in demineralisation of the enamel, which is the first stage of dental caries.

The caries process can be expressed as a formula:

Bacterial plaque + Carbohydrates
= Acid + Time + Susceptible tooth surfaces
= Dental caries

The four essential factors for the production of dental caries are:

❶ susceptible tooth surfaces;

❷ dental plaque;

❸ carbohydrates; and

❹ time.

Dental caries is a dynamic process in which both demineralisation and re-mineralisation are taking place beneath the plaque, as can be seen in Figure 12.1. Demineralisation is caused by acid produced within the plaque. Re-mineralisation repairs the damage by replacing the lost minerals with new ones, which come from either the saliva, from various forms of fluoride or from re-mineralising gels.

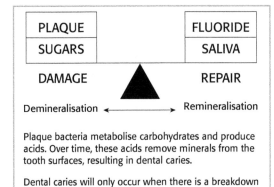

Plaque bacteria metabolise carbohydrates and produce acids. Over time, these acids remove minerals from the tooth surfaces, resulting in dental caries.

Dental caries will only occur when there is a breakdown in the balance between damage and repair.

Figure 12.1 The process of caries formation

The location and appearance of dental caries

The three sites at which dental caries occur most frequently are:

❶ in the depths of the pits and fissures found on the occlusal surfaces of molars and bicuspids, and pits or fissures on the buccal or palatal surfaces of some molars (caries occurring in the lingual pits of the maxillary anterior teeth is now relatively uncommon);

❷ on the proximal surfaces of adjoining teeth, commencing just below the contact points — these lesions are difficult to detect clinically when small but are well demonstrated on bitewing radiographs; and

❸ on the gingival one-third of the buccal and lingual surfaces of anterior or posterior teeth, the so-called gumline cavities.

All these sites are ones where effective plaque removal is difficult to achieve.

Early smooth surface caries appear as a chalky demineralised area that resembles the surface produced by acid etching. There is no cavity, and this early subsurface decalcification is reversible by using re-mineralisation techniques, improving oral hygiene, and dietary modification.

Fissure caries may show up as a bluish-grey shadow around the actual fissure, but a black or brown fissure may simply be stained and not carious.

Radiographs are used to estimate the depth of penetration of the carious lesion into the enamel. Restorative treatment is usually not commenced unless half the thickness of the enamel has been penetrated.

Once the enamel has been breached, caries continue in the dentine. This lesion is soft, rubbery and brown in colour due to the lower mineral content in dentine.

The prevention of dental caries is discussed in Chapter 27.

Diseases of the dental pulp

When we speak of toothache and abscesses, it implies the presence of pulp disease, resulting from either the caries process or from trauma to the tooth.

Healthy pulp

Healthy pulp means either that there is no caries or possibly some early enamel caries. As there are no nerve endings in enamel, no pain is experienced at this stage.

Early pulpitis

In early pulpitis the pulp will react painfully to hot, cold and sweet stimuli but the pain does not last long and will cease when the stimulus is withdrawn. This may be reversible. The pulp may recover.

Irreversible pulpitis

In irreversible pulpitis the pain becomes more severe, and pain may be present without any stimulus. The patient may be kept awake at night. The pulp will not recover. The pain may sometimes be described as throbbing. This pain is intensified by heat, and may be partly relieved by cold.

Further progression from irreversible pulpitis will result in necrosis [death] of the pulp, and the patient may report that the pain 'got better'.

However, a necrotic pulp will eventually progress to other pathological conditions such as acute periapical abscess, chronic periapical abscess, or cellulitis. If the chronic abscess becomes walled off by fibrous tissue it is often described as a periapical granuloma. This commonly appears as an 'area' on radiographs.

In some cases, these lesions may develop into radicular or periapical cysts. See Figure 12.2.

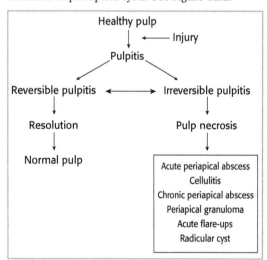

Figure 12.2 Diseases of the pulp

Diseases of the dental pulp and their treatment are discussed in depth in Chapter 33.

Periodontal diseases

Dental caries and periodontal disease have different causes. Dental caries is caused by acids produced by bacteria in the supragingival plaque. Perio-dontal diseases are chronic infectious diseases caused by an inflammatory response to subgingival plaque bacteria.

Gingivitis

If supragingival plaque is allowed to accumulate undisturbed at the gingival margin for a period of 14–21 days, it will lead to the development of a subgingival plaque, and produce a superficial inflammation of the gingiva, called 'gingivitis'.

Gingivitis is:

- superficial — only the gingiva is affected;
- non-destructive — there is no permanent loss of tissue; and
- reversible — if the plaque is removed, the condition will resolve; resolution means complete healing and a return to normal tissues, without scarring.

The gingiva becomes red and swollen. It also becomes soft and no longer hugs the necks of the teeth. It will bleed on probing or when brushing or flossing the teeth. The patient will have bad breath — **halitosis**.

Periodontitis

Periodontitis implies destruction of the alveolar bone, loss of periodontal ligament and changes to the cementum. It develops in about 35 per cent of patients with untreated gingivitis. See Figure 12.3.

The most significant sign of periodontitis is the presence of periodontal **pockets** that bleed on probing. One wall of the pocket is inflamed gingival epithelium. The other is biologically unacceptable cementum that has absorbed bacteria and their toxins. Pockets often contain subgingival calculus.

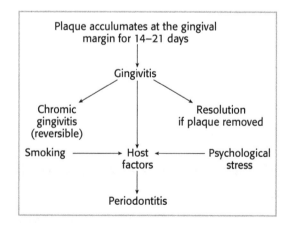

Figure 12.3 Development of periodontitis

■ **halitosis:** unpleasant breath.
■ **pocket formation:** an abnormal space developing between the tooth root and the gum

Some or all of the signs and symptoms of gingivitis may be present in periodontitis. In addition, in severe cases of periodontitis there may be:

- mobility of the teeth due to loss of attachment;

- migration of the teeth, with spaces opening up;

- suppuration from pockets; and

- **recession** may be present, exposing the cemento-enamel junction and the cementum.

Periodontitis affects the deep supporting tissues and is destructive and irreversible. However it can be treated and its progress arrested. The treatment of periodontitis is discussed in Chapter 31.

Salivary dysfunction

Functions of saliva

Some of the functions of saliva are to:

- lubricate the oral mucosa;

- assist in swallowing the food bolus;

- dilute and flush away food debris;

- provide the first line of defence against micro-organisms;

- provide minerals for the repair of erosion and demineralisation, and to neutralise acids; and

- assist in taste and speech.

Specific biochemical and microbiological tests are available to measure resting and stimulated saliva flow, the buffering (acid neutralising) capacity of saliva, and the levels of certain cariogenic bacteria.

Salivary dysfunction

Numerous dental problems are associated with disturbances in the saliva flow or changes in the quality of the saliva.

Xerostomia is the term used to describe severe reduction in quantity of saliva or the complete absence of saliva. Unfortunately, patients with xerostomia may be tempted to suck acid-type sweets or drink acidic carbonated beverages (fizzy soft drinks) in order to gain some relief and this will contribute to tooth erosion and dental caries.

Some degree of xerostomia occurs due to ageing. A far more common cause is the effects of many different types of commonly used prescription medications and the use of illegal narcotic type drugs.

A severe form of xerostomia occurs following radiotherapy to the head and neck region, if it involves the salivary glands.

Severe exercise results in temporary dryness due to dehydration. This deprives the oral cavity of the protective effects of saliva. Consumption of acidic and carbonated sports drinks by athletes is a major contributor to tooth erosion.

Saliva flow is substantially reduced at night. This is one of the reasons why it is recommended that at-risk patients do not raid the refrigerator at night after they have brushed their teeth. It is also the reason that denture wearers are strongly advised to leave their dentures out at night.

Some of the dental effects of salivary dysfunction are:

- chronically painful, uncomfortable mouth;

- increased caries rate, including recurrent caries around existing restorations, and root caries in older persons;

- dental **erosion**;

- difficulty in retaining dentures due to lack of suction;

- denture sore mouth due to friction and more particularly due to chronic fungal infection with candida albicans;

- hoarseness;

- difficulty in swallowing;

- increased severity of periodontal disease; and

- painful mucosal lesions.

Depending on the severity of the problem, some of the strategies for assisting patients with xerostomia are to:

- undertake a medical review of medication;

- avoid alcohol or mouthwashes based on alcohol (dehydration effect);

- control consumption of coffee, tea and cola drinks which cause dehydration by diuretic effect;

- encourage consumption of water, particularly if fluoridated;

- modify consumption of acidic drinks and citrus fruits;

- use specially formulated low detergent toothpaste;

- use sugar-free or re-mineralising chewing gum;

- carry an atomiser to spray water into the mouth whenever required;

- use saliva substitutes, particularly under dentures;

■ **erosion:** loss of tooth substance due to chemical causes and not bacterial or frictional causes. A common cause is excessive consumption of acidic drinks, juices or sports drinks. It can also occur from acid regurgitated into the mouth in bulimia, anorexia and gastric reflux. In some cases erosion occurs for unknown reasons. This is known as idiopathic erosion. ■ **recession:** the gradual shrinking back of the gums leaving the tooth cervix, and part of the root, exposed.

- use additional fluoride preparations as prescribed; for example, neutral sodium fluoride mouthwash, high concentration fluoride toothpaste;
- use re-mineralising gel;
- maintain a balanced diet and avoid frequent snacking;
- ensure dentures are left out at night; and
- have water available at all meals.

Some non-carious oral conditions

There are a number of non-carious causes of loss of tooth substance, such as attrition, abrasion, erosion and resorption.

Attrition

Attrition means wearing away of tooth substance by friction from direct tooth-to-tooth contact. Some degree of attrition is considered physiological, due to normal chewing, and becomes more evident with age. Pathological attrition occurs in excessive tooth grinding (bruxism) and wear facets may be seen on the teeth.

The process is accelerated when the enamel is worn away and the dentine exposed. Concurrent erosive factors will also hasten this destructive process.

Abrasion

Abrasion is the wearing away of tooth structure by friction from external sources. It may be caused by habits (chewing hard objects), or by poorly fitting retainers on removable appliances. The most common cause is the over vigorous use of hard toothbrushes or abrasive toothpastes. Abrasion can occur if the teeth are brushed directly after contact with acidic drinks, when the enamel is still softened by the acid.

Toothbrush abrasion lesions usually have very sharp edges, are often wedge-shaped, and are located at the gingival margin. Abrasion is also caused by habits such as holding pins, pipes or nails between the teeth.

Erosion

Erosion means loss of tooth substance due to chemical and not bacterial or frictional causes.

Common causes are excessive consumption of acidic drinks, juices or sports drinks. It can also occur from acid regurgitated into the mouth in bulimia, anorexia and gastric reflux.

In some cases, erosion occurs for unknown reasons. This is known as idiopathic erosion.

Resorption

Resorption means removal of tooth structure by the body's own cells. Internal resorption begins from the inside of the tooth from the pulpal surface. Advanced cases will show up a 'pink spot' in the crown of the tooth. The most common cause is pulpal inflammation.

External resorption involves the exterior of the root surface from the cementum into the dentine. The usual cause is some form of trauma such as excessive orthodontic force or severe bruxism.

Replanted avulsed teeth are at extreme risk of both internal and external resorption.

In some cases, resorption occurs for unknown reasons.

Two developmental conditions which may occur are supernumary teeth and diastema.

Supernumerary teeth

Supernumerary teeth are additional or extra teeth beyond the normal complement. They are often small, pointed and peg shaped. Fourth molars are not uncommon. The most common location for a supernumerary tooth is between the upper central incisors, when it is called a 'mesiodens'. Some supernumeraries erupt normally, and others are detected during radiography.

Diastema

Diastema is the term applied to naturally occurring spaces between teeth, and commonly occurs between maxillary anterior teeth, particularly the central incisors.

Other oral diseases

Pericoronitis

Pericoronitis simply means inflammation (itis) of the soft tissues around (peri) the crown (coronal portion) of an erupting or impacted tooth. It is a condition frequently associated with impacted or erupting third molars.

Traumatic mouth ulcers

These are the most common type of oral ulcer and are mainly due to mechanical trauma such as that caused by jagged teeth, rough or over-extended denture margins, tooth brush abrasions, hard and sharp food particles, and cheek or lip biting; for example, after local anaesthesia.

Oral ulcers can also be caused by physical trauma such as excessive heat due to hot foods, irradiation for cancer or electrical burns but these are less common forms of ulcers. Burns may be sustained from overheated handpieces, or from recently sterilised instruments that have not had time to cool down.

Recurrent oral aphthous ulceration

These ulcers are also called aphthous ulcers and aphthae. They can vary in severity from small, single ulcers to extensive ulceration involving large areas of the mouth. The ulcers recur at regular or irregular intervals of days, weeks or months and usually heal in five to seven days without residual damage to the oral mucosa. The pain can be severe and for those patients who are never free of ulcers, the disease can be debilitating. A characteristic feature is that the ulcers mainly appear on non-keratinised mucosa (cheeks, floor of the mouth, soft palate) and do not occur on keratinised mucosa such as the attached gingiva.

Acute primary herpetic gingivostomatitis (APHG)

This is the primary infection of the epithelial cells of the lips and oral mucosa by the herpes simplex virus. The primary infection usually occurs in children, or in young adults below the age of 30. The acute infection lasts 7 to 14 days with typical viral symptoms such as malaise, fever and enlarged lymph glands.

The condition affects the lips, cheeks, tongue, gingiva and the soft palate and fauces. Swallowing is extremely difficult and painful.

Acute primary herpetic gingivostomatitis is readily communicable. The saliva is highly infectious, and can cause lesions such as herpetic paronychia (whitlow) or a very painful conjunctivitis.

Acute necrotising ulcerative gingivitis (ANUG)

Acute means a condition of sudden onset. Necrotising means that there is death in some tissue. Ulcerative means that ulcers are present. Gingivitis refers to an inflammation of the gingiva.

Acute necrotising ulcerative gingivitis was once a common condition. It is now most commonly seen in profoundly immunosuppressed patients; for example, organ transplant recipients, those with HIV/AIDS, or persons in the acute stage of drug withdrawal. It is associated with heavy smoking, which is both locally and systemically immuno-suppressive. In addition, smoking compromises the gingival blood supply, because nicotine is **vaso-constrictive**.

Clinical features of ANUG are intense pain, very rapid onset, profound and spontaneous gingival bleeding, foul taste in the mouth and severe halitosis. Small, punched-out ulcers affect the tips of the interdental papillae, and the attached gingivae become covered with a slough. Systemic symptoms such as lymph gland enlargement and malaise may occur. The condition progresses very rapidly to a destructive periodontitis.

Oral carcinomas

A small proportion of carcinoma, about 4 per cent, occurs in the mouth and is commonly associated with tobacco smoking. This cancer, which is predominantly squamous cell carcinoma, frequently presents in the mouth as a raised fungating mass, or as an ulcerating lesion with rolled margins and a hard base. The lateral surface of the tongue is a common site for the lesion to occur.

Cancer of the mouth metastasises very early by lymphatics and blood vessels to other parts of the body (e.g. lymph nodes of the neck) and it is essential that it be detected and treated before this occurs. Treatment of oral cancer is either by surgery, chemotherapy or irradiation or by a combination of these methods.

Oral carcinoma has a good prognosis (outcome), but early detection is essential if the patient is to have a reasonable chance of survival. Dentists have an important role to play in this regard as they regularly inspect the mouths of patients and are in a unique position to diagnose early malignant change in the oral mucosa.

■ **vaso-constrictive**: causing blood vessels to constrict (tighten) and reduce blood flow.

Oral fungal infections

The most common fungal infection of the mouth is thrush, which is caused by the fungus candida albicans. It is more correctly called oral candidiasis or moniliasis.

A severe thrush infection appears as white plaques covering large areas of the oral mucosa. These plaques can be scraped off to leave a bleeding surface.

Such infections can occur from incorrect use of steroidal inhalants for asthma control, or after the administration of antibiotics. Much more common are less obvious infections such as denture sore mouth and angular cheilitis. In denture sore mouth, the oral mucosa is reddened and inflamed over the area covered by the denture. In angular cheilitis the patient suffers from fungally infected moist creases radiating out from the corners of the mouth onto the skin.

Both of these conditions are associated with poor denture hygiene and the wearing of dentures at night when the protective effect of saliva is reduced or absent.

White lesions of the mouth

There are a number of diseases in which white patches or lines are seen covering areas of the oral mucosa. Some are hereditary, such as white sponge naevus in which white patches, like rippled sand, are seen in the floor of the mouth or the cheeks. Others, such as lichen planus, in which white patches or crisscrossing white lines occur, are epithelial conditions of unknown **aetiology**.

An important group are those in which the white patches are an excessive build-up of keratin on the surface of the oral mucosa either due to friction (e.g. from an ill-fitting denture) or to excessive smoking (smoker's keratosis). The last condition is particularly serious because it can become cancerous and the patient must be warned against continued irritation of the oral mucosa by smoking.

The appearance of reddened areas within the white patch may indicate that the lesion is developing malignant potential.

Summary

An understanding of oral pathology is crucial if you are to effectively assist with procedures in the surgery. It will also allow you to better understand the effects that oral pathology can have on the general health of the patient.

■ **aetiology**: the causative factors which produce a disease.

chapter thirteen
dental pharmacology.

Introduction

Pharmacology is the branch of medical science relating to **drugs** and their properties, their uses and effects. In this context, a drug is a substance applied or administered to a patient for **therapeutic** purposes. That is, we use drugs in dentistry to cure disease, prevent suffering and to maintain health. Many drugs are used in dentistry, often as drug mixtures containing more than one drug. Most drugs used in dentistry are extremely safe.

However, drugs may interact with other drugs being taken by the patient for therapeutic or social reasons. Even simple drugs such as aspirin may give rise to undesirable response in some patients, either due to overdose or possible interaction with another drug.

For this reason, it is important for you to know about the range of drugs used in dentistry, their effects and side effects and methods of administration. This will help you to maintain accurate, up-to-date medical histories of patients.

As patients often equate the word drug with narcotic or illicit drugs it may be preferable to use the word medicine when discussing substances with a patient.

You should never attempt to prescribe any drug. This is not the legal right or responsibility of a dental assistant. However, you can and should:

- ensure that an adequate medical history is taken that may reveal previous episodes of some allergy or adverse drug reaction — these should be prominently displayed on the patient's card, often noted with a diagonal red stripe drawn across the card;
- observe all patients receiving any drug in the surgery and immediately report any adverse reaction; and
- maintain fresh emergency drugs, know the practice first aid protocol and keep emergency telephone numbers prominently displayed.

Drug laws

The states and territories of Australia legislate to control the supply and use of drugs. The laws are similar in all states and territories but some variations do occur and you should check local legislation to ensure that you understand the laws that apply to your workplace.

The *Therapeutic Goods Act* divides drugs and poisons into scheduled (S) numbers S1 to S8. Only S1, S2, S3, S4 and S8 are relevant to dentistry. Three groups of drugs that are of particular interest are Groups 1, 2 and 3.

Group 1 (S1, S2, S3) drugs are usually described as pharmacy medicine on the packet and include substances that may be purchased from pharmacists and stores without a prescription (for example, some mild pain killers). These Group 1 drugs are usually safe drugs for minor ailments but should still be used strictly as directed.

Group 2 (S4) are described as 'prescription medicines' and are restricted drugs available from a pharmacist only with a prescription written by a medical practitioner, dentist or veterinary surgeon (for example, **antibiotics**, **tranquillisers** and **hypnotics**). Supply without prescription is illegal.

Group 3 (S8) are the dangerous drugs or drugs of addiction (narcotics). These are strictly controlled. In some states, these drugs can be administered but not prescribed by the dentist. In all states a record must be kept of drugs held and used, names and addresses of patients treated and dosages given. A **Drug Register** is required for this purpose. It must contain the patient's name, name of the drug

■ **drugs:** chemical compounds, either naturally occurring or synthetic, administered to alter the function of the body or of an invading pathogen. ■ **therapeutic:** using pharmacological knowledge to prevent or treat disease, and for the relief of pain. ■ **antibiotics:** drugs that alter the action of invading micro-organisms, either by destroying them (bacteriocidal action) or by interfering with their metabolism or reproduction (bacteriostatic action). ■ **tranquillisers:** drugs that relieve anxiety. ■ **hypnotics:** drugs that alter body function by acting on the central nervous system. They induce sleep. ■ **Drug Register:** a record of drugs kept, when used and to whom administered or given.

used, date administered and amount administered. It must be signed by two responsible people. Supply without authority or possession without prescription is illegal. These drugs must be kept under lock and key.

S5, S6 and S7 are chemicals produced for domestic or agricultural use.

Drug dosages and toxicity

Dosages

A therapeutic dose is the amount of a drug that must be administered to bring about the desired medicinal effect. A toxic dose is an amount that produces symptoms of poisoning.

The wider the difference between the therapeutic dose and the toxic dose, the safer the drug. If the difference between the therapeutic dose and the toxic dose is very small, special care is required in estimating the dosage and the patient must be carefully observed after the administration of the drug.

For each patient, the therapeutic dose may vary greatly from the average dose. Factors that must be considered include the patient's age, mass (body weight), sex, time of administration (e.g. in relation to mealtimes), patient's state of health, patient's metabolism, the history of previous use and any concurrent or recent medication. Dosage is also influenced by the expected rate of elimination from the body and by the route of administration of the drug.

Toxicity

The use of any drug is a carefully calculated risk. All pharmacologically active compounds (drugs) can be toxic. There are two major forms of toxicity.

❶ Overdose toxicity is by far the most common form of toxicity. Such toxicity results from an exaggeration of the clinical effects produced by the drug. The symptoms of poisoning (toxic effect) are due to the medicinal action of the drug.

❷ Drug **idiosyncrasy** is an unpredictable allergic or hypersensitive response. It is not as frequent or as predictable as overdose toxicity and is not related to the size of the dose. Even a very small amount may produce an exaggerated response in a susceptible person. Most idiosyncrasies are based on an immune response as a reaction to a foreign substance. Possible reactions are local

dermatitis, generalised skin rash (hives), purpura (bleeding spots), serum sickness, asthmatic or other breathing symptoms. These usually respond to withdrawal of the drug and antihistamines.

The most severe reaction is **anaphylactic shock**, a potentially life threatening emergency of very rapid onset. It most commonly occurs in patients receiving their first intramuscular injection of an antibiotic, such as penicillin, without being aware that they may be allergic to it. Some preservatives in food and wine (e.g. metabisulphite) can also be responsible. Latex rubber in gloves can also cause this type of allergic reaction.

Patient assessment

A patient should be assessed physically and medically before dental treatment begins. The patient's recent history form, which includes details of recent and current medication and medical status, is crucial to patient assessment and must be kept up to date.

Before administering drugs it is necessary to know of any other drugs being taken concurrently or recently as many drugs can either interact with (increase or produce a side effect) or antagonise (decrease the effectiveness) each other in the body.

Drug interactions can cause serious problems.

Patients taking anti-coagulants may have had a coronary thrombosis and their increased bleeding tendency needs to be considered before treatment. The addition of paracetamol or aspirin can increase their clotting time and consequently there is a risk of serious bleeding following extractions.

Cortisone therapy, if prolonged, can cause potentially serious complications during general anaesthesia and surgery, even when the cortisone is discontinued many months previously.

Anti-depressant and anti-hypertensive drugs, which are taken by a large number of apparently healthy people, have a potential for causing serious reactions, such as collapse, when used with some local anaesthetic agents. They may also cause a dry mouth (xerostomia) due to a reduction in saliva flow.

Prolonged antibiotic treatment may change the resident oral bacterial population and cause the fungal infection called thrush.

From these examples it is clear that a good medical history of each patient is essential. It is also essential to check whether patients are taking any compli-

idiosyncrasy: a tendency, individual peculiarity or characteristic.
anaphylactic shock: an extreme form of allergic reaction associated with sudden swelling of the throat and oral cavity.

mentary medicines such as herbal or other remedies. Some of these have also been known in certain situations to cause problems of drug interaction.

Unintended effects of drugs

Drugs can have unintended effects as well as their intended effects. Unintended effects can be very serious. Some of these, such as **anaphylaxis** and allergic reactions, are discussed in Chapter 22 in the section on medical emergencies in the surgery.

Patients can also become drug tolerant or drug addicted. When a drug is taken for a long time, it may lose its effectiveness and the patient becomes tolerant and receives no benefit from the drug. In this case, the dosage might need to be increased or the drug changed. Extended use of the drug may lead to dependence (addiction) and if the patient stops taking the drug they might develop physical symptoms of withdrawal.

There are other less significant but more common side effects such as drowsiness and hyperactivity, dizziness and thirst. Patients should be warned of these potential side effects and cautioned against operating machinery or undertaking tasks that might have legal implications, such as signing legal documents or deciding on financial matters.

You should *never* attempt to advise the use of, or prescribe, any drug. This is not the legal right or responsibility of a dental assistant. However, you can and should:

- ensure that an adequate medical history is taken, which may reveal previous episodes of some allergy or adverse drug reaction (these should be prominently displayed on the patient's card, often noted with a diagonal red stripe drawn across the card;
- observe all patients receiving any drug in the surgery and immediately report any adverse reaction to the dentist; and
- maintain fresh emergency drugs, know the practice's first aid protocol and keep emergency telephone numbers prominently displayed.

Safety considerations

Drug potency

The effectiveness of a drug may be influenced by many factors. Simple precautions will ensure that freshness and effectiveness are maintained.

Many drugs have a shelf life. When this is exceeded they should be destroyed. Some drugs can become poisonous past a certain age, e.g. local anaesthetic solutions.

When ordering, do not maintain excessively large stocks that could deteriorate. Rotate stock so that older packets are used up first, before they exceed their shelf life. Write the date of receipt on the outside of the packet as a reminder.

Heat, light and radiation may affect some drugs. Absorbed moisture may dilute a drug and cause chemical degeneration. It is commonsense *not* to store any medications or chemicals near a steriliser or a hot windowsill.

Drugs should be stored in a cool, dark, dry place and bottles should be well sealed.

Other safety considerations

Drugs should be labelled clearly and kept in a locked cupboard, preferably with one responsible key holder. Drug containers should be thrown away when empty and not reused for other purposes, even if relabelled. Drugs should always be kept in the original container and not transferred to other containers. Accidental injection of the wrong substance can be very serious.

No drug should be administered without good reason. Few drugs only have one effect and undesirable side effects can be harmful and sometimes deadly.

Sterile drugs in ampoules, rubber stoppered vials and cartridges must be handled with care and cleanliness to prevent contamination.

Any unused drug left in a single-dose container should be disposed of according to local regulations.

Drug names

Drugs may be referred to by their generic (chemical) name, or by proprietary (brand) name. For example, acetylsalicylic acid is the chemical name of the drug aspirin, while one of its brand names is Aspro. Each drug may have many brand names. For example, lignocaine, a local analgesic agent, is marketed as Nurocaine, Xylocaine, Xylotox and Vicaine.

It is best to try to remember the generic name and to always double and triple check the label before passing the drug to the dentist.

■ **anaphylaxis:** sudden onset of allergic reaction which can include shock, cardiac and respiratory failure and which can be fatal.

Methods of drug administration

The methods of administration are described here in general terms. For more information about pain control, anaesthesia and sedation in dentistry, see Chapter 20.

Oral administration

The most convenient route of administration is by mouth. Drugs taken in this way are usually in the form of tablets, capsules, powders and mixtures. **Absorption** occurs in the stomach and intestines. There are some disadvantages of this route of administration.

- It is not the most accurate way of administering an exact dose as absorption may be irregular or slow in the presence of food.
- The drug can also be diluted or inactivated by the gastric juices.
- Patient compliance may be a problem, especially in the elderly.
- There could be failure to complete the full course of treatment, e.g. antibiotics.
- The medication is relatively slow acting.

Topical administration

Some drugs are applied to the skin or mucous membranes as ointments, pastes or solutions and produce an effect at the site of application. There are also some drugs that, when applied to the skin or mucous membrane in the form of transdermal patches, are absorbed in large enough quantities to produce a **systemic effect**.

Inhalation

The inhalation of medicinal gases, such as nitrous oxide, or the vapours of volatile liquids, such as fluothane, is an efficient method of administering these drugs. As the lungs have a very large absorptive surface, a high concentration of the drug can be obtained rapidly. Additionally, as these gases are discharged unaltered via the lungs (breathed out) the concentration in the blood can be reduced reasonably quickly and a rapid clinical recovery occurs.

Administration by injection

Infiltration means that the drug is deposited under the skin or mucous membrane and from there infiltrates surrounding tissues and bone. Absorption by these methods is reliable, reasonably fast and the effect may be local or systemic depending on the drug used. Submucous injections deposit drugs beneath the mucous membrane of the mouth and subcutaneous injections deposit drugs under the skin.

Intraosseous injection is sometimes used to deposit a local analgesic solution within the bone near a tooth to be treated. This gives instant effect without wide areas of tissue numbness.

Intramuscular injection (IM) involves injection into a suitable muscle to administer larger doses of drugs when the oral route is unsatisfactory. For example, it is used when penicillin is needed for fast and/or prolonged action before treatment commences to prevent any possible infection. Aqueous (water based) solutions allow uniform absorption of the drug while oily solutions are used if a slow rate of absorption is desired.

Intravenous injection (IV) involves injection directly into the blood stream via a vein. It gives almost instant effect and is often used to induce general anaesthesia or administer emergency drugs. The administration of drugs by the intra-venous route can be an effective way of assessing a critical dosage. The drug is injected slowly, in increments, every minute or half minute and the patient's reaction is assessed continually. Certain methods of sedation employ this technique.

Intraligamental injections are injections directly into the periodontal ligament and sometimes used to numb an area around a mandibular tooth where a block injection is not required. (A block injection is a type of injection used to anaesthetise most mandibular teeth. The mandibular bone is thick and dense and this makes it difficult for the anaesthetic to diffuse through it. Instead, the anaesthetic is injected near the nerve and this numbs half of the lower jaw.)

Drugs affecting the nervous system

Analgesics

Analgesics are drugs employed for the relief of pain. Most analgesics exhibit a ceiling dose effect. This means that if the maximum therapeutic dose is not effective then increasing the dose will not produce more analgesia. In such cases it is necessary to employ a more **potent** analgesic, as well as investigating the patient's level of anxiety as it may be a contributing factor to pain.

■ **absorption:** soaking up of a substance through the mass of another. For example, a stone cast, placed in water, will absorb the water.
■ **systemic effect:** for example, nitroglycerine tablets placed under the tongue are absorbed through the mucosa and dilate the coronary arteries of the heart.
■ **potent:** strong, powerful.

Commonly used analgesics are:

- Aspirin — the drug most commonly used for the relief of mild to moderate pain. Aspirin is also **anti-pyretic** and in large doses has **anti-inflammatory** properties that are useful in the treatment of gout, arthritis and rheumatic conditions. A common brand name is Disprin.

- Paracetamol — an aspirin-like drug used for mild to moderate pain. It is both an analgesic and anti-pyretic agent. It does not cause gastric irritation. Paracetamol is available as Panadol and is a constituent of preparations including Panadeine, Codral Red and Mersyndol.

- Codeine — an analgesic chemically related to morphine but not as potent. It is prescribed for pain of moderate intensity. Side effects are dose-related and include dizziness, nausea and constipation.

Sedatives

Sedatives reduce excitability and may induce sleep when given in higher doses. Drowsiness and lack of coordination are likely complications of all sedative drugs so patients should be warned not to drive or conduct business requiring responsible judgment during the post-operative period. Sedated patients attending the dental surgery should be accompanied by a responsible adult. Barbiturates are the most common sedative-hypnotics. They are also popular for pre-operative dental sedation.

Tranquillisers

These are anti-anxiety agents. That is, they are drugs that calm without making the patient unduly drowsy. Examples are:

- Valium (diazepam), which in small doses exhibits good calming effects and muscle relaxation and is relatively safe due to the wide margin of safety between the therapeutic and toxic dose (elimination from the body is relatively slow);

- Serepax (oxezepam) also reduces anxiety and tension; and

- Atarax and Phenergen, which are a class of drug commonly used to treat allergic conditions (anti-histamines). Many of them have a significant tranquillising or sedative effect and so they are sometimes used clinically for sedation.

All anti-anxiety drugs are capable of producing sleep if given in excess and all can be dangerous if taken concurrently with other central nervous depressants such as barbiturates or excessive alcohol.

Narcotic drugs

Drugs such as morphine and heroin, which have both pain relieving and sleep inducing properties, are not likely to be encountered in the dental surgery. They are Schedule 8 drugs because they are classified as drugs of addiction.

Nitrous oxide/oxygen

Nitrous oxide, also known as happy gas, has been used as a general anaesthetic for over a century. In relatively recent years it has been used in combination with oxygen to produce a state known as relative analgesia during which the patient is relaxed and cooperative. This is really a light form of sedation that reduces anxiety. The active agent, nitrous oxide, is administered in low concentration (25 per cent) by inhalation. An advantage of using it in dentistry is that it reduces the gag reflex in susceptible people and recovery is relatively fast with administration of 100 per cent oxygen for a short period.

There are some disadvantages for patients such as nausea, dizziness and perspiration, and disadvantages for dental staff due the patient giggling and laughing, or talking excessively. There is particular disadvantage especially for female staff members because studies have proven that unless strict precautions, such as **scavenger units**, are attached to the equipment, constant use in the surgery may bring on spontaneous abortions. Some staff members have also developed allergic reactions to the gas.

General anaesthetics

General anaesthesia produces loss of consciousness, loss of protective reflexes and loss of sensation in the patient. Complete unconsciousness is experienced.

Drugs used to induce anaesthesia, in appropriates dosages, include short-acting barbiturates (Brietal or Pentothal, for example), nitrous oxide, chloroform, ether and halothane. Atropine (to dry out mucous secretions) and various muscle relaxants may be given to facilitate treatment during anaesthesia.

Local anaesthetics

Local anaesthetics (local analgesics) are drugs used to eliminate pain sensation in a particular region of the body by prevention of transmission of nerve impulses to the central nervous system. A solution of local anaesthetic may be injected into

anti-pyretic: reduces fever. ■ **anti-inflammatory:** decrease the effect of inflammation on certain tissues of the body; for example, pain caused by arthritis in joints. ■ **scavenger unit:** an exhaust system used to eliminate any stray fumes while using nitrous oxide.

one or more sites around the operative area or it may be applied topically in solution or ointment directly to the site required.

Some local anaesthetics are:

■ Lignocaine (Nurocaine, Xylocaine) — its onset of action is fast, duration is reasonably long and the depth of anaesthesia is profound. It is an effective topical anaesthetic.

■ Prilocaine (Citanest) — this is a more recent drug with a potency and toxicity similar to lignocaine. It does not require as much vaso-constrictor as lignocaine and in 4 per cent solution is used without vaso-constrictor to give short duration anaesthesia. It is generally used for patients with known or suspected heart conditions and elderly patients.

■ Bupivacaine (Marcain) — this is a longer acting local anaesthetic used for long dental procedures such as oral surgery or prosthodontic procedures.

The toxicity of a local anaesthetic can be greatly increased, whether due to the vaso-constrictor or anaesthetic base, by accidental injection into a vein. This causes the solution to be rapidly carried to the heart, brain and all parts of the body and a toxic reaction (faint, collapse or convulsions) may occur quite rapidly. To avoid inadvertent intra-venous injection, an aspiration test is performed. This is achieved by the operator pulling back slightly on the plunger of an injection syringe. If blood is found in the barrel it may be in a vein and the needle needs to be repositioned.

Vaso-constrictors in local anaesthesia

A vaso-constrictor is a drug that causes the blood vessels to contract, decreasing their diameter and reducing the amount of blood flowing through them. Most anaesthetic preparations include vaso-constrictors for three reasons.

❶ Firstly, the reduced blood flow prevents the local anaesthetic being removed too quickly, and so deepens and prolongs the anaesthesia.

❷ Secondly, the reduced blood flow delays the diffusion of the anaesthetic agent to the rest of the body, which reduces the chance of toxic reaction.

❸ Thirdly, they prevent any possible infection from spreading to the rest of the body.

Agents that have been used as vaso-constrictors include:

■ Adrenaline — this is used in very small quantities to contract the peripheral blood vessels. It tends to increase the blood pressure and pulse rate. This is sometimes noted in patients as transient palpitations. It enlarges the vessels supplying blood to the heart.

■ Noradrenaline — this contracts peripheral blood vessels but has little effect on the vessels of the heart. It can increase blood pressure more than adrenaline in local anaesthetics.

■ Fellypressin (Octapressin) — this is an alternative vaso-constrictor that is free of most of the undesirable side effects of adrenaline and noradrenaline. Fellypressin is used in combination with prilocaine under the brand name Citanest with Octapressin.

Chemotherapeutic drugs

Chemotherapy is the treatment of systemic infections using chemical substances that attack the disease-producing organisms.

Sulphonamides

The sulphonamides are drugs that were first used in about 1936. They are chemically similar to some industrial dyes, tend to inhibit the growth and reproduction of many bacteria rather than killing them and they are inactive in the presence of pus. The sulpha drugs, as they are sometimes called, are likely to cause harmful side effects of many kinds and for dental treatment they have largely been replaced by antibiotics.

A modern drug marketed as Bactrim or Septrin contains a sulpha drug. This drug is interesting as each of its individual components merely inhibits bacteria growth but in combination they destroy a wide spectrum of organisms.

Antibiotics

These are also chemotherapeutic agents. They are chemical substances that may be produced by living organisms, such as moulds, and that have an antibacterial action. They may be **bactericidal**. They include:

■ Metronidazole (Flagyl) — this is effective in treat-ing the acute stage of acute necrotising ulcerative gingivitis (ANUG) if taken for four to five days.

■ Nystatin (Nilstat) — this is an antibiotic for use against fungal infections such as candida infection. As nystatin is only used locally it

■ **bactericidal:** capable of destroying bacteria.

should be applied topically or the tablets slowly dissolved in the mouth.

- Penicillin — this was the first antibiotic introduced (in 1940) and is still the most commonly used. Nowadays it is produced in many forms. Penicillin is potent, virtually non-toxic and active in the presence of pus. Unfortunately, allergic reactions to penicillin are relatively common and care must be taken to avoid administering any form of penicillin to persons who have had an allergic reaction to the drug. Reactions can be serious, even fatal because each administration increases the allergic response.

- Erythromycin — this is an antibiotic active against a similar range of organisms to penicillin. Erythromycin is both **bacteriostatic** and bacteriocidal and is often used against bacteria that are resistant to other antibiotics. The incidence of side effects is low although a few cases of jaundice have been observed. Erythromycin is a suitable alternative to penicillin for pre-operative cover for patients with a history of heart valve damage. This is called antibiotic prophylaxis and is the use of antibiotics with uninfected patients to reduce the risk of bacterial infection.

- Teracyclines — these are bacteriostatic antibiotics effective against a range of micro-organisms (broad spectrum) and usually taken by mouth. Mouthwashes are also used for some cases of oral ulceration. The use of tetracyclines in children can result in permanent staining of the teeth developing at the time. The preparation Ledermix contains ledermycin, a tetracycline, and a cortisone drug that reduces pain in inflamed dental pulps.

- Lincomycin — this is an antibiotic used dentally only where infections of bone are likely or being treated. It appears to have an affinity for bone. It is sometimes used to combat bone infections after radiotherapy for oral cancer.

Other chemotherapeutic agents in dental use

Other chemotherapeutic agents in dental use include:

- Idoxuridine (Stoxil) — this ointment is an antiviral agent used to treat herpes infection (cold sores). To be effective it should be applied as soon as the itchy symptoms develop and be continued hourly.

- Acyclovir (Zovirax) — a newer, more effective treatment for herpes simplex.

- Amphotericin (Fungulin) — this is for the treatment and control of **thrush**.

Antiseptics and disinfectants

An antiseptic is a substance that inhibits bacterial growth. They are mostly used to clean the skin in hand washes (e.g. chlorhexidine), as antiseptic gargles and mouthwashes (iodine) or as topical paints or creams (nystatin).

Disinfectants are substances that destroy bacteria in non-sporing state. These substances are commonly used for cleaning equipment. It is important to remember that chemical disinfection is not the same as sterilisation.

Miscellaneous drugs

Corticosteroids

Cortisone-based drugs such as triamcinolone acetonide combined with antibacterial or anti-fungal agents are used for symptomatic relief of some painful oral ulcerations by reducing inflammation. These sorts of preparations are either applied as an ointment or dissolved slowly in the mouth.

Eugenol

Eugenol, or oil of cloves, is one of the essential oils and is both antiseptic and pain relieving. It is often present in toothache cures as it has a **palliative effect** on pulpal pain. Eugenol is also a basic ingredient in many dental lining materials and impression pastes (for example, Kalsogen). It must not be used under glass ionomer cements (GICs).

Desensitising agents

These are applied to sensitive dentine and cementum and include sodium fluoride paste, potassium nitrate, strontium chloride and sodium monofluorophosphate. They are applied directly to the ends of the dentine tubules by the dentist during cavity treatment or in combination with toothpaste for home use, to reduce hypersensitivity of teeth.

Haemostatic agents

Gingival retraction for impression taking is carried out by the careful insertion of light cord or cotton into the gingival crevice. To prevent gingival seepage or bleeding, the cord can be pre-treated by soaking the cord with an astringent (ferric sulphate)

■ **thrush**: candida albicans or monilia.
■ **bacteriostatic**: inhibits the multiplication of bacteria.
■ **palliative effect**: providing pain relief.

or aluminium chloride. This is a short-term treatment because prolonged application may cause tissue damage.

Fluorides

These include sodium and calcium fluoride and stannous fluoride and have been proven to reduce dental caries when applied topically to strengthen tooth enamel. Consequently, many preparations of fluoride are marketed in toothpastes, mouthwashes and gels for home and professional application, and in tablet form. Tablets are normally prescribed when young people have an inadequate dietary intake of this essential element. If fluoride is available to developing teeth during their formation, caries has been shown to be reduced by up to 60 per cent compared with teeth that are deficient in fluoride. The protection gained is lifelong.

Calcium hydroxide

Calcium hydroxide (e.g. Dycal, Pulpdent) is used as cavity liner to act as a barrier against chemical or thermal shock and to encourage the formation of secondary dentine.

Hydrogen peroxide (H_2O_2)

Acts as a topical anaesthetic, antiseptic and, in strong concentrations, bleaches teeth.

Summary of drugs used in dentistry

Analgesics

These alter body function by acting on the central nervous system. They relieve pain.

Sedatives

Sedatives alter body function by acting on the central nervous system. They relieve apprehension and anxiety.

Anaesthetics

These alter body function by acting on the central nervous system in producing loss of sensation, loss of consciousness, amnesia and loss of protective reflexes.

Local anaesthetics

Local anaesthetics alter body function by acting on the nervous system in producing loss of sensation in the area to be treated.

Narcotics

These alter body function by acting on the central nervous system. These are the drugs of addiction. They relieve anxiety and pain, can induce sleep and a general feeling of wellbeing. These drugs are capable of causing loss of consciousness.

Vaso-constrictors

Vaso-constrictors are used in local anaesthetic solutions to prevent the anaesthetic agent from rapid systemic distribution by constricting the blood vessels near the injection site. By keeping the anaesthetic localised they prolong the analgesic effect of the solution and decrease bleeding in the treatment area.

Antibiotics

These drugs alter the action of invading micro-organisms, either by destroying them (bacteriocidal action), or by interfering with their metabolism or reproduction (bacteriostatic action).

See Table 13.1 for additional information.

Other chemicals used therapeutically in the dental practice

This list is not exhaustive. However, Table 13.2 contains a summary of chemicals commonly used as therapeutic agents in the dental surgery.

Prescription drugs that may affect dental treatment

Each patient's medical history should identify prescription drugs the patient is using. Some of the commonly used prescription drugs that may affect dental treatment are shown in Table 13.3.

Type of drug	Common Examples	Mode of action
Analgesics (Note: those prescribed for severe pain are often mixtures so they are classified as either S3 Pharmacy Medicine or S4 Prescription Only Medicine.)	• Panadol, Dymadon, Tylenol (paracetamol S2) • Solprin, Disprin, (aspirin S2) • Nurofen (ibuprofen S3) • Codral Forte (aspirin and codeine S4)	Act on the central nervous system (CNS) to prevent or relieve pain.
Anti-anxiety agents (tranquillisers)	• Serepax (oxazepam S4) • Valium (diazepam S4) when given in small doses, in pill form	Act on the CNS to reduce anxiety and tension.
Sedatives	• Valium (diazepam S4) — given intravenously	Same as tranquillisers, but induce drowsiness and quickly reduce tension and muscle spasm.
Narcotics (rarely used in dentistry). These drugs are addictive.	• Morphine (derivative of Heroin S8) • Pethedine (S8)	Act on the CNS to relieve severe pain. Cause drowsiness and depression of the respiratory system.
General anaesthetics; used for major surgical procedures, usually in operating theatres, initially intravenously, then maintained by inhalation.	• Pentothal (thiopentane sodium S4) • Fluothane (halothane S4) • Nitrous oxide (S4)	Act on the CNS to produce unconsciousness, i.e. loss of sensation, reflexes, muscle control and amnesia.
Local anaesthetics (also used for epi-dural blocks and spinal anaesthesia).	• Xylocaine (lignocaine S4) • Citanest (prilocaine S4) • Marcain (bupivacaine S4) long acting, used for very long oral surgery procedures	Act on the peripheral nervous system (PNS) to produce local loss of pain sensation.
Vaso-constrictors (used in dentistry combined with local anaesthetic agents).	• Adrenalin (S4) • Noradrenalin (S4) • Octopressin (felypressin S4)	Act to constrict local blood vessels in order to localise the anaesthetic solution.
Antibiotics	• Amoxil (amoxycillin S4) • Pensig (penicillin S4) • Mysteclin (tetracycline S4) • Erythrocin (erythromycin S4) • Flagyl (metronidazole S4)	Act to destroy micro-organisms (bacteriocidal). Act to hinder the growth and spread of bacteria (bacteriostatic).
Antiseptics, germicides and topical anti-infective agents.	• Betadine (providone iodine S2) • Chlorohex, Savacol (chlorhexidine)	Antiseptic paint or gargle and antiseptic mouthwashes.
	• Zovirax (acyclovir S4)	Treatment for herpes simplex.
	• Nilstat (nystatin S4) • Fungilin (amphotericin S4)	Control of thrush (candida albicans or monilia).
Topical corticosteroids; powerful anti-inflammatory agents that will worsen existing infections unless used in combination with antibiotics.	• Kenalog in Orabase (triamcinolone acetonide S4)	Reduces inflammation from some ulcers.
	• Ledermix (triamcinolone acetonide and tetracycline S4)	Controls inflammation of the pulp.
	• Corlan pellets (hydrocortisone)	For treating inflammation caused by aphthous and mucosal ulcers.

Table 13.1 Summary of drugs used in dentistry

Type	Common Examples	Use
Sedative/analgesic lining or temporary dressing materials	• Zinc oxide powder • Eugenol (oil of cloves)	Widely used for dressings and temporary fillings.
Calcium hydroxide	• Dycal • Pulpdent, Life	Analgesic to pulp and dentine, used in combination with zinc oxide for dressings and root canal filling paste.
Hydrogen peroxide	• Hydrogen peroxide (H_2O_2 S2)	Acts as a topical anaesthetic and antiseptic. Bleaches teeth in stronger concentration.
Fluorides	• Floran (stannous fluoride S2) • Phos-flur (APF S2) • Bifluoride (sodium and calcium fluoride S2)	Prevents dental caries by strengthening tooth enamel and reduces dentine sensitivity – (in toothpastes, mouthwashes and varnishes).
Desensitising agents	• Potassium nitrate • Strontium chloride	Reduces hypersensitivity of teeth.
Haemostatic agents	• Astrigident (ferric sulphate) • Ultradent • Haemodent (aluminium chloride)	Used to control gingival bleeding, often used to soak retraction cords.

Table 13.2 Summary of chemicals used therapeutically in the dental practice

Type	Examples	Effects on treatment planning
Anti-angina agents	• Adalat • Isoptin • Angenine • Nitradisc	Patient should bring medication to each appointment. Appointments should be short. Special care is needed with local anaesthetic.
Anti-coagulants	• Cardiprin • Dindevan • Heparin • Coumarin • Aspirin	Risk of severe haemorrhage. Consult patient's doctor before any invasive procedure. Not to be prescribed any extra aspirin.
Anti-psychotics and anti-depressants	• Anatensol • Allergon • Modecate • Stelazine • Sinequan • Tryptanol	Possibility of inappropriate behaviour. Xerostomia may be present. Good communication skills and patience required. Care with local anaesthetic.
Corticosteroids	• Celestone • Prednisone • Cortisone	Increased risk of infection. May need antibiotic cover for dental treatment. Risk of collapse if stressed.
Hormones	• Insulin • Daonil • Rastinon	For diabetic patients. Risk of infection. Poor tolerance of stress.

Table 13.3 Some commonly used prescription drugs that may affect dental treatment

Summary

You will not prescribe drugs for patients but you will be involved in preparing some drugs for use in the surgery. You may also be asked by patients about drugs they require and, with the dentist's permission, may explain to patients the basic function of drugs. You may also be responsible for collecting information from patients for their medical and dental histories and must understand that all drugs (prescribed, over the counter, or illicit) may have implications for treatment. By understanding this you are in a better position to clarify exactly which substances the patient needs and is using and to record this on the medical history form.

Section 3

Clinical dentistry

Dentistry shares with all of the health professions a common obligation to ensure the welfare of the patient. As part of the dental team, you play an important role in patient care.

In the surgery you:
- prepare the surgery for each patient;
- assist the dentist during clinical procedures;
- prepare equipment, materials and instruments for procedures;
- monitor and assist in the care and comfort of the patient;
- are responsible for the maintenance of good infection control practices;
- maintain and file patient records; and
- prepare laboratory work orders, and assist with radiography.

This section describes these duties.

Surgery protocols and procedures

Every surgery should have a set of written procedures for:
- decontaminating/cleaning the surgery each morning, between patients and at the end of the day;
- hand washing;
- sterilising area set-up;
- immunisation schedules;
- use of personal protective equipment;
- the flow from contaminated to clean items;
- care, cleaning and loading of sterilising equipment;
- cleaning, sterilising and storing reusable instruments;
- equipment maintenance;
- handpiece care and sterilisation;
- disinfection (if absolutely necessary) of reusable, non-autoclave items;
- use and handling of disinfectants;
- handling sharps and dealing with needle-stick injuries;

- radiographic procedures;
- patient record keeping;
- procedures involving lasers and air abrasion;
- laboratory procedures (sending work to the dental laboratory);
- handling patient emergencies;
- managing blood spills or exposure to blood or body fluids;
- cleaning and decontaminating office furniture/equipment;
- keeping of staff immunisation, injury and exposure records; and
- any other procedure followed in the surgery.

You should consult those procedures regularly for a better understanding and reminder of the duties you perform in your place of work.

chapter fourteen
infection control

Introduction

Infection control is a series of procedures carried out in dental practices (and in all health establishments) to prevent the transmission of disease.

Dental health professionals are exposed to a wide variety of micro-organisms. Some viruses and bacteria can be transmitted through the blood and saliva of patients. Examples of these are herpes, hepatitis B and C, and HIV. Others, spread by **aerosols** created in the surgery, cause infectious diseases such as colds, chickenpox, pneumonia and tuberculosis. At present most of the guidelines for infection control procedures are aimed at preventing the spread of blood and other body-fluid borne viruses (e.g. hepatitis B and C, and HIV) but we must not forget other conditions that can be transmitted by **droplets** or the **faecal-oral route**.

Who is responsible for infection control?

Dentists, whether in private practice or heads of public dental health clinics, have the responsibility to establish, implement and monitor infection control policies. They should be thoroughly familiar with safe practices, malpractice issues and laws of negligence. They should ensure that they comply with all relevant local and national standards and legislation.

All staff members involved in the treatment of patients and the implementation of infection control procedures should have an understanding of the hazards associated with the spread of disease and appropriate training in all aspects of infection control.

Each dental practice should have a written infection control policy consistent with both government regulations and the National Health and Medical Research Council (NHMRC) Commonwealth

infection control guidelines for the prevention of transmission of infectious diseases in the health care setting. Copies of these are available from government publishers and WorkSafe organisations in your state or territory. A list is available in the appendix.

Staff training

It is an employer's duty to ensure that all staff members receive training (initial and ongoing) that allows them to work safely. This training should enable staff to anticipate and manage any health-threatening situation such as exposure to infectious organisms or chemical spills. Contact your local occupational health and safety office for information about workplace training programs.

There should be a routine for training staff whenever a new member joins the team, a new piece of equipment or material is introduced to the surgery, or if there are changes in regulations or standards that have consequences for surgeries. A record should be kept of all training undergone by each staff member, whether that training was supplied in-house or through another provider.

Means of transmission of infection

Although we are in constant contact with micro-organisms, most of them are harmless. Only some of these micro-organisms are pathogens and cause injury to tissue. We call this tissue injury disease.

Cross-infection involves the transfer of pathogens from one person to another. In some cases, the second person will become a **carrier**. In other cases, the second person will become actively infected.

Infection results when micro-organisms gain access to the body's tissues and then multiply (despite, or

■ **aerosols:** materials suspended in vapour or gas. For example, the fine spray created by the spinning of a high speed hand piece containing blood, saliva and micro-organisms. ■ **droplets:** minute particles of moisture expelled by talking, sneezing or coughing and which may carry infectious micro-organisms. ■ **faecal-oral route:** transfer of organisms from faeces to the mouth (usually because of lack of adequate hand washing). ■ **carrier:** a person who carries a pathogenic organism but who does not necessarily become sick. A person who has had a disease and recovered can be a carrier. Carriers can still pass the disease on to other people.

due to, the failure of the body's defence mechanism). As a result, injury to tissue occurs.

The three major groups of organisms that are sources of infection and are of principal concern in the dental surgery are:

❶ viruses;

❷ bacteria; and

❸ fungi (moulds and yeasts).

Prions are also of concern.

For these micro-organisms to be transmitted from one person to another there must be both:

■ a means of transmission; and

■ a portal of entry.

Transmission by direct contact

Many organisms are unable to survive for very long outside the environment of their host and must be directly transmitted; for example, by kissing or sexual contact. Venereal diseases and herpes virus infections are examples of this.

Transmission by indirect contact

Organisms that are able to exist outside the body are easily transmitted. Contaminated food or drink, non-sterile instruments and needles can all result in infections. Hepatitis, food poisoning and wound infections are examples.

Transmission by droplet spray

The micro-organisms responsible for respiratory tract infections can be transmitted by the fine spray or aerosol that results from coughing or sneezing. This is a very common mode of transmission, especially in close communities. Another kind of aerosol encountered in the dental surgery is the fine spray caused by the spinning of a high-speed handpiece, an ultrasonic scaler or a triplex syringe. See Chapter 16 for more information about these pieces of equipment.

Self-infection

Under some circumstances, organisms that usually live in the body without causing disease can begin to do so. For example, if a micro-organism that is usually found on the skin gets into the bloodstream, it can cause problems.

Portals of entry

There are five main ways by which micro-organisms can enter the body. Possible routes to cross-infection in the dental surgery are shown in Figure 14.1.

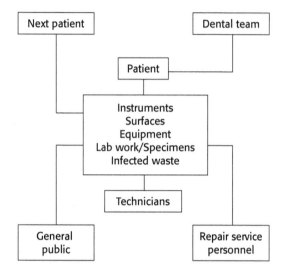

Figure 14.1 Routes to cross-infection in the dental surgery

Inhalation

The moist surfaces of the respiratory tract trap many of the micro-organisms that we breathe in. However, some can still cause infections such as the common cold, influenza, measles and tuberculosis (TB).

Ingestion

Food and drink can contain micro-organisms that cause food poisoning or dysentery; for example, salmonella.

Implantation

The intact skin is usually a barrier to infection but if skin or the mucous membranes are damaged, organisms can be implanted in deeper tissue and cause infection; for example, an infected wound after surgery.

Injection

Vectors (biting insects, such as mosquitoes and ticks) can inject micro-organisms into deeper tissues; for example, in the case of malaria. Contaminated needles or solutions are other ways in which infection can be spread by injection.

■ **prion:** a protein capable of causing disease.
■ **vector:** an organism such as a fly or mosquito that carries disease from one sick person to another.

Congenital infection across the placenta

A pregnant woman can pass a disease to her unborn baby. German measles is an example of this.

Preventing cross-infection

There are a number of components of an effective infection control procedure. Each of these components will be dealt with separately in the following sections of this chapter.

However, as an overview, these components include:

- a two-tiered approach to infection control involving standard precautions and transmission-based precautions;
- aseptic techniques;
- instrument cleaning and sterilisation;
- safe storage;
- environmental cleaning and surface decontamination;
- equipment care and asepsis;
- laboratory asepsis;
- radiography asepsis; and
- safe disposal of surgery waste.

Figure 14.2 shows how each component helps to create a barrier to cross-infection.

Other components crucial to effective infection control are personal hygiene and personal protective equipment (PPE). These will be covered in Chapter 15.

Barriers that prevent cross infection in the dental surgery are shown in Figure 14.2.

Standard and transmission-based precautions

The only way to protect the health and safety of patients and the dental team is to regard everyone who enters the dental practice as if they were potential sources of infection. When a patient walks into your surgery you have no way of knowing whether or not that person has an infectious disease. In fact some patients may themselves be unaware of their infectious status (as is often the case of a hepatitis B or C carrier).

Transmission-based precautions are the second tier of infection control.

Standard precautions

Standard precautions constitute best practice in infection control. They are a routine of clinical safeguards that are used for every patient regardless of their perceived infectious status.

Standard precautions apply to:

- blood;
- all body substances, secretions and excretions (except sweat) regardless of whether or not they contain visible blood;
- non-intact skin; and
- mucous membranes.

Standard precautions also apply to dry blood. Copies of standard precautions for your state or territory can be obtained from government publishers in your capital city. A list of these is available in the appendix.

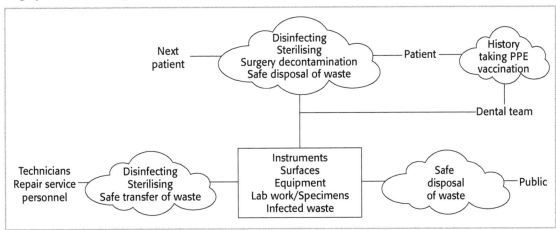

Figure 14.2 Barriers to cross-infection in the dental surgery

As an approach to infection control, standard precautions are essential because:

■ infectious patients may not manifest any signs or symptoms of infection that would be detected in the course of routine history taking or a medical/dental examination;

■ infectious status is often determined only by laboratory tests that cannot be completed in time to provide emergency care;

■ patients may be infectious before laboratory tests are positive or signs of disease are manifested (the window period); and

■ staff and patients may be placed at risk of cross-infection from those who are symptomless but infectious.

The introduction of standard precautions has meant that no patients need feel discriminated against because of their presumed infection status. Every person who enters a health establishment is considered potentially infectious.

However, medical and dental histories still need to be obtained. They provide essential information for the dentist and protection for the patient. A complete medical history can identify any conditions that may compromise the patient's health during dental treatment. It can also help to identify any communicable disease from which a patient may be suffering and be aware of but may not consider relevant to the dentist.

Although the responsibility for assessing a complete and thorough medical/dental history will always remain with the treating dentist, you have a very important role in getting patients or guardians to provide the necessary information and to help them with any difficulties they may have completing the forms. It is also your role to reassure patients that this procedure is for the their own protection and that absolute confidentiality of the information is guaranteed.

Transmission-based precautions

Transmission-based precautions are the second tier of infection control.

They apply to those situations where standard precautions may be insufficient to prevent transmission of infection and are used in addition to the standard precautions. These precautions are most likely to be required in hospital settings. As a general rule, people who are acutely ill with an infection are unlikely to make routine dental appointments. However, emergencies can occur where an infectious patient requires dental treatment and in

this instance transmission-based precautions may be required.

Transmission-based precautions are used in situations where patients are known or suspected to be infected (or colonised) with highly transmissible pathogens that can cause infection:

■ by airborne transmission (e.g. mycobacterium tuberculosis, measles and chickenpox virus);

■ by droplet transmission (e.g. mumps, rubella, pertussis, influenza);

■ by direct or indirect contact with dry skin, or with contaminated surfaces (e.g. colonisation with MRSA — multi-drug resistant staphylococcus aureus); or

■ by a combination where micro-organisms have multiple routes of transmission.

Transmission-based precautions include:

■ masks with extra filtration (particulate masks) for airborne diseases such as TB or chickenpox;

■ gowns;

■ minimisation of aerosols; and

■ isolation for very infectious cases.

Additionally, these patients should be prioritised ahead of other patients and their movement through the practice should be limited as much as possible. Appointments should be avoided at the busiest time of the day. Only the emergency should be treated and routine work should be completed when the patient is well. Single-use equipment must be used whenever possible.

Whenever transmission-based precautions are required, standard precautions must also be used.

These precautions are not required for patients with blood-borne viruses such as hepatitis B, C or HIV, unless there are complicating factors present, such as pulmonary TB.

An exception

The emergence of 'Mad Cow Disease' (Bovine Spongiform Encephalitis) and the human equivalent, Creutzfeldt-Jakob Disease (CJD), has created new hazards for the dental team. This disease is transmitted by a prion (a protein). It is a 'slow' infection characterised by:

■ a prolonged incubation period, thought to be 15 years or longer;

■ a brief, progressive clinical course which is ultimately fatal; and

■ lesions confined to a single organ (e.g. the brain).

To date, there is no established set of precautions for prion diseases. The agents transmitting the prion diseases are not readily destroyed by conventional sterilisation, including autoclaving. Some autoclaves now come with a prion cycle but research into their effectiveness is inconclusive.

In principle:

- the patient should be treated in a hospital environment;
- single-use equipment must be used;
- if single-use equipment is not possible, equipment should be sterilised at 134°C for 18 minutes; and
- all waste should be incinerated.

However, procedures for your surgery will need to be developed by the clinician based on all available, up-to-date information.

Asepsis

Asepsis is the condition of being free from pathogenic organisms.

The chain of asepsis or the sterile chain is a set of procedures that starts with sterilisation and then continues with procedures that keep articles sterile until they are used. The chain is only as strong as each individual link. If it is broken at any stage, cross-infection may occur.

Whatever method is used to achieve sterilisation it is essential to handle reusable instruments in an orderly and systematic manner. Used or contaminated instruments must be kept completely separate from sterile ones.

Single-use equipment and instruments (e.g. scalpel blades) must be disposed of.

Remember, it is impossible to judge by appearance whether an article has undergone sterilisation. A clean, shiny instrument may be more heavily contaminated than an item carrying obvious signs of use.

Working zones or the zone of activity

The zone of activity is the working area around the patient that is occupied by you and the clinician. It can also be called the zone of contamination. It is the area that requires special attention when decontaminating the surgery between patients.

Aseptic techniques for use during four-handed dentistry

The teamwork in four-handed dentistry allows good aseptic techniques to be used and these are the ideal way of minimising cross-contamination. These techniques ensure that sterile items do not come in contact with contaminated items. See Procedure 14.1 (overleaf) for more information.

Flow

Separate areas, well removed from one another, should be available for the collection of soiled instruments and the placement of sterilised items. The flow in the designated sterilising area should always be in one direction, i.e. from contaminated to sterile. Infective or contaminated material can be placed on contaminated surfaces but contaminated material should never be placed on clean or disinfected surfaces.

Cleaning and sterilising areas

The cleaning and sterilisation area should have:

- plenty of bench space with smooth, non-porous surfaces and be free from crevices;
- good lighting and ventilation;
- hand washing facilities separate from the cleaning sink;
- containers for waste disposal;
- plenty of storage space for equipment and materials; and
- a dedicated storage area for sterile instruments.

The recommended layout for a processing area is shown in Figure 14.3 (page 139).

Environmental cleaning

The cleanliness of the surgery, the sterilising area and laboratory is your responsibility. Remember that dust can harbour many micro-organisms and is a potential source of infection. Horizontal surfaces should be kept free of dust at all times. See Procedure 14.2 (page 139) for more information.

Procedure 14.1 Aseptic techniques for use during four-handed dentistry

Preparing for a procedure

■ Pre-determine needs by checking on the patient's treatment plan and prepare all instruments and equipment for each procedure. Leave equipment bagged until the patient is seated and ready for treatment.

■ Prepare patient's bib, protective drapes and goggles. Place a plastic-backed tray, mat or other barrier on the bracket table.

■ Pre-dispense disposables (cotton rolls, pellets, pledgets, wedges, matrix bands, retraction cord, articulating paper, etc.) and place them on a bracket table or assistant's trolley. Keep this covered until required. There must be a fresh, clean, sterilised pair of tweezers available for every patient for the clinician and the assistant to retrieve any additional materials or instruments.

■ If possible, pre-dispense materials and medicaments required for each procedure and place them within easy reach before patient contact. Follow manufacturers' recommendations on how light-sensitive materials may be pre-dispensed safely.

■ If possible, also pre-set light and chair positions. If adjustments are needed during treatment, only touch clearly defined points of contact. If possible, cover these points with disposable plastic wrap and change the wrap between patients. Use disposable plastic bags as covers for chair controls and x-ray units. Only touch lights by their handles.

■ Volatile materials or medicaments (e.g. isopropyle alcohol) may need to be dispensed at the time of use.

■ Reduce the contamination of clean surfaces by using sterilisable trays to collect used instruments. Alternatively, use disposable plastic-backed paper and change it between patients.

During treatment

■ Charting should be carried out by the dental assistant and checked by the clinician without contaminating the patient's records. Any additional notes can be written on a separate pad and recorded on the patient's chart by the dentist at the completion of treatment. Non-disposable and non-sterilisable materials, for example, charts, radiographs and bulk materials, should be placed only on 'clean' surfaces (this includes the interior of cabinets and drawers).

■ Use efficient high volume aspiration to minimise splatter and aerosols created by handpieces, ultrasonic scalers and the like.

■ Use uncontaminated gloves or over-gloves when mixing impression materials, as well as when handling curing lights, amalgamators, etc. Clean hands, without gloves, are acceptable when there is no direct contact with the patient.

■ Wipe the mixing spatula and any plastic instrument.

■ Adjust the operator light to aid visibility to reduce the risk of contamination.

■ Injection syringes, if used more than once during a procedure, should be re-sheathed by the clinician using a single-handed technique.

After treatment

■ Wear utility gloves and face protection for clean-up.

■ Place all non-reusable 'sharps' into the designated puncture resistant 'sharps' container. The person who generates the contaminated sharp is responsible for its disposal immediately after it is used. This is almost always the dentist.

■ Separate re-usable instruments and burs from all disposables.

■ Place all sterilisable instruments and equipment (e.g. triplex syringes and aspirator tips) into a puncture-resistant container for removal to the sterilising area.

■ Remove barrier wraps.

■ Flush handpieces, triplex syringes, scalers and suction lines.

■ Discard all non-hazardous waste.

■ Change gloves.

■ Wipe surfaces with a neutral detergent mixed to the correct dilution.

■ Dry all cleaned equipment with a lint-free cloth.

■ Wash utility gloves and hang them to dry.

■ Remove personal protective equipment (PPE).

■ Wash hands.

■ If possible, use one sink as a scrub sink for non-contaminated personal use and a second, deep, flush sink for cleaning contaminated instruments.

■ Unused diluted detergent should be discarded at the end of each day.

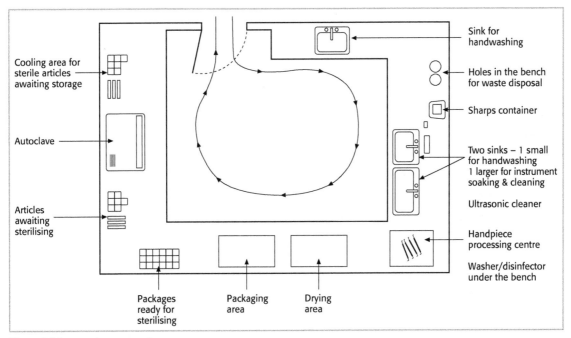

Figure 14.3 Layout for a processing area

Procedure 14.2 Environmental cleaning

- Surgeries should be damp-dusted first thing in the morning, before patients arrive, at the end of the morning session if time permits, and again at night before closing down the surgery.

- Use a neutral to slightly alkaline detergent for general cleaning. Disinfectants should not be used for general cleaning. Check manufacturers' recommend-ations for cleaning detergents to be used on the dental chair and unit.

- Do not use alcohol wipes for cleaning surfaces. Alcohol wipes are not **viricidal** (they do not kill viruses). Additionally, alcohol can make blood and body fluids adhere to some surfaces. However, they are very useful for drying surfaces quickly after the surfaces have been wiped with water and detergents.

- Water and detergent are very effective in removing **bio-burden**.

- Do not spray surfaces indiscriminately. Spray the detergent into the tissue or cloth that you use.

- Use disposable cloths (e.g. Chux) or tissues for wiping surfaces. The cloth should be thrown away after use. Re-usable cloths and sponges harbour, and become a great breeding ground, for micro-organisms and therefore should not be used.

- After cleaning, a dry cloth should be used to thoroughly dry all surfaces and electrical components.

- Clean work surfaces regularly. Surfaces should be cleaned immediately following spills or when visibly soiled. (This includes walls, dental chairs and all dental equipment.)

- Mop vinyl floors if they are soiled (and especially if there is acrylic powder residue after a denture adjustment).

- Have air-conditioning units (particularly filters) regularly inspected and cleaned.

- Wear general purpose gloves when cleaning.

If there is likelihood of splashing during cleaning, a fluid-repellent gown and eyewear should be worn.

Surface decontamination

After dismissing the patient, all contaminated items and materials should be systematically removed. Because of the difficulties associated with some disinfectants, authorities recommend wiping most surfaces (unless they have been grossly contaminated with blood products) with a neutral pH detergent. This will clean as well as decontaminate.

Equipment asepsis

All areas touched (i.e. the zones of contamination) by either you or the dentist must be decontaminated between patients. As well as decontaminating surfaces, there are some pieces of equipment that need special attention. This equipment includes, but is not limited to:

- the dental light handles and switches;

■ **viricidal**: capable of killing viruses.
■ **bio-burden**: any contamination that adheres to a surface. Also referred to as biofilm.

- the suction line;
- curing lights;
- ultrasonic scalers;
- spittoons and sinks;
- filters;
- chairs, cupboards and handles;
- handpiece caddies;
- x-ray machines;
- triplex syringes, if not autoclavable;
- triturators (material mixers); and
- relative analgesia machines.

Where **environmental wrapping** is used, the procedure is simpler and faster. A careful routine must be developed for systematic removal of all plastic covering. Special purpose plastic bags and covers are available from dental houses but these are relatively expensive. Freezer bags, probably cheaper, are available from the supermarket and can in some instances be utilised instead.

If there is any suspicion that the plastic wrap has been compromised, all surfaces beneath them should be wiped with an appropriate detergent.

Note that cleaning and sterilisation of specific pieces of clinical equipment and instrumentation are also discussed in Chapter 16.

Instrument cleaning

Instruments and equipment are divided into three categories, based on the degree of risk of infection associated with their use. Examples are listed in Table 14.1.

Before instruments can be **sterilised** they must be properly cleaned. If an item cannot be cleaned, it cannot be sterilised. The **cleaning** process must:

- remove blood, saliva and pus, dried on cements and other materials from the instrument;

- not damage the item; and
- not further contaminate any item (e.g. by using dirty water).

The result must be a clean article with no residue of detergent, soap or brush bristles. The physical methods you use to remove the bio-burden are essential to the subsequent process of sterilisation.

Remember, it is impossible to sterilise dirty instruments. There is no such thing as sterile dirt. Saliva, blood, pus, oil or grease can encapsulate micro-organisms and protect them from the sterilising process. Alkaline material from ordinary soap may also protect bacteria, therefore thorough rinsing is essential. No method of sterilisation is able to penetrate materials adhering to surfaces.

The two methods of cleaning discussed here are manual cleaning and mechanical cleaning. Manual cleaning is most effective/essential for all articles such as mouth mirrors and handpieces, which could be damaged by being placed into an ultrasonic cleaner or washer/disinfector.

Mechanical cleaning in ultrasonic cleaners and washers/disinfectors is recommended for all other instruments as a very effective means of removing bio-burden.

Manual cleaning of instruments

Full personal protective equipment including domestic gloves must be used when cleaning instruments. As soon as possible after use instruments should be:

- collected — the task of cleaning cements and other filling materials is made easier if instruments are wiped immediately after use; if unable to wipe the instrument, keep the material pliable (soft, not set) by placing the instrument into a container with cold water until the end of the procedure;

Category	Application	Process	Example
Critical	Instruments and equipment which enter, or are capable of entering, tissue that would be sterile under normal circumstances.	Sterilisation	Instruments and equipment covered by this category include surgical instruments, implants, dental handpieces, ultrasonic scalers, stainless steel syringes, and matrix bands.
Semi-critical	Instruments and equipment which come into contact with non-sterile tissue (other than intact skin).	Disinfection	Instruments and equipment covered by this category includes prosthetic dental appliances, impression trays, impressions, one-way breathing valves, mouth props,
Non-critical	Instruments and equipment which come into contact with intact skin.	Cleaning	Instruments and equipment covered by this category include dental chairs, benches and linen.

Table 14.1 Three categories for processing reusable instruments

- dismantled or opened (scissors, for example) if possible;

- thoroughly rinsed in warm (not cold or hot) water to remove visible blood and body substances — cleaning with warm water assists in mechanical removal of soil and reduces the bio-burden;

- soaked, if necessary, in warm water and detergent that has been diluted to the manufacturer's recommendation; where there is gross contamination of instruments with proteins such as blood, an enzymatic cleaner may be utilised (this is not recommended for routine cleaning);

- scrubbed, if necessary, under cold or tepid (not hot), running water with the scrubbing action going away from the body;

- rinsed under hot (50–60°C) running water to initiate self-drying;

- inspected for left-over debris; and

- dried in a drying cabinet or with a lint-free cloth before sterilising.

Instruments should be washed in a deep sink to avoid splashing and aerosol spray. A long-handled dishwashing brush is ideal for preventing injuries when cleaning sharp instruments.

Selection of a detergent for cleaning

Check the label of any detergent you use. A good detergent should *comply with Australian/New Zealand Standard (AS/NZS) 4815* and be mildly alkaline in the *pH range of 8.0 to 10.8*. It should be:

- biodegradable;

- non-corrosive;

- non-toxic;

- low foaming;

- free rinsing;

- free from perfumes, emollients or lanolin; and

- detergent only and not a disinfectant/detergent mix.

Hand-washing liquid or household detergent are not suitable for cleaning instruments because they have a high volume of suds and can shorten the life of instruments quite dramatically.

Used diluted detergents should be disposed of at the end of the day. Spray or squeeze bottles must be completely dry before being refilled, to reduce the risk of microbial contamination. At the end of each day, any buckets used must be rinsed and turned upside down to dry.

Avoid abrasive cleaners. They scratch instruments and leave a residue.

Ensure you have material safety data sheets (MSDS) on all products.

Special cases for manual cleaning

Some articles are not suitable for ultrasonic cleaning and must be manually cleaned, such as:

- plastics and rubber that may be weakened;

- soldered instruments, as the solder gets eaten away in mechanical cleaners;

- instruments with lights or lenses that may be damaged or even fractured;

- glass (e.g. mouth mirrors, which will pit and flake); and

- fibre optics, which are very fragile.

Mechanical cleaning of instruments

Mechanical cleaning of instruments can be done by ultrasonic cleaners and/or washer/disinfectors.

Ultrasonic cleaners

Ultrasonic cleaners, if available and used properly, are efficient in removing bio-burden from the jointed and serrated instruments and burs used in dentistry.

Ultrasonic cleaners work by subjecting instruments to high-frequency, high-energy sound waves. These create tiny bubbles which, when they come into contact with a surface, implode. This creates a slight sucking action that causes soil to be dislodged from instruments. The soil then drops to the bottom of the tank or is sufficiently loosened to be removed by the rinsing process.

No part of the operator's body should be immersed in the detergent solution while the ultra-sonic cleaner is turned on. It can cause serious damage to tissues and is harmful to bone marrow.

Ultra sonic cleaners are not suitable for:

- rubber, soft plastic or wood;

- instruments that are plated;

- glass;

- instruments with solder or cement; or

- instruments with lights or a lens.

See Procedure 14.3 for more information.

Procedure 14.3 Using, maintaining and testing ultrasonic cleaners

- Manufacturers' instructions for the use and maintenance of ultrasonic cleaners should be strictly followed.

- Efficacy tests, such as the lead pencil or aluminium foil test, must be done daily and documented. Refer to manufacturers' instructions for details.

- Use only the recommended detergent, to the correct dilution, and follow manufacturers' instructions.

- De-gas the cleaner following manufacturer's instructions.

- Rinse all items thoroughly before placing them into the ultrasonic cleaner.

- Where possible, dismantle or open instruments before cleaning.

- Do not over-fill the container with instruments or it will not do its job properly.

- Lower instruments into the tank slowly so air is not reintroduced to the tank.

- Use a special receptacle for burs and other small items to facilitate retrieval. Special stands for diamond burs are recommended as they can prolong the life of the bur.

- Follow manufacturers' recommendations for the timing of the cleaning cycle. The time set for cleaning depends on the number of items placed in the ultrasonic cleaner. The larger the load, the longer the cycle.

- Always rinse and inspect the instruments carefully on completion. All blood and other matter must be removed.

- All instruments must be dried thoroughly with a lint-free towel (or in a drier, if available) before placing them into any type of steriliser.

- Change detergent and water at least daily and more frequently if visibly soiled.

- Make sure lids are in place before turning the machine on as the high sound frequency could possibly cause damage to hearing. The lid will also prevent aerosol from escaping from the tank.

- Most importantly, do not submerge any part of your body in the ultrasonic cleaner during operation. This can be harmful to the tissues of the hand and to the bone marrow.

The exterior of the tank, the lid and the gaskets should be cleaned daily. Water strainers and filters should be drained and checked daily.

Washer/disinfectors

There are small thermal washer/disinfectors on the market for use in dentistry. These are similar to domestic dishwashers but reach very high water temperatures. There are special trays and containers for holding instruments. Instruments/utensils must be positioned to ensure surfaces are exposed to the action of the water spray without dislodgement, and to allow drainage. Complete cassette systems, if used in the practice or clinic, can be placed into these machines.

Many of the same rules apply for the use of these machines as for ultrasonic cleaners. For example, instrument washers need to be regularly cleaned and maintained to prevent colonisation and formation of **biofilms** that could contaminate the instruments being processed. Manufacturer's instructions for operation and maintenance should be strictly followed.

A recommended detergent should be used as a cleaning agent. Enzyme cleaners should only be considered for articles heavily soiled with protein matter.

Successful cleaning removes all of the visible contaminants and approximately 80 per cent of the microbial population on instruments and equipment. The effectiveness of sterilisation depends on thorough cleaning.

Sterilisation methods

Sterilisation is the destruction of all forms of microbial life, including bacterial spores. It is an absolute term. An instrument or article is either sterile or it is not. There are no degrees of sterility. As an example, after a dental probe is soaked in a disinfectant solution for a few minutes we may speak of it as being decontaminated but micro-organisms may still be present on it, so it is not sterile.

The two principal methods of ensuring the sterility of instruments involve heat. This can be in the form of dry heat or, more effectively, dependably and economically, moist heat under pressure. This second method is called autoclaving and is discussed in more detail later in this chapter.

There are other means of effective absolute sterilisation and these are discussed briefly below. Although it is unlikely that any of these methods will be used in dental practice, they are useful to know about.

Dry heat sterilisers

These work using hot, dry air, just like baking ovens. A typical cycle is 160°C for 60 minutes, plus **penetration time**. The higher the temperature, the shorter the cycle. The disadvantage of dry heat ovens is that they are slow compared to autoclaves and time must be allowed for instruments to cool before use. Another disadvantage is that the high heat may damage sterilising bags and instruments.

Using dry heat sterilisers

- Always use the recommended temperature setting as specified in AS/NZS 4815 or AS/NZS 4187 because high heat can scorch and damage articles and instruments.

- Clean all debris from instruments before sterilising. Baked on cement could result in the instrument not being sterile.

- Thoroughly dry all instruments to be heat sterilised. This will prevent rusting and staining. Instruments should be dried in a drying cabinet or with a lint-free cloth.

- Correct loading is essential. The hot air must be able to circulate between all items.

Ethylene oxide

This is used to sterilise heat-sensitive items that cannot withstand temperatures greater than 60°C. These items usually come to the surgery pre-packaged and clearly labelled sterile. For example, silastic implants (e.g. breast implants), paper points and gutta percha points, sterile gauze squares and acrylic appliances (such as dentures) are sterilised in this way. Ethylene oxide sterilisers are often used in large hospitals. Because of their slow cycle (approximately six hours) they would not be considered useful in the dental setting.

Low temperature hydrogen peroxide plasma sterilisation

This is used to achieve low temperature/low moisture sterilisation.

Low temperature peracetic acid

Moist, low temperature peracetic acid is used to achieve low temperature sterilisation in an environmentally sealed chamber. It is designed to process instruments for immediate use but is rarely used in dental practices.

Nuclear or gamma radiation

Nuclear radiation is sometimes used commercially for items such as gauze that cannot withstand heat or gases.

Sterilisation by autoclaving

Autoclaves are sterilising machines that use moist heat, in the form of saturated steam under pressure, to sterilise. They are similar to a domestic pressure cooker or a car radiator. Under ordinary conditions water boils at 100°C. Increasing the temperature only increases the boiling action of the water. To raise the temperature at which water boils it is necessary to increase the pressure. The autoclave does this by preventing the steam from escaping. Autoclaves are recommended for all reusable articles because no living thing should be able to survive 15 minutes direct exposure to steam under pressure at 121°C heat.

Manufacturers' instructions for the use, maintenance, cleaning, calibration and testing of autoclaves should be strictly followed at all times.

Please refer to your local occupational health and safety authority for rules on the use of pressure vessels.

Types of autoclaves

There are two types of autoclaves available for use in office-based practices.

Portable (benchtop) steam sterilisers

These are the most commonly used autoclaves in dental practice. They are **downward displacement** steam sterilisers (classified as N class) usually in the form of an electrically operated bench-top unit. During each cycle, a volume of (de-ionised) water is boiled within the chamber space. The steam generated in this way expels the chamber air and heats the chamber and contents to the required sterilising temperature. Modern steriliser units have a drying cycle incorporated. Instrument packs (pouches, bags or wraps) can only be sterilised in autoclaves that have a drying cycle.

Pre-vacuum sterilisers

These sterilisers (classified as B class) remove air from the chamber before pumping in steam. They operate between 134° and 136°C. They provide a more effective method of air removal, providing a faster operating cycle and greater productivity. However, they require daily testing additional to that required by downward displacement sterilisers. See Procedure 14.4 for more information.

■ **downward displacement:** steam gradually replaces any air in the autoclave.

Packaging and wrapping items for sterilisation

The wrapping and packaging of items allows them to maintain their sterility by providing them with a barrier against contamination. The packaging and wrapping materials should allow air to be removed from the pack and steam to penetrate. The packs should not be so large that steam cannot penetrate all parts of all instruments in the pack or not allow the instruments to dry effectively. Autoclave pouches are available in different sizes and the appropriate size must be used for the size of the contents. If the contents of packs are wet after completion of sterilisation, then sterilisation has not been successful.

All instruments should be disassembled or opened prior to packaging. If a tray is used to package the instrument it should be a perforated tray to allow steam to circulate and to allow drying. Items should not be stacked within a package. Hollow items and items such as kidney dishes should be laid on their side and all facing the same direction. Items should not be able to move inside the packaging.

The different types of packaging materials and sterilising tape for sterilising reusable medical and surgical equipment are listed in the Australian/New Zealand Standard AS/NZS 4815 — 'Office based practice: Cleaning, disinfecting and sterilizing reusable medical and surgical instruments and equipment, and maintenance of associated environments in health care facilities'. Contact the local Standards Australia office for a copy.

Batch labelling and tracking

Each pack should be labelled with a soft, felt-tipped marking pen, rubber stamp or labelling gun. The label should include:

- a list of contents, and
- batch information which is the date, autoclave number (if there is more than one in the practice) and cycle number.

Procedure 14.4 Procedures for the use of autoclaves

- All autoclaves have specific instructions for use, maintenance, cleaning, calibration and testing. Manufacturers' instructions must be strictly followed at all times. Keep an operator's manual in the vicinity of the steriliser.

- Thoroughly clean and dry all instruments before they are packaged to go into the autoclave. Open instruments (scissors, for example) if possible.

- Items are packaged for sterilisation to allow aseptic removal of the contents of the pack from the steriliser when the cycle is complete.

- Laminated pouches are best positioned on their side in a rack to allow air or condensate to exit and to allow the entry of the sterilising agent (steam). Packages should not touch the walls of the autoclave.

- If a rack is not available, place instrument pouches carefully in a single layer, paper side down, to allow heat/steam penetration of all surfaces of all trays and instruments. Correct loading is essential for successful sterilisation. Crowding of instruments may result in incomplete sterilisation.

- Follow the manufacturers' instructions for cleaning, oiling, purging, packaging and temperature settings when sterilising handpieces.

- Monitor and validate the sterilising process constantly. A record book should be kept even if there are printouts available for the autoclave. All types of monitoring recommended by the Department of Health, NHMRC, and Standards Australia should be followed. Include chemical indicators with every package in every load.

The following table gives the recognised international temperature/pressure/time relationships for steam-under-pressure sterilisation.

°C	kpa	psi	Holding time (in minutes) plus safety factor
121	103	15	15
126	138	20	10
132	186	27	4
134	206	30	3

- Penetration time must be established and added to these **holding times**. Holding time is the length of time required for sterilisation after penetration time has been reached. Penetration time is the time required for the autoclave and its load to reach the correct temperature to achieve sterilisation. This time varies for each machine. The manufacturer's recommendations should be followed carefully to establish penetration time.

The sterilising process must be constantly monitored and validated. This is now compulsory under the Australian Standards. Contact local Standards Australia organisations to obtain copies of appropriate testing schedules and procedures.

Care should be taken with marking pens or rubber stamps that penetration of ink into the packet does not occur. For this reason, bags should be marked on the front laminate. Sharp-tipped, water–based or ballpoint pens should not be used as they may compromise the pack integrity.

Monitoring sterilisation

Sterilisation of dental equipment is so critical to an infection control program that a routine monitoring program is essential in every surgery. Such a routine should detect sterilisation failures as soon as possible after they occur so any equipment involved can be re-sterilised before it is used.

There is a wide range of specific tests to monitor the sterilising process. Depending on the type of autoclave in your practice, these tests could include:

- leak rate test;
- Bowie Dick type air removal test;
- air detector function test;
- air detector performance test;
- chemical indicators;
- biological indicators;
- enzymatic indicators;
- process challenge devices;
- data loggers; and
- thermocouples and digital readout thermometers.

These tests are described in more detail in Australian/New Zealand Standard AS/NZS 4815. You should have a copy of this standard in your practice and should refer to it, and to the manufacturer's instructions for your autoclave, to determine the correct tests and frequency of testing to be carried out.

The most commonly used tests are explained below.

Mechanical indicators

These are the charts, timers, gauges, printers and lights that are part of the sterilising equipment. However, these indicators only tell you about whether the machine has functioned or not, and cannot tell you whether any particular item is now sterile.

Chemical indicators

Currently, AS/NZS 4185 recommends that every tray of unwrapped items have a chemical indicator included and every wrapped item have a chemical indicator on or in the item. These indicators change colour according to whether one or more conditions of the sterilisation process were met (exposure to steam sterilisation conditions, for example).

Biological/enzymatic indicators

These indicators test all the variables of the sterilisation process and can show whether or not the conditions were sufficient to achieve sterilisation. These indicators contain live resistant spores. When these spores are killed it is safe to assume that other organisms in the load were also killed.

There are different types of biological indicators available and their instructions for use should be carefully followed. The type of indicator should also be selected according to the types of steriliser and load being processed.

The Bowie Dick type and leak rate tests

These tests are used before the first batch of the day in pre-vacuum sterilisers.

Record keeping

Australian/NewZealand Standard AS/NZS 4187 requires that daily records be kept of all monitoring processes undertaken in the surgery.

Flash sterilisation

Flash sterilisation is a process of putting unwrapped, un-bagged articles through a cycle in the autoclave. It should only be considered as an emergency measure for instruments that will be used within 20 minutes of being processed.

When using this method, instruments must be clean and dry, placed on the tray in a single layer and not touching. This sterilising cycle is not suitable for handpieces, which must always be bagged and autoclaved on the specially recommended cycle.

Flash sterilisation should never be used as an alternative to purchasing additional instruments or as a general time-saver. This is stated clearly in health department regulations.

In order to avoid any injury to patients, flash sterilised instruments must be completely cooled before being used.

Sterilisation problems

Certain articles and instruments pose special problems in sterilisation. Manufacturers of dental products are overcoming these and most items now come to us packaged and pre-sterilised. However, there may be occasions when some package is accidentally damaged or there has been a spillage (e.g. gutta percha points), so we need to know how to deal with these situations effectively.

Currently, Australian and New Zealand Standard AS/NZS 4187 states:

> Grossly soiled or damaged store packs should not be accepted. Dust shall be wiped from the store pack before it is opened. Sterile items shall be removed from the store pack before being brought into a clean area. Sterile items from external suppliers shall be inspected for cleanliness or damage to the unit packs or their contents.

Gauze squares, cotton rolls and pellets are not usually pre-sterilised. In fact, in some countries where they are manufactured there are no strict laws on aseptic procedures. For surgical, periodontic and endodontic procedures these items can be safely autoclaved in special bags or wrapped in calico. Dry heat can also be used but care must be taken to lower the temperature and to allow extra time to complete the cycle. All endodontic instruments, reamers, files and paper points can be dealt with in the same way.

Gutta percha points are easily contaminated in their small vials. They cannot be heat sterilised but should at least be immersed in isopropyl alcohol (70 per cent) for a few minutes before use.

Instrument disinfection

Disinfection is an extension of the cleaning process. It progressively reduces **pathogenic load**. However, disinfection is not a substitute for sterilisation. It is suitable if the instrument does not invade normally sterile tissue. It is not suitable for invasive (sharp) instruments (such as dental probes and matrix bands), which must be sterilised.

Disinfection is achieved by either thermal (heat) or chemical methods. Chemical disinfection may only be used where thermal methods are unsuitable or unavailable. Nowadays there are very few items for dental use that are not autoclavable or disposable.

Thermal disinfection

Two methods can be used for this process. They are:

❶ washer/disinfectors (as described previously in this chapter); and

❷ boiling water.

Many people believe boiling water to be an old-fashioned method of disinfection as it used to be the means of achieving sterilisation before the advent of autoclaves and dry heat sterilisers. However, it is recognised by Standards Australia as an efficient and cost-effective method of disinfection when used appropriately. It is not a method of sterilisation.

For thermal disinfection to be effective, all items must be clean before the disinfection process takes place and the temperatures and times specified in AS/NZS 4185 must be achieved.

Chemical disinfection

This method should only be used when it is impossible to sterilise or use thermal disinfection techniques (e.g. for soaking plastic instruments and appliances that cannot be heated). For the process to be effective, all items must be clean and dry before immersion in disinfectant.

A disinfectant specified in the Australian Register of Therapeutic Goods must be used and all relevant manufacturers' instructions followed. It is critical that the manufacturer's instructions for each individual chemical are followed. These instructions are not interchangeable for different chemicals.

Special lifting forceps (such as cheatles) should be used for lifting items out of chemical and thermal disinfectants. These forceps should be stored (not soaked) in a dry, dust free, covered container.

See Procedure 14.5 for more information.

Safe storage of instruments

Safe storage of instruments is another vital link in the chain of asepsis. Sterile items must be stored and handled in a manner that maintains the integrity of the packaging and prevents contamination from any source. This applies equally to items sterilised in the surgery and to the items purchased in pre-sterilised packages.

All instrument packs should be dated and inspected regularly for any damage to the packaging. Packs must only be handled with clean dry hands.

Sterile stock should be rotated systematically. This is why labelling that includes the date of sterilisation is so important.

Procedure 14.5 Using chemical disinfectants

- Thoroughly clean, rinse and dry all instruments to be disinfected before immersing them in the disinfectant. The presence of blood, pus, tissue fluid, soap or detergent seriously reduces the efficiency of even the best chemical disinfectant.

- Completely immerse objects to be disinfected for the length of time and at the concentration recommended by the manufacturer.

- Regularly wash containers used to store the diluted disinfectant. Solutions must be changed as recommended or if contaminated by debris.

- If still using disinfectants containing glutaraldehyde, ensure that they are used only when there is local exhaust ventilation.

- Follow manufacturers' instructions exactly. These chemicals have been designed to kill micro-organisms. If not handled with care they can cause great damage to humans. There have been many

cases of permanent allergies caused by the use and misuse of these products. Remember that stronger is not necessarily better but it can certainly cause more harm.

- Always make sure that the supplier encloses a material safety data sheet (MSDS) and study it before commencing use. Ask your dental supplier for a MSDS if one is not included with your order. Material safety data sheets are required by law and contain much valuable information about the product. Make up a folder of all these sheets for quick reference. Read them often to refresh your memory.

- Do not store instruments in solution. Immersion for the recommended time will destroy certain micro-organisms but instruments should then be removed, rinsed, dried and stored in a covered or sealed container. Dry storage is far more conducive to maintaining a disinfected status. Microbes generally need a liquid environment to thrive and survive.

If carefully stored under the right conditions, these items should be safe for use as long as the packaging has not been compromised.

Factors that compromise sterile stock include:

- incorrect cleaning procedures in the storage area;
- damaged or opened packaging;
- moisture and condensation;
- incorrect temperature;
- excessive exposure to sunlight and other sources of ultraviolet light;
- vermin or insects;
- inappropriate packaging materials;
- incomplete sealing;
- sharp objects or rough handling that may cause damage to the packaging materials; and
- incorrect handling during transportation.

In multi-member practices, procedures for careful storage, rotation and handling of sterile packages is essential. All staff must be trained and educated in handling sterilised items. Protocols and procedure manuals are mandatory.

See Procedure 14.6 (overleaf) for more information.

Laboratory asepsis

Impressions and prosthetic appliances can also be a source of cross-contamination. Impressions and appliances should be thoroughly cleaned and disinfected before being sent to or returned from

the laboratory. Some type of tag or sticker should be attached to the container to signify that the impression has undergone an acceptable form of disinfection.

Thorough, careful rinsing to remove saliva is the first essential step. Most impressions, alginate, rubber base or other material, can be effectively soaked in hypochlorite (household bleach) at the recommended dilution (2 per cent) for up to ten minutes but supplier's instructions for each individual material should be checked first. (Note that although hypochlorite can be used for disinfecting impressions, it is *not* registered by the Australian Register of Therapeutic Goods for disinfecting instruments.)

Procedures for in-house denture adjustments must also be developed. Full dentures can be safely soaked in hypochlorite. Chrome partial dentures may, depending on the **alloy** used, become tarnished or black if left in hypochlorite for a long time. Bite registration rims and try-ins also need to be decontaminated to avoid contaminating models and articulators. Polishing mops and cloths can be laundered and disinfected, even autoclaved.

Fresh pumice should be used for each new adjustment. Fully autoclavable surgery denture adjustment kits are available. These obviate the need for brushes and pumice.

Impression trays should either be disposable or must be thoroughly cleaned after soaking in a recommended solution for the removal of impression materials. Most trays are autoclavable.

- **alloy**: any mixture of metals. A silver/tin/copper/zinc alloy is used as a dental filling material when mixed with mercury.

Procedure 14.6 Handling and storing sterile stock

- The storage area should be cleaned using the correct procedures. Hands should be clean and dry when handling sterile equipment.

- Packaging should be checked for holes, moisture or other damage.

- Items should be rotated to ensure that those processed earlier are used before those sterilised more recently.

- Indicators must be checked to ensure that the packs have been through the steriliser.

- Packages should be kept dry. They should be cooled before placing in storage to prevent condensation forming.

- Packages should be protected from exposure to sunlight and other sources of ultraviolet light and from vermin or insects.

- Appropriate packaging materials should be used and packs should *not* be secured with staples, rubber bands or anything that could damage packaging.

- Packages should be checked to ensure that seals are complete.

- Take care during transportation of sterile items to avoid damaging packaging.

- Open shelving should be at least 250 mm above the floor and 440 mm below ceiling fixtures.

- Unwrapped items that will be used for invasive techniques must be re-cleaned and re-sterilised immediately prior to use.

- Instruments should not be stored in cardboard boxes as these are porous and can harbour micro-organisms and dust.

Instruments should be re-sterilised if:

- they are incorrectly wrapped or the wrapping or packaging is damaged or opened;

- the contents of the package are still wet when the cycle is complete or the package comes into contact with moisture;

- the package comes into contact with a dirty surface;

- there is no labelling on the package and it cannot be shown to have been sterilised;

- the storage area is not clean;

- the package has been exposed to sunlight or other ultraviolet light or to vermin or insects;

- the package is handled incorrectly or sharp objects in the package compromise the packaging;

- the wrong packaging materials are used; or

- the package is incompletely sealed.

Acrylic trimming burs and handpieces used for denture adjustments also need to be sterilised.

Single-use containers (e.g. a well-washed takeaway container) or sterilisable plastic containers are best for transporting impressions to and from the laboratory.

Laboratories must also disinfect the job that is being returned to the surgery. Some form of label, signifying the disinfection process has taken place, must be affixed to the parcel.

If you have a laboratory in the practice, it may also be your responsibility to keep it clean and tidy. The same rules apply as in caring for the surgery. Dust should be kept to a minimum and good exhaust and ventilation systems are essential.

Radiography asepsis

Research has shown that dental radiographic procedures can result in cross-contamination from one patient to another or to dental staff. It has also been demonstrated that some potentially pathogenic organisms can survive automatic processing.

Operators are usually well protected but infection control of the working environment (equipment, surfaces, etc.) is often neglected. It is essential that we follow infection control procedures in radiography so that any infection risk is 'as low as reasonably achievable' (the ALARA principle). The application of standard infection control procedures and commonsense will ensure that the risk of any cross-infection as a result of dental radiographic procedures is very greatly reduced.

See Procedure 14.7 for more information.

Reception and waiting room asepsis

These areas in the practice or clinic are often neglected but are just as important as the surgery. Remember, the patient's first impression of the practice is the waiting room and this impression must be favourable, providing confidence in the hygiene and the treatment given in the establishment. The office and reception area should also be neat and dust free and have the minimum of clutter.

Damp dusting should be carried out at least daily (first thing in the morning) but preferably at the completion of the morning session as well.

Any used cups need to be removed, water should be changed in vases with fresh cut flowers, carpeted areas should be vacuumed daily and vinyl floors should be swept and mopped.

The telephone receiver needs to be wiped over at least daily with a neutral detergent or antiseptic. Remember, more than one person is likely to use the telephone.

Office equipment such as computer keyboards must be wiped over regularly.

Any member of the dental team leaving the surgery should remove their gloves. Contaminated gloves and masks must be discarded and gowns should be removed before leaving the surgery area. Ensure that patient records are not handled with contaminated gloves.

Procedure 14.7 Maintaining radiography asepsis

Physical facilities and equipment

- Avoid touching walls and other environmental surfaces with contaminated gloves. Treatment rooms should be cleaned on a regular basis or as circumstances dictate (e.g. if contamination is known to have occurred, disinfection procedures should occur).

- Keep materials or instruments on surfaces that are either covered or satisfactorily disinfected. Think about equipment disinfection or wrapping of relevant surfaces.

- Cover all ear rods, chin rests, head positioners (and similar items that cannot be removed for cleaning and sterilisation) with a protective wrapping material or decontaminate them with a satisfactory surface disinfectant or neutral detergent.

- Set out supplies necessary for the procedure beforehand. Seat the patient, cover the patient with the lead apron and set the exposure before you glove up. All materials used during the procedure should be disposable or sterilised before using again.

- Carry out all bagging and disposal of all contaminated supplies in accordance with policy and regulations at national and local government levels.

Operative procedures

- Keep patient records well away from any contamination source.

- Wash hands both before and after wearing gloves. Appropriate decontamination procedures should be used for faucets and soap dispensers. Foot controls, and other methods to avoid hand contact, should be considered when new equipment is being installed.

- Wear gloves during all radiographic procedures and while handling all contaminated film packets, supplies and instruments. Gloves should also be worn during clean-up procedures.

- Use disposable wrap to cover work surfaces such as control panels, beam applicators, exposure switches, chair controls, ear rods, head stabilisers, etc. Surfaces that cannot be so protected should be decontaminated with a neutral detergent.

- Set out beforehand all film packets and necessary instruments. If additional films or other items are necessary these should be obtained from a co-worker or gloves should be changed. Do not put contaminated fingers into the bin holding unexposed film.

- Use plastic disposable film envelopes with attachable paper and bite tags.

Darkroom procedures

- Routinely clean all surfaces that may be contaminated by film packs.

- Use a disposable container such as a paper cup or paper towel to carry contaminated film packs to the darkroom. Access to the darkroom should not involve contamination of doors, door handles or other environmental surfaces.

- Wear gloves while handling contaminated film packs. If film packs are in barrier bags they can be dropped onto a clean covered surface and then processed with un-gloved hands once the barriers have been removed. Note that barrier bags are now available for most Kodak films, and this is the method of choice.

- If films are not in barrier bags they should be washed under running water to remove any adherent matter. They could then be placed in 2 per cent hypochlorite solution for three minutes, washed off again in water and processed. This is not a suitable technique for paper-backed (non-plasticised) film packets. Ensure that soaking bowls are covered or sealed to minimise solution vapour.

- The use of daylight loaders is not recommended since contamination is very difficult to avoid. If film packs are not removed from barrier bags before the daylight loader is used, the following procedure should be used.

  - Remove gloves and wash hands before using the loader.
  - Place gloves and the contaminated film packets inside the loader through the removable cover.
  - Put the hands into the loader and put on the gloves before handling the film packets.

- Remove gloves before hands are withdrawn.

- Do not wear gloves while receiving and mounting processed radiographs or while handling paperwork.

Disposal and recycling of surgery waste

The principle of all waste disposal is 'the generator of the waste is responsible for its disposal'. All states have legislation regarding general waste disposal. Some water boards have regulations for disposal of liquid waste from the surgery and all practices must make themselves familiar with these.

In waste disposal, each surgery needs a set of procedures that:

- prevent the spread of disease;
- protect the environment from the damage our waste products can cause; and
- protect the safety of the people who have to handle the waste.

Chemical disposal

All chemicals must be disposed of through a licensed waste disposal contractor. Check with local authorities.

Recycling

To be a really 'green' surgery there are many things that can be recycled. All packaging, cardboard, glass jars and bottles can be sorted. Silver recycling companies will collect used **amalgam** that has been carefully stored under water or spent x-ray fixer. They may also take radiographic developer and fixers that contain silver and are very toxic to our waterways. Local water authorities have regulations for disposing of chemicals used in the practice. The local councils will collect general waste.

Clinical waste

Clinical waste is waste that has the potential to cause sharps' injury, infection or offence. Clinical waste includes:

- sharps;
- human tissue (excluding teeth, hair and nails);
- blood; and
- visibly blood-stained body fluids and visibly blood-stained disposable material and equipment (e.g. cotton rolls and swabs after extractions).

Clinical waste should be collected in strong yellow plastic bags clearly labelled as infectious waste or carrying the bio-hazard symbol. Special contractors generally collect clinical waste. Special yellow bins are also required in some areas for collecting clinical waste.

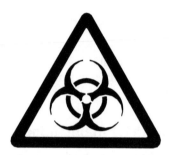

Figure 14.4 Biohazard symbol

Make sure you contact local authorities to determine legislation relating to the disposal of all waste generated by the surgery.

Disposal of sharps

Not all waste will be infectious but there are items we discard (e.g. injection needles, matrix bands and scalpel blades) that can be a hazard to those who handle them. The Occupational Health, Safety and Rehabilitation Council has laid down guidelines for the handling and disposal of 'sharps' in health facilities. This includes dental practices.

- Sharps containers should be made of rigid, impermeable material that can be sealed. These containers must meet AS/NZS 3825.
- Containers should have a wide mouth so that sharps can easily be placed in them but not so wide that a child could get a hand into the mouth. The size of the containers will depend on the needs of the practice.
- Containers should never be more than three-quarters full, to avoid accidental spillage.
- Containers are usually bright yellow in colour (the universal colour used to denote hazardous waste).

In any event, sharps containers must carry a label with a yellow background and black lettering with the wording 'Contaminated Waste — Sharps Only'. Sometimes you will find the international biohazard symbol on them as well.

Summary

Perhaps your most important responsibility in the surgery is the prevention of cross-infection. The best way to achieve this is to have in place, implement and adhere to a sound, comprehensive infection control program that is observed by all members of the dental team.

■ amalgam: any alloy in which one of the metals is mercury.

chapter fifteen
occupational health and safety

Introduction

There are national and state Occupational Health and Safety Acts that aim to protect the health, safety and welfare of people at work.

These Acts lay down general requirements that must be met at places of work in Australia and in each state. The provisions cover every place of work, self-employed people, employers and employees.

The National Occupational Health and Safety Commission (NOHSC) is a statutory body, with government, employer and employee representatives. Its mission is to lead and coordinate national efforts to prevent workplace death, injury and disease in Australia.

Penalties

It is an offence not to comply with an Act and it can result in a hefty fine, or the issuing of an improvement or prohibition notice. Some states and territories can issue on-the-spot-fines. It is important to know that a breach of an Act does not have to result from a person being injured. Not meeting the requirements of an Act constitutes a breach even if no injury occurs.

Penalties differ between states/territories but can be several hundred thousand dollars for companies and several thousand dollars for individuals.

Appendix 1 lists places where you can get a copy of the Acts that apply to your state or territory.

All employers and employees should be aware of their obligations under these regulations.

Employers' duties under the Act

Duty of care

Occupational Health and Safety Acts require employers and employees to exercise a 'duty of care'. This means they must anticipate possible causes of injury and illness and do everything reasonably practicable to remove or minimise these.

Employers must:

- provide and/or maintain equipment and systems of work that are safe and without risk to health;
- provide information, instruction, training and supervision necessary to ensure the health and safety at work of employees;
- maintain places of work under their control in a safe condition and provide and maintain safe entrances and exits; and
- make available adequate information about research and relevant tests of substances used at work.

Employers must not require employees to pay for anything required to meet specific requirements made under the Act.

Employers and self-employed people must also ensure the health and safety of people visiting their place of work who are not their employees.

In summary, employers must ensure:

- safe property, which includes premises (safe access and exit), safe plant and equipment, materials and substances (raw materials, chemicals, products, stock, etc);

- safe systems of work, which includes your work practices, standard operating procedures and administration procedures; and

- safe staff, which includes providing them with suitable information, instruction, training and supervision. For example, staff who know the safe use of plant and equipment, materials and chemicals and information about the working environment and health and safety generally.

Employers may be breaching the Act if they:

- do not provide adequate resources and training to improve health and safety;

- ignore medical opinion reports of work-related injuries including overuse injuries or stress-related illnesses;

- ignore or do not take seriously a complaint about safe practices from employees or patients;

- require an employee to complete a new job task without first assessing if there is a risk to that employee's health and safety; and

- do not provide employees with safety and health information about a chemical they are using.

Employees' duties under the Act

Employees also have duties. They must:

- be in good health and have a high standard of personal hygiene;

- take reasonable care for the health and safety of persons who are at their place of work;

- be aware of protocols following exposure to blood and body substances;

- co-operate with their employer in making sure that the employer does not breach the Act or any other safety provisions;

- not intentionally or recklessly interfere with or misuse anything that has been provided in the interest of health and safety; and

- not aid or abet any other person in breaching the Act.

Note that it is a duty of the employer to provide training to employees so that employees are aware of the responsibilities and procedures they must follow.

Written safety rules should be issued to all employees and a signed acknowledgment of receipt of the safety rules should be kept with employee records.

Keeping records

Legislation requires that you keep records regarding OHS practices in your workplace. Employer associations, unions and state or territory OHS organisations should be able to tell you what records need to be kept and for how long. All employees should know these record-keeping requirements.

A first aid kit is obligatory in the workplace. An injury register should be kept with it. This register should list every injury that occurs and contain medical certificates if required, workers compensation forms if required, relevant reports to government authorities, etc.

Developing protocols and procedures

Protocols are lists of procedures that are to be carried out in the same way every time they are performed. By following the same, safe routines each time, you reduce the chances of cross-infection.

There are many protocols required in the dental setting. Some examples are provided in this text but each workplace will need to develop sets of protocols that meet local needs, while still conforming to sound infection control practices and local legislation.

Changing procedures

Any changes that occur in the workplace have an impact on employees and may require changes in the protocols. Each change (e.g. new suppliers of chemicals or new chemicals, new staff, new equipment) should be considered in light of its implications for health and safety, and protocols should be updated as required.

Some safety symbols you will see in the dental setting are shown in Figure 15.1.

Occupational health and safety in the dental surgery

Issues of concern in the dental setting

Some of the risks in the dental setting are:

- exposure to infectious diseases;
- handling hazardous substances;
- use of gasses (e.g. nitrous oxide);

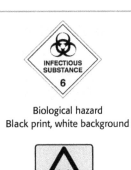

Biological hazard
Black print, white background

Non-flammable, non-toxic gas
Black print, green background

Toxic chemicals
Black print, yellow background

Caution, risk of ionising, radiation
Black print, yellow background

No smoking
Black text, red circle

Not drinking water
Black text, yellow circle

Do not enter; No access
Black text, red circle

Laser beam
Yellow print, black background

No sharps to be placed in this receptacle
Black print, yellow background

Figure 15.1 Safety symbols in use in the dental setting

- exposure to radiation;
- respiratory system damage;
- occupational overuse injuries;
- back injury;
- foot and leg injuries;
- industrial deafness;
- stress; and
- latex allergies.

The risks due to exposure to infectious diseases and the methods that can be used to reduce those risks are covered in detail in the previous chapter.

The other risks listed are discussed briefly in the following pages. Remember that each state and territory has different legislation dealing with safety in the workplace and you should contact one of the organisations listed in Appendix 1 to get information specific to your own working conditions.

Personal hygiene and protective apparel

Personal hygiene and personal protective equipment (PPE) are integral to Standard and Transmission Based Precautions. All dental staff have to adhere to a very high standard of personal hygiene and presentation. You and the dentist should wear:

- Gloves for all patient treatment — new gloves should be worn for each patient and torn gloves should be replaced. Gloves should be removed before touching charts, records, phone, etc. Hands must then be re-washed and new gloves put on.

- Protective eyewear — in the form of plastic glasses with side flaps, or a full face shield if undertaking procedures that produce aerosol spray.

- Masks — which must be changed after each patient and more often if the wearer has a cold or the mask becomes moist.

- General purpose household gloves — to be used when cleaning instruments. These can be washed and reused but should be discarded when they become peeled, cracked, discoloured, torn or punctured.

- Protective gowns — clothing contaminated with blood or body substances should be removed as soon as possible.

- Shoes — sturdy, enclosed shoes with non-slip soles should be worn.

If there is a likelihood of splashing or contamination with blood or other body fluids during a procedure (e.g. implant surgery) a fluid-resistant gown or apron made of impervious material must be worn.

Do *not* wear:

- jewellery on hands or wrists, even under gloves (pinned-on watches are preferable to wrist watches);
- cardigans or jumpers with loose, dangly sleeves;

- protective clothing, such as gowns or 'pop-overs', outside the treatment area; or
- work uniforms when travelling to and from work.

In addition:

- hair should be clean and, if long, tied back;
- fingernails should be kept short and clean with no nail polish and no artificial nails; and
- any cuts or open sores must be covered with a suitable waterproof dressing.

Hand-washing

Hand-washing is the single most important procedure for preventing cross-infection.

See Procedure 15.1 for more information.

Procedure 15.1 Effective hand-washing

Essential steps are:
1. Palm to palm.
2. Right palm over left dorsum, left palm over right dorsum.
3. Palm to palm, fingers interlaced.
4. Backs of fingers to opposing palms with fingers interlaced.
5. Rotational rubbing of right thumb clasped over left palm and left thumb over right palm.
6. Rotational rubbing backwards and forwards with clasped fingers of right hand in palm of left hand and vice versa.

Rub hands and wrists until the end of a 30-second period.

Note: Number of strokes in each step is five.

Hands must be washed:
- before and after patient contact;
- each time gloves are changed;
- before leaving the surgery;
- after handling soiled or contaminated items;
- before meals, and
- after using the toilet.

Meticulous attention should be paid to washing the nails and **interdigital spaces** for a minimum of 15 seconds. Any shorter time has the effect of increasing the bacterial count. (This does not occur with a bactericidal skin cleanser. However, all products used must be suitable for repetitive use.)

Re-usable bristle nail brushes are not recommended, even for nails.

Liquid soap must always be used. Bar/cake soap must never be used as the slimy coating on wet soap left for a while is actually a layer containing gram-negative bacteria.

Soap containers should never be topped-up. All soap should be used and the container and pump thoroughly cleaned and dried before the container is re-filled.

To dry hands, disposable paper towels must always be used.

Hand basin taps can be foot or infra-red controlled to avoid contamination. If not, taps should be turned off using an elbow or paper towel.

A protective hand lotion or cream that is compatible with the hand-washing solution can be used before and after work to prevent chapped and cracked skin but should not be applied during the working day.

Diseases of concern to dental assistants

There are a number of diseases that are or primary concern to dental assistants as they are the diseases most likely to be transmitted in the dental setting.

HIV/AIDS

HIV is a disease that weakens the immune system. It is a virus and is blood-borne. A person with the disease may have no symptoms and may not be aware that they have the disease. When symptoms develop, the carrier of the disease is said to have AIDS. Patients with HIV are often more susceptible to other diseases and may also have diseases such as hepatitis.

Hepatitis

There are many different forms of hepatitis and they have different severity. All affect the liver in some way. Hepatitis can be caused by viral infection as

■ **interdigital spaces**: the spaces between the fingers.

well as by drug reactions and by other diseases. The viral forms are of most concern in the dental setting.

Herpes virus

There are four different forms of the herpes virus. It is spread through contact with the lesions that are formed, often in or around the mouth or nose. Gloves will protect the hands, although there is also some risk through aerosols produced by the handpiece. Protective glasses should always be worn because an infection in the eye can cause blindness.

Other diseases of concern

These include tetanus, measles, mumps, rubella, tuberculosis, syphilis and legionnaires' disease.

Immunisation

Immunisation (vaccination) can help to prevent disease and all members of the dental team should be immunised against preventable diseases.

Diseases that currently have vaccinations available include hepatitis B, measles, varicella, mumps, rubella, tetanus, tuberculosis (TB) and influenza.

Immunisation for hepatitis B requires a series of vaccinations and a post-vaccination test to ensure that the treatment has been successful. There is no vaccine for hepatitis C at the current time.

If working in an area where there is a risk of TB infection, staff should also be immunised against TB. See Procedures 15.2 and 15.3 for more specific information.

Procedure 15.2 Dealing with blood and body substance spills

The Department of Health Infection Control policy is as follows. In the event of spills, staff involved in the management should immediately:

- Don protective apparel including gloves.
- Confine and contain the spill. Cover the spill with paper towels to absorb the bulk of the blood or body substances.
- Treat debris as clinical waste.
- Clean the spill site with neutral detergent and water. If there is carpet in the practice and a spill has occurred it is likely that the products necessary to clean will cause damage. Spills on carpets should be managed as follows:
  - Mop as much of the spill as possible using disposable towels.
  - Clean with a neutral detergent and arrange for the carpet to be shampooed with an industrial carpet cleaner as soon as possible.

Procedure 15.3 Dealing with exposure to blood or body fluids

If anyone in the surgery is exposed to blood or body fluids, the following should occur immediately.

- If the skin is penetrated, the area should be washed thoroughly with soap and or water. If water is not available, alcohol-based rinses or foams can be used.
- Any blood on the skin should be washed well with soap and water.
- If fluids get into the eyes, the open eyes should be thoroughly rinsed with water or normal saline.
- If blood gets in the mouth, it should be spat out and then the mouth should be rinsed with water several times.

The accident should be reported to the dentist in charge immediately and an accident form filled in, stating:

- the date and time of exposure;
- the type of exposure (instrument and/or body substance involved, whether PPE was worn, etc.);
- how the accident occurred; and
- the name of the source individual (if known).

If the patient is known to have HIV or hepatitis, the person exposed to the body fluids or blood should be immediately assessed by a doctor with experience in this area.

Employers' responsibilities

Employers should:

- Ensure that the exposed area has been washed thoroughly and an accident report form filled in.
- Arrange for the employee to attend a healthcare facility where the risk can be assessed, counselling offered and a blood test arranged if there has been possible or definite parenteral exposure. The results of the employee's blood test are not required to be disclosed to the employer.
- Contact the source to organise for blood to be taken (informed consent required), to be tested for HIV antibody, hepatitis B surface antigen (ABsAg) and hepatitis C antibody (anti-ACV).
- Ensure that the employee gets professional support and counselling.
- Notify the insurer as for any other workplace injury. The details of the employee's medical record and blood test results do not need to be disclosed to the insurer unless there is a later acquisition of an infection.

These procedures are based on procedures outlined by the National Occupational Health and Safety Committee and WorkCover Australia.

Hazardous chemicals

Dental surgeries use a range of chemicals for disinfecting, sterilising, processing x-rays and treating patients. All of these chemicals can be absorbed by the body and if absorbed in large enough quantities, can be harmful. The harm may be immediate, if a large amount of chemical is absorbed in a short time, or the harm may be cumulative. That is, the effects may build up over a long period — maybe even years. In some cases, the build up of chemicals can cause cancer, have an effect on fertility, affect the development of foetuses, or cause other illnesses.

Some chemicals may be fire risks or may be dangerous if mixed with other chemicals. Some chemicals are corrosive. That is, they can burn skin or other surfaces. Chemicals should be kept in a cool, dry place where they are not exposed to sunlight. Container lids should be tightly closed. The minimum number of chemicals should be stored. Chemicals should be kept away from flames and heat.

It is possible for chemicals to be absorbed by the body through:

- inhalation (that is, the chemicals in the form of vapour, dust or gases are breathed in);
- skin contact (normally, skin is a good barrier but some chemicals can be absorbed through the skin); and
- ingestion (chemicals are accidentally swallowed).

The best method of protection is to block the chemicals from entering or coming in contact with your body.

To prevent inhalation of chemicals, a mask should be worn when working with chemicals. The mask should be fluid repellent and should allow easy breathing. Good ventilation is necessary and some surgeries require special exhaust systems in the darkrooms and sterilisation areas.

To prevent skin contact, thick rubber gloves should be worn when handling chemicals. The latex gloves used for treatment of patients are not sufficient protection. Depending on the chemical, it may also be necessary to wear a thick rubber apron to prevent staining or burning. Hands should be washed immediately after gloves are removed.

Safety goggles should be worn whenever handling chemicals. An eye wash unit should be available for emergencies and all employees should be trained in its proper use.

It is possible to accidentally ingest chemicals by eating without washing hands first, or eating in an area where chemicals are used. There should be no eating, drinking or applying makeup in areas where chemicals are used.

Material safety data sheet (MSDS)

Each chemical supplier should also supply a material safety data sheet (MSDS). Material safety data sheets contain information about the handling, use, storage and disposal of industrial chemicals, especially those classified as hazardous substances.

An MSDS should contain:

- identifying information about the product;
- complete health hazard information;
- precautions for use; and
- safe handling instructions.

These sheets should be stored in a folder and additional copies should be kept with each chemical.

An inventory of all chemicals should be kept in addition to MSDSs. Contact your local National Occupational Health and Safety Commission office for copies of the guidelines about MSDSs. Manufacturers' instructions for the use of chemicals should always be followed. Read the instructions carefully and do as directed.

All containers should be clearly labelled with the name of the chemical, any associated hazards and a use-by date. Some chemicals change over time and lose their effectiveness so a use-by date should be clearly written on each chemical container.

Most manufacturers' labels have this information but if the chemical is transferred to another container, that container should also be labelled, even if the transfer is simply the dilution of fresh disinfectant to go in a squeeze/squirt bottle. Chemicals should not be mixed with other chemicals unless the result is known.

Chemical containers should be disposed of appropriately. Remember that empty containers can be dangerous as they hold residues that may explode. Your MSDS should contain information about the best way to dispose of the container. Other materials should never be poured into empty containers because of the risk of reaction with residues in the container.

Contact state authorities for information about legislation and services relating to chemical disposal.

Other chemical risks

Handling mercury

Mercury is a potential health hazard in the dental surgery. The risk comes from mercury vapour in the air and from handling mercury or mercury-containing compounds because they can be absorbed through the skin and the lungs.

Mercury is extremely toxic. Even very small levels of exposure are dangerous, especially for pregnant women. Inhalation should be avoided completely. For example, when amalgams are polished, small particles of mercury become airborne. A mask should be worn to prevent the inhalation of these particles.

All staff involved in the handling of mercury should understand the necessity for observing careful mercury hygiene practices.

The workspace should be well ventilated. Air filters, such as those in air-conditioners, may act as mercury reservoirs and should be replaced periodically.

Water spray and high volume evacuation should be used when removing old, or finishing new, amalgam restorations. Appropriate masks should be worn to prevent the inhalation of amalgam dust.

Amalgam or mercury must *never* be heated. All instruments contaminated with amalgam must be thoroughly cleaned before autoclaving.

There should be no skin contact with the mercury and the vapour should not be inhaled. The cover of the amalgamator should be closed before starting the machine. A no-touch technique should be adopted with mercury and amalgam at all times. Skin accidentally contaminated by mercury should he washed thoroughly with soap and water.

Mercury should be stored under water in tightly sealed, unbreakable containers. It should be stored somewhere cool and dry, and out of the reach of children.

Waste systems into which amalgam scrap may enter (e.g. cuspidors, sinks, suction systems) should be provided with plastic traps from which the scraps can be recovered and stored. All amalgam scraps and left-over amalgam from capsules should be collected and stored in a tightly closed container (strong plastic with a narrow neck) under spent (used) radiographic fixer. Scrap amalgam that has been removed from dental unit traps should be disinfected in bleach and water and then placed in the scrap container. Any waste contaminated with mercury or amalgam should be placed in a polyethylene bag and sealed.

Only capsules that remain sealed during amalgamation should be used. (The seal can be tested by wrapping sticky tape around the join in the capsule.) An amalgamator with a completely enclosed arm should be used. The capsules should be re-assembled immediately after dispensing the amalgam mass (to reduce the spread of mercury vapour from the capsule).

Any spilled mercury must be cleaned up immediately. Appropriate procedures should be used to clean mercury spills. Mercury can be collected with narrow bore tubing attached to the low volume aspirator of the dental unit, or sucked up into a syringe through a wide bore needle. Household vacuum cleaners and high-volume evacuators should not be used.

Sticky tape wrapped around the hand, sticky side out, is useful for picking up small droplets. Sulphur made into a paste of sulphur and lime can be spread in areas that are difficult to reach. However this produces only a film coating and will be effective only while the mercury droplets remain undisturbed.

(The information provided in the above section was developed from NHMRC recommendations on dental mercury hygiene.)

Using nitrous oxide

Nitrous oxide is used in the dental surgery to calm patients. It is possible for members of the dental team to be exposed to dangerous levels of the gas while it is being administered to patients.

Long-term exposure can lead to a range of diseases such as kidney and liver disease and cancer. Nitrous oxide exposure can also cause spontaneous abortion.

As nitrous oxide is inhaled by the patient through a mask, it is possible to have a scavenger system attached to the mask. This catches the escaping nitrous oxide as the patient breathes. Additionally, levels of nitrous oxide in the room should be monitored.

Exposure to radiation

Occupational exposure to radiation is the accidental exposure to radiation at work. In the dental surgery, radiation is used to produce dental x-rays (radiographs).

There is no reason why you should be exposed to unsafe, or indeed any, levels of radiation if all appropriate precautions are taken.

Pocket dosimeters

These are small badges that are worn by the person taking radiographs or at any risk of exposure. The badge measures the levels of occupational exposure to radiation. These badges are processed by the company that provides them and a report is given showing the employee's recent and accumulated radiation levels. This report should be kept with the employee records.

The instructions provided by the manufacturer should be followed carefully.

X-ray machines

These must be monitored to ensure that there is no radiation leaking from broken components. Each machine should come with instructions for how to monitor it for leakage and all employers should be aware of their duties in relation to monitoring equipment. Annual inspection by the radiation branch of the Environmental Protection Agency (EPA) is mandatory.

Physical barriers

These can provide protection from radiation. For example, some surgeries have a lead wall that x-ray machine operators can stand behind. In other instances, the operator can be safe by leaving the room.

If the operator must stay in the room, they must not stand in the line of the primary beam. The safest place to stand is at a right angle to or behind the primary beam, at least two metres from the x-ray unit.

Remember, frequent exposure to radiation can cause you harm if you do not take the necessary precautions to avoid exposure.

The National Health and Medical Research Council (NHMRC) has published a Code of Practice for Radiation Protection in Dentistry. It can be obtained from the NHMRC and relates to intra-oral radiography, periapical, bitewing and occlusal views, panoramic radiography, intra-oral tube radiography and panoramic topography, radiography of the complete skull and of certain parts of the dento-maxillo-facial region.

The code states requirements for:

- allocation of responsibility and need for clinical assessment of the indications for radiography;
- provision of appropriate equipment, film and processing facilities; and
- adoption of procedures to minimise exposure to radiation.

Ergonomic issues

Ergonomics

The science of ergonomics uses an understanding about how the human body works to design products and environments that are comfortable, safe and efficient to use. Good workplace design and work habits can reduce the risk of occupational hazards such as neck and shoulder pain, headaches, back pain and foot pain. The workplace should be organised so that bending, twisting, reaching, and extension and flexion of the wrist and shoulder, are kept to a minimum.

Dental stools should be adjustable and should have a proper back support. They should allow the whole body to turn in order to reach equipment, rather than just the head and shoulders. Equipment and instruments should be placed in positions that allow them to be reached without straining or twisting.

Occupational overuse syndrome

Occupational overuse syndrome (OOS) is also known as repetitive strain injury (RSI). It is caused by repetitive movement of the arms or the maintenance of awkward postures and causes pain in muscles, tendons and soft tissues in the back, neck, shoulder, elbows, wrists, hands or fingers.

Carpal-tunnel syndrome can also be a problem for dental assistants. The tendons that run through the carpal tunnels in the wrist become swollen and inflamed by repetitive motions.

These kinds of injuries are painful, can be disabling and can result in substantial workers compensation claims. They are also common in the dental surgery. This is because dental assistants are often sitting or standing in twisted or contorted positions in order to assist the dentist. However, proper surgery design and good work habits and posture can alleviate or avoid many of the headache, neck and shoulder and back pains.

Workplaces should be designed to allow comfortable and safe work practices. Chairs and equipment should be designed and placed at the correct height and in positions that reduce strain and repeated movements. Stools should be ergonomically designed and equipment and materials should be easily accessible and not require twisting or stretching to reach or operate.

Repetitive and non-repetitive activities should be interspersed where possible and if a job cannot be varied there should be frequent short breaks.

State and territory OHS organisations have information sheets about preventing OOS.

Other potential sources of injury

Handling sharps

- Use a puncture-resistant tray or kidney bowl to pass sharp instruments from hand to hand.
- Pass injection syringes out of sight of the patient with the sheathed needle away from the operator.
- Only recap needles if absolutely necessary and keep them well away from other instruments on the bracket table.
- If re-capping is the policy of the practice, it should be done by the operator. If re-sheathing is required too, the following rules apply.
  - The needle must be properly recapped.
  - The sheath must not be held in the fingers.
  - Either a single-handed technique or long forceps, or a suitable guard designed for the purpose, should be used. Preferably, this should be done by the dentist.
- Dispose of non-reusable sharps in puncture-resistant containers immediately after use.
- Place reusable sharps in a puncture-resistant container immediately after use and keep them in there until ready for cleaning and sterilising.
- Some practices have adopted the rule 'the person who uses, disposes of sharps', with good results. Each person handling sharps has responsibility for their correct management and disposal.
- Sharps containers should be made of rigid, impermeable material that can be sealed.
- Containers should have a wide mouth so that sharps can easily be placed in them but not so wide that a child could get a hand into it. The size of the containers will depend on the needs of the practice.
- Containers should never be more than three-quarters full, to avoid accidental spillage.
- Containers are usually bright yellow in colour (the universal colour used to denote hazardous waste).

In any event, they must carry a label with a yellow background and black lettering with the wording 'Contaminated Waste — Sharps Only'. Sometimes you will find the international bio-hazard symbol on them as well.

Industrial deafness

Industrial deafness results from repeated exposure to excessive noise over a period of time and is permanent. Noise can be caused by equipment in the dental surgery and can be continuous or sporadic.

Contact your state or territory OHS authority for information and assistance in establishing a noise control program.

Respiratory damage

Damage to the airways can sometimes be caused by exposure to chemicals. Applying good principles of occupational health and safety can minimise the risks.

Latex allergies

Some dental assistants develop hypersensitivity to the latex rubber in gloves and other pieces of equipment in the surgery. In some cases this takes the form of dermatitis where the skin becomes cracked, irritated, red and sore. Other forms of allergy can be much more serious and can result in death, as they involve the immune system.

There is currently no treatment for latex allergies and if they are suspected it is necessary to see a doctor to confirm the allergy, and contact with latex in all forms should be avoided.

Eye damage

Infection and injury of the eyes can take place where care is not taken to protect the eyes. Wear protective eyewear with side shields to minimise the risk of damage to the eyes and be sure that an eyebath is available in the first aid kit and all members of the dental team are aware of how to use it.

Foot injury

Enclosed shoes should be worn at all times in the surgery to reduce the risk of injury should equipment be dropped on the feet or chemicals spilled.

Non-dangerous spills

Materials that may be spilt in the dental surgery, and which are not necessarily dangerous, include:

- Cavity varnish — this may be difficult to remove. Use trial and error methods. Try using various solvents (e.g. ether, alcohol).

- Iodine —stains may be removed from clothing with x-ray fixer, followed by washing in water.

- Impression materials — the worst of these from the point of view of staining are the lead dioxide-containing, rubber-based (polysulphide) materials. Solvents such as dry cleaning spirits should be used before the material sets.

- Inlay wax — this can be removed with a hot instrument and blotting paper over the material. The blue colour may remain and should be removed with chloroform.

- Silver nitrate — wash immediately with a solution of common salt in water, and follow this with x-ray fixer, and then wash with an ample flow of water.

- X-ray developer — solutions can be made up by a pharmacist to help remove the stains.

- Hypochlorite — this can bleach colour from clothing.

Summary

There is a wide range of OHS risks in the dental setting. These were described in general terms in this chapter. For specific information regarding legal requirements, refer to the appropriate organisation in your state or territory, as listed in the Appendix.

The NOHSC website (*http://www.nohsc.gov.au/*) has information about Acts and regulations regarding occupational health and safety in Australia. The website also has a great deal of information about identifying hazards in the workplace and solving workplace safety problems.

chapter sixteen
surgery equipment and its maintenance

Introduction

There is a range of equipment and instruments that you will use in the surgery; from large items such as the dental unit or x-ray processor, to small items such as matrix bands and burs. You will need to be familiar with the use of these items as well as their maintenance and care.

Equipment maintenance

Dental equipment must be properly maintained both to extend its life and to ensure that it does not become a means of spreading infection. If there is more than one dental assistant working in the practice, routines should be developed and tasks designated to ensure that maintenance is done on a regular basis.

Surgery equipment (sometimes referred to as plant) is expensive and it should not be neglected or treated carelessly. If in doubt about cleaning of equipment or its maintenance, refer to your employer. Do not leave it because you do not know how to do it.

Surgery equipment must also be cleaned properly as part of infection control in the surgery.

Surgery equipment

The functional operating stool

For comfort while in the seated position, your feet should rest on the foot bar provided on the assistant's chair, with your thighs horizontal. An operating stool must be adjustable to the correct height for vision. You should be seated at least 5 cm higher than the dentist.

You should hold your back as upright as possible while working and, to reduce strain on the back muscles, the backrest of the stool is often designed to be turned around to the front to support the upper body around the waist. It is often called a 'belly bar'.

The stool must be mobile. For this purpose, most stools are equipped with castors.

The contour dental chair

To provide good access and vision for a seated dentist, the patient's head should be virtually in the dentist's lap, with the mouth opening almost vertically upwards. Modern dental chairs provide this by enabling the patient to be placed in the supine position (horizontally on the back) and by supporting the body comfortably along its whole length. For most dental procedures the chair should be inclined so that the patient's nose is at the same level as the patient's knees. This position is far more comfortable and relaxing for most people than the upright position. It is only contraindicated for a few dental procedures, and in the case of patients with some uncommon illnesses, or elderly patients who are used to a seated position and who are uneasy lying down.

The inclination of the chair to the correct angle may be made when you have seated the patient. The raising or lowering of the chair to the correct height is usually carried out by the dentist after he or she is seated. Apart from adjustments of the chair as a whole, the patient's head can be positioned at different angles to facilitate work on different parts of the mouth. For treatment of the upper arch, the head is generally tilted back further than for the lower arch. Rotation of the head to one side often gives improved access to different areas.

Learn to adjust the chair smoothly and efficiently. If the seat pad is removable, lift it out each week and dust the surrounds. Wipe over the armrest and head rest after each patient. If disposable head rest napkins are used, they should be changed after every patient.

Cleaning the dental chair

Switches and buttons on the dental chair, even if covered in plastic, should be wiped between patients. In fact, the whole chair should be wiped down. Once again, a neutral detergent is recommended unless the manufacturer instructs otherwise. Using the wrong cleaning agent for chairs may void the guarantee by the manufacturer. Make sure detergent does not get into the joints and moving parts of the chair as it can cause corrosion and breakdowns. Do not spray indiscriminately — spray or use a squirt bottle into a cloth or paper towel.

Foot controls

Foot controls should be clean and free of dust. Keep the controls close to the foot of the operator with the cord untwisted and away from your stool and the dentist's stool.

The functional dental unit

The dental unit consists of the mechanics that operate the handpieces, saliva aspirator and the air-water (triplex) syringe. It usually carries attachments for the handpieces, too. The unit also contains the controls that allow each piece of equipment to be adjusted. The type of dental unit used in the surgery will depend on the design of the surgery and the preferences of the dentist.

In most units there is a bracket table or tray attached to a jointed arm so that it may be brought close to the operating area. This is usually:

- mounted on the tray bracket or a similar arm;
- fitted in a separate mobile unit on the right of the chair; or
- fitted in a cabinet behind the chair.

Every unit has a master switch. This must be turned off every night, and turned on first thing every morning. Failure to do this can result in a short circuit with consequent damage to a valuable piece of equipment or even a fire.

Most dental units no longer have engine arms and cords. Handpieces are driven by miniature air-driven or electric motors mounted as part of the handpiece itself and these are connected to the unit by flexible hoses or cords. Manufacturer's instructions regarding cleaning and maintenance must be followed closely because these instruments run at very high speeds and thus can be rapidly damaged if lubrication is inadequate. Care must be taken to avoid damage to the flexible hoses and cords.

Water lines

The unit contains water lines that feed the handpieces and air-water syringe. These must be properly maintained to ensure there is no build-up of pathogens in the lines. Many dental units are fitted with bottled, filtered water for use in water lines. To try to reduce the risk of contaminated water entering the patient's mouth, the handpieces should be run for 30 seconds after each use. All manufacturer's instructions for cleaning and care of the unit should be carefully followed. The water lines should be run for several minutes at the beginning and end of each day.

Air-water syringes/triplex

These pieces of equipment have removable heads made either of metal or plastic. The metal heads can be sterilised after each patient but the plastic heads should be disposed of after each patient. The tip used by both the clinician and the assistant to retract the lip must be sterilised.

Ultrasonic scalers

Ultrasonic scalers must also be purged for 20 seconds, the scaler tips removed and autoclaved after thorough cleaning. Their handles, if not removable, must be carefully wrapped or wiped. Scalers are involved in invasive procedures and could easily be contaminated by blood.

Ultrasonic scalers should not be cleaned in the ultrasonic cleaner.

Bracket arm and table (if fitted)

Avoid coarse abrasives. Dust under the bracket table and along the supporting arm each day. After each patient, wipe down the bracket table as part of your decontamination routine.

Suction devices

There are two types of suction:
❶ high velocity–low volume, and
❷ low velocity–high volume.

High velocity–low volume

This is a fine bore sucker used to suck up small amounts of fluid (for example, when a root canal is being irrigated or during oral surgery when you need fine control). The saliva ejector, placed into the patient's mouth under their tongue, falls into this category.

The saliva ejectors are single-use items and must be disposed of after use.

Low velocity–high volume

This wide bore aspirator is usually used by the dental assistant during routine intra-oral procedures. It removes debris, blood, saliva and water.

Most high volume evacuators now use single-use, disposable tips.

The tip of reusable wide bore aspirators must be sterilised after each patient. They should be scrubbed with a bottlebrush before sterilisation.

Cleaning the suction unit

Because this piece of equipment carries a high cross-infection risk, particular care needs to be taken during cleaning. Manufacturer's instructions should be followed. Cleaning includes:

- flushing a cup of water through the line between patients;

- flushing the suction lines with the recommended disinfectant each day to ensure the hoses are clear and to prevent the build-up of debris;

- cleaning the traps that catch the debris removed from the mouth (bits of amalgam, etc.) at the end of each day — the waste should be discarded according to instructions and the trap cleaned with water and a long-handled brush.

You should wear personal protective apparel while undertaking these tasks.

The mechanical parts of the evacuation system (the compressors and other parts) should be maintained by carefully following manufacturer's instructions.

Spittoon (or cuspidor)

This is used for patients' rinsing during and after procedures. In older dental units this is connected to the water main and at the base of each unit there is a master tap that must be turned off each night.

The spittoon bowl is usually mounted in rubber and it is easily broken at the point of entry into the outlet drain. Move it aside whenever necessary by holding the outlet drain, not by pushing the bowl.

Decontaminate the bowl after each patient by rinsing it with a cup of water. The rim should be wiped with detergent on a paper towel. Clean the filter at least once every day.

Many modern units no longer have spittoons. This is more hygienic and reduces the risk of cross-contamination.

X-ray machine

Dust daily. Wipe the head carefully after use. Move this equipment carefully to avoid bumping the head of the x-ray machine and damaging the tube. Switch the unit off when it is not in use.

Efficient lighting

To illuminate the mouth in four-handed dentistry, an operating light must be placed over the patient, a little further forward than the head. Some arrangements include two lights, one directed at the upper arch and one at the lower arch, or a single light may be moved backwards and forwards to suit particular procedures.

The most effective way to prevent cross-contamination is for you to make sure that you always have the light adjusted for the operator as required.

Frequent readjustments of the eyes from brightly lit to dimmer areas is a certain source of eye strain. To minimise this, the overall lighting in the surgery should be of sufficiently high intensity so that there is not a great contrast between the brightly lit interior of the mouth and the objects around it.

Some lights are wired to an individual switch and this must also be turned off at the completion of the day's work. Ensure the glass cover on the light, and the dome at the back, are regularly cleaned (when the light is cool) to remove splatter. At least one spare light globe should be kept in stock and a new one obtained as soon as the spare globe is used.

Cleaning and maintaining lights

Some practices use plastic wrap, stick-on plastic covers or specially designed plastic bags around light handles. For this to be effective the bags need to be changed between each patient. There are autoclavable handles available but this could be very expensive where there is a high turnover of patients. Wiping the light handle and switch with a neutral detergent between patients will generally be sufficient.

The light should only be cleaned when cool. They become extremely hot when lit and break easily. Ensure that a broken bulb has cooled completely before changing bulbs. The globe must never be touched with bare hands as it contaminates the bulb and can make it prone to fracturing. A tissue or gauze square should be wrapped around the globe before handling.

Curing lights

These are used to harden or set some composites and bonding agents. They must be working efficiently at full power for the materials to cure properly. Manufacturer's instructions for cleaning and testing the light must be followed.

Curing lights are a hazard to eyes. A protective shield filtering UV light emissions must be used while the light is turned on.

Curing lights are also a potential transmitter of infection. Even if wrapped, these lights need to be wiped down with the rest of the equipment (when the light has cooled). Sterilisable or disposable tips are available.

Autoclaves and ultrasonic cleaners

Memorise the operating instructions for the autoclave in your practice and follow them exactly. An instruction booklet is supplied with each machine. A wall chart, hung near the unit, is an effective reminder of the routines to be followed. Autoclaves and ultrasonic cleaners are discussed in depth in Chapter 14.

Air compressor

If care for the air compressor is your responsibility, then drain off the water each day and change the oil according to instructions.

Dental amalgamators/triturators

These are electrically operated mechanical devices that rapidly combine the measured proportions of mercury and dental amalgam alloy, and GIC or other cements. It is important to remember that mercury vapour is toxic and the lid of the amalgamator should be kept closed during operation. The amalgamator must be kept scrupulously clean and spillages avoided.

The components of the mix are placed into a small plastic or metal capsule (or come already pre-dispensed in disposable capsules). The capsule is fitted to the machine and trituration (mixing) is carried out for the required time. If reusable capsules are employed, clean out all traces of set amalgam. It tends to collect particularly in the end of the capsules. Plastic capsules are likely to cause most difficulty in this respect. Improper closure will result in mercury spillage.

Most amalgams are now supplied in disposable capsules containing pre-measured amounts separated by a suitable diaphragm. Just before use, the capsule is squeezed to rupture the diaphragm and this allows mixing of mercury and alloy in the amalgamator. A similar method is used for all capsulated materials.

Prosthetic equipment

All pieces of equipment that are placed in or around the patient's mouth should be properly decontaminated. This includes metal impression trays, facebow, mould and shade guides, stones, burs or wheels used in denture adjustments, etc.

Mould and shade guides should be soaked in a disinfectant solution.

Cabinets

Even with the use of prepared trays, some additional items are needed for each procedure. The cabinets holding these should be placed where they are most convenient to the seated operating team. If the dental chair is correctly sited in relation to the walls of the room, built-in cabinets on the left and behind the chair will be within easy reach. The tops of the cabinets will provide working space for preparation of materials, etc. A small mobile cabinet, wheeled into position on the left of the chair after the patient is seated, is very useful for holding items needed frequently by the dentist, such as sandpaper discs and strips, dental dam clamps, spare instruments, and so forth, which you pass to the dentist as required.

Items you need, such as lining and filling materials, slabs and spatulas, are kept in this cabinet, convenient to your position. Small bottles of cement and so forth can be held in a bottle rack within a drawer. Larger bottles of medicaments need to be kept in a cupboard, but a turntable (obtainable in kitchen hardware departments) can be used to make those medicaments at the back accessible.

All drawers and shelves should be kept as dust free as possible. Do not line the drawers with paper napkins as this encourages bacterial contamination.

Some important principles of storage are:

- The most frequently used items should be placed in the most convenient drawers and cupboards. The more awkward places should be used for the less frequently required items.
- The cabinets around the chair should not be used to store any bulk supplies. These should be kept in another part of the room or in a different room altogether.
- Heavy bulk items (e.g. large containers of disinfectant) should be stored on low shelves.
- All items should be grouped according to function, so that slabs and spatulas are kept in the same drawer as cements and liners. Dental dams in pre-cut sheets should be kept in the same drawer as the dam punch, clamps, clamp forceps, lubricant, frame and scissors for removal.
- Every item should have a particular place in a drawer or cupboard, so that it can be found without delay. For example, dental dam clamps may be kept in a plastic ice cube tray. It is suggested that each hole in the tray be labelled with the number of its clamp. The most frequently used clamps are kept in the corner holes where they can be located instantly.

In multi-surgery practices, try to store the same items in the same location in each surgery, so all staff members can find items when moving from surgery to surgery.

Additional equipment

Each practice has its own additional equipment and gadgets. It is possible that your surgery will have lasers, a computer-operated ceramic restoration unit and air abrasion machine. Ensure that you follow the manufacturer's instructions for their maintenance.

Do not forget the triturator, any medicament bottles or applicators, patients' protective glasses and the lead apron. It is your responsibility to care for all of these items.

In cooperation with all other staff members, a cleaning and decontamination protocol should be established that encompasses all areas of infection control and can be easily adhered to by all concerned. Procedures manuals are essential. A protocol should also be established to retrieve additional equipment or instruments during a procedure.

Glass slabs

A separate slab should be kept and used for GIC (glass ionomer cement) and composite cement only. Wash, disinfect and dry it after use and avoid scratching it with metal instruments. Slabs used for mixing cements with eugenol must not be used for GICs because the oil contaminates the mix and makes it unusable.

Laboratory equipment maintenance

Most dental practices have a small laboratory equipped with basic items to perform routine laboratory work. Depending on the type of practice, the dental assistant may or may not be required to perform simple laboratory procedures, such as pouring of models.

The laboratory is considered a clean area and all prosthetic items must be decontaminated before entering the laboratory.

Laboratory equipment may be divided into heavy and light equipment. Heavy equipment includes such items as the vibrator, dental lathe, model trimmer, bench dental engine, mechanical invester, inlay furnace and casting machine.

Light equipment is easily moved and includes many hand instruments. The light equipment includes such items as the plaster bowl, mechanical spatulator, bunsen burner, balance, articulators, water bath, gas-air blowtorch, inlay rings and an assortment of laboratory knives, pliers and spatulas. It is important that these are not scattered around the laboratory but returned to the correct storage place after use.

The care of laboratory equipment may also be your responsibility. Laboratory equipment usually does not need the same delicate care as some equipment in the operating room. Each manufacturer supplies maintenance information with the equipment. You should become familiar with this material and follow the suggestions to preserve efficiency and life of the equipment.

Always turn off water, gas or electricity when the appliance concerned is not in use.

Laboratory equipment is just as vital to productivity as the equipment in the surgery. It must be kept clean and the easiest way to do this is to clean each piece of equipment as soon after use as possible. This prevents the accumulation of debris that in time will be difficult to remove. Procedure 16.1 should be adhered to.

Procedure 16.1 Laboratory equipment maintenance

- Spread paper on workbench tops before using lab equipment. After the work is completed, gather this paper, along with the debris, and dispose of it.

- Clean instruments containing wax or any thermoplastic material on them by heating gently over a bunsen burner and then wiping with paper towel.

- Instruments that cannot be heated may be cleaned with suitable solvents.

- Place a paper towel over the vibrator table before use.

- Clean any gypsum product from spatulas, brushes and mixing bowls immediately after use, before the material sets. Do not allow a large amount of unset gypsum material to be flushed down the drain, as it may set in the drain pipes and cause an expensive blockage. Rather, collect the waste in a bin, or on a piece of paper.

- Flush the model trimmer thoroughly with water immediately after use.

- Place an inlay ring and contents in a pan or bowl of water, rather than in the sink, following a casting. All used mops must be washed and disinfected, or autoclaved if sterilisable.

- Pumice paste used for polishing acrylic dentures must be renewed for every new case. Ideally, a 1.5 per cent solution of sodium hypochlorite should be used to mix the pumice to the required consistency.

Articulators

In the fabrication of prosthetic appliances and cast restorations, models or casts are made that duplicate the dental arches. Any appliance is unsatisfactory unless it is compatible with the tissues of the opposing arch. If the appliance is too high, the patient cannot close their mouth and if it is malpositioned, the patient cannot chew properly. Casts are made and placed on an articulator, which simulates the jaw (arch) relationship and movements. The articulator helps to maintain properly established relationships.

There are many types of articulators of various sizes, shapes and complexity. There are two general types; simple (or plain-line) and adjustable. The simple type works as a hinge and allows for only the opening and closing movement while the adjustable articulators can simulate lateral and protrusive movements of the mandible.

Articulators must be kept clean. After the completion of an appliance, all traces of plaster, wax and debris should be removed. Moving parts should be lightly lubricated and mounting plates should be covered with a light coat of lubricant or petroleum jelly. The more complicated the articulator, the more maintenance it must receive.

Summary

Correct cleaning and maintenance of all surgery equipment is absolutely vital. These pieces of equipment are expensive and often fragile. Incorrect maintenance will lead to early replacement.

Surgery equipment cleaning and disinfecting is also mandatory as part of a good infection control regime.

chapter seventeen
patient management and clinical assistance.

Introduction

The duties of a dental assistant are many and varied. Your day starts with preparing the surgery for the first patient and continues with clinical, reception and office duties. Your role as an assistant in clinical duties is discussed in this chapter.

Preparing the surgery for the day

When you arrive at the dental practice, the day should commence with the immediate preparation of the surgery, as it is essential that a surgery is always ready for use. The surgery should be spotless. Follow the procedure set out below.

■ Walk into the surgery as if you were a patient and look around critically. Seat yourself in the chair, look up at the ceiling, and, if fitted, look under the bracket table for dust. Look at the outside, and into, the spittoon and note if there are any traces of debris. Check around the base of the unit and chair and foot controls for dropped items or dust.

■ Fill and switch on the steriliser or autoclave. Run autoclave tests if required. Prepare chemical disinfecting solutions if used. (Used solution should be discarded at the end of every day and the container thoroughly washed and drained to dry.) Fill the ultrasonic cleaner with recommended detergent, de-gas and perform daily tests.

■ Turn on air, water and gas connections and flush water lines.

■ If an airconditioner is used, switch it on and adjust it to the climate.

■ Take particular care with damp dusting, starting at the highest point and working downwards, cleaning the hand basin/s, spittoon, the dental chair and all other equipment.

■ Wipe all areas which the dentist's hands come in contact with during treatment (e.g. cabinet handles, operating light handle and chair adjustment switches). Wipe them with an appropriate solution and, if practicable, wrap them with plastic wrap or a plastic freezer bag to reduce the risk of cross-infection. This must be repeated before each patient.

■ Prepare handpieces and the bracket table, or tray set-ups, for treatment of the first patient of the day.

■ Collect from the office the day sheet showing the day's patients, appointment times and treatment plans. These should be placed in the surgery with all treatment cards, radiographs, study models and prosthetic items that will be needed during the day.

■ If a tray set-up system is used, (that is, a special tray is prepared for each clinical procedure) have a duplicate day sheet from which to work.

■ Keep odours in the surgery to a minimum. A patient entering a surgery can be affected by these. A strong odour of medicines and cleaning solutions does not present an agreeable atmosphere, although many of these are difficult to control. Where practicable, and acceptable to the dentist, the occasional use of a scented room spray or aromatherapy oil burner is effective. (However, the possibility of a patient being allergic to perfumes should also be considered.)

■ Damp dust the reception area and waiting room, and clean the telephone receiver with an appropriate detergent. Tidy magazines, books and toys in the waiting area.

Preparing the surgery between patients

Between patients, it is necessary to make the change-over quickly and this requires a routine that will alter for different surgeries. The important thing is to have a routine of procedures that everyone follows and which becomes practically automatic.

All evidence of the previous treatment is removed before the next patient is admitted. Wearing full personal protection equipment (PPE):

- flush a cupful of water through the spittoon (or cuspidor) and through the suction equipment before removing attachments from the line;
- sort and remove non-reusable sharps to the appropriate, puncture-proof sharps container;
- sort clinical waste and clear the bracket table;
- remove all used instruments from the working area and place them in the sterilising area (to be cleaned and sterilised later when the patient is settled);
- if recommended by the manufacturer, purge the handpiece/ultrasonic scaler for 10–20 seconds before removing it;
- change gloves;
- clean and wipe, with a suitable neutral detergent solution, the bracket table or work trolley, light handles and switches, the spittoon bowl and any area touched by you or the dentist during treatment, and wipe the headrest and chair, or change the headrest cover, and remember:
  - that spray bottles should not be used (solutions should be squeezed into a cloth or paper towel);
  - to start with the least contaminated items/area and work towards the most contaminated; and
- remove gloves, mask and glasses. Decontaminate glasses, wash hands and set up for the next patient.

Patient management

Greeting the patient

This is covered in more detail in Chapter 5. Always greet the patient by name. Don't forget to introduce yourself and the dentist to a new patient you have not met before.

The reception room should be checked for appearance by whoever escorts the patient to the chair. If a clean-up is needed in the reception room, it should be done after the patient is seated in the dental chair and prepared for treatment.

Positioning the patient

One of the first responsibilities of the good dental assistant is to make sure that the patient is correctly seated, is comfortable and placed in the right position for the dentist to operate.

Although the need for light conversation is most important to relieve tension during the first few minutes that the patient has in the surgery, it is important not to talk for too long as this will delay the treatment. Avoid any discussion of other patients' treatment, religion or politics. It is important not to be over-curious about a patient's personal life. A little interest does a lot of good, but too much is harmful.

You should adjust the headrest (if it is adjustable) to support the base of the skull. Bib or drape the patient in accordance with your surgery's practice and give the patient a pair of protective glasses.

The angle of the chair should be adjusted so that the patient's teeth are approximately on the same level as the legs, but this may vary somewhat according to the particular dentist. Some dentists prefer to do this adjustment themselves when they first welcome the patient. Always ensure that the person you are working with is happy for you to adjust the chair and warn the patient before you alter the position of the chair. Some dentists prefer the patient to sit up until treatment is commenced. Immediately after the patient is seated and in the preparation stage:

- place the patient's treatment chart in its designated place and put any radiographs on the viewer;
- put on glasses, mask and clinical gown;
- a fresh mouthwash, if used, should be placed in position in the patient's presence, as this leaves no doubt regarding possible earlier use;
- wash your hands and put on gloves;
- adjust the light as required.

Dismissing the patient

If the dentist has not assisted the patient out of the chair at the end of the appointment, gently push the tray or bracket table aside, move the operating light away and adjust the chair (upright and lower), allowing an easy exit. Before you adjust the chair, inform the patient that you are going to do so.

Remove the patient's dental napkin. Offer a tissue and a hand mirror if some dental material is left on the skin or lipstick has been smudged, or wipe the face if necessary for an elderly person or child.

Assist older patients from the chair if they require help. If the patient has a bag, accessories, a coat, an umbrella, a mobile phone and so forth, then pass these items to the patient ensuring nothing is left behind in the surgery. Depending on the practice protocol, escort the patient to reception to make the next appointment. It is important to dismiss the patient with an air of friendliness. In some practices the dentist escorts the patient to reception to allow the DA time to clean the surgery.

When at the front desk, always mention the next appointment or check-up time; 'See you next week/on the 24th /in six months' or similar. Never neglect to say goodbye to a patient.

If a patient is over-talkative when the time comes to leave the surgery, you should break into the conversation politely with a reasonable excuse for interrupting. The object is to terminate the conversation but not to offend by making the patient feel they are being 'pushed out'.

You should waste no time in decontaminating and preparing the surgery and seating the next patient. A system should be developed for cleaning the surgery after treatment but care should be taken that the system is well ordered, no traces of the previous procedure remain and no shortcuts are taken.

Chair-side assisting

Setting up

Select the necessary instruments for the bracket table according to the patient's treatment (as shown on the day sheet) or select the tray set-up required for the patient's treatment.

When these have been arranged, add:

- a bur stand;
- a sterilised pack with a selection of burs;
- the required handpieces;
- an aspirating tip;
- a triplex syringe; and
- any necessary medicaments.

Where possible, instruments should be kept out of the patient's vision and bagged, to be opened in front of the patient. This reassures the patient that the instruments have been sterilised and have not been used before.

Assisting

During the procedure, you must know exactly what your duties are. You should know what the dentist will be doing, anticipate which instruments and materials will be required and in what order. Instruments and materials should be prepared before they are needed so that they are ready for use as soon as they are required. In some cases however, the treatment plan may change and you need to be adaptable and (observing all infection control protocols) select and prepare the additional instruments and materials as required.

You may be required to participate in the dental procedure by preparing and helping with the placement of a **dental dam**, by handing each instrument to the dentist as it is required and by preparing and mixing materials. You may use the high velocity evacuator, retract the cheeks or lips and remove debris from the mouth during treatment. If the person you are working with utilises four-handed dentistry (see below), you will also pass and receive instruments, medicaments and other items to and from the dentist and operate the air and water syringe while assisting.

Surgery conduct

Unless it cannot be avoided, the dentist should not be spoken to while working on a patient, although some dentists prefer some light conversation with the patient to put them at ease. If the dentist is needed somewhere else, the patient should be told in a clear, low voice or shown a note that is held out behind the patient's head. Patients appreciate the undivided concentration of the dentist so this should always be done in a controlled manner. Never whisper in the presence of the patient as it could cause undue concern to the patient. Whispering can be distressing to a fearful patient.

If, during treatment, the amount of mixed material is getting low, inform the dentist so that additional material may be mixed, ready for use. Do not wait until there is no material before planning an additional mix.

You should anticipate when the dentist needs the next instrument and should rarely need to be told what to pass or when.

dental dam: a thin sheet of rubber or other non-latex material used to exclude moisture and maintain a sterile field during cavity preparation and endodontic procedures.

Four-handed dentistry

The design of modern dental surgeries allows efficient and comfortable teamwork. It allows the dentist to make as few movements outside the patient's mouth as possible and even these movements are over a very short range. Most instruments and materials are passed between the dentist and assistant. The assistant also maintains a clear, dry field in the mouth for the dentist to operate.

This method of working is called four-handed dentistry. It allows safe transfer of dental equipment between you and the dentist. This allows the dentist to work smoothly and uninterrupted. It enables you to remove excess moisture (saliva, blood and water) and debris from the patient's mouth. This in turn is beneficial to the patient as it decreases their discomfort and reduces the length of time for each procedure.

The clock concept of operating zones

As well as increasing the efficiency and comfort of the dental team and patient, four-handed dentistry is also a crucial part of effective infection control as it reduces the risk of contaminated materials coming in contact with clean materials. Four-handed dentistry is based on a clock concept, as shown in Figure 17.1.

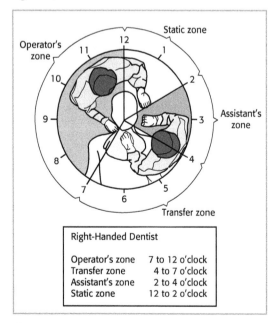

Right-Handed Dentist	
Operator's zone	7 to 12 o'clock
Transfer zone	4 to 7 o'clock
Assistant's zone	2 to 4 o'clock
Static zone	12 to 2 o'clock

Figure 17.1 The clock concept

The dentist sits in the operator's zone. The area over the patient's chest is the area where instruments are passed. You sit in the assistant's zone. There is a zone behind the patient where portable equipment might be placed. There might be some movement around these zones depending on the area of the mouth being worked on or if the dentist is left-handed.

Passing instruments

Under new occupational health and safety laws it is not permitted to pass sharp contaminated instruments to the dentist's hand. They have to be placed into a firm, puncture-proof container and not passed over the patient's chest.

Any instrument or piece of equipment that does not have a sharp point, for example, a ball burnisher or amalgam gun, should be placed firmly in the dentist's hands in the direction of use (i.e. put into the dentist's hand in the way in which it will be used). Ideally, the instrument will be handed to the dentist in such a way that the dentist does not need to look away from the operating area.

With practice, it is possible to hold the instrument to be passed with your thumb and first two fingers and to remove the used instrument by hooking it with your little finger. In this way, the other hand can be used to hold the aspirator or another piece of equipment.

Continuous chair-side assistance

Some dentists prefer to work using two chair-side assistants; a left-side assistant and a right-side assistant. This technique is also called six-handed dentistry.

Left-side assistant

The left-side assistant's duties normally include the following.

■ Evacuation of fluids and debris from the mouth. This should be done during cavity preparation, during all restorative procedures, and examination and scaling procedures.

■ Washing and drying of teeth and soft tissues with the triplex syringe. When the dentist pauses to inspect the cavity during tooth preparation, you should partially dry it with a short blast of air. At the completion of the preparation, you may wash and partially dry the cavity to prepare it for filling placement. Frequent flushing and evacuation during scaling procedures will eliminate the need for the patient to rinse. Some dentists find it helpful for you to direct a blast of air on to the mouth mirror to keep it clear during the preparation of upper teeth.

- If an amalgam restoration is being placed in a position accessible to you in the right mandibular quadrant, you may insert the amalgam into the cavity with the amalgam carrier, while the dentist condenses it.

Right-side assistant

The right-side assistant is normally responsible for the following.

- Preparation and transfer of materials. To maintain a chain of asepsis, most materials are mixed by the right-side assistant and passed to the dentist.

- Transfer of instruments. Although a dentist may pick up instruments directly from the tray, it is possible to work more smoothly if you have them ready to hand to the dentist. The new instrument should be held close to the mouth, in the direction in which the dentist will use it; that is, generally parallel to the instrument being used before it. The little finger of the same hand may be extended to receive the old instrument when the dentist is ready to change over. If you are not sure which instrument will be needed next, you can ask or hold out the three or four instruments that the dentist is most likely to use. Instruments frightening to the patient, such as anaesthetic syringes or extraction forceps, should be transferred out of the patient's line of sight, preferably behind their head, in a firm container such as a kidney dish.

- Changing of burs. The first bur should be placed in the handpiece before work is commenced, and burs should be changed by you as directed.

- Preparation and transfer of dental dams, medicaments, matrices, wedges, etc. These items should always be passed to the dentist ready-to-use; for example, dental dam clamps passed on the clamp forceps, varnish passed on a cotton pledget held in tweezers, matrix bands already fitted to the matrix retainer, and so on.

In practices where only one chair-side assistant is employed, the dentist will probably carry out some of the above tasks but you should still look for every opportunity to assist. It is important for the chair-side assistant to be familiar with the operating procedures of the dentist in order to anticipate the next step.

Some dentists use the routine of the right-hand side assistant being a 'clean' person to reduce the chance of cross-contamination. In this case, the right-hand assistant would not touch any items that had been in contact with the patient. There is also less clean-up required as items (medicaments, curing light, amalgamator, etc.) have only been touched by clean hands.

Precautions for four-handed dentistry

There are certain dangers inherent in this method of working, as in all methods. You should be aware of these and take the precautions set out below:

Great care must be used when handling very small items in and around the patient's mouth. If dropped into the back of the throat they may be swallowed or inhaled. Most restorative procedures and all root canal therapies should be carried out with a dental dam in place.

Bottles or dishes containing caustic drugs, or indeed any liquids, should never be passed or held over the patient.

The patient's eyes are especially vulnerable, and the possibility of injury by instruments or drugs must always be borne in mind. The patient must wear protective glasses at all times during treatment. Tinted safety goggles help reduce glare from the operating light and at the same time afford protection from accidentally dropped instruments or materials or splashes from aerosol spray. When turning away from the patient suddenly, you must be careful not to bump the patient or the dentist with an elbow or with an aspirator tube, etc.

If the chair is operated by foot controls, you must avoid accidentally kicking or stepping on these. A sudden movement of the chair can be dangerous. Warn the patient when you are about to adjust the position of the chair. Some elderly and arthritic patients may need to have their head supported.

Take care when seated on the operating stool that your feet are resting on the foot bar and do not come into contact with the dentist's feet or foot pedals, especially when alighting from the chair.

Make sure you sit in your assistant's chair correctly, with the 'belly' bar supporting your waist and your feet firmly on the foot support.

Controlling moisture in the mouth

This is one of your most important roles during any procedure. It involves keeping the mouth clean of debris, blood, saliva and excess water from the triplex syringe. It is an important role because:

- many procedures (for example, restorations) require a dry, clean working field;
- it allows the dentist clear vision of the working area;
- it reduces the patient's need to 'swallow' excess water; and
- it reduces the risk of transmission of infection.

Cotton rolls

A common form of moisture control is the placement of cotton rolls. Cotton rolls can be placed between the teeth and the cheeks and between the teeth and the tongue in the lower jaw.

The dentist will place the cotton rolls as appropriate. It is important that they be damp when they are removed because a dry roll may stick to the oral mucosa and damage it. A quick squirt with the water syringe will make removal more comfortable.

Suction devices

These pieces of equipment and their maintenance are also mentioned in Chapter 16.

High velocity–low volume

These suction devices help to keep the working area free from moisture during shorter procedures and allow some materials time to set. They can be used under a dental dam to prevent saliva and water from accumulating and causing the patient discomfort.

Low velocity–high volume

With the patient supine, saliva, debris and the water used for cooling high speed cutting instruments collect at the very back of the mouth, where the tongue falls back across the throat.

The tube of this wide bore aspirator should be held so that the opening is close to and facing the tooth being prepared, and, if possible, just below the occlusal plane. In this position it can serve the additional purpose of retracting the cheek or tongue.

This should be done in a way that the evacuator tube does not obstruct or hinder the dentist.

Care should be taken not to suck soft tissue into the high volume aspirator as this may damage the tissue. You need to be aware that the noise the high volume aspirator makes if it touches the cheek or tongue may frighten the patient. You may need to reassure the patient that this does not cause any harm.

The aspirator also reduces aerosol caused by the high-speed handpiece.

Dental dams

Dental dams are a barrier formed by a thin, stretchable (usually latex) material. When the dam has been put in place, one or more teeth are exposed but the rest of the mouth is covered by the latex. Non-latex dams are also available for patients with a latex allergy.

The dental dam is used for:

- Moisture control — moisture may encroach into the working field from saliva or the gingival crevice. The dental dam is the only method of adequately controlling moisture entry.
- Patient protection — the dental dam prevents the aspiration (inhalation) of instruments used in endodontics. It also prevents irritating and bad-tasting irrigating solutions from getting into the patient's mouth.
- Isolation of the operating field — the operating field is cleared by retraction of the lips, cheeks and tongue. Additionally, all other teeth are kept out of view, enabling the dentist to more effectively focus on the interior of the tooth that matters.
- Patient control — the dental dam eliminates the desire and need of patients to rinse and spit. Conversation is discouraged and the oral mucosa and tongue do not get dehydrated.

Depending on state regulations, dental assistants are not allowed to place dental dams, but are expected to assist in the preparation of the dam by creating the required hole or holes with a dental dam punch.

A plastic template or rubber stamp can be a guide for the holes. A large hole is made for a molar; half size for other teeth.

The notched beaks of forceps are placed in the clamp. The bow of the clamp (unless it is of double bow design) should be to the distal for posterior teeth, and to the left for right incisors if the dentist is right-handed.

The whole assembly is then handed to the dentist, who applies the clamp to the designated tooth.

The patient is given an antiseptic mouth rinse before the dam is placed. Before the dam is placed, the teeth to be exposed must be cleaned of plaque and debris and the patient should be checked for latex allergies.

Equipment used in the application of a dental dam consists of the dental dam material clamps, holder, punch and forceps. A dental dam tray set-up is shown in Figure 17.2.

The dental dam material is supplied in rolls or in pre-cut sheets (125 × 125 mm or 150 × 150 mm). It is available in light or dark colours and in various thicknesses: thin, medium, heavy, extra heavy and special heavy. There are also many different sizes and shapes of clamps available. They should be placed in separate receptacles, properly labelled, in the operating cabinet drawer. This will facilitate rapid selection of a clamp.

Holes are punched in the dental dam. These holes allow exposure of the teeth that require work. Dental dam punches allow the punching of holes of different sizes. These holes must be punched cleanly and care should be taken that the punch is not damaged by being used when poorly aligned.

The dam is held in place by an external frame that keeps it clear of the patient's face. Some dentists also like to use a lubricant (such as vaseline or KY jelly) to ease the dam into the interproximal spaces and to ensure that the dam does not stick to the patient's lips. It is also possible to put a disposable pad under the dam to absorb moisture. If the saliva ejector is being used under the dam, it should be placed on the opposite side of the mouth from the working area. This may be your responsibility so you need to check with the dentist which tooth needs to be exposed.

Sometimes, due to abnormal anatomy of the tooth, the clamp and dam may not fully seal around the neck of the tooth, therefore a sealant may be used.

The dental dam should be routinely used in endodontic procedures. See the example in Figure 17.3.

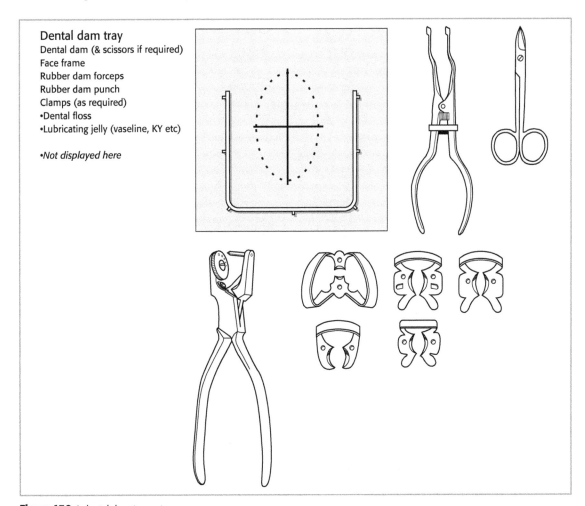

Dental dam tray
Dental dam (& scissors if required)
Face frame
Rubber dam forceps
Rubber dam punch
Clamps (as required)
•Dental floss
•Lubricating jelly (vaseline, KY etc)

•*Not displayed here*

Figure 17.2 A dental dam tray set-up

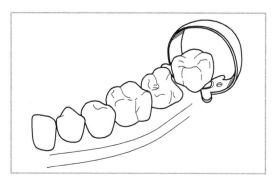

Figure 17.3 A dental dam in place

In some states this is legally obligatory. Its use ensures that no instrument will drop into the patient's throat, or medicaments or solutions be swallowed. It also inhibits the flow of saliva into the cavity.

The dam must be removed carefully and inspected to ensure that no piece of it is left under the free gingiva.

A range of different dental dam clamps is shown in Figure 17.4.

Preparing for the next day

When all the patients have left at the end of the day, there are still many tasks to be completed, including:

- thoroughly cleaning the surgery, putting away all items from bench-tops and covering the bracket tray;
- discarding all mixed disinfectants and cleaning the container in which the disinfectant is kept;
- running a prescribed cleaner/disinfectant through the suction system;
- purging all dental unit water lines;
- putting all sterilised instruments into their correct place;

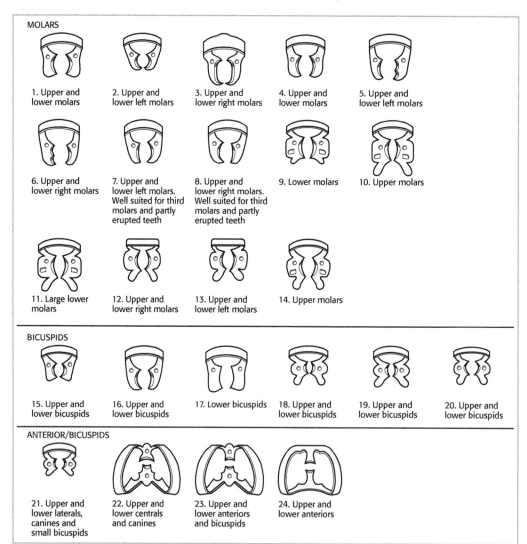

Figure 17.4 Dental dam clamps

- turning off all equipment, including the air conditioner, triturator, the dental unit, compressor (open the release valve to drain if required), autoclave and radiographic processor;

- cleaning all used instruments, drying and bagging them, ready for sterilising (if unable to do this, place them into a safe container under water and detergent, ready to be sterilised the next day);

- emptying and cleaning the ultrasonic cleaner, which must be done every day;

- correctly storing or filing all records from the autoclave for the day, as well as any other equipment assessment records such as autoclave printouts (these are printed on thermal paper and will fade if incorrectly stored; if all information has been correctly documented on a log these printouts can be disposed of or, alternatively, photocopied and pasted into a book);

- processing and mounting any radiographs;

- filing all patients' cards and radiographs from the day;

- finding patients' cards for the next day and putting them in the order in which the patients will arrive;

- checking the expected treatment for each of the following day's patients and, if appropriate, checking that all necessary laboratory work for the next day's appointments has been received;

- making enough copies of the next day's day sheet to have one in each of the major working areas;

- backing up the computer files;

- phoning patients for appointment confirmation or to remind them that they are due to make an appointment; and

- setting the answering machine and fax to take incoming messages.

Most practices will have additional routines to carry out before the surgery can be closed down for the night.

Additional duties

Laboratory work orders

Instructions for laboratory work to be undertaken by a dental technician are written down in full detail and set out on a laboratory work order form. The dentist may draw the design of a denture for the sake of clarity. This avoids any confusion as to exactly what work is required.

There are many varying designs of laboratory work orders. A somewhat similar card with relevant details is used for crowns, bridges, inlays, study models, repairs and other items that are passed to the technicians. See the sample laboratory forms in Figures 17.5 and 17.6.

Figure 17.5 Sample laboratory form for crown and bridges

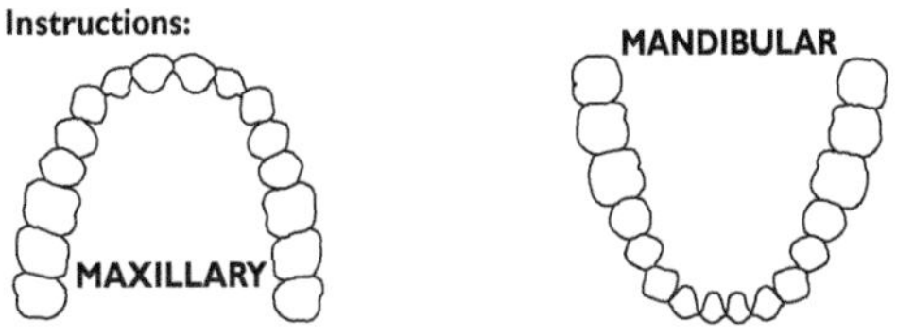

Figure 17.6 Sample laboratory form for dentures

Spare time duties

When all other duties are completed or the dentist is away, many chores can be simplified by doing them before the demand becomes urgent. For example, in the surgery, some pieces of equipment can only be serviced when the surgery is not in use for a period of time. It is also possible to check stock and enter shortages in the order book, clean out cabinet drawers, clean any special equipment, oil and service equipment, rearrange supplies, cut wedges, fill crown form boxes, set up endodontic packs, sharpen instruments (if you are expected to do this), prepare the month's recalls and follow up recalls, etc.

In the office you can:

- check files for patient record cards that are in the wrong position;
- check inactive files to see if any unpaid accounts were filed by mistake;
- check files to see if any patients with unfinished work are coming in for appointments;
- tidy desk drawers;
- change printer cartridges (if necessary) and clean all business machines.

In the x-ray room, or if automatic processors are used, chemicals should be changed at set intervals. A record of dates of preparations and solutions should be kept in the processing room. When the time comes to change the developer and fixer, both tanks are removed, emptied and cleaned. Similarly, the water-wash tank should be cleaned. Make a list of the duties in the surgery that require regular attention and check this list with the dentist; for example, radiographs may need to be processed twice a day and developing solutions should be changed at least every two to four weeks, depending on use. All cleaning and sterilising equipment needs maintenance.

Summary

There are many duties that you must fit into your day. The clinical duties and chair-side assisting are only a small part of your duties. In a practice where there is more than one assistant, systems need to be in place to allot and record duties, to avoid doubling up.

chapter eighteen
oral examination, diagnosis and treatment planning.

Introduction

The ultimate success or failure of a treatment usually stems from the preliminary examination. An examination involves the systematic gathering and recording of information on which a diagnosis may be based.

The dental assistant plays an important role in this aspect of dental care.

Treatment planning is the active treatment that is proposed to the patient after diagnosis and prognosis. Diagnosis is the process of determining the nature of the problem based on the patient's signs and symptoms and the results of any tests. A prognosis is an assessment of the probable future course of disease, including the estimated time for, and outcomes of, treatment.

A complete and careful examination involves:

■ taking a full medical and dental history;

■ noting the patient's chief complaint; their signs (the aspects of a disease process that the dentist finds during an examination, e.g., redness, swelling, ulceration, bleeding, etc.) and symptoms (the aspects of a disease process that the patient complains of but that are not visible, e.g., pain, nausea, headache, ear-ache, etc.);

■ detailed clinical examination including an external and internal oral examination such as probing (also periodontal probing), mobility testing (jaw and teeth), percussion, muscle palpation, listening to joint clicking, olfactory (smelling), soft tissue examination, radiography; and

■ recording of findings. The examination findings must be accurately recorded, legible and clearly set out on the patient's treatment card. You will record these findings and must take care as there can be no ambiguity, error or omission. What you record *must* always be checked and initialled by the dentist who dictated the findings.

Following examination, the diagnosis, prognosis and plan for treatment will be outlined. Before any treatment is performed, the patient must be informed of:

■ what work is required;

■ how they can be treated, with options discussed;

■ the number of appointments that may be needed;

■ possible outcomes and contra-indications described; and

■ the likely cost.

The patient is then required to sign a statement that they have been informed of, and have understood, the detailed treatment plan and consent to having the work done. The patient may be given a copy as well. This is essential to avoid future misunderstanding and is the dentist's proof in case of litigation. This is called 'informed consent'.

The object of the examination of a patient's oral condition is for the dentist to gain an overall assessment of treatment to be carried out.

Treatment planning aids the dentist in estimating the time and cost of the necessary treatment. It gives the dentist a record of the case for future reference and allows the dentist to discuss the case with another dentist or physician.

You should never question or pass an opinion about treatment being carried out.

General oral examination methods

Visual examination

The whole of the oral cavity is inspected with emphasis on the tongue, floor of the mouth, tonsillar areas and the alveolar mucosa. Externally, the lips, the face and the neck are inspected. You can assist by correct positioning of the patient, supporting the head of infants and invalid patients and adjusting the light source as required. You should monitor the patient for any signs of distress and reassure them.

Tactile examination (that is, by feeling)

Teeth may be pressed with an instrument handle to test for mobility or looseness, whilst tapping with a mirror handle will often determine sensitivity. Tooth surfaces are probed to detect 'catches' in small cavities, whilst swellings and suspect soft and hard tissue areas are felt to determine their consistency.

You should ensure that all necessary instruments and equipment are handy. All required protective clothing should be worn and standard and transmission-based precautions observed.

Audible examination (sound)

This includes listening to the sounds associated with tooth tapping, speech, breathing and the movement of the jaws and joints. When this examination is carried out you should reduce background noise in the surgery.

Examination by smell

Some diseases produce distinctive odours that you may be the first to observe when settling the patient in the chair. You should acquaint the dentist of your suspicions. Acute necrotising ulcerative gingivitis (ANUG) and diabetes are two such examples.

The intense local examination

A complete examination of each tooth and its supporting structures is performed and the findings are recorded graphically on a dental chart.

Entries involve the number of teeth present, plaque and calculus deposits, restored teeth, carious teeth, missing teeth, periodontal problems and frank pathology.

You should ensure the examination tray contains a mouth mirror, probe, college tweezers, periodontal probe, dental floss and, if it is your dentist's preference, plaque disclosing solution.

Special clinical tests

Pulp vitality tests

Pulp vitality tests are carried out by thermal (heat or cold) means, by tapping, gutta percha testing, carbon dioxide testing or by the use of an electric pulp tester. You should be aware of which method the dentist uses and have it available.

Evaluation of occlusion

The evaluation of occlusion involves assessment of the movements of the mandible. The patient should be relaxed during this test. You should ensure that distractions are kept to a minimum in the surgery. Articulating paper, indicator and bite waxes should be on hand.

Laboratory tests

Laboratory tests include blood tests, smears (cytological and microbiological) and biopsy. If, after all these tests have been performed, further consultative assistance is required from the patient's physician then you should check that stationery is available for the dentist. Where you have to arrange a referral appointment you should have the name, address and telephone number of the referred patient ready before placing the call. The patient must also be requested to sign a release of information form, so that the referral form and details can be sent on.

Records

Records are essential in diagnosis and to ascertain any future changes that may occur. Records may consist of accurate charting of all the teeth and their supporting soft tissue, full arch impressions for the construction of study models, tooth form and colour, and radiographs. Clinical photographs are often useful records.

The treatment plan

The treatment plan lists the treatment in the order of priority and allows the dentist and dental assistant to intelligently plan the necessary appointments. It allows the dentist to answer the patient's questions.

- What is the problem?
- How can it be fixed? (Are there options?)
- How long will it take and how successful is the treatment likely to be?
- How much is it going to cost?

When the examination is complete, active treatment can be commenced and you should now discuss with the dentist which appointments will be required and the time per visit. Treatment plans usually follow the order:

- emergency relief of pain;
- scaling and cleaning, oral hygiene instruction, and home care in addition to active chair-side treatment;
- oral surgery if necessary;
- preventive dentistry;
- restorative dentistry and endodontics;
- prosthetic dentistry; and
- a recall program.

Basic examination tray set-up

The set up for an examination consists of:

- mirror (magnifying or plain);
- college tweezers;
- explorers of various kinds (straight, right angle, sickle probe, right and left curved); they must be kept sharp and correctly shaped;
- periodontal probe;

- a suction tube and triplex syringe; and
- dental floss (to test contact points and detect overhanging margins).

The dentist expects you to have these items on each tray set-up, as shown in Figure 18.1.

Mouth mirrors

The dental mirror is used for:

- viewing areas of the oral cavity;
- reflecting light on dark areas;
- retracting lips, cheeks or tongue for better visibility; and
- protecting this tissue from injury in case an instrument slips off the working surface.

An example is shown in Figure 18.2.

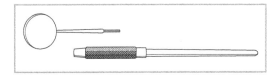

Figure 18.2 Mouth mirror and single-ended cone-socket handle

Some dentists use dental mirrors that are magnifying. Others use plain mirrors or front-surfaced mirrors. Dental mirrors also come in various sizes. You must know the dentist's preferences and ensure that there are always additional mirrors stocked in the supply cupboard. Front surface mirrors are more expensive and do not have the reflective 3D effect.

Mirrors are usually detachable from their handles by unscrewing them. This feature saves the expense of the handle when it becomes necessary to discard the mirror. The handles used are called cone-socket handles and the mirrors are mounted on a cone-socket stem.

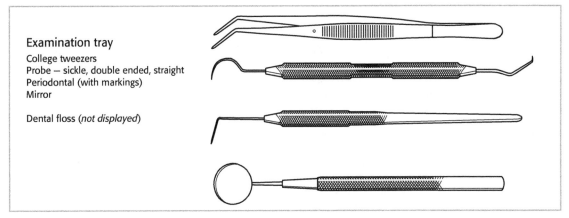

Examination tray

College tweezers
Probe – sickle, double ended, straight
Periodontal (with markings)
Mirror

Dental floss (*not displayed*)

Figure 18.1 Examination tray set-up

You must be constantly alert to the condition of the dental mirrors. Replacing old mirrors with new ones when they are badly scratched, permanently fogged or smeared with varnish is your responsibility.

Care has to be taken to prevent rust occurring in the handle or in the cone socket where the mirror is inserted. Mirror heads should be removed from the handle before the handle is placed in the ultrasonic cleaner.

Probes (or explorers)

The dentist uses explorers to examine teeth through the sense of touch. These instruments are used in the initial examination of the teeth and during the entire cavity preparation and restoration procedures. They are used to locate decay and check the walls and angles of the preparation as well as the margins of the restoration. These instruments are made of steel, have sharp tines and come in many different shapes.

The most commonly used types are the curved and right-angled explorers. You are expected to maintain a few of each of the dentist's preferred explorers in the supply cupboard as replacements for those that are broken or become blunt.

See the examples in Figure 18.3.

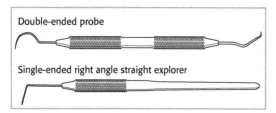

Figure 18.3 Sickle explorer with hygienist or No 17 on the opposing end and No 6 explorer

Surgery tweezers (or dressing tweezers)

Tweezers are available in several designs. See the example in Figure 18.4. Locking tweezers are also quite popular for items that need to be held firmly. College tweezers are used to convey objects such as cotton pellets, cotton rolls and small lengths of wire to and from the mouth.

The beaks of tweezers may distort easily if they are used incorrectly.

Since these tweezers are used in the mouth, they should never be placed over an open flame. This will destroy the temper or springiness of the metal and discolour the tips, making them unsightly.

There are other tweezers of similar design that can be used in conjunction with open flames.

Handle tweezers gently to avoid damage to the beaks.

Solutions such as cavity varnish adhere strongly to the beaks but can be removed by either wiping or immersing in spirit.

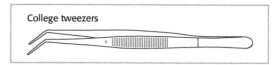

Figure 18.4 Tweezers

Prophylaxis instruments and accessories

The examination or first visit is usually accompanied by a prophylaxis. In fact proper examination is only possible after a prophylaxis. A prophylaxis tray set-up is shown in Figure 18.9.

The periodontal probe

The periodontal probe has a blunt point with millimetre measurements marked along the tip of the probe, as shown in Figure 18.5. It is used to locate and measure the depth of periodontal pockets.

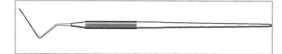

Figure 18.5 Periodontal probe

Scalers

Scalers are used to remove calculus from teeth. The morse scaler is widely used and has a detachable scaler tip for easy replacement. The head or the tip is available in different shapes and sizes. Scalers must be kept sharpened to be efficient in their action. This is done by stroking them gently on a fine oilstone. An example of an anterior sickle and morse scaler is shown in Figure 18.6.

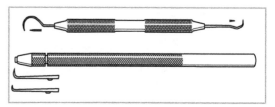

Figure 18.6 Anterior sickle and morse scaler

Prophylaxis rubber cups

Rubber cups are used with an abrasive paste for polishing teeth and prophylaxis. Types available are screw for handpiece prophylaxis, and latch for handpiece latch heads. See Figure 18.7.

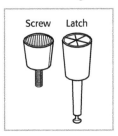

Figure 18.7 Rubber caps – screw and latch

Bristle brushes

Bristle brushes are for plaque and stain removal, like rubber cups, but they are made from natural bristles. They are available in various sizes and types, such as screw, snap on, or latch, as shown in Figure 18.8.

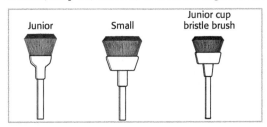

Figure 18.8 Some different bristle brushes

Scissors

Keep coarse scissors for coarse jobs (e.g., cutting cotton rolls). Fine scissors must be sharp and capable of cutting a wisp of cotton wool without any dragging or removing of sutures.

Records

The patient's dental card

The dental treatment card is the information centre for the dentist. It should provide all necessary information, written or typed, large enough to be read easily. The design of the chart should provide for the patient's name, address, both residential and business telephone numbers, date of birth, contact details for next of kin, guardian, occupation, who referred the patient, their physician's name and address and health fund (if any). Old cards should be attached or a note made of where they are filed.

Names with unusual pronunciation should be spelt out phonetically and nicknames of children should be noted. The card should show information of dental treatment carried out, dates of treatment and a record of radiographs taken.

Where practical, the card should show general information about the patient and their health history. Most important are any special emergency notations, such as an allergic reaction to certain drugs (e.g., an antibiotic), or any other allergy or condition due to past or present illness. The medical–dental history form and informed consent form must be attached.

Primarily, the card is used to record work proposed to be done and so has a diagrammatic chart of all the teeth and their surfaces. A treatment plan and

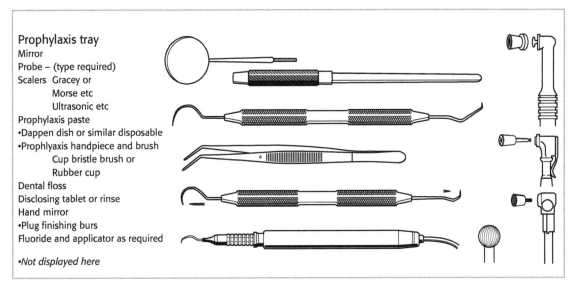

Prophylaxis tray
Mirror
Probe – (type required)
Scalers Gracey or
         Morse etc
         Ultrasonic etc
Prophylaxis paste
•Dappen dish or similar disposable
•Prophlyaxis handpiece and brush
         Cup bristle brush or
         Rubber cup
Dental floss
Disclosing tablet or rinse
Hand mirror
•Plug finishing burs
Fluoride and applicator as required

•Not displayed here

Figure 18.9 Prophylaxis tray set-up

appointment schedule should be shown along with the treatment done at progressive appointments.

Most treatment cards have a space for recording fees charged, fees paid, and the method of payment. Some dental offices use a separate card for financial records or a family card for several members of the one family.

Many practices now use computerised systems for dental records.

Charting

As the dentist examines a patient, you chart the proposed treatment on the card and add any comments the dentist makes concerning any condition in the mouth.

You should practise charting so that there is no hesitation. To avoid mistakes you must be familiar with general anatomical terms used in relation to the mouth.

Charting the mouth

In Chapter 9, the different types of charts and methods of charting were discussed. To reiterate, there are two types of dental charts, anatomical and diagrammatic. Both are in common use. There are two methods of notation, Palmer's and International (FDI). Both are in common use and both can be used on anatomical or diagrammatic charts.

A number of examination circuits of both arches are made by the dentist. Using a lead pencil, you mark the charts to show restored and carious teeth or unsatisfactory restorations, as dictated by the dentist.

Decayed or carious cavities in teeth are usually divided into five types, as shown in Figure 18.10.

Class I (shown here in tooth 14) cavities occur in occlusal or chewing surfaces. These appear in pits and fissures of molars and premolars. They are also referred to as occlusal cavities. Class I cavities also are found in lingual pits of anterior teeth.

Class II cavities (shown here in tooth 16) appear on proximal surfaces and can be mesial (M) or distal (D). Cavities often involve the occlusal surfaces (O) of molars and premolars and are written as MO or DO cavities. If all three surfaces are involved the tooth is scored as MOD.

Class III cavities (shown here in tooth 12) are those that involve the proximal surfaces of anterior teeth but do not involve the loss of the incisal angle.

Class IV cavities (shown here in tooth 11) refer to anterior teeth where the incisal edge has been lost.

Class V cavities (shown here in tooth 13) are all cavities that appear on the gingival third of the labial, buccal or lingual surfaces of any tooth.

Abnormal tooth positions in the arch, such as over-erupted teeth, un-erupted teeth, missing teeth, drifted, tilted or rotated teeth, can also be charted. You should, with practice, be able to detect such changes from observations of the study models and radiographs.

Gingival tissue abnormalities may include gingivitis, **hypertrophy**, **hyperplasia**, recession and pocket formation. Abnormal tooth surfaces such as **hypoplastic enamel**, erosion, abrasion and attrition areas may also be noted. These conditions are described in Chapter 12.

Charting abbreviations

These abbreviations indicate a surface of the tooth or multiple surfaces, as shown in Figure 18.11.

Charting symbols

The symbols shown in Table 18.1 are commonly used when charting. The symbol is drawn over the appropriate teeth on the charts, using a lead pencil. Check with your dentist for any symbols used in your surgery. Some sample charts are shown in Figures 18.12 and 18.13.

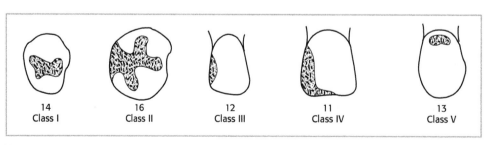

14
Class I

16
Class II

12
Class III

11
Class IV

13
Class V

Figure 18.10 Classifications of cavities

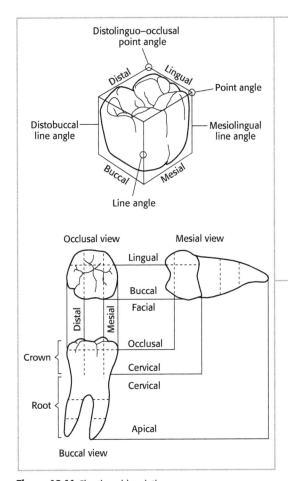

B	buccal
M	mesial
D	distal
Li	lingual
O	occlusal
I	incisal
P	palatal (lingual of maxillary teeth)
F	facial (also labial/buccal)
La	labial anterior teeth
BO	buccal-occlusal
DO	disto-occlusal
MO	mesio-occlusal
LO	linguo-incisal
DI	disto-incisal
MI	mesio-incisal
DL	disto-lingual
MOD	mesial occlusal distal
MODB	mesial occlusal distal and buccal

Figure 18.11 Charting abbreviations

Summary

All successful dental treatment planning relies on good diagnosis. As a dental assistant you have an important role and responsibility in preparing all the necessary instrumentation and equipment for the initial examination.

You now have the necessary knowledge to play your part in the accurate charting of the oral condition of patients. This is essential if treatment planning is to be successful.

Restoration present	Cavity	RC Recurrent caries	Root filling required	Root filled tooth	# Fracture
/ To be extracted	X Extracted	Missing tooth	FC Full crown required	Full crown present	Bridge required
Bridge present	___mm Pocket depth	F/- Full upper denture	/P Partial lower denture	↑ Erupting mandibular	↓ Erupting maxillary
UE Un-erupted	Space closed	↻ Tooth rotated	→ Tooth drifted	OH Overhanging margin	V Vital (after testing)
NV Non-vital (after testing)	³/₄ crown	Cantilever bridge	SS Sub-surface lesion for SnF₂ application (Stannous Fluoride)	RR Retained root	IMP Impacted (written above or below the tooth)

Table 18.1 Charting symbols

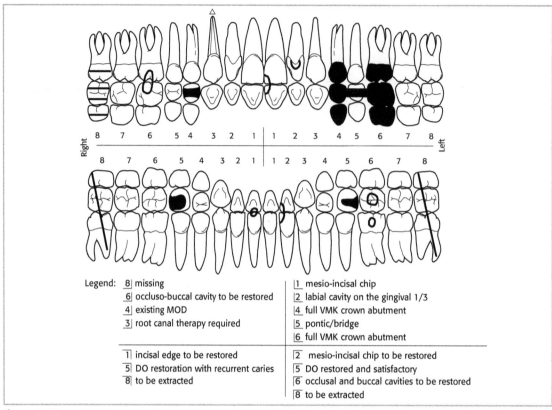

Legend: $\underline{8|}$ missing
$\underline{6|}$ occluso-buccal cavity to be restored
$\underline{4|}$ existing MOD
$\underline{3|}$ root canal therapy required

$\underline{|1}$ mesio-incisal chip
$\underline{|2}$ labial cavity on the gingival 1/3
$\underline{|4}$ full VMK crown abutment
$\underline{|5}$ pontic/bridge
$\underline{|6}$ full VMK crown abutment

$\overline{1|}$ incisal edge to be restored
$\overline{5|}$ DO restoration with recurrent caries
$\overline{8|}$ to be extracted

$\overline{|2}$ mesio-incisal chip to be restored
$\overline{|5}$ DO restored and satisfactory
$\overline{|6}$ occlusal and buccal cavities to be restored
$\overline{|8}$ to be extracted

Figure 18.12 Sample chart using Palmer's Notation

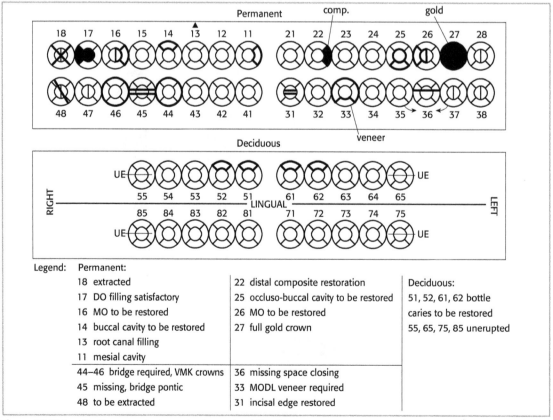

Legend: Permanent:
18 extracted
17 DO filling satisfactory
16 MO to be restored
14 buccal cavity to be restored
13 root canal filling
11 mesial cavity

44–46 bridge required, VMK crowns
45 missing, bridge pontic
48 to be extracted

22 distal composite restoration
25 occluso-buccal cavity to be restored
26 MO to be restored
27 full gold crown

36 missing space closing
33 MODL veneer required
31 incisal edge restored

Deciduous:
51, 52, 61, 62 bottle caries to be restored
55, 65, 75, 85 unerupted

Figure 18.13 Sample diagrammatic chart using International Notation

chapter nineteen
instruments and accessories

Introduction

This chapter provides an overview of the instruments, appliances and accessories most commonly used in the dental surgery including:

- hand tools and their components;
- handpieces and burs; and
- other instruments, appliances and accessories in common use.

Instruments and set-ups that are used primarily in areas of specialist dentistry (e.g. periodontics, oral surgery, etc) are discussed in Section 6.

Pre-prepared instrument trays

To save time and to allow for continuity during procedures, all the instruments and accessories that might be needed for the procedure are set out in advance. Most surgeries do this through the use of pre-prepared trays. The use of these trays is also good infection-control practice.

At the beginning of the appointment the prepared tray of instruments is put in position. When the operation is finished the tray is removed together with all dirty instruments, and after decontamination of the surgery it is replaced with a new tray that has been prepared for the next patient. In this way, the changeover time between patients is greatly reduced.

This system requires at least two trays but most practices use multiple trays, with the instruments stored in the trays as complete set-ups. If sufficient storage space and instruments are available, it is possible to provide enough prepared trays for a half or even a whole day's work, so that sterilising need only be done only once or twice a day. To provide for any likely half-day appointment schedules a typical practice may require, for example, six examination and prophylaxis trays, six filling trays (amalgam, or composite resin), one crown and bridge tray, one cementation tray, one endodontic tray and one surgical tray. Spare sterile instruments should be available in a convenient cabinet in case an instrument is dropped or changed.

With this system, all the instruments belonging to a particular set can be identified by a narrow band of instrument-coding tape placed around the handles, but the use of coding tape is not recommended by Australian Standards. A strip or strips of the same colour should be attached to the outside of the tray itself if this system is used.

A set of burs is required for each filling tray. These should be kept in bur-blocks with each hole marked by an abbreviation for a particular bur. In this way a required bur can be picked up without delay. The burs should be bagged and sterilised separately and opened in front of the patient.

Hand instruments

Component parts

The component parts of hand instruments are:

- the shaft;
- the blade; and
- the shank.

These are shown in Figure 19.1.

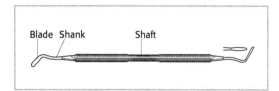

Figure 19.1 Component parts of hand instruments

Hand instruments can be single-ended (SE) or double-ended (DE). See Figure 19.2. A double-ended instrument is more efficient as it eliminates the need for two separate instruments.

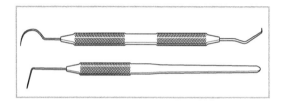

Figure 19.2 Double and single-ended instruments

The shaft

The handle of the instrument is sometimes called the shaft. It is about the same size as a pencil. This is the part where the instrument is gripped and it may have a smooth or a rough finish. The rough finish enables a firmer hand and finger grip.

Some handles have a cone socket so that the working end of the instrument can be replaced. See Figure 19.3.

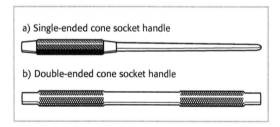

a) Single-ended cone socket handle

b) Double-ended cone socket handle

Figure 19.3 Single and double-ended cone socket handles

The blade

The blade is the functional end of the instrument and is sometimes called the nib.

The shank

The shank is also referred to as the shoulder of the instrument. It is often angled to provide access to various areas and surfaces of the mouth and the teeth, as shown in Figure 19.4.

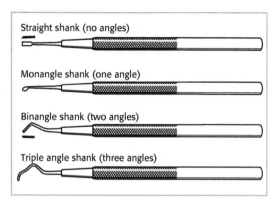

Straight shank (no angles)

Monangle shank (one angle)

Binangle shank (two angles)

Triple angle shank (three angles)

Figure 19.4 Shanks

Some hand instruments are used regularly by most dentists. Each dentist will have preferences for instruments and you must become familiar with the instruments commonly used for each procedure.

Hand-cutting instruments

Hand-cutting instruments may be used in cavity preparation to remove carious dentine and to smooth, prepare and finish surfaces for restorations. Hand-cutting instruments are made of any one of three types of alloys — stainless steel, high-carbon steel or tungsten carbide alloy. Not all dentists use hand-cutting instruments.

Hand-cutting instruments made of high-carbon steel retain their cutting edges better than those made of stainless steel alloys. However, they are subject to rust and corrosion if they are left sitting in water. Rust inhibitors help prevent this reaction but the hand-cutting instruments are best dried, bagged in autoclave packaging and sterilised in an autoclave with a drying cycle. This will help to preserve the sharp cutting edge.

It is essential that these instruments be kept sharp. Blunt instruments are more liable to slip and cause damage than sharp ones. These instruments are sharpened on an oilstone. Most dentists prefer to do this themselves, however, you may be asked to do this. If this is the case, ensure that the dentist gives you appropriate training beforehand. Any damaged instruments should be reported to the dentist and replaced.

The angle of the shank changes according to the function of the tool. An instrument for a buccal surface will have a smaller angle than an instrument used inter-proximally, for example. The parts of a hand-cutting instrument are shown in Figure 19.5.

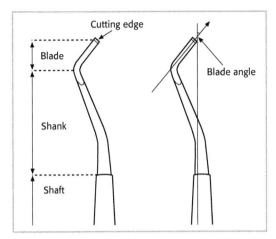

Figure 19.5 The parts of a hand-cutting instrument

In order to standardise instruments, manufacturers produce hand-cutting instruments in accord with an instrument formula. This formula appears on the instrument handle as a number or series of numbers. These numbers actually indicate measurements of the blade. When more than one number appears, the first figure represents the width of the blade in tenths of a millimetre. The second figure indicates the length of the blade in millimetres and the third figure designates the angle the blade forms with the long axis of the handle.

These numbers should not be confused with the manufacturer's stock number appearing near the end of the handle. The formula numbers aid in obtaining the correct instrument when ordering new instruments, and identification between dentist and assistant.

Hand-cutting instruments may be classified as excavators, gingival margin trimmers, chisels, hatchets and hoes.

Spoon excavators

Spoon excavators are commonly used for the removal of soft caries and other soft materials, including excess cement bases or cavity liners. Some excavators have a rounded cutting edge that resembles a spoon or disc (discoid). Others have a claw-like edge (cleoid) and these are also used for carving amalgam. See an example in Figure 19.6.

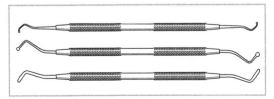

Figure 19.6 Spoon excavator

Gingival margin trimmers

The gingival margin trimmer is a special type of chisel used for placing bevels on enamel margins at the gingival edge of Class II cavities. The blade is similar to that of an enamel chisel but is slightly curved and the cutting edge is at an angle with the blade. These instruments are made in pairs for either the mesial or the distal surface of the tooth, as well as for narrow (premolar) and wide (premolar).

See an example in Figure 19.7.

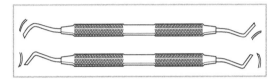

Figure 19.7 Gingival margin trimmers

Chisels

Dental chisels are similar to carpenter's chisels. They may have a straight shaft or it may be bent. The cutting edge is at right angles to the handle, as shown in Figure 19.8.

The chisel is used for planning and cleaving enamel.

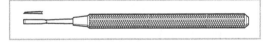

Figure 19.8 Chisels

Hatchets

Hatchets are similar in size to chisels but the cutting edge is in line with the handle, rather like the hatchet used in cutting wood.

These instruments are designed to use on the internal surfaces of cavity preparations mainly to prepare retentive areas and to sharpen internal line angles. Some of them may be bevelled on both sides of the blade. See Figure 19.9.

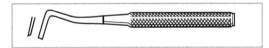

Figure 19.9 Hatchets

Hoe

The hoe is used for the removal of hard caries and to form line angles in anterior teeth. See Figure 19.10.

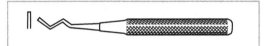

Figure 19.10 Hoe

Handpieces

Handpieces attach to the dental engine and hold the bur for the purpose of cutting cavities in teeth. They are available in a number of different shapes and sizes — straight, contra-angle (when the head is angled with respect to the shaft) and miniature. See the example in Figure 19.11.

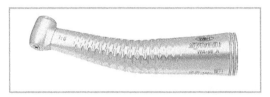

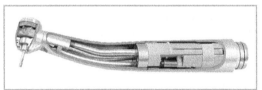

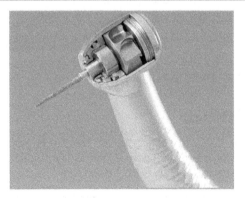

Figure 19.11 Handpieces

Handpieces are valuable and highly sensitive pieces of equipment. They are precision instruments containing many gears. Read the instruction manual carefully and follow the instructions implicitly. Regular lubrication and cleaning is essential and should be done after each use. However, over-lubrication can also damage the handpiece. Proper cleaning before sterilisation is essential to prevent the build-up of debris. A summary of handpiece maintenance is provided under a separate heading below.

Special handpieces should be set aside for use with prophylaxis paste as this material can enter the handpiece gearing and, being abrasive, can cause considerable wear. Some handpieces are lubricated with an aerosol spray or there are special lubrication machines that can do the job. Read and carefully follow the manufacturers' instructions regarding the maintenance of the handpieces used in your surgery. Be sure the unit is turned off each evening.

High-speed handpieces

High-speed handpieces are used to remove decay, old restorations or tooth structure in the preparation of the tooth for a new restoration. As the revolution (speed) of the bur is very fast, the cutting of tooth structure means that the bur creates heat. To keep the working area cool these handpieces are equipped to send a fine spray of water onto the working surface. This keeps the tooth and the tool cool and helps to keep the working surface free of debris. The 'finishing' work is then done using a low-speed handpiece.

Low-speed handpieces

Low-speed handpieces are used for removing soft decay, working close to nerve, finishing, contouring and polishing. The reduction rate of slow speed handpieces varies according to the purpose of the handpiece.

Handpiece maintenance

Handpieces should be cleaned, lubricated and prepared strictly according to the manufacturer's instructions. Thorough cleaning of both internal and external surfaces needs to be carried out. Proper care will prolong the life of this very expensive, but vital, piece of equipment.

There are special handpiece cleaning and purging units available that accomplish the whole purging and lubricating procedure.

Note that handpieces are a potential source of cross-infection and proper sterilisation techniques must be used.

Additional to manufacturer's instructions, note the following.

■ Handpieces must be purged (run for 30 seconds) before removal from the unit to discharge water and to allow air to flush out any gross debris that may have entered the turbine and air or water lines. Care should be taken to minimise aerosol dispersion during this procedure.

■ Some handpieces should not be run without a dummy bur. Check the manufacturer's instructions.

- Do not use a wire brush to clean the handpiece sheath. Wipe it clean with detergent on a damp cloth. A soft toothbrush may be use to clean the textured finger grip area.
- Do not place the handpiece in an ultrasonic cleaning device.
- Take care not to drop the handpiece as it may cause serious damage.

Handpiece lubrication

Follow the handpiece manufacturer's instructions. Lubrication cleans the working parts of the handpiece as well as lubricating them. It is important to check that the handpiece is not expelling dirt or black particles. To check this, place a tissue over the head of the handpiece and lubricate it, then inspect the tissue.

If there are visible black particles or dirty lubricant patches on the tissue, repeat the process until no dirt is expended from the handpiece. In the case of slow-speed or prophy handpieces this may require disassembling the head and lubricating each component or bearing separately.

Wipe excess lubricant from the handpiece.

Handpieces must be bagged separately for autoclaving to prevent contaminating other items with any left over lubricant.

Autoclave at 134°C for seven minutes, but check the manufacturer's instructions on required temperatures.

Dental burs

Dental burs are instruments used in the handpiece to cut tooth structure in cavity preparation. They are available in a variety of different sized shanks (the part which is gripped in the handpiece) depending on whether they are to be used in a straight, contra-angle, miniature or friction-grip handpiece. They also have different shaped and sized cutting heads. The sizes increase from the smallest (000) to 00, 1, 2, and up to 10 or more. They are made from tungsten carbide or steel. Some have diamond heads.

Burs come in different shapes — round, inverted cone, wheel, flat fissure, tapered fissure, round-ended fissure and pear, as can be seen in Figure 19.12.

Burs have different cutting edges depending on what they are designed to cut. Acrylic and bone-cutting burs have coarse open blades, while plug-finishing burs, used for minor trimming of restorations, have many fine blades. Diamond burs are also produced in similar shapes and are more efficient in the high-speed handpieces.

The shape and size of the cutting head will be selected depending on the cavity preparation or procedure (e.g. denture adjustment) to be performed by the dentist. For the same type of cavity, the dentist will often routinely use the same type of bur. You must know what the dentist is going to do for the patient so that the correct instruments can be selected. You must be able to recognise burs at a glance.

Unmounted stones or discs are attached to a mandrel by a screw or friction grip for use with a handpiece.

Cleaning burs

Burs should be kept clean and sterilised at all times, and if showing signs of wear they should be replaced. Diamond burs, when cleaned ultrasonically, should be placed into special bur stands. This avoids the burs bouncing in the ultrasonic bath, which can damage them and shorten their lives. Debris is removed from diamond burs by brushing with a nailbrush. A rubber eraser is also useful for removing debris from diamond instruments and will not damage the diamond chips.

Steel burs can be cleaned ultrasonically and autoclaved but single use, slow-speed steel burs are preferred.

Other instruments, appliances and accessories

Ultrasonic scaler unit

The ultrasonic instrument is not a rotary instrument and is not used to cut tooth structure. An example is shown in Figure 19.13. This type of instrument converts electrical energy into mechanical energy in the form of tiny mechanical vibrations. This energy activates a metal tip to move back and forth within a distance of 25 micrometres at speeds up to 25,000 times per second. The tips that are mounted in a handpiece are available in various sizes and shapes. The instrument can be a self-contained unit, light in weight and portable or may be like a handpiece that is clicked onto a handpiece coupling.

Patients with pacemakers should not be treated with ultrasonic scalers.

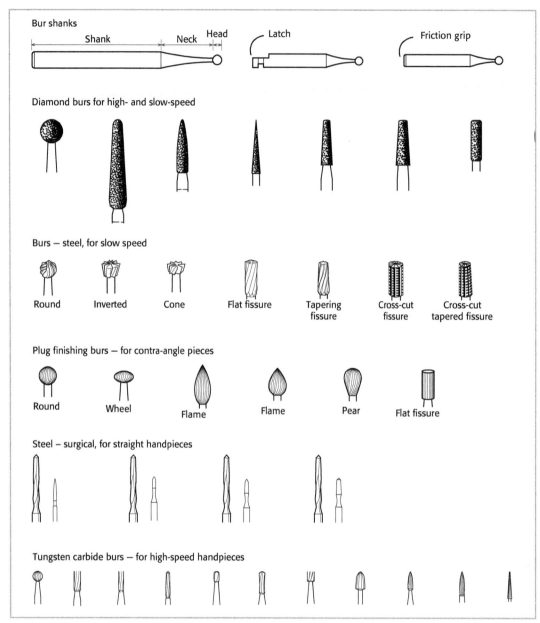

Figure 19.12 Bur heads and shanks

The primary function of the ultrasonic instrument is in oral prophylactic procedures and in minor periodontal procedures. During these procedures, water is passed over the activated tip in order to keep the work area cool.

Refer to manufacturer's instructions for cleaning and sterilisation. Some ultrasonic scalers cannot be placed in ultrasonic cleaners. Proper sterilisation of the tips is the dental assistant's responsibility.

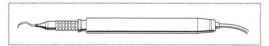

Figure 19.13 Ultrasonic scaler tip

Prophy-jet

A combination of air/water and sodium bicarbonate powder is sprayed from the prophy-jet onto the tooth surfaces. This creates a sandblasting effect that assists in the effective removal of plaque and staining. The prophy-jet tip should be disinfected after each use.

Miscellaneous accessories for restorative dentistry

Spatulas

Spatulas come in many shapes and sizes for mixing cements, temporary fillings and impression materials.

Alginate spatulas, available in metal or plastic, are large-bladed implements, flexible to manipulate and they prevent air being incorporated in the alginate mix.

Articulating paper forceps

Articulating paper forceps, as shown in Figure 19.14, are used to hold the articulating paper in place when checking occlusion. They are also known as Millar's forceps. This procedure is done after the completion of restorations, during the fabrication of dentures and for the analysis of occlusal patterns of the natural dentition.

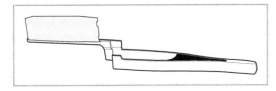

Figure 19.14 Articulating paper forceps

Syringes

Modern syringes are used in combination with sterilised disposable cartridges and needles, and are often of the aspirating type. Be sure the adaptor is fitted correctly to avoid leakage at the needle. To avoid the risk of disease transmission and needle fracture, a pre-sterilised new needle must be used for all patients. A new cartridge must be used for each patient. Any remaining analgesic solution must be discarded with the used cartridge. Types of syringes include aspirating and regular syringes. More information about syringes can be found in Chapter 20.

Summary

There are hundreds of instruments that you might work with in the course of your regular duties. Each dentist will have a preference for particular instruments.

You should be able to instantly recognise the instruments that the dentist uses and be able to provide them without delay by anticipating the dentist's requirements. Knowing the instruments will also simplify the process of preparing tray set-ups and allow you to sort and store sterile instruments easily and efficiently.

chapter twenty
pain control in dentistry

Introduction

Many people associate a trip to the dentist with pain. This might be because they present to the dentist with a history of pain requiring relief. Alternatively, the treatment provided by the dentist may cause pain at the time of operation or result in pain as a sequel to the treatment. For most patients, though, the degree of discomfort during and after treatment is minimal. Excellent methods are available to virtually abolish pain sensation during dental treatment.

Because many patients do experience pain during dental procedures it is necessary to understand what pain is.

Pain is totally subjective in the sense that it can only be registered and described by the person feeling it. Since there are important factors that vary the pain sensation and its recognition, it is important to understand some important points about the pain process.

The perception threshold

The point at which pain is first perceived as a sensation is often referred to as the perception threshold. This will vary from one individual to another and in the same individual from one time to another. It is influenced by emotional states and other factors. This is why it is best for patients to be treated sympathetically, in a quiet and restful, and generally comfortable, environment.

Previous pain, fear and anxiety, adverse climatic conditions or other disturbing factors will lower the point at which pain is detected. Therefore, any measures that will raise this pain threshold are

important not only in the general handling of a patient but in relation to the response to the dental procedure, including the administration and effectiveness of local anaesthetics.

Interpretation and localisation

Another stage in the pain process is the interpretation and localisation of the pain. People experiencing pain will place their own interpretation on the cause of the pain and will record the type of pain that is being felt; for example, stinging, burning, or deeper, nauseating pain.

The reaction to pain

The point at which a person will react to pain may also be described as a threshold point. This will tend to vary with the individual and to some extent with emotional states.

The importance of the emotional state of the patient is obvious. Much of the pain process can be controlled by careful handling and conditioning of the patient. Local anaesthetics are much more effective in a patient who is relaxed and less fearful.

Anaesthesia and sedation in dentistry

Local anaesthesia (analgesia)

Analgesia is the elimination of pain. **Anaesthesia** is the elimination of all sensation. Although different, the two are often used in dentistry as meaning the same. An important point about all clinical anaesthetic methods is that the effects of the agents should be reversible and should leave no residual harmful effects on the patient's tissues.

Administration of local anaesthetics

Topical or surface anaesthesia

Topical or surface anaesthesia is obtained by the application of a suitable agent to an area of skin or mucous membrane. The agents do not penetrate skin or mucous membrane readily but act on superficial nerve endings. Topical agents are mostly used in dental practice to produce surface anaesthesia of the mucous membrane before injection into the underlying tissues, or for incision of a soft tissue abscess. The agents used are often in the form of a spray or ointment containing lignocaine hydrochloride.

Infiltration anaesthesia

With infiltration anaesthesia, small terminal nerve endings in an area are flooded with solution, producing anaesthesia of the localised area served by these nerve endings. Infiltration injections are used in regions where the overlying bone is thin and porous enough to allow the solution to diffuse through the cortical plate of bone to reach the nerves, mostly in the upper jaw.

There are two special types of infiltration anaesthesia that may occasionally be used by dentists if there is a difficulty achieving patient comfort by conventional means. Intra-osseous injections go into the bone adjacent to the tooth to be anaesthetised. This gives instant effect without wide areas of tissue numbness. Intraligamental injections are injections directly into the periodontal ligament and sometimes used to numb a specific area around a mandibular tooth where a block injection is not required or is inadvisable.

Inferior mental nerve block or regional block anaesthesia

For inferior mental nerve block, or regional block anaesthesia, the anaesthetic solution is deposited adjacent to the sheath of a main nerve trunk before it enters the bone. This prevents impulses from beyond that point travelling to the brain. Regional block anaesthesia is used more commonly in the lower jaw because the posterior areas of the body of the mandible have a hard dense outer layer of bone that is not porous and thus not easily penetrated by anaesthetic solutions. This has the effect of anaesthetising (numbing) one side of the mandible to the midline.

Composition of local anaesthetic solutions

Commercial local anaesthetic solutions consist of:

- a local anaesthetic drug;
- a vaso-constrictor drug;
- a physiological saline solution; and
- other additives designed to maintain the stability of the solution.

Dental local anaesthetic solutions deteriorate with prolonged storage or under unfavourable storage conditions. The date marked on the package should be carefully checked for currency.

Dispensing local anaesthetic solutions

Local anaesthetic solutions are marketed in the form of cartridges (carpules), designed for use with a dental cartridge syringe, or as ampoules. The cartridge is the recommended form for use in dentistry since the risk of contamination of the solution is greatly reduced.

A dental cartridge or carpule, as shown in Figure 20.1, consists of a glass tube containing the solution. It is sealed at one end with a soft cap and at the other end with a plunger. The glass or polypropylene tube is carefully manufactured to have a uniform inside diameter. The sealing cap may be all rubber or may consist of a rubber disc with an aluminium cap crimped or bent over a collar in the glass of the carpule. The plunger is used to expel the contents of the tube.

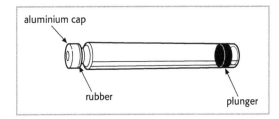

Figure 20.1 Anaesthetic carpule or cartridge

Discomfort to the patient is minimised if cartridges are warmed to body temperature (37°C) prior to injection.

A cartridge that is not completely used in an injection must be thrown away and never used on another patient. It is possible, with the pressure used in injecting and with sudden release on stopping the injection, to suck back tissue fluids. Therefore, if the cartridge is reused on another patient it is possible to transmit infectious disease from one person to another (e.g. serum hepatitis, HIV).

It is preferable to store the dental cartridge in a cool, dark place to give a maximum shelf-life. Manufacturers specifications must be followed.

The expiry date on local anaesthetic cartridges needs to be closely observed. Out-of-date solutions can become toxic or become ineffective.

Syringes and needles

Types of syringe

The four types of dental syringes are:
❶ cartridge syringes (end- and side-loading);
❷ aspirating (auto-asp) syringes;
❸ intraligamentary syringes; and
❹ disposable syringes.

An example of an intraligamentary syringe and an aspirating syringe is shown in Figure 20.2.

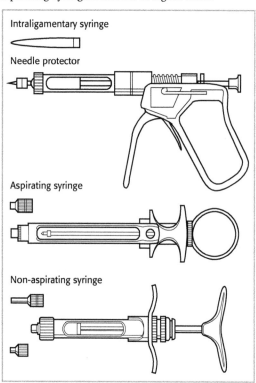

Figure 20.2 Aspirating syringe

End-loading and side-loading cartridge syringes

The most widely used hypodermic syringe in current practice is the standard cartridge syringe, which may be either an end-loading type or a side-loading type. This consists of a metal barrel and plunger united by a spring-loaded hinge mechanism. A threaded hub at the lower end of the barrel permits the attachment of a double-ended needle. Opening of the hinge mechanism (end-loading) permits the insertion of the glass cartridge containing the sterile anaesthetic solution. The side-loading patterns provide for the insertion of the cartridge into the side of the barrel.

Aspirating dental cartridge syringe

The aspirating dental cartridge syringe differs from the standard cartridge syringe in that the piston is designed to engage the rubber plunger of the cartridge so that on withdrawal of the handle, the syringe can be made to suck back or aspirate. If on aspiration blood appears in the cartridge, it is assumed that the end of the needle is in a very vascular area and the injection will not be given without withdrawing the needle and repositioning it.

Intraligamentary syringes

Intraligamentary syringes are designed to provide anaesthesia directly into lower anterior teeth instead of giving a block injection. Although not very widely used, they may be the choice of a dentist with specific training and experience with the specialised technique of using intraligamentary syringes.

There are different types and shapers of intraligamentary syringes but as a standard their barrels are usually shorter, utilising smaller cartridges. The nozzle may be inclined for ease of depositing the anaesthetic. The plunger works on a trigger system because steady pressure is needed to inject into the periodontal ligament.

Disposable dental syringes

Disposable syringes, that is, units consisting of a plastic syringe with needle and barrel full of anaesthetic solution, are also available. Using this equipment, an injection can be given and the whole unit, syringe and needle, thrown away after use.

The parts of a hypodermic syringe (hypodermic means literally under skin) are the:
- barrel;
- plunger; and
- handle.

Needles

Hypodermic needles used with the dental cartridge syringe are of the double-ended type and are available in varying gauges and lengths.

The **gauge** of the needle denotes the thickness of the diameter of its shaft or **lumen** and gauges

gauge: the diameter of the tube through which the solution passes into the tissues.
lumen: the bore or inner width of a tube.

range from 20 to 30. The lower the number, the thicker the needle. 14G is wider than 23G and much more solution can be administered quickly into the tissues. Fine gauge needles (e.g. 27G, 30G) tend to be used in dentistry to minimise pain on injection. For example, 30G needles can only be used with intraligamentary syringes. In medical emergencies, such as severe blood loss, wide bore needles are used to administer as much fluid as possible in a short time. This may be life-saving. In routine work, anaesthetists have their personal preferences but may use 18G or 20G.

A needle consists of three parts: the hub, the shaft and the bevel. The hub will vary with the type of syringe with which the needle is to be used.

Needles for dental use are made in two lengths. Short needles (usual length = 25 mm) are used mostly for infiltration injection. Long needles (usual length = 41 mm) are used mainly for block anaesthesia. It is recommended practice that the long needles should not be of the very fine gauge 30, but rather 26 gauge or, at the most, 28. This is because the heavier needles are not so likely to be deflected by the tissues or bent during use.

Hypodermic needles for dental use are disposable. The needles are packaged and sterilised by radiation before dispatch. The needle is used once and then discarded. This reduces the risk of transmitting disease. Many needles have a silicone coating, which allows for easier introduction of the needle through the tissues.

Any needle that is bent when setting up a syringe should be immediately discarded because it is dangerous to straighten a needle after it has been bent. Bending causes the metal to work harder and the needle then fractures easily.

Rules for syringe use

The syringe should not be removed from the sterilising pouch until the local anaesthetic (LA) is required. The non-touch technique is essential for this procedure so the cap of the cartridge, through which the needle is inserted, is not contaminated.

The needle is fitted to the barrel of the syringe before loading with the local anaesthetic cartridge, the needle sheath being left in position.

The cartridge is pushed carefully down on to the needle. This ensures that the needle pierces the cartridge diaphragm cleanly in order to obtain a good seal and avoid leakage of the solution at the point of puncture.

The plunger of the aspirating syringe should engage the rubber plunger in the cartridge.

Anaesthetic syringes should only be prepared as required and must never be pre-prepared for the whole day's procedures. The moment the cartridge is pierced by the needle there is a risk of contamination. The solution expiry date should be checked before use.

Possible complications during administration of local anaesthetic

Systemic complications include:

- fainting — this is unlikely if the patient is treated in the supine position; and
- allergic reactions — hypersensitivity reactions to injected modern local anaesthetic solutions are rare. Procaine tended to cause reactions more frequently.

Local complications include:

- haematoma — the formation of a haematoma or bruise at the site of the injection in the oral tissues is more often associated with the nerve-block type of injection than with infiltration injections; delayed discomfort and partial **trismus** may result but the haematoma is usually absorbed within a few days with no further complications (the use of the aspirating type of syringe minimises the possibility of haematoma formation);
- breakage of a needle — this complication has become infrequent since the introduction of sterile disposable needles which are used once only;
- lip trauma — children, especially those who have had a mandibular block injection, should be warned of the danger of eating or drinking hot foods or of biting the lower lip until the anaesthetic effect has disappeared (trauma may also result from the injudicious use of cheek or lip retractors or other instruments by the dentist or the assistant, or by instrument burns);
- pain on injection;
- facial paralysis (Bell's Palsy);
- visual disturbances (local anaesthetic deposited in wrong site);
- infection at injection site; and
- blanching of surrounding tissues.

All these conditions are very rare in modern dental practice.

trismus: inability to open mouth fully.

195

Sedation and anaesthesia

Psycho-sedation

Factors influencing psycho-sedation include:

- pleasant office décor;
- background music;
- friendly, considerate staff;
- airconditioning;
- unhurried efficiency; and
- calm, reassuring talk.

An increasing number of dentists now use hypnosis as a major aid to anxiety and pain control.

Oral premedication

Tablets and syrups are the easiest way to give a patient a tranquillising drug. The main disadvantage of this technique is that the results are not predictable as to the time of onset of the effect or the depth of sedation.

The more commonly used drugs in this group are diazepam (Valium) and phenergan.

These tablets (or for children, syrups) are given some time before the dental appointment and usually result in more peaceful operating conditions. Sometimes, however, no sedative effect is noted at the time of treatment and the effect is only noticed some hours later. Because of this possibility, it is recommended that the patient be accompanied by a responsible adult and be advised against driving a car or operating any machinery, or making any important decisions for the remainder of the day. The elimination of diazepam from the body is very slow and can take up to 24 hours.

Sedation techniques

Sedation in dentistry should be conscious sedation; that is, where rational verbal communication with the patient is maintained throughout. The following methods are used in dentistry. (See the earlier pages on routes of administration for additional information.)

Note that combinations of these forms can be used.

Oral sedation

Oral sedation is simple and safe. However, the effect can be variable, due to unpredictability of absorption from the gut.

Relative analgesia (nitrous oxide sedation)

The mixture of nitrous oxide and oxygen is sometimes called happy gas and is an effective anti-anxiety agent, which helps eliminate fear and relax the patient. Relative analgesia is well accepted by children. They relax very quickly.

In this technique, small amounts of nitrous oxide gas, mixed with oxygen and sometimes air, are administered to the patient via a nose mask from an analgesia machine. Patients can control the effect to some degree by breathing through their mouth. They will feel relaxed and tension is lowered. As a result the pain threshold is often raised. It is sometimes possible to carry out some simple dental procedures without local anaesthesia, though it is usual to supplement relative analgesia with local anaesthesia.

This is safe and easy to use, with minimal training. There is good patient acceptance of this technique and it reduces the gag reflex. Some specialised equipment and facilities are required, and a post-operative escort for the patient is desirable.

Post-operative recovery is very quick with administration of 100 per cent oxygen for a short period (two minutes approximately). However, there can be some **anterograde amnesia**.

The relative analgesia machine differs from an anaesthetic machine in that, when switched on, the relative analgesia machine delivers a minimum flow of oxygen of three litres per minute, and it has a failsafe device which, in the event of oxygen failure, automatically cuts off the nitrous oxide flow and opens a valve, allowing air to enter the system.

This technique should not be used on patients with nasal congestion, any advanced nasal pathology (emphysema), the common cold, pregnancy (especially in the first trimester), epileptics or people with psychiatric problems.

A small number of patients may find relative analgesia ineffective or unpleasant.

There may be some side effects such as nausea, dizziness, excessive perspiration, excessive talking and giggling, and palpitation.

anterograde amnesia: forgetting events that occurred after the anaesthetic was used.

Long-term effects on staff as a result of surgery pollution have been reported as liver damage, spontaneous abortions, effects on sperm and foetuses. Although these are very rare, all necessary precautions are advisable. There is more information on this topic in Chapter 15.

Intravenous sedation

Intravenous (IV) conscious sedation involves the administration of anti-anxiety medication that produces a degree of sedation while retaining a level of consciousness. The patient retains continuous and independent ability to maintain an airway and to respond appropriately to physical or verbal stimulation. This technique is enormously valuable in the right hands, enabling some people to have dental treatment who might not otherwise attend. However, it is potentially dangerous in the wrong hands.

Accredited training (Diploma in Clinical Dentistry) is now required before this kind of anaesthesia can be used.

Some patients do not like a needle in the back of the hand and are therefore resistant to IV sedation.

Patients should be assessed for this procedure and this should include:

- a concise, current medical history;
- informed consent for the procedure (see the example in Figure 20.3); and
- appropriate written instructions for preparation (at least six hours of fasting), information about the procedure and post-operative instructions and explanation of possible after-effects.

Considerable amounts of equipment and facilities are necessary to perform intravenous sedation.

Hypnosis

Hypnosis is used with great success by a small number of practitioners. Something you can do is simply to speak calmly and quietly to reassure the patient and to ensure that they are comfortable to the extent of becoming relaxed.

General anaesthesia

General anaesthesia is a complete state of unconsciousness in which there is a loss of all muscle control and protective reflexes, including the ability to maintain an airway independently and to respond appropriately to physical stimulation or verbal command.

Request for procedures using intravenous sedation

I _____

Of _____ address
following a discussion about my present dental status and the treatment options with
Dr _____, request the following treatment/procedure

_____

be carried out using intravenous sedation.

I also request and consent to other forms of treatment normally associated with this procedure and deemed necessary to achieve an optimal result.

Although this procedure will be carried out with all due professional care and responsibility, I understand that in some circumstances the expected result may not be achieved.

I also understand that complications may occur with any procedure and accept the possible risks associated with this procedure.

Signature of patient _____

Signature of witness _____

Name of witness _____

Date _____

In the case of surgery being performed under general anaesthetic, this consent form does not replace the standard hospital form which must also be completed.

Figure 20.3 Sample consent form for intravenous sedation

This form of sedation is rarely used in dentistry. However, it is a speciality of medicine very useful for the most apprehensive patients and children who need to undergo large amounts of treatment. Large amounts of specialised equipment and facilities are required to perform general anaesthesia.

General anaesthesia must be administered by a qualified anaesthetist. It is usually performed in fully equipped day surgery units.

Your role during intravenous sedation and general anaesthesia

Your role will largely depend on the practice in which you work and your employer's requirements. It is very important that the dentist never be left alone in the surgery with the patient (to minimise litigation risks).

Before the treatment, ensure all equipment and materials are close at hand. It is useful to have a checklist on hand.

As soon as the patient arrives, check the patient's identity, give a warm welcome and reassure the patient, as most will be apprehensive.

Check that:

- the patient has had nothing to eat or drink for at least six hours before the procedure;
- the consent form is signed; and
- that the patient has made arrangements to be collected after treatment.

During the treatment, carry out procedural duties as required. Constantly observe the patient and if you have concerns make this known in an appropriate manner. Nursing duties required of you in the surgery will be explained to you by the dentist.

After treatment the patient is monitored closely until normal reflexes return. The patient should not be left unattended while regaining consciousness. Attend to their needs during the recovery phase as required. Give written post-operative instructions and preferably explain them to the patient's escort.

Possible systemic complications

As with all procedures that involve administering drugs, there are possible systemic complications. They could include:

- myocardial infarction (heart attack);
- cardiac arrest (heart stops beating, i.e. no pulse, unconscious);
- allergy (especially anaphylactic shock, which can be fatal); and
- post-operative complications.

Fortunately these complications are rare.

Other medical conditions to be aware of, as they may complicate the procedure, include:

- diabetes mellitus;
- epilepsy; and
- those conditions for which patients take corticosteroids.

Emergencies during drug administration

Precautions during drug administration

Ensure that:

- the correct drug is being used (check label on vial/syringe);
- the drug has not passed the expiry date;
- the patient is not allergic to the drug;
- the patient is not taking other drugs that may interact;
- the patient does not have a medical condition which could be worsened by administration of the drug;
- needle-stick injury is avoided by following established protocols;
- all emergency equipment and telephone contact numbers are close at hand and prepared for immediate use; and
- members of the dental team regularly practice emergency protocols to ensure every member knows their role and responsibility during an emergency, no matter how small.

Maintenance of emergency equipment

- Regularly check expiry dates on local anaesthetic and re-order as necessary.
- Check at least monthly, preferably weekly, that the emergency oxygen cylinder is full.

- Check expiry dates on emergency drugs (for example, adrenaline) and drugs used for sedation.
- Check resuscitation equipment regularly with special attention to perished tubing.

Cardiopulmonary resuscitation certification

Dental assistants should have cardiopulmonary resuscitation (CPR) certification. This should be kept up to date.

For a Dental Assistant Certificate III the national requirement is a Level I First Aid, previously known as a Senior or Industrial First Aid Certificate.

Emergency equipment list

Clinical equipment

- Oxygen with tubing and mask
- Resuscitation mask — oropharyngeal airways
- Suction
- Intravenous cannula or butterfly needle for venous access
- 5 ml and 10 ml syringes
- 21G needles
- Stethoscope and blood pressure measuring equipment
- Pulse oximeter
- Tourniquet.

Drugs

- Adrenaline(strongly advised)
- Hydrocortisone
- Diazepam
- Dextrose or sugar lumps (for diabetes).

Administrative information

Ensure your emergency contact list is placed in an obvious location. Time may be critical. The list should contain:

- telephone numbers of ambulance, a nearby medical practitioner, police and fire brigade and poisons information centre; and
- a simple statement of your location (e.g. '15 Wattle Street, Acacia, dental surgery opposite the Shell service station').

Try to speak clearly, avoiding repetition.

Cranio-mandibular pain dysfunction syndrome

Cranio-mandibular pain dysfunction conditions are relatively common. Symptoms range from a joint 'click' or other sound on opening or closing the jaw to very severe facial pain and headaches. This problem is an increasing part of dental practice, probably due to:

- better recognition of the problem by dental and medical practitioners;
- teeth being retained for most of a person's life because of better dental awareness and care; and
- increased stresses of modern life. In a great majority of cases, stress is a factor.

Pain and functional problems may arise with:

- one or both temporo-mandibular (TM) joints;
- muscles involved in mastication or head posture; or
- a combination of the above.

The temporo-mandibular joint

For a description of the temporo-mandibular joint (TMJ), see Chapter 8.

The TMJ is a very complex and relatively easily damaged joint. Injury may result from yawning, attempting to chew things too large or too hard, general anaesthetics, prolonged dental procedures, trauma or from dysfunction in the masticatory complex.

The inter-articular disc may be displaced or may be perforated.

This joint tends to be less afflicted by arthritis or rheumatism than other joints. However, painless conditions that are left untreated can proceed to traumatic arthritis and considerable discomfort.

Muscular pain

Muscle tension or spasms are caused by a disturbance of information flow from the nerve supply to the muscles of the joint. This may cause severe pain, headaches or migraine and limitation of opening the mouth.

These muscular problems typically result from disturbances in occlusion and are exaggerated by stress and habits such as bruxing, clenching, tongue thrusting, and so forth.

Hobbies and occupations such as scuba diving, or playing wind, brass or stringed instruments (such as violins and violas) may also play a part.

Some occlusal problems can be **iatrogenic**. For example, bridgework or orthodontics may produce disturbances in occlusal function. Premature tooth loss with rotation or tipping of teeth can be factors.

Treatment

Treatment for cranio-mandibular pain dysfunction conditions is aimed at returning the function of the masticatory complex as much as possible. Treatment is usually by splint therapy but there are other methods used, too. Regardless of the method used, when pain relief is obtained and is longstanding, other methods may be used to stabilise the pattern of muscle activity.

Joints may be helped by manipulation and exercise in the case of disk derangement.

With some severe cases, orthodontics or surgery involving jaw repositioning may be used.

Summary

Fear of pain and the experience of pain can cause patients to avoid dental treatment with the result that minor conditions become quite serious. Effective pain relief influences the patient's perception of the quality of dental care received.

Although side effects are rare, some patients do experience them and you should be prepared to act appropriately should they occur. A thorough understanding of pain relief techniques and drugs will assist you to do this.

■ **iatrogenic:** brought about by (dental or medical) treatment. Treatment-related condition.

chapter twenty-one
dental radiography.

Introduction

When discussing radiographs, nearly everyone refers to their 'x-rays'. In reality these x-rays should be called radiographs. A radiograph is a picture in which the teeth and jaws appear as shadows. The traditional method of producing these pictures is to expose a piece of radiographic film to x-rays and then develop (chemically process) the film. However, with today's digital equipment, an image receptor and computer are often used instead of film. Either method produces a 'shadow image' that shows the teeth, bone and other structures. From these images, the dentist can determine if there are any pathological conditions or abnormalities within the teeth and jaws.

Good quality radiographs are essential to good diagnosis and treatment planning. Without radiographs, some serious pathological conditions may be hidden from the dentist.

From the dentist's point of view, radiographs:

- are an essential aid to diagnosis and treatment planning;
- are an essential aid during treatment; for example, endodontics, difficult extractions;
- allow a post-operative follow-up of completed treatment by allowing an assessment of the effectiveness of treatment and healing;
- provide a permanent record of the patient's dentition, both before and after treatment;
- minimise patient trauma; for example, by revealing how close a carious lesion is to the pulp, the risk of accidental pulpal exposure can be minimised; and
- provide an invaluable legal record of treatment should there be a legal dispute about the standard of care. Radiographs can record the patient's condition both before and after treatment.

From the patient's viewpoint radiographs:

- permit early detection of carious lesions (early detection often minimises the amount and cost of any necessary treatment);
- permit early detection of underlying disease (oral pathology); for example, bone loss due to periodontal disease, cysts, missing or un-erupted teeth, etc;
- ensure thoroughness of treatment;
- minimise the chance of unexpectedly complex and often painful procedures and the risks associated with them;
- reveal the unexpected. These are known as 'incidental findings'. For example, a radiograph may reveal supernumerary teeth, un-erupted teeth, cysts, root resorption, malignancies or some other dental or general pathology.

Additionally, dental radiographs can be used for positive forensic identification of people after accidental or suspicious death.

Uses of radiographs

Restorative dentistry

- To detect interproximal caries, especially at the initial stage. The advantage of early detection is that damage to tooth enamel, if discovered early enough, may be remineralised by fluoride treatment. This means that no restoration is needed and the loss of tooth structure from operative procedures is avoided.
- To detect cavities too small to be seen even by careful visual examination. Small cavities do require smaller, less expensive restorations and because there is less loss of tooth structure, the strength of the tooth is preserved. Smaller restorations also last longer.

- To diagnose occlusal caries. If left untreated, these caries may penetrate deep into the tooth structure.
- To detect recurrent caries around or beneath existing restorations, which may be impossible to diagnose without radiographs.
- To gauge the depth and extent of large carious lesions.
- To assess tooth anatomy (e.g. root structure for bridge or partial denture work).
- To detect faulty contours on restorations (e.g. overhanging margins).
- To assess the relationship to neighbouring teeth.
- To determine the state of development of both the deciduous and permanent dentitions.

Periodontics

- To assess the health of alveolar bone and the degree of any bone loss. Important features such as cementum and bone cannot be properly assessed without the assistance of radiographs.
- To detect subgingival calculus.
- To assess the health of the periodontal membrane.
- To assess the effectiveness of treatment.

Endodontics

- To detect pulpal involvement from caries.
- During treatment, to assess root length and the shape of root canals during root canal therapy.
- To visualise the condition of the periapical tissues before endodontic treatment.
- Post operatively, to assess periapical healing.

Oral pathology

- To detect periapical lesions; for example, chronic abscess.
- To detect the presence of cysts.
- To detect changes in tissues and abnormal growths, such as tumours.
- To detect and aid in the treatment of fractures; for example, fractured teeth, fractured jaws.

Oral surgery

To aid in the treatment of pathological conditions (for example, bone growths) or to assist in the localisation of foreign bodies (for example, bullet wound, industrial or car accidents).

- To provide essential information prior to potentially complex extractions; for example, impacted wisdom teeth. Dental radiographs allow the dentist to determine the relationship of impacted or un-erupted teeth to other anatomical structures, such as the maxillary sinus or inferior dental canal. This reduces the risk of complications or trauma during surgery.
- To check post-operative healing of tissues.

Orthodontics

- Some patients appear to have missing or un-erupted teeth. A panoramic radiograph, to determine if this is the case, is essential in planning orthodontic treatment.
- To ascertain the precise position of malpositioned teeth.
- To relate the position of teeth to the dental arch and adjacent teeth.
- To assess the upper and lower jaw relationship (cephalometric radiograph).
- To assess and predict future growth patterns, especially of the teeth and jaws (cephalometric radiograph).

Prosthodontics

- To detect root remnants. Radiographs may also show root fractures caused by accidents, violence or sporting injuries.
- To assess the status of the alveolar bony ridges.
- To relate the denture-bearing area to other structures; for example, the mental nerve.
- Essential in assessment for implant procedures.

Dental assistant's role in taking radiographs

In some states of Australia it is possible for a dental assistant who has completed a post-certificate course in dental radiography to take dental radiographs. You should check local legislation to see what is permitted in your location. Even if you are licensed, you may only take radiographs under the dentist's supervision/prescription.

Unless you have successfully completed a dental radiography course, you are not permitted to take radiographs or even to push the exposure button.

Depending on your workplace you may be required to:

- drape the patient with a lead apron;

- set the exposure time (this can only be done if you have a licence);

- press the exposure button (again, this can only be done if you have a licence);

- explain procedures to the patient;

- process the exposed x-ray film;

- sort and mount radiographs;

- record information on the radiographs; and

- maintain good infection control practices in all procedures relating to the taking of dental radiographs.

It is essential that radiographs are of good quality. A poor quality radiograph is useless as both a treatment aid and a legal document and the procedure will need to be repeated. Consequently, you must follow procedures correctly to ensure the radiograph is of the best possible standard.

Also, although dental radiographs involve very low doses of radiation, you should wear a personal monitoring device if you work in a practice where large numbers of radiographs are taken.

One of the most significant roles you have is ensuring that asepsis is maintained throughout the radiograph procedure and you may also be responsible for processing and mounting radiographs if required (i.e. if digital radiographs are not taken). See Procedure 21.1 for more information. Maintaining asepsis in radiography is discussed in detail in Chapter 14.

Consent

Consent should always be obtained prior to the taking of dental radiographs. Minors (children under 18 years) require the consent of a parent or guardian. See the section overleaf for more information about legal implications for radiography.

Procedure 21.1 Preparing a patient for radiography

- If asked, and the dentist is not present to do so, explain the procedure to the patient. Some patients will be very nervous and will require comfort and support.

- Make sure the patient has removed any spectacles, dentures, and jewellery (including body adornments such as piercings) that would be in the path of the x-ray beam. These things can render a radiograph unusable for diagnosis as they cast 'shadows' on the film.

- To ensure that good infection control can be practised, be prepared before the procedure starts. Have environmental wraps already covering equipment, and have the patient's chart ready. Also have available cotton rolls, paper towel and containers to receive exposed films.

- Place the lead apron on the patient.

- When all of the above has been completed, you should put on fresh gloves.

- If the patient requires assistance holding a film in place, the helper should be shielded by a lead apron and should *not* be a member of staff. In the case of a young child, the parent may have the child in their lap during radiography. Alternatively, special film holders may be utilised.

- Mark the exposed film with a felt pen. This is to ensure that the film is not accidentally exposed a second time. A felt pen will not damage the film emulsion but a pencil or ball-point pen might.

- Have a container ready to place exposed (and contaminated) films in, away from any risk of radiation exposure.

- Make sure that used film holders are not placed directly on exposed benches. They should always be placed in a sterilisable tray or on paper towel.

- Take all exposed films to the darkroom or processor.

- Change gloves and decontaminate the film. If the film is in a barrier bag, use clean gloves to remove the barrier bag and drop the film onto a clean surface (e.g. a paper towel).

- With clean hands, process the film and then return processed films to the dentist in a clean container. If presenting films to the dentist on a hangar ensure infection control protocols are followed at all times.

- Equipment should be kept clean using environmental wrapping put in place before the patient arrives. At the end of the treatment, this wrapping should be removed. Make sure you are wearing gloves when you do this. If environmental wrapping is not used, all contaminated surfaces should we wiped with disinfectant wipes. Paralleling devices should be sterilised or at least disinfected between patients.

- Film holders should be sterilised.

- After you remove your gloves, wash your hands.

- If digital equipment is being used, thought must be given to avoidance of contamination of the computer keyboard and other components. The sensors should be barrier-protected and decontaminated as recommended by the manufacturer.

Legal implications for dental radiography and radiographs

Ownership of radiographs

Radiographs form part of the patient's permanent record of treatment and must be kept on file with other medico–legal documents.

They are the property of the dental practice. The patient is not paying for the radiograph but rather for the dentist's interpretation of the radiograph.

Sometimes patients request that they be given the radiographs as they are moving away and wish to avoid further irradiation and cost at their new dental practice. It is preferable that the dentist forward the radiographs to the patient's new dentist rather than handing them to the patient. The dentist should still maintain a copy of the radiographs on file.

It is possible to take a photocopy of radiographs if required. Copies of radiographs can also be made at x-ray laboratories. An alternative is to use double film packs routinely, which results in two sets of radiographs being available. Digital radiographs are easily copied or forwarded.

Keeping radiographs

Legally, radiographs and all other dental records should be kept for seven years after the last attendance by the patient (except for patients under 18 years of age in which case they should be kept until the patient is 25 years old). However, although the dentist is not legally obliged to do so, it is wise to *keep patient records indefinitely* as courts on occasions have extended the statute of limitations by many years. The implication of this is that radiographs must be processed correctly or they will deteriorate and be useless as a legal record.

Safety

There are Australian Standards for electrical, radiation and workplace safety and all x-ray units used for dental radiographs should comply with these standards. New machines can only be installed by suppliers where these standards are met. In addition, all x-ray units not only have to be registered but, as required by regulations, must have a compliance certificate as evidence that they comply with current standards.

Everyone who operates an x-ray unit, be they a dentist, assistant or any other person, must have a current radiography licence which has to be renewed annually.

You should also be informed of:

■ the hazards implied in working with radioactive substances and radiation apparatus;

■ ways to protect yourself from these hazards and to minimise risk (see later in this chapter for more information); and

■ the name of the radiation safety officer to whom you should go if you have questions or problems.

Further information about any occupational exposure to ionising radiation (x-rays) that is of relevance to dental assistants is provided below.

X-rays

Although the science behind radiography can be complex, it is important to have a basic understanding of x-rays in order to be able to adequately protect the patient and the dental team from unnecessary exposure.

X-rays are a form of energy called electromagnetic radiation. This is a form of energy where little particles, called photons, travel in waves at the speed of light. Photons are invisible and weightless.

Other examples of electromagnetic radiation are light, microwaves, television and radio waves. Figure 21.1 shows how different forms of electromagnetic radiation are used and how their wavelengths vary.

As already mentioned, x-rays are comprised of little packets of energy called photons. The amount of energy the x-ray photons have (how well they penetrate substances such as human body tissues) depends on the wavelength of the x-ray. X-rays have a range of wavelengths but all of them are very short. So the shorter the wavelength the greater the x-ray photons energy and penetrating power. The x-rays used in medicine and dentistry to produce radiographs are in a range of wavelengths around $1/10$ billionth of a metre.

Forms	Wavelengths	Uses
	$\dfrac{1}{100,000}$	Radiotherapy
	$\dfrac{1}{10,000}$	
X-rays and gamma rays	$\dfrac{1}{1,000}$	
	$\dfrac{1}{100}$	
	$\dfrac{1}{10}$	Dental radiography
Soft x-rays	1	
Ultraviolet rays	10	
	100	Sun
Visible light	1,000	Photography
Infrared rays	10,000	
Measured in nanometers	100,000	Microwave
Measured in meters	$\dfrac{1}{1,000}$	
	$\dfrac{1}{100}$	Radar
	$\dfrac{1}{10}$	
	1	Television
	10	
Radio waves	100	
	1,000	Radio
	10,000	
	100,000	

Figure 21.1 The electromagnetic spectrum

The properties of x-rays

X-rays penetrate solid objects

Because of their short wavelengths, x-rays can penetrate solid objects that normally absorb or reflect visible light. As mentioned previously, how much they penetrate depends on:

- the energy of the x-ray (which depends on the wavelength);
- the density of the object; and
- the thickness of the object.

In the mouth the enamel, dentine, bone and some types of restoration absorb more x-rays than the soft tissues.

X-rays expose photographic film

X-rays work to expose photographic film or affect digital image receptors in much the same way as light enters the camera and exposes a film when you take a photograph. The difference is that the film in a camera records light rays *reflected* from an object, radiographic film records x-rays that pass *through* an object.

How easily the x-rays penetrate the tissues depends on the nature of the tissue. These differences in the ways x-rays are absorbed is known as 'differential absorption'. For example, because bone absorbs much of the x-ray, the film behind the bone is less exposed than the film behind the soft tissue. Therefore, bone appears white on the processed film and soft tissue is grey. (Exposing the x-ray film is only half of the process. The potential image [called the latent image] needs to be made visible by chemically processing [developing] the film. If digital technology equipment is being used after the image receptor is exposed, the image is produced by the computer.)

X-rays cause some substances to fluoresce

This means that the substances glow in the dark. That is, a combination of light and radiation on the film dramatically reduces the exposure time necessary to produce the diagnostic image. This is the case when cassettes with intensifying screens are used, such as in the production of panoramic and cephalometric radiographs.

X-rays cause secondary radiations

When an x-ray hits a solid object, such as a patient, not all of the x-ray goes through to the film. Some photons are absorbed and secondary radiations are then produced, emanating from the object in all directions. This is called 'scatter radiation'. It is important to understand this when protecting yourself from unnecessary exposure to radiation.

X-rays can cause biological changes

This is the reason why x-rays are sometimes used in radiotherapy (for example, in the treatment of some forms of cancer). However, these changes can be harmful. This is why, for your own safety and the safety of the patient, you must understand the process and be cautious when undertaking these procedures. The potential hazards and ways of minimising them are discussed in the following pages.

The effects of radiation

One of the properties of x-rays, as noted previously, is that they may cause biological damage. This is because x-rays are ionising radiations. They can cause an atom to lose or gain an electron.

In the early years of x-ray use in medicine, this was not well understood and some patients and early clinicians received huge doses of radiation that later caused severe medical problems, and even death. However, the doses that patients now receive when having a radiograph taken are very small. In fact, the background radiation you receive during your life (e.g. ionising radiation received from the environment) is very much higher than the radiation you receive from having medical and dental radiographs taken.

The ALARA principle

Despite the dosage from dental radiographs being very low, it is still important to take care with any radiographic procedure. We do this by following the ALARA principle, which states that any exposure to radiation should be kept 'as low as reasonably achievable', compatible with achieving a good quality radiograph.

The biological effects of radiation (somatic and stochastic)

Somatic effects

A somatic effect is one that involves a change in the body or a cell. The severity of the change is dependent on the dosage received. An analogy is spending to much time in the sun; the longer the time, the worse the sunburn. For example, people exposed to high radiation after a nuclear accident lose their hair and have their skin peel as the initial symptoms of radiation poisoning.

Stochastic effects

Stochastic effects are random. That is, any exposure may not have any effect at all or have an adverse effect, usually either as a genetic effect or the development of a **malignancy**. The typical radiation

induced malignancy is leukaemia as can happen after a nuclear explosion or accident.

However with the diagnostic use of x-rays the risk of any such event occurring is extremely low. Every hour human cells undergo *at least 50 to 100 times more* spontaneous or naturally occurring damaging events than would result from the absorbing of ionising radiation from literally hundreds of dental radiographs. This damage is routinely repaired by the body hour by hour, day by day, year after year.

The latent period and cumulative effect

The effects of radiation exposure may not show up for many years. The length of time before any clinical effect becomes apparent is called the latent period. The length of time could be hours, years or generations depending on the type of exposure and the type of effect.

These effects are cumulative. Each time tissues are exposed to radiation, some damage occurs. While most of the tissue can repair itself, some will remain changed. These changes add up with each exposure. As an example of cumulative effect compare the skin on your hands with the skin on parts of your body that are always covered.

Radiation sensitivity of different tissues

Not all tissue types are very susceptible to damage caused by radiation. For example, very specialised tissue, such as heart muscle tissue, is not very likely to suffer damage from exposure. See Table 21.1 for more information.

Table 21.1 shows the tissues that are most sensitive to radiation exposure. It is worth noting those tissues that are most likely to be affected by dental radiography (i.e. the eyes, the skin and the oral mucosa). However, any risk is negligible.

Monitoring your radiation exposure at work

You will find information about pocket dosimeters in Chapter 15. These are small badges used to monitor exposure to radiation. These devices are called thermoluminescent dosimeters or TLDs.

They are made of materials that are sensitive to ionising radiation and every 12 weeks are sent away to be analysed by a monitoring company. Normally,

Tissue	Result
Embryonic tissue (cells of the developing foetus)	Birth defect
Bone marrow	Leukaemia
Gonads (ovaries and testes)	Genetic changes
Glandular tissues (thyroid gland, salivary gland)	Malignant tumour
Skin	Skin cancer
Intestinal mucosa	Cancer
Oral mucosa	Cancer
Lens of the eye	Cataracts

Table 21.1 Radiation sensitivity of different tissues

the company returns a report showing exposure for the testing period as well as accumulated quarterly, yearly and lifetime dosages. When compared with a control, they show any occupational exposure above that received from workplace background radiation. If your TLD shows an abnormally high exposure to radiation, it is possible that the x-ray machine in your practice is faulty, or that you or your dentist are taking insufficient care to protect yourselves from unnecessary exposure.

The exposure reports should be kept with your staff files.

Dosimeters should not be worn outside or when you yourself are having dental or medical radiographs taken. They are meant to record only occupational exposure above background radiation levels in the workplace.

Safe radiography

Because there is a risk involved, no matter how small, you are morally and ethically bound in the taking of radiographs to protect the patient, yourself and other staff as much as possible. The best way to do this is to observe the ALARA principle by:

- using the smallest radiation exposure possible that will still allow good quality radiographs; and
- protect yourself and the patient with the use of shielding.

Minimising the radiation dosage

There are a number of things that can be done to reduce unnecessary radiation exposure for the patient. Most obviously, only essential radiographs should be taken. Radiographs should not be taken on a 'just in case' basis. The correct exposure time should also be used, as should fast films to reduce the necessary exposure time.

Digital equipment will also enable shorter exposure times.

By applying the best possible technique, from exposure to processing and mounting, it is possible to ensure that the first set of radiographs are of good quality. This ensures that it is not necessary to take a second set.

All equipment should comply with safety standards and should be checked regularly to ensure it complies with current standards requirements.

Although there is evidence that lead aprons for patients are unnecessary for dental radiography because of the very low doses involved, there is both a medico–legal requirement implication and a best practice implication. It also makes patients feel better. Staff should be protected, with shielding, where practicable.

Radiography of pregnant patients

Many pregnant patients are concerned about the risks of having radiographs taken. However, the National Health and Medical Research Council (NHMRC) states that necessary *dental* radiography poses no risk to the baby or the mother and there is no reason to defer it.

Similarly, pregnant dental assistants have no cause for concern if all care is taken in the production of radiographs.

Shielding

In the section on the properties of x-rays it was noted that some portion of the radiation will bounce off the patient and scatter in every direction (scatter radiation). To be properly protected, you and the dentist should stand behind a lead-lined barrier. Alternatively, it is possible to protect yourself by standing far enough away from the unit. This is because the strength of the x-ray, and therefore its ability to penetrate the body, rapidly diminishes the further it travels.

A safe position (Figure 21.2) away from the x-ray unit is a distance of two metres at an angle of 135 degrees to the path of the primary beam. As it is obligatory that the exposure cord to an x-ray unit is a minimum of two metres, it should be possible to do this in any instance where a lead-lined partition is not available.

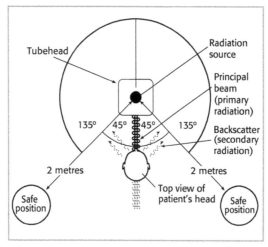

Figure 21.2 Safe position from the x-ray unit

Lead aprons

Patients must (by regulation and NHMRC recommendation) be shielded with a lead apron. These aprons should:

- be properly positioned on the body of the patient;
- have a high collar to protect the thyroid gland;
- cover the body and gonads;
- meet all safety standards and be regularly tested for compliance as required by the relevant regulations; and
- be properly stored, lying flat or hanging from two hooks. They should never be folded. See Figure 21.3 for an example.

Infection control

Infection control during radiography is covered in depth in Chapter 14. The following is a brief summary of that information but you are encouraged to revise that chapter.

Some bitewing and periapical films come in barrier envelopes that can be discarded after the film has been in the patient's mouth. Alternatively, plastic wrap can also be placed around an intra-oral film and disposed of after use.

Most films come encased in a moisture-resistant plastic packet and after exposure these should be washed in running water and then soaked in hypochlorite for a couple of minutes or cleaned by a disinfectant wipe or spray. Paper-backed films (such as occlusal films) cannot be disinfected in this way but may be placed in a plastic bag or wrap.

The image receptors used in digital procedures should be protected by a disposable sheath or cleaned as recommended by the manufacturer.

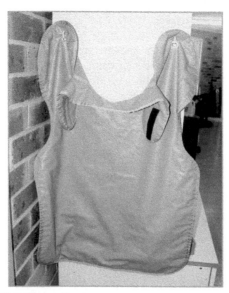

Figure 21.3 Storage of lead aprons

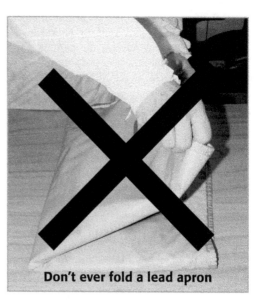

Don't ever fold a lead apron

Environmental wrapping of equipment is the fastest and simplest method of keeping equipment clean. Plastic wrap, freezer bags or purpose-made sleeves can be used to cover the control panel, cone and any other parts of the x-ray machine that will be touched during the procedure. Areas not protected should not be touched.

Paralleling devices should be sterilised or disinfected between patients.

Film holders and bite-blocks that have been in the patient's mouth should be sterilised or disinfected according to manufacturer's instructions.

Infection control in the darkroom is covered in Chapter 14. This is an area of infection control that is often overlooked and, because it represents risks to patients and staff, you are urged to review the information in Chapter 14.

X-ray units used in dental radiography

Radiographs can be intra-oral or extra-oral, and depending on the type of equipment used, the image produced may be either a conventional radiograph or a digital image. Most equipment takes either conventional radiographs or digital ones. However, some brands of equipment allow the option of taking either digital or conventional radiographs.

The three main components of an x-ray unit are the tube head, the extension arm and the control panel. The tube head contains the x-ray tube and is constructed to prevent any radiation escaping, other than that necessary to produce the radiograph.

On an intra-oral unit, the extension arm can rotate through 360 degrees. It is used to hold and position the tube head correctly. It also contains the wires that run between the tube head and the control panel.

Extra-oral radiographs in dentistry are mainly panoramic or cephalometric (Figure 21.4). On panoramic units, the patient's head is fixed in a set position and the tube head rotates around behind the patient's head. In cephalometric radiography, the patient is positioned in a cephalostat, which is located on an extension arm fixed to a panoramic unit, and the tube head is locked into place. These types of radiography are discussed later in this section.

The control panel is preferably located outside the room in which the x-rays are taken or behind a lead shield partition, and the patient monitored through a suitable glass window. The control panel holds the master switch, exposure timer, the milli-

amperage selector and the kilovoltage selector. You should not adjust these settings unless you are a certified dental radiographer and even then you must be supervised by a dentist. Regardless of where the control panel is situated, the exposure timer must be outside the room or located in a safe position.

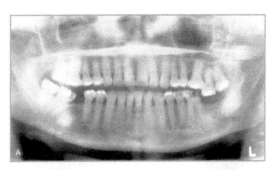

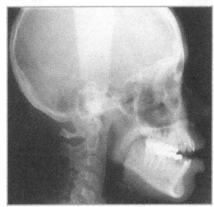

Figure 21.4 Panoramic and cephalometric radiographs

Intra-oral radiographs

Intra-oral radiographs are the most common type of radiograph used in dentistry. Typically these are periapical, bitewing or occlusal. A range of different types and sizes of films can be exposed using these units.

These units (Figure 21.5) are less expensive to purchase than digital imaging equipment. However, images produced by conventional units are subject to operator error. Examples of this are incorrect exposure times and faulty processing procedures. Any such errors will result in poor quality images. Operator error is discussed in more detail later in this section.

When film is used with these units it is processed in a darkroom or using daylight-loading film automatic processors. This means that images are not as immediately available for diagnosis as are those obtained by digital sensors connected directly to a computer. With computer technology, images appear almost immediately on the visual display unit (VDU).

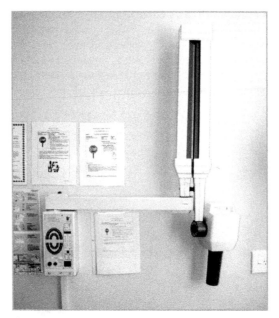

Figure 21.5 A typical intra-oral x-ray unit

Extra-oral radiographs

Panoramic radiographs

Also commonly called OPGs, panoramic radiographs are one form of extra-oral radiograph. These radiographs show the whole maxilla and mandible and associated structures on one film. They require a special unit (Figure 21.6) in which the film (or receptor) and the tube head rotates around the outside of the patient. With these units it is also possible to produce radiographs of individual quadrants, the temporo-mandibular joints or cross-sections of the jaw.

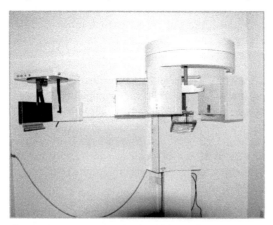

Figure 21.6 A typical panoramic x-ray unit

The units use only a low radiation dose to collect a lot of information and sometimes provide information about pathological conditions that are not seen on intra-oral films.

The image clarity (in other words the definition) of panoramic radiographs is not as good as that on an intra-oral film. They are commonly used in conjunction with bitewing and periapical radiographs and can indicate where additional periapical or other radiographs are necessary.

Cephalometric radiographs

Cephalometric radiographs give a repeatable true lateral view of the whole skull with the right and left sides superimposed on each other. They are taken using a device called a cephalostat (Figure 21.7), which is attached to the panoramic x-ray unit by an extension arm.

Cephalometric radiographs are used by orthodontists to assist in predicting growth patterns of a patient and in order to both plan and monitor treatment.

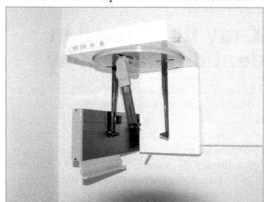

Figure 21.7 A cephalostat

Other types of extra-oral imaging

Other types of extra-oral imaging include lateral jaw films, lateral, postero-anterior or antero-posterior radiographs of the skull, and radiographs of the temporo-mandibular joint (TMJ). With the exception of the examinations that can be performed by OPG (panoramic) and cephalometric units, these must be done in a medical radiological practice.

In the case of TMJ examinations, the traditional method was the transcranial radiograph. This method involved placing a cassette against the side of the ear and projecting x-rays through the skull to produce an image of the side placed against the cassette. Modern panoramic units have programs that provide excellent images of the TMJ and other cranial structures and are less technique-sensitive than conventional methods.

Arthography is a form of radiography involving the injection of a dye into the joint space, and is used to obtain images of the TMJ. Another method for obtaining TMJ images is to use a special tomographic unit (hypocycloidal axial tomography). The method that gives the most information about the TMJ is magnetic resonance imaging (MRI) where such equipment is available.

Computerised tomography (CT) examinations are particularly useful for implant dentistry and in the treatment of malignancies of the head and neck.

Ultrasound examination is also being used as a diagnostic aid; for example, in the examination of the parotid gland.

Digital imaging

The process for producing computer or digital images is similar to that for producing film images. However, the image is captured by an image receptor and the result is viewed on a computer screen rather than on film. In some systems the radiographic image appears on the computer screen almost immediately after the exposure, but with others the receptor must be laser scanned before the image appears on the VDU.

Although digital systems are more expensive than the conventional tube/film equipment described previously, digital imaging technology can reduce patient radiation exposure by up to 80 per cent. This is because a shorter exposure time is needed (depending on the type of sensor and the speed of the film that is being used) to produce the radiographic image even though, at the present time, the receptors have a smaller range of sizes and shapes than film.

Digital systems have many other advantages. For example, the images can be manipulated, enabling digital enhancment, magnification, the contrast increased and areas of interest enlarged. This aids diagnosis and can also be extremely useful for patient education.

Images can be easily stored, duplicated, printed and readily transferred over the internet (teleradiography) should another opinion be required. Care must be taken to store images correctly and, as with all computer records, back-up copies should be kept in case of computer failure.

In some systems the image can be converted to a three dimensional one, to further enhance diagnosis. There are computer programs that can accurately measure the length of root canals in the practice of endodontics.

There are many different digital systems available and you will need to be given specific instruction in the systems at your place of work.

Radiographic film

Intra-oral radiographic film

Film has a colour-coded panel according to its speed. You should learn these codes and the speed of the film being used. The faster the film speed, the shorter the exposure time, although the slower film — 'D' speed — produces better contrast. 'E' speed films are almost twice as fast as 'D' speed films and so require about half the exposure time. Film speeds are as follows:

- Green = D speed single film (ultraspeed)
- Grey = D speed double film (ultraspeed)
- Royal blue = E speed single film (ektaspeed plus)
- Apricot/pink = E speed double film (ektaspeed plus)
- Mauve = F speed single film (insight; not as fast as E speed)
- Beige = F speed double film (insight).

Intra-oral film comes in five sizes numbered 0–4:

- Size 0 — 22×35 mms for:
  - periapical radiographs of the deciduous teeth
  - bitewing radiographs of the deciduous teeth
  - lower anteriors of the permanent dentition.
- Size 1 — 24×40 mms for:
  - bitewing radiographs of mixed dentitions
  - periapical radiographs of permanent anterior teeth.
- Size 2 — 31×41 mms for:
  - occlusal views of very small children
  - periapical radiographs of permanent molars and premolars
  - bitewing radiographs of the permanent dentition.
- Size 3 — 27×34 mms for long bitewing films, not recommended for use by the NHMRC.
- Size 4 — 57×76 mms for occlusal views of adults and children. May also be used for lateral jaw views of children in some circumstances.

Films have a use-by-date but that can sometimes be extended by keeping the film in the refrigerator. However films should be removed from the refrigerator and allowed to reach room temperature before use otherwise condensation could cause problems. If beyond their expiry date, the film's usefulness can be checked by processing an unexposed film. It should be completely clear with no background fogging.

If not refrigerated, film must be stored in a cool, dry place away from vapours (such as formalin, hydrogen sulphide, hydrogen peroxide, ammonia, etc.) as these may fog the film.

Extra-oral radiographic film

In extra-oral radiographs (panoramic or ortho-pantomograms, cephalometric films, skull and facial projections, etc.), the film is a large sheet held outside the mouth in a light-proof cassette that must only be opened in the darkroom.

The cassette is also fitted with two intensifying screens. These screens have a coating that fluor-esces or, in other words, glows when it is irradiated. This assists in the formation of the radiographic image and therefore greatly reduces the exposure time necessary to produce a diagnostically acceptable film. The fluorescence can be blue, green or violet depending on the screen manufacturer. It is very important to match film to the screens being used. For example, blue sensitive film must be used with blue emitting screens and so on. If screen and film do not match, an underexposed image will result.

Felt or foam pressure pads hold the film tightly in between the intensifying screens. The films are loaded into the cassettes in the darkroom.

Screens should be kept free from stains, abrasion and dust, dirt and lint. Chemicals such as fluoride are very damaging. Any imperfection on the screens will show on every film taken. As they are very expensive, care must be taken with their mainten-ance, and they should always be cleaned according to the manufacturer's instructions. The cassette should be left open in a dust-free place to dry, and must be completely dry before being reloaded.

The cassettes should only be opened when neces-sary. They can be wiped clean on the outside with a damp cloth.

Cassettes must be very carefully handled as they are easily damaged or warped, especially if drop-ped, and any damage could result in light leakage that leads to fogging of the film. See Procedure 21.2 for more information.

Procedure 21.2 Ordering, storing and handling radiographic film

- Film can go foggy if stored in a hot or humid place. It should be stored in a dark, cool place, and if possible in the refrigerator. This increases the life of the film (even past the expiry date).

- However, take care not to keep too much film in stock. Large stocks may well see film beyond its expiry date. It is best to keep 4–6 weeks supply. The principles of stock rotation and ordering used for other stock should also be used for film. Old stock should be used first. If you receive film from the supplier that is near the use-by-date you should return it and ask for replacement film.

- Boxes of film should be stored on their edges to minimise the risk of pressure point artefacts, which show up as black marks on the processed film. Film should be kept in a plastic bag to guard against condensation.

- Ensure that film is kept away from chemicals that may contaminate it and from liquids such as water and coffee.

- Film should also be kept well away from any radiation source. Film stored in the treatment room or near the x-ray machine should be stored in an appropriate metal container. Lead-lined boxes are no longer recommended from an occupational health and safety point of view.

- Keep room and processing temperatures within an acceptable range.

- Ensure that the darkroom does not have white light leaking into it.

- Extra-oral film must be compatible with the intensifying screens or the resulting film will be underexposed and will not be clinically adequate.

If the intensifying screens are green light emitting, the film must be green light sensitive.

Handling intra-oral film

- Store film carefully, away from wet surfaces.

- If film is stored in the refrigerator, allow it to return to room temperature before use.

- Keep the film flat. Do not bend or crease it as this causes a crease artefact or shadow that may interfere with good diagnosis.

- Check the film speed as this is crucial to exposure time.

- Keep unexposed films separate from exposed films. For example, write the patient's name on a paper cup and drop the exposed film into the cup before selecting the next film for exposure.

- Preferably, use the no-touch technique when preparing the film for processing.

- Be careful not to process double films together. They should be separated before processing.

Handling extra-oral film

- Fingers on the film can cause finger print artefacts that can interfere with good diagnosis. Do not handle the flat surface of the film. Lift the film by its edge and hold it at the corners.

- Be particularly careful not to touch the film surface when removing the film from the cassette.

- Loading or removing the film too quickly can cause static electricity that produces either dark patches or lightning strike artefacts.

Radiograph quality

A good quality radiograph is essential to diagnosis. The quality is dependent on the **density** and **contrast** of the image as these determine the amount of detail that can be seen on the radiograph. The image also needs to be free from distortion and to be processed correctly.

Radiographs are black and white images, or more correctly, are made up of:

■ black (air);

■ white (metal restorations); and

■ grey scale — a range of different shades of grey (tissue, teeth and other anatomy), from very light grey to very dark grey.

Density

Density refers to the general darkness or lightness of the image and is determined by the degree of exposure of the film. It can be affected by the distance that the radiation has to travel to reach the film, the processing times used and even how thin the patient is.

Contrast

The difference between the lightest and the darkest greys is the contrast. The amount of contrast is determined both by the exposure time and the temperature of the developer.

Distortion

Images can be distorted if the distance between the source of the x-ray and the object being x-rayed are unfavourable. For intra-oral radiography the distance from the x-ray source to the skin is required by regulation to be at least 20 cm. The object (the teeth or jaws) of the examination should be as close to the film as possible. Distortion also occurs if the film is not parallel to the object being x-rayed, and blurring will occur if the patient, film or x-ray machine tube head moves during the exposure. Bending of the film will cause blurring in the apical region.

Dental assistant's role in producing good quality radiographs

Setting up and exposing the radiograph will not be your role. However, you will probably be responsible for developing the film. You will find more information about good developing procedures later in this chapter.

Intra-oral radiographs

There are three types of intra-oral radiograph. These all involve radiographs where the film is placed inside the mouth and the x-rays are directed at the film through the part to be x-rayed (the area of interest) on to the film.

The films used in this kind of radiography have an embossed dot on one corner. The raised side is always placed towards the x-ray machine. The film is also placed in the mouth so that this embossed dot is not situated in an area of diagnostic interest.

The films come in light-proof, moisture-resistant packaging that facilitates the use of the no-touch technique when processing is being done, and which consists of:

■ an outer wrapping sealed against light and saliva;

■ an inner fold of black paper to further protect the film from light;

■ the film (either single or double); and

■ a lead foil backing sheet.

The lead foil partially absorbs the rays after they have registered on the film. The film packet must be placed so that the foil is away from the tube, otherwise the x-ray has to travel through the foil before it registers on the film. This causes a herring-bone pattern on the exposed film.

Periapical radiographs

Periapical means 'around the apex'. These radiographs show the whole tooth and the supporting and surrounding tissues. They are used to determine the anatomy of the tooth and its surrounding tissues and to detect any pathology in the crown, root or supporting tissues and bone.

Bitewing radiographs

Bitewing radiographs are also called interproximal radiographs but are known as bitewing radiographs because the patient bites on a tag that projects at right angles from the film cover. This holds the film in place while the exposure is made. The exposed film shows the crowns and part of the roots of the upper and lower bicuspids and molars of one side of the mouth. These are useful to determine the presence of interproximal and occlusal caries, and any pathology relating to the tooth pulp. They can also demonstrate the presence of overhanging margins on restorations and give an indication as to whether or not there is any loss of supporting bone.

■ **density:** the overall blackening or darkening of the radiograph when viewed by transmitted light such as from a viewing box.
■ **contrast:** the difference in densities in adjacent areas of the film; for example, dentine and enamel. Some areas are very dense, some are not dense.

Occlusal radiographs

A large size film is used here to show most of the upper or lower arch on one film. Various views can be obtained depending on the placement of the film and direction of the x-ray beam.

Intra-oral positioning devices

There are a number of positioning devices that assist in the correct positioning of the film so that it is parallel to the tooth. This is necessary to obtain a distortion-free image.

Processing radiographs

Radiographs can be processed manually and automatically.

Manual processing is cheaper than automatic processing and requires relatively little equipment. However, it is more prone to operator error and this might make radiographs clinically unusable.

Automatic processors are a much more regulated system than manual processing. They offer the ability to standardise processing and ensure better quality control.

To process the films, they are:

- placed in a developer for the recommended time;
- placed in a stop bath to stop the action of the developer and to remove the developer;
- placed in fixer for twice the developing time, to remove remaining undeveloped emulsion; and finally
- washed for 15 to 20 minutes in running water to remove any residual chemicals, to prevent any subsequent discolouration and deterioration.

Working with radiographic chemicals

The chemicals used in developing and fixing radiographs are extremely toxic and should always be handled with care. Misuse can lead to respiratory distress, skin and eye damage and can permanently stain clothing. Protective clothing should always be worn.

Never mix developer and fixer together as the resulting gas is very noxious and the solutions rendered useless.

Always dispose of chemicals properly. Every state and territory has a set of procedures that must be followed. The local water authorities (such as Sydney Water) have printed guidelines that can be obtained that describe procedures to be followed. Contact your local council and water boards for information about procedures that should be used in your surgery.

Silver rich solutions such as fixer must never be poured down the sink and you and your employer can be fined significant amounts of money for doing so. Some states require that a silver recovery unit be used and silver-rich solutions (fixer) be collected by a licensed transporter. Some states require that large practices have special waste water permits.

Remember that these chemicals are toxic and they should be disposed of in a way that protects the environment. There is more information about disposing of chemicals in Chapter 14.

Generally, developer and rinse water can be poured down the drain but you must find out what your local regulations are and check that this can be done. The procedure to be followed may vary according to the volumes of solutions used. Remember that there are penalties for not disposing of these chemicals properly. See Procedure 21.3 for more information.

Manual processing

It is crucial that the correct combination of time and temperature is used when processing radiographic film. The higher the temperature of the developer and fixer, the shorter the processing times. If it is desired to keep processing solutions at a constant temperature, aquarium thermostats are a simple and effective means of temperature control.

It is essential that you have:

- an accurate thermometer to take the temperature of the developer;
- a timer that is easy to set; and
- a time and temperature chart that allows you to simply calculate the length of developing needed according to the temperature of the developer. These charts are available from the suppliers of radiographic films and chemicals.

As a general rule, films should be fixed for twice as long as they take to develop, and washed in running water for at least 15 to 20 minutes.

Improper processing of films will result in staining and deterioration that makes them useless as a treatment and legal record. See Procedure 21.4 for more information.

Procedure 21.3 Preparing chemicals

- The laboratory should have a set of personal protective clothing (apron, mask, goggles and gloves) for use while preparing radiographs. Make sure you always use them. Also make sure that the ventilation system is working efficiently so fumes are removed from the room.

- Always follow the manufacturer's instructions. Refresh your memory by reading the instructions on a regular basis. Most chemicals come to you pre-mixed but you may need to add water.

- Replenish the chemicals daily. This extends the life of both the developer and fixer by reactivating the processing chemicals and minimises the risk of the processing chemicals levels being incorrect. If the baths are full you may need to draw off some of the old chemicals. Dispose of these chemicals appropriately. Do not pour them down the sink.

- Stir the chemicals before use to reactivate the processing chemicals and mix up the layers into which the chemicals tend to settle. Do not use the developer-stirring spatula in the fixer or vice versa.

- Check the temperature of the chemicals and if necessary bring them to the appropriate heat.

- When the chemical baths are not in use they should be covered. This helps to keep the chemicals uncontaminated by water, air and each other, minimises fumes in the room and helps to maintain the temperature. Developer left open to the air will markedly deteriorate in as little as an hour.

- When pouring chemicals to replenish the baths, be sure to avoid any fixer contaminating the developer as just a few drops will contaminate the solution and render it useless.

- Safety issues relating to the preparation and use of radiography chemicals are discussed in Chapter 15.

Procedure 21.4 Manual processing of radiographs

- Whenever possible, use the 'no-touch' technique and avoid touching the film. It is particularly important that you do not touch the flat surfaces of the film as this can leave finger print artefacts on the processed image. Instead, peel the film packet back, clip the hanger clip directly onto the film and use the hanger clip as a handle with which to pull the film from its packet.

- Have fresh developer *stirred* and ready for use.

- Use the thermometer to check the temperature. If the developer is too cold, some of the ingredients in the solution will not function properly. If the developer is too hot, the emulsion on the film may be damaged. If the temperature of the developer is too hot or cold, do not meddle with the solution. Instead, the temperature of the surrounding bath should be either warmed or cooled.

- Use the time and temperature chart to determine the correct developing time.

- Set the timer.

- Always ensure that the film is never exposed to any white-light until it has been developed and then placed in the fixer for two minutes.

- Clip the film onto the hanger using the 'no-touch' technique described above. Be sure the film hangers are clean and dry.

- Put the film into the developing solution and agitate it slightly to remove air bubbles.

- Turn on the timer.

- When the timer rings, remove the film, shake it slightly to remove excess developer and put the

film in the stop bath to stop it from further developing. The solution in the stop bath is usually water or water with a trace of weak acid (often acetic acid).

- 'Fix' the film, usually for twice the developing time. A film that is not properly fixed will go smoky and be difficult to interpret.

- The film must be thoroughly washed to remove all chemicals. Residual fixer will stain the film and render it useless as a treatment record. The suggested washing time is 20 minutes in running water.

- The following graph is a guide to determining developing time.

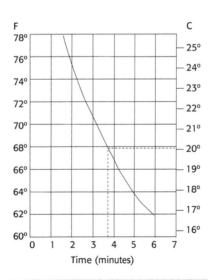

Time (minutes)

Darkrooms for manual processing

The requirements for a darkroom suitable for the manual processing of films are:

- a simple light-tight room, lockable or with a warning light — the room must have good ventilation and temperature control, and if the darkroom is lockable, some alternative method of entry must be available;

- a bench large enough to provide a wet and a dry area (separated by a splash barrier) and, for safety, with rounded corners;

- processing chemicals and stop baths that are easily cleaned and not affected by the chemicals (made of non-corrosive materials);

- a sink with fresh, running water so that films can be properly washed after processing;

- protective clothing and glasses;

- decontaminating solution container for exposed intra-oral films if barrier envelopes are not used;

- white light, safelight, and power point(s);

- timer with audible alarm;

- time/temperature chart appropriate for the films and processing chemicals being used;

- a Centigrade or Fahrenheit thermometer according to which type of time/temperature chart is being used;

- solution tanks labelled according to their contents;

- water bath/stop bath;

- thermostat to control the temperature of solutions;

- stirring rods (labelled for fixer and developer);

- sink with hot and cold running water;

- clean film hangers;

- drying racks;

- cool storage cupboards for film processing chemicals and other solutions;

- a dry and cool separate storage area or cupboard for films;

- paper towel dispenser;

- manufacturers' safety data sheets for all chemicals; and

- a film viewer.

The room must be white-light proof. Occasionally you should enter the darkroom, leaving lights on outside. Turn off all lights in the darkroom, wait for a few moments until your eyes adjust and then search the room for light leaks.

Although the room must be white-light proof, it must have the appropriate safe-lights that allow the room to be used safely. The bulb wattage, filter and the height of the safelight above the working area should comply with that specified by the manufacturer. Manufacturers of safe lights supply instructions as to their installation, maintenance and use.

A safe-light can be tested to see if it is functioning correctly by unwrapping a film, sitting a coin on top of it and leaving it exposed to the safe-light for a minute. If the outline of the coin is visible after processing, then the safe-light is not safe.

Darkrooms must comply with occupational health and safety requirements, particularly regarding ventilation and temperature control. It is essential that venting be in place to remove glutaraldehyde and ammonium fumes, both of which are toxic.

The room must be maintained at a constant, cool temperature to ensure that film stock stored in the room does not deteriorate and to keep the developer temperature at an appropriate level.

Figure 21.8 demonstrates a film being prepared for processing.

Automatic processing

Chemicals in automatic processors need to be replenished daily (unless replenishing is done automatically) and replaced every two weeks or sooner if there is a high film throughput.

Automatic processors can either be used in darkrooms or as free-standing units that have daylight

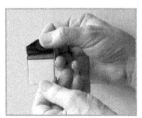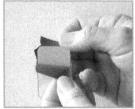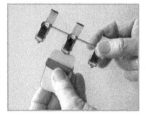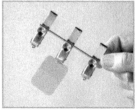

Figure 21.8 Preparing a film for processing

loaders attached. They contain a series of rollers or a belt system that carry the film through the developing and fixing solutions for processing.

Care must be taken to avoid contaminating the equipment by touching it with contaminated gloves. For example, if you touch the uncontaminated, exposed film and then put your hands in the daylight loaders, the sleeves of the loader will be contaminated. See Chapter 14 for information about maintaining good infection control techniques while using automatic processors. See Procedure 21.5 for more information.

Procedure 21.5 Automatic processing of radiographs

- If your infection control technique involves the use of gloves when processing, ensure that they are clean before touching any part of the processor, including the buttons and switches. Otherwise, the processor will need to be decontaminated after use. *Only powder-free gloves should be used.*

- Turn on the machine to start the drive mechanism. This is usually the simple matter of pushing a button.

- Ensure that the film you are loading into the processor has been decontaminated and that you are wearing clean, powder-free gloves or are glove-free, with clean hands. While holding the film, put your hands inside the daylight loader.

- Put the film into the feed slot. If several films are to be processed, use alternate feed slots. Allow at least 15 to 20 seconds after feeding a film into the slot before inserting another film.

- Press the start button again to start the full cycle of operation.

Maintaining automatic processors

Maintenance is particularly important because these processors are easily damaged and expensive to repair and replace. They are particularly sensitive to powder and can be damaged by the powder that comes from powdered gloves.

It is very important that all manufacturer's instructions regarding the use and maintenance of automatic processors are followed. Most manufacturers recommend that a system cleaner be used every three months and particularly if the developer module shows a build-up of oxidised reducing agent. System cleaner stains clothes and skin and should be used with caution.

The chemicals used in the processor should be regularly checked and replaced or refilled as required.

The racks (or modules) for each cycle (there are four of them) should be removed and inspected once a week to ensure that the teeth on all cogs, the meshing gears, nylon belts, and drive cogs are in good condition. Some parts may require lubrication.

Mounting and storing radiographs

Legally, radiographs must be kept for three-and-a-half years but are more usually kept for at least seven. Recent court cases have led to some practices storing radiographs and dental records indefinitely so that such records are always available. This is because of the possibility of litigation arising many years after treatment was carried out. Radiographs are also useful (and often crucial) for the identification of bodies in forensic examinations. For these reasons radiographs must be properly developed and fixed as well as properly mounted and stored.

Each radiograph should be identified with:

- the patient's name, age and date of birth (or with a dental record number if that is the practice routine); and

- date of examination, the examined region shown by quadrant and tooth number, and right and left sides marked.

Every dental practice will, in its policies and procedures manual, describe the routine to be followed when mounting radiographs. They can be mounted in commercial film mounts that are available in various formats, or laminated, or carefully stapled on clear plastic sheets. If you use the stapling method, take care not to staple over any details of vital structures shown in the radiograph.

Whether the radiograph is mounted dimple-side up or dimple-side down depends on the dentist's preference. Those dentists using International Notation require that the radiographs be dimple-side up. That is, if you look at the radiograph, the patient's left side is on the right of the radiograph (as though you were standing in front of the patient). However, some dentists prefer to look at the radiographs from the patient's viewpoint — as though you are behind the patient, looking over their head. The patient's left is on the left of the radiograph and therefore the dimple must be facing down.

It is important that all radiographs are mounted consistently using only one system. In some practices you may be required to place sticky labels saying 'left' and 'right' on the radiographs to confirm their orientation.

Sorting the films

If the films have always been placed in the mouth with the dots to the distal when radiographs are being taken, sorting is made simpler.

- Place them all on a viewing box and if the International Notation is being used, turn the embossed dots up. Decide which are films of the upper teeth and separate them from those of the lower teeth.

- Select those showing incisor teeth and place them in the centre, so that the upper teeth point downwards and the lowers upwards.

- Next, select all films showing cuspids and bicuspids so that the cuspids come next to the incisors and the bicuspids are towards the distal. Films showing molars are then put into place with the first molar next to the second bicuspid, and the last molar to the back of the mouth.

- Then you will have the films showing the teeth of the patient's left side on your right side, and those of the patient's right on your left.

Once sorted, the films are then ready to be mounted (Figure 21.9). The mount should be marked clearly to indicate the patient's left and right sides.

Recognising teeth in radiographs

To mount films correctly, some knowledge of the anatomical landmarks to be found on intra-oral films is required. You must be able to recognise the various teeth as described in Chapter 9 and decide which teeth belong to the upper jaw (maxilla), and which are those of the lower jaw (mandible), which are films of the patient's left side and which of the right side. Taking the anterior teeth first — you will notice that, of the four incisor teeth, the two central incisors are generally bigger than the next two (lateral incisors). The crowns are longer and wider and the roots are longer and thicker. The four lower incisors are much the same size, and are all much more slender than the corresponding upper teeth.

In the upper jaw, two large radiolucent areas may appear above the roots of the incisors. These represent the anterior portion of the nasal cavity and between these large dark areas is a white line caused by the bone of the nasal septum. A dark area sometimes shows between or near the tips of the roots of the two central incisors. This is the incisive foramen, an opening through which nerves and blood

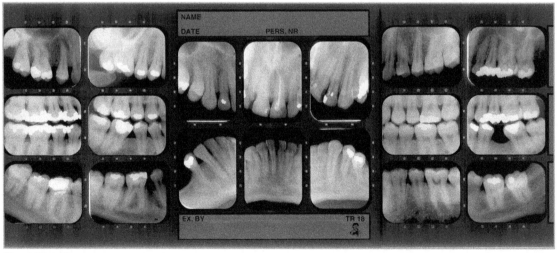

Figure 21.9 Film mounted in film mount

Upper molars	Upper premolars	Upper canines/ lateral incisors	Central incisors	Lower canines/ lateral incisors	Upper premolars	Upper molars
Molar bitewing	Premolar bitewing				Premolar bitewing	Molar bitewing
Lower molars	Lower premolars	Lower canines	Lower anteriors	Lower canines	Lower premolars	Lower molars

(Figure 21.9 Legend)

vessels pass. Anatomical features which help to identify the other teeth are detailed below.

- Canines. The next teeth in the arch are the cuspids (canines). The uppers are larger than the lowers and much larger than any of the incisors. In young patients these are pointed but they become flatter with age.

- Premolars. Next are the two bicuspids (premolars) in each side and in each jaw. It is more difficult to decide which are the upper and which are the lower bicuspids. However, in most films of upper bicuspids there is a portion of thin white line above the roots. It may be in the corner of the film. This is part of the floor of the antrum.

- The lower bicuspids usually have a small dark area between or near the tip of the roots. This is caused by the mental foramen, the point where the mandibular canal ends. The mental nerve and blood vessels reach the surface through this foramen.

- Molars. There are possibly three molars on each side, upper and lower. The third molar is the wisdom tooth. Most films of upper molars show the white line of the floor of the antrum and usually the large dark (radiolucent) area above the roots, which is the cavity of the antrum itself. Over the first molar there is often a white or radiopaque area in the shape of a 'V' or perhaps only a small lower portion of it. This is the shadow cast by the zygoma or cheek bone.

- Upper molars generally have three roots, but they are often not clearly separated in the radiograph. Lower molars have two roots, which are often well separated, especially in first molars, and the roots show a tendency to turn distally or towards the back of the mouth. Behind the last molar, the bone of the mandible can be noticed curling upward to become the ramus of the mandible. Below the lower molars a long dark area is usually seen running parallel to the border of the mandible. This is the shadow of the mandibular canal.

Causes of faulty radiographs

There are a number of errors made in the handling, and processing of radiographs that will result in the radiograph being of poor clinical quality. If radiographs are of poor quality then sound diagnosis will not be possible.

Processing faults

You will need to be able to recognise and correct processing faults in order to prevent them from occurring again. A normal radiograph can be seen in Figure 21.10. The three main faults you are likely to see will be:

- an image too light;

- an image too dark; or

- mechanical damage of the film.

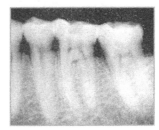

Figure 21.10 A normal radiographic image

Light images

Light images (as seen in Figure 21.11) can be caused by:

- the film being underexposed;

- the distance between film and tube head being too far, leading to underexposure;

- under-development, which is itself caused by the film not being in the developer for long enough, or the developer being too cold or too old;

- the film being left in the fixer for a very long time;

- the film being back to front in the mouth, in which case there will be a herringbone effect on the film; or

- the film being incorrectly fixed, the result of too short a time in the fixer, or the fixer being too cold or too old, in which case the film will be smoky in appearance.

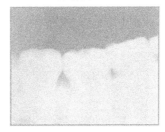

Figure 21.11 A light radiographic image

Dark images

Dark images (as seen in Figure 21.12) can be caused by:

- the film being overexposed;

- the film being double exposed; or

- over-development, which is itself caused by the film remaining too long in the developer, or the developer being too hot.

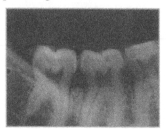

Figure 21.12 A dark radiographic image

Film fog

If the film appears 'fogged' (as seen in Figure 21.13) it may be:

- light fog — white light has fogged the film, due to either the film being opened in daylight, the leakage of white light into the darkroom, or the use of a faulty safelight;

- chemical fog caused by developing for too long, the developer being too hot, the solutions being too old, or the developer being contaminated with drops of fixer;

- storage fog due to the effects of heat, chemical vapours or radiation (film may be kept in the refrigerator provided it is allowed to reach room temperature before use); or

- age fog — if the film is past its use-by date.

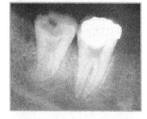

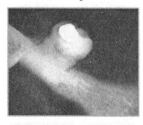

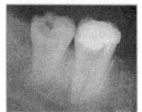

Figure 21.13 Fogging

Mechanical and other damage

Artefacts

- Black lines (as seen in Figure 21.14) can be caused by over-bending or crimping of the film in an attempt to fit a large film into a small space, or by rough handling.

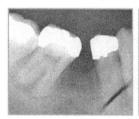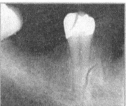

Figure 21.14 Black lines

- Touching the flat surface of the film can leave fingerprints, especially if you have hand cream, hair product, sweat, and so forth on your fingers.

- For reasons of good infection control, your fingernails should be kept short and clean. However, if you have long fingernails and hold a film too hard, this can leave half-moon shapes in the film similar to those caused by bending of the film.

- Films can be easily scratched by being brushed against fingernails, film hangars, sharp surfaces in the darkroom, the tank wall, or dropping the film (especially if wet) on a bench top or floor, etc.

Bubbles on the film during development can leave artefacts as can unclean hangers, dirty intensifying screens and inadequate washing. Air bubbles clinging to the surface of the film in the developer prevent the developer from reaching the emulsion beneath the air bubbles. An air bubble allowed to remain on the film causes a spot on the radiograph.

The round white spot on the root of the left central incisor on the radiograph in Figure 21.15 is the result of an air bubble on the surface during development.

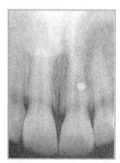

Figure 21.15 Air bubble

Static electricity

Apart from the fogging mentioned above, film can also be fogged by static electricity (see Figure 21.16). This can be caused by loading or unloading films into cassettes too quickly, or by electrostatic charges you carry, caused by walking on synthetic floor surfaces. Such problems are more common on very dry, warm days.

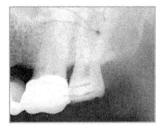

Figure 21.16 Static electricity fogging

Fixer splashes

Fixer solution, splashed onto the film before it is processed, will show up as white blotches on the radiograph (see Figure 21.17). Careful handling of all solutions is an absolute *must* in the processing room.

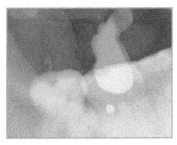

Figure 21.17 Fixer splash marks

Other types of faults

Film packet back to front

If the film packet is accidentally placed back to front in the mouth, the image of the lead foil backing is superimposed over the resultant very pale images, as seen in Figure 21.18.

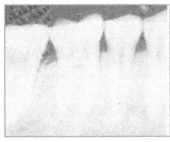

Figure 21.18 Superimposed image caused by film packet back to front

Clip lines

If clip lines appear on a radiograph, it means that the clip has not been properly washed after previous immersions in fixing solution. The dried fixer chemicals dissolve in the developer and run down the surface of the film. The result is a radiograph showing lines such as those seen in Figure 21.19. The remedy is better cleaning of equipment. A similar problem can occur with automatic processors if the equipment is not routinely cleaned and maintained.

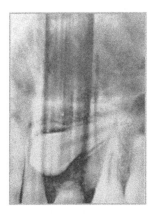

Figure 21.19 Clip lines

Fluoride stains

Some fluoride compounds, notable stannous fluoride, will produce black artefacts on the radiographs as shown Figure 21.20.

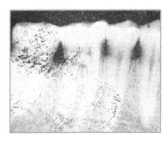

Figure 21.20 Fluoride stains

After the hands have become contaminated with the fluoride compound, even thorough washing with soap and water will not remove the contamination. Wiping the hands with a mild acid, such as vinegar or lemon juice, followed by soap and water will effectively remove the fluoride compound contaminant.

Double exposure

Figure 21.21 shows a film which has been accidentally exposed twice.

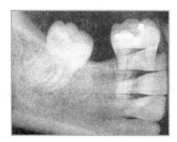

Figure 21.21 Double exposure

Blurred images

Blurred images are caused by one or a combination of the following:

- movement of the patient;
- movement of the tube; or
- movement of the film by the patient during exposure.

Partial images

- Cone cutting is the result of film and cone not being properly aligned. As seen Figure 21.22, a clear area with a circular edge will be visible on the side of the film.

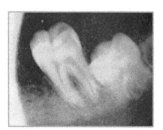

Figure 21.22 Cone cutting

- If solution levels are not checked, this may result in the film being only partially submerged in the developer. Accordingly, the image is only partially developed, as seen in Figure 21.23.

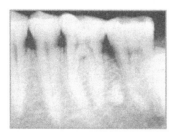

Figure 21.23 Partial submersion

- Films can also be damaged by coming in contact with each other when wet. This can happen quite easily in automatic processing unless care is taken loading the films. Films may also touch the side of the tank when manually processing. It can also occur if paper from the packet sticks to the film.

Summary

Dental radiography plays an essential role in successful diagnosis and treatment planning. Radiographs are also vital pre- and post-treatment records. They must therefore be diagnostic, correctly labelled and stored with the patient's history and treatment records.

chapter twenty-two
first aid and emergencies

Introduction

Though very rare, emergencies can arise in dental practice. They fall into two main groups; medical and dental. Some emergencies may constitute the reason for patients presenting for dental treatment, for example:

- a fractured tooth;
- an **avulsed** tooth;
- a bleeding tooth socket; or
- dental pain/toothache.

Other emergencies may develop unexpectedly during the course of treatment or while the patient is in the surgery, and may be the result of dental treatment or due to unrelated causes. Your surgery should have a set of protocols in place that list staff responsibilities in times of emergency. These protocols must include a list of emergency telephone contact details, positioned close to the telephone, for ambulance, doctors and the nearest hospital.

Medical emergencies

Assessment of collapse

Collapse is a general, non-specific term that refers to a sudden deterioration of a patient's condition, which may or may not result in the patient becoming unconscious. When confronted with a patient who has collapsed, it is important that no time is wasted. Your immediate reaction should be to:

- Look for dangers and either remove the danger or remove the patient from the danger and call for help. If necessary, lift the patient (with assistance) out of the dental chair on to a level surface (the floor).

- Check the A-B-C
  A — is the airway clear?
  B — is the patient breathing?
  C — is there a carotid pulse?

  If the answer is NO to any of these observations, then you must commence cardio-pulmonary resuscitation (CPR) immediately.

The first observation to make is whether the patient is conscious or unconscious. This may be done by squeezing the patient by the shoulder, asking their name, and giving a simple command; for example, 'Squeeze my hand. Let it go'. If the patient is conscious they will answer to the spoken word and respond to their shoulder being squeezed.

If the patient does not regain consciousness in a few seconds:

- you should turn the patient on their side;
- open their airway with a backward head tilt and jaw support;
- remove any vomitus or foreign material; and
- check their pulse.

If the patient is breathing, they are left lying on their side in the lateral or 'recovery' position. Pulse and breathing are checked after one minute and at least every two minutes thereafter. If the patient is not breathing, appropriate basic life support should be given.

Syncope (fainting)

Fainting is a very common occurrence. Apprehension and pain may result in a sudden fall of blood pressure and a slowing of the pulse. Warning signs consist of restlessness, pallor, coldness, sweating, sighing and vomiting. If the patient does not lie down, there will be a loss of consciousness, depression of breathing and perhaps brief con-

■ **avulsed:** knocked out.

223

vulsive movements. The patient should be placed into the supine position with the head lower than the feet. If there is further delay and the patient is not placed in a horizontal position, cardio-respiratory arrest could occur.

Treatment

All work must stop. Any tight clothing the patient is wearing should be loosened (e.g. ties and belts). Keep the patient warm and observe them for any changes in their condition. Do not try to give them a drink.

Once in progress, this sequence of events takes place in a matter of 4–5 seconds. Recovery is usually rapid when the patient is horizontal. Consciousness is regained, colour returns to the face, normal breathing returns and the pulse rate increases. If vomiting takes place, the patient should be turned onto his or her side and the vomitus wiped or sucked away. After recovery, the patient should not be moved for 10–15 minutes.

More serious emergencies may lead to a sudden fall of blood pressure and therefore give the appearance of fainting, for example:

- hypotensive side effects of sedatives, narcotics and tranquillisers;
- toxic effects of local anaesthetics;
- coronary occlusion; or
- anaphylactic shock.

In these emergencies, the pulse may be very rapid or very slow. Chest pain suggests coronary occlusion, and rashes and facial swelling suggest a severe drug reaction. Initial treatment is the same as for fainting. However, after the patient is placed in the horizontal position, recovery may not be as rapid as it is after a fainting spell.

If the patient does not regain consciousness in a few seconds, the airway should be opened with backward head tilting and jaw support, and respiration and pulse should be checked. You should provide appropriate basic life support.

Tetany (hyperventilation)

Tetany is a condition resulting from anxiety and in this regard is similar to syncope. It is characterised by spasm of the hands and feet (carpopaedal spasm) and is usually due to 'over-breathing' in a nervous patient.

When the patient breathes too deeply and too quickly, the carbon dioxide levels in the blood are reduced. It can immediately be reversed by reassurance and having the patient breath directly into a paper bag. The increased carbon dioxide content in the air that is re-breathed remedies the situation very promptly.

Usual treatment is to:

- stop all work;
- place the patient in a seated position;
- reassure the patient by speaking softly and calmly; and
- encourage slower breathing.

If normal breathing does not return, it could be more serious than hyperventilation. In this case, you should get help!

Cardiorespiratory arrest

Cardiopulmonary resuscitation is needed when, in acute collapse, a patient has suffered a cardiac arrest. Primary cardiac failure may be caused by:

- coronary occlusion;
- electrocution;
- drug reaction (due to inadvertent intravascular local anaesthetic injection);
- secondary or untreated hypotension;

or may be due to primary respiratory failure caused by:

- respiratory obstruction;
- inhalation of blood, teeth, dental material or vomitus; or
- drug overdose (e.g. sedatives, narcotics) causing respiratory depression.

Diagnosis of cardiac arrest is dependent on three criteria. The patient is:

❶ unconscious;
❷ not breathing; and
❸ has no carotid pulse.

Treatment

The management of cardiac arrest is the maintenance of airway, breathing and circulation.

Angina pectoris (cardiac pain)

Extreme anxiety or fluctuation in blood pressure may precipitate **anginal pain** in patients with **ischaemic** heart disease. Angina may be indicated by:

- complaint of central chest pain, spreading to shoulders, arms or jaw;

anginal pain: a suffocating pain in the chest produced by an inadequate blood supply to the myocardial (heart) muscle.
ischaemic: a localised lack of blood supply to a tissue causing it to look blanched.

■ pallor and sweating; or

■ frequently, a fall of blood pressure and pulse rate.

Treatment

■ Stop all dental treatment.

■ Do not lay the patient in a completely supine position.

■ If the patient has had angina before, they are likely to have tablets, or spray of glyceryl trinitrate or similar medication. Allow the patient to suck one tablet, and if the pain does not go in two minutes, ask the patient to suck a second tablet.

■ Give oxygen therapy with a facemask.

■ Reassure the patient.

■ If the patient starts to lose consciousness, place them in the horizontal position, continue oxygen therapy and prepare for further basic life support.

■ If the patient develops cardiorespiratory arrest, start CPR immediately, obtain the assistance of a medical practitioner and arrange for immediate transport to hospital.

If the pain does not pass in 15 minutes, the patient is likely to have a coronary occlusion (or myocardial infarction). Do not allow the patient to move. Arrange immediate transport to hospital and continue oxygen therapy.

Respiratory obstruction

Respiratory obstruction occurs when an object becomes caught in the airways and restricts breathing. Constant vigilance and meticulous attention to good technique will prevent respiratory obstruction. Failure to clear any obstruction of the upper respiratory passages may lead to inhalation of foreign matter, **hypoxia** and cardiorespiratory arrest.

Obstruction can be caused by:

■ the tongue;

■ vomitus or blood;

■ foreign bodies, e.g. teeth, dental packs or small instruments;

■ depression of the mandible in the unconscious supine patient or during dental manipulations; and

■ impaired protective laryngeal and pharyngeal reflexes due to administration of sedatives, narcotics, regional anaesthesia or general anaesthesia.

Signs of respiratory obstruction include noisy breathing, no escape of air from the mouth or nose during exhalation and laboured respiration. **Cyanosis** is a late sign.

Treatment

To treat respiratory obstruction, turn the patient on their side (the lateral position). Remove any foreign bodies, using suction if necessary. Put the head in the maximum backward tilt with jaw support, or elevate and protrude the mandible (jaw thrust).

Respiratory arrest

Respiratory arrest may be primary respiratory failure due to:

■ drug overdose (narcotic or sedative);

■ respiratory obstruction (soft tissue obstruction by the tongue); or

■ inhalation of foreign material, e.g. tooth fragments or fillings, blood or vomitus;

or it may be:

■ secondary respiratory failure, due to cardiac arrest.

In respiratory arrest, there will be *no* respiratory movement and this condition must be distinguished from respiratory obstruction, which may lead to respiratory arrest if not detected.

Treatment

Once respiratory arrest is suspected, the airway must be opened and ventilation commenced. Obtain the assistance of a medical practitioner and arrange for immediate transport to hospital.

Convulsions

A patient who has convulsions (fits), other than a known epileptic, requires investigation to determine the cause. Fitting can be generalised or local (e.g. face or one limb) and may involve loss of consciousness.

Fits can be caused by:

■ low blood pressure;

■ hypoxia;

■ IV local anaesthetic (e.g. lignocaine), although this is very rare;

■ epilepsy (poorly controlled);

■ hyperventilation; or

■ hypoglycaemia.

■ **hypoxia**: a state of reduced oxygen in the blood.
■ **cyanosis**: the bluish appearance of skin and mucous membrane caused by insufficiency of oxygen in the blood.

Treatment

- Place the patient flat.
- Clear the airway and maintain an open airway.
- Protect the patient from injury during convulsion.
- Administer oxygen.
- Do *not* put padded spoons or other instruments into the mouth.
- Do not attempt to inflate the lungs during a fit.
- Do *not* attempt to restrain the patient in any way.
- On recovery, a patient who has had a fit should be allowed to rest for some time and always be discharged into the care of a responsible adult.

Dyspnoea (shortness of breath)

Dyspnoea may be caused by sudden congestion and oedema of the lung, or bronchospasm. The symptoms and signs of dyspnoea are:

- laboured respiration; or
- paroxysms of coughing often accompanied by restlessness, flushing, cyanosis and sweating.

Treatment

- Reassure the patient and permit sitting in the most comfortable position.
- Give oxygen therapy with a face mask.

Closely observe the patient's state of consciousness, respiration and pulse. If the patient becomes pale and loses consciousness, lay the patient in the horizontal position, continue oxygen therapy and prepare for further basic life support.

Asthma attack

Asthma attacks can be caused by strong chemical smells, vapours, aerosols, and glove powder as well as other causes. The same treatment should be used for asthma attack as for dyspnoea.

The asthmatic patient will know if they are having an attack of asthma. Allow the patient to take two metered inhalations from their pressurised bronchodilator aerosol.

Treatment

Treatment is the same as for shortness of breath. If the attack does not subside after use of the inhalant, arrangements should be made for the patient to be taken to hospital.

Hypertensive response

A **hypertensive** response may be indicated by:

- complaints of pounding headache, chest pain, palpitations or dyspnoea;
- extreme pallor, coldness, muscular tremor and sweating;
- high blood pressure, rapid or irregular pulse; and
- cardiorespiratory arrest.

Treatment

- Stop all dental treatment.
- Place the patient in the semi-recumbent position.
- Give oxygen therapy with a facemask.
- Reassure the patient.
- Closely observe the patient's state of consciousness, respirations and pulse.
- If the patient starts to lose consciousness, place the patient in the horizontal position, continue oxygen therapy and prepare for further basic life support.

If cardiorespiratory arrest is suspected or confirmed, start CPR immediately, obtain the assistance of a medical practitioner and arrange for immediate transport to hospital.

Diabetes

Diabetes is relatively common and dentists must frequently treat patients suffering from this condition.

Insulin shock (hypoglycaemia)

This is caused by too much insulin and insufficient sugar and food. Symptoms include:

- hunger;
- nervousness and weakness;
- muscle spasms (e.g. in the calf);
- abdominal pain and nausea;
- sweating; and
- periods of unconsciousness and dizziness (the patient may appear to be intoxicated).

Later, convulsions, coma and finally death may follow if untreated.

Treatment

Give glucose/sugar (two or three teaspoons) by mouth if the patient is conscious. Otherwise, seek immediate medical aid.

hypertensive: abnormally raised blood pressure.

Diabetic pre-coma (hyperglycaemia)

Diabetic pre-coma may occur in the diabetic patient who has not taken the necessary insulin. Symptoms include:

- gradual onset of nausea and/or vomiting;
- acetone smell on the breath (diabetic acidosis);
- increased heart rate;
- dry skin;
- collapse;
- coma; and, if untreated,
- death.

A patient with diabetic acidosis and pre-coma will not generally present as an emergency but as a sick, dehydrated person smelling of acetone. Before dental treatment always ask the patient if they had their medication or insulin injection.

In the diabetic, an abscess or similar acute infection may aggravate the diabetic state and produce the generalised signs of the disease described above.

Anaphylaxis (an extreme allergic reaction)

Anaphylaxis may occur in patients unaware of their susceptibility but is most common in patients with a history of allergy. The most common precipitating agents are penicillin, muscle relaxants, iodine containing contrast material (sialography) and all products containing serum.

Anaphylaxis may present as:

- complaints of itching;
- the appearance of hives, weals or blotching;
- swelling of the face, eyelids, mouth, tongue and throat;
- an asthma-like attack with dyspnoea, wheezing and cyanosis;
- sudden fall in blood pressure (shock) leading to syncope and perhaps unconsciousness, or
- cardiorespiratory arrest.

In dental practice, anaphylaxis rarely occurs, and the most common and outstanding sign is rapidly developing (i.e. over a period of seconds) severe difficulty in breathing, syncope, leading to unconsciousness and cardiac arrest.

Treatment

The treatment of anaphylaxis should be the provision of basic life support.

There is an 'anaphylactic kit', containing hydrocortisone and adrenalin in injection form, available on prescription. This should be in the first aid kit of every surgery. The hydrocortisone should only be administered by the dentist or staff legally entitled and qualified to do so. It is important to regularly check the use-by date on these drugs and, when necessary, replace immediately with fresh supplies.

Accidents in the surgery

Accidental poisoning

Many of the fluids used in the dental surgery and home are extremely dangerous if swallowed (e.g. fluoride solutions). The correct treatment of such cases is very important. In each capital city there is immediate expert telephone advice on the emergency treatment of poisoning. The specified telephone number should be readily available, near the telephone, in case of emergency.

Spillage of materials

Spillage of dangerous fluids can be avoided if consideration is given to the prevention of such accidents.

Bottles should never be left where they can spill on patients or staff if they are overturned. Dangerous fluids should be stored away from dentist/patient areas and dispensed from small-capacity bottles with well-fitting lids so that only a small volume of the liquid enters the potential accident zone.

Remember, prevention is better than cure. Careful work practices will eliminate the risk of spillages and other preventable accidents in the surgery.

Procedures for dealing with emergencies

Your practice should have procedures in place for dealing with emergencies. These procedures should outline who is responsible for:

- calling emergency services (ambulance, fire, etc.) in case of emergency (appropriate phone numbers should be kept by the phone);
- remaining with the patient;
- performing CPR;
- remaining with other patients;
- collecting the first aid kit, oxygen unit, portable defibrillator, emergency drug kit, or any other piece of emergency equipment kept by the practice; and
- any other duties that might arise.

It is an OHS requirement that staff undertake regular training and emergency drills to practise what they would do in such an emergency situation. Each state and territory has different requirements for emergency drills.

When the emergency is under control, the dentist and all members of the team involved in the emergency should write a report about the condition of the patient and any action taken.

Use of simple apparatus

Artificial ventilation with simple apparatus may be undertaken when it can be achieved without interrupting basic life support. Most dental surgeries use relative analgesia equipment and would therefore have oxygen available that can be administered by using a mask. Appropriate airway or manually triggered oxygen pressure devices may also be utilised. However, correctly performed basic life support is always superior to oxygen equipment used late or any other equipment used ineffectively by untrained people.

Training and retraining

You will receive Level I First Aid training as part of completing the Dental Assistant Certificate III course. All staff should at least have training in CPR. The technique of CPR is learned only by repeated practice on manikins, under expert supervision. Once learned, the technique requires regular practice, if it is to be effective in an emergency. Fortunately, the average person working outside a hospital encounters cardiac arrest rarely. However, to approach resuscitation with confidence, practice must be frequent and thorough. First aid certificates must be renewed every three years with a refresher course in CPR undertaken every 12 months.

Dental emergencies in and away from the surgery

Dental pain/toothache

When a patient calls the surgery complaining of toothache, a number of questions need to be asked to establish the urgency of treatment. These include:

- Is the pain worse with hot or cold drinks or food?

- Has it been aching for a long time?
- Does it react to sweets?
- Is there an obvious cavity?
- Is there any oral or facial swelling?
- Does the patient have a temperature?

If the answer is yes to any of these, the patient should be seen immediately to establish the cause.

Fractured teeth

Fractured teeth can be the result of an injury sustained during sport or other accident. Extensive fractures may involve pulp exposure, therefore they will need immediate attention to save the vitality of the tooth.

Avulsed teeth

A permanent tooth that has been knocked out by accident can be saved by prompt action. The quicker the tooth is replaced, the greater chance that it will survive.

Teeth that are replaced within half an hour have a 90 per cent chance of being saved. See Procedure 22.1 for the steps to take for saving a tooth.

Soft tissue trauma

Soft tissue trauma includes any injury to the gingiva, lips and mucous membrane. If bleeding is severe, the patient should be seen immediately by the dentist.

Bleeding tooth socket following an extraction

A rolled up gauze swab held firmly over the socket may be sufficient to stem the flow of blood. Suturing may be required if bleeding continues.

A dry socket

This is an extremely painful inflammation/infection of the tooth socket following extraction. It is usually caused by the loss of the protective blood clot that forms in the base of the socket. Hot food or too vigorous rinsing of the site can be the cause. Patients should be advised and instructed on home care following an extraction. See Chapter 32 for a sample instruction sheet.

Procedure 22.1 Avulsed teeth

Avulsion means that a tooth has been completely dislodged out of its socket, as in being knocked out by trauma. Not only has the blood supply to the pulp been severed and the periodontal ligament compromised, but the ligament remaining on the tooth root has probably been contaminated by dirt and bacteria, and is also at risk of drying out, which would kill off the cells on the root.

Emergency procedure

An avulsed tooth can be replanted; that is, replaced directly back into its socket. If this procedure is successful then the tooth will eventually be restored to normal appearance and function. (Avulsed deciduous teeth are not usually replanted because of treatment difficulties and the risk of damage to the developing permanent successor.)

Time is a crucial factor in the success of replantation and a tooth that is replanted within 30 minutes of avulsion has the best chance of survival.

- Stay calm and find the tooth.
- Handle the tooth by the crown only. *Do not* touch the root.
- If, or when, the tooth is clean, replant directly into the socket.
- Get immediate dental treatment.
- If the tooth is dirty, replant it after rinsing in milk, or get the patient to suck it clean first. Water is not ideal.

If it cannot be replanted immediately, ask the patient to bring the tooth directly to the dentist either completely submerged in milk, in the patient's mouth, or in plastic wrap with some of the patient's saliva. Do not place in water or in a matchbox, etc.

Dental treatment

Following replantation, the dentist should:

- order a tetanus prophylaxis;
- prescribe antibiotics; and
- temporarily splint the tooth into place, usually with some composite resin, glass ionomer, wire or nylon fishing line.

The dentist may also:

- take a radiograph to check for fractures in bone and adjacent teeth; and
- treat for soft tissue injury.

Follow-up treatment

The root of an avulsed tooth is very susceptible to resorption or ankylosis. In addition, degeneration and death of the pulp inevitably occurs, except in young children. For these reasons it is usual to carry out endodontic treatment on teeth which have been avulsed, and this is often commenced at least a week after replantation.

Secondary bleeding

Following any major surgical procedure in the oral cavity there is a chance that secondary bleeding might occur. Although it is very rare and you may never come across it, you should know how to respond. The bleeding can be quite severe and very frightening for the patient. Make an appointment for them to be seen immediately. Recommend that they fold a piece of clean cotton (such as a hand-kerchief), place it over the bleeding area and bite down hard. The site will most likely need suturing.

Summary

The majority of emergencies will not be serious but they must all be treated promptly and correctly so that the occasional serious emergency will be recognised and treated effectively. When you complete your first aid certificate course you will learn what to do in these situations. They are discussed briefly in this chapter as a reminder and a reference. However, you must constantly refresh your knowledge and keep your skills up to date. If there is a real emergency you will not have time to check your textbook or surgery protocols for instructions!

Section 4

Restorative dentistry

The aim of restorative dentistry is to return a tooth to normal function or to replace the tooth with a functional and cosmetically pleasing replacement. Much of your work will be related to restorative dentistry.

New techniques, equipment and materials for restorative dentistry change and are introduced regularly. Therefore it is impossible to include them all in this text. Your workplace should have a procedure in place that ensures you receive proper training whenever a new technique, instrument or material is introduced to your surgery. Keep a folder of instructions close to hand as a quick reference.

The most commonly used techniques and materials are described in Chapters 23 to 26 in this section.

chapter twenty-three
restorative materials.

Introduction

A crucial part of your job is the correct preparation of materials used in the restoration of teeth.

The materials used must be able to withstand harsh conditions in the mouth. They must be able to withstand high pressures caused by chewing, and rapid changes in temperature caused by eating or drinking hot and cold foods. They might be exposed to foods that make them corrode or dissolve. Incorrect preparation will weaken the restoration.

It is essential that you know:

- the manufacturer's recommendations for the preparation of materials;
- what equipment is required to prepare materials; and
- what equipment is required for the dentist to apply them.

Different restorative materials work in different ways and the main features of each material are described in the following pages. In summary though, restorative materials need to set (harden). Most are mixed to form a paste and after the paste is applied the material sets either by:

- self-curing (because a chemical reaction in the paste makes it harden);
- light-curing (by being exposed to a curing light); or
- some combination of these two methods.

Restorative techniques

Cavity lining

A tooth that has suffered decay and had a cavity prepared has been traumatised. The dentine and pulp require protection from further injury. In this respect, a tooth is just like any other wounded tissue. Therefore, it may be necessary to cover the exposed dentine with a sedative dressing to help reduce and overcome any irritation of the pulp.

Dentine is made up of a mass of microscopic tubules running more or less at right angles to the surface of the tooth. These have direct access to the pulp chamber and bacteria can gain entry to the pulp along the tubules. Injurious chemical substances contained in some filling materials can affect the pulp in a similar manner. Additionally, the rapid transfer of temperature changes across metallic fillings can adversely affect the pulpal tissues and cause pain to the patient.

Cavity liners and dental cements are used to prevent or reduce the effects of such harmful stimuli.

The most common materials used for cavity liners or bases are:

- glass ionomer cement (GIC);
- cavity varnish;
- calcium hydroxide;
- polycarboxylate cement;
- zinc oxide-eugenol (ZOE); and
- ledermix cement.

Restorations

Restorations are used to treat carious lesions and to restore the normal function of damaged teeth.

Sometimes they are also performed for cosmetic reasons. The most common restorations are amalgam and composite resin restorations. These materials are described below and the techniques are described in Chapter 24.

Fissure sealing

Fissure sealing is a technique used to provide a physical barrier that prevents bacteria and food from entering the fissures in the teeth, especially the grinding surfaces of molars. Before the sealant is placed, the tooth is acid etched (see below), rinsed and dried.

Additional techniques and materials

Additional techniques and their related materials (e.g. acid etching, bonding agents and dentine adhesives) are described later in this chapter.

Materials for direct tooth restoration

Some general guidelines for mixing materials

- All manufacturer's directions should be implicitly followed.
- Many of the materials now used in direct tooth restorations come in capsulated form and must be mixed in an amalgamator/triturator/capsule mixer.
- Some materials are dispensed from specially designed tubes.
- If mixing materials on a slab, the temperature of the slab can affect the setting times. Ensure that the slab is the correct temperature for the material being mixed.
- Use the appropriate mixing pad recommended for each material.
- Cleanliness of the slab and spatula is crucial.
- The slab must be completely dry. The manufacturer has carefully controlled the water content of the cement liquid and if the slab is not carefully dried, the water taken up from a wet or damp slab will adversely affect the properties of the set cement, particularly setting time and strength.
- To avoid evaporation, do not dispense liquids until ready to commence mixing.

- Cement liquids will either lose or gain water if the bottle is left open, depending on whether it is a dry or humid day. Loss of water will cause slow setting while gain of water speeds up the reaction. If either occurs, the rest of the physical properties also deteriorate. The bottles must be kept well stoppered when not in use.
- The top of most liquid bottles are designed to act as a dropper to dispense drops of liquid. The dropper must be kept scrupulously clean and must be wiped after each dispensing or the size of the drops will vary.
- If consistent volumes or drops of liquid are to be dispensed, the dropper must be used correctly with the dropper point vertical and the drops must be allowed to fall freely under their own mass and not be forcibly squeezed out of the dropper.
- Mixing times must be adhered to.
- In all cases, premature contact of the setting cement with moisture adversely affects the properties. Never add liquid to a mix that is too thick. Start a new mix. Discard any unused powder on the slab. Never return it to the powder bottle as this will contaminate the powder in the bottle.
- Clean the spatula and slab immediately, before the cement sets.
- Whenever possible, only materials that appear on the Australian Dental Association List of Certified Products should be used.
- The various brands of powders should never be mixed with different liquids. Combinations of powders and liquids are formulated to react one with the other for each brand, and mixing different combinations can lead to vastly inferior properties.

Specific requirements for materials are described below, as are some general guidelines for the mixing and handling of materials.

Cavity liners

Cavity varnish

Properties

Various resins, either natural (such as copal) or synthetic, when dissolved in a solvent, such as ether or chloroform, produce a fluid material resembling nail polish.

Clinical uses

The varnish is painted on the freshly cut dentine and after the solvent evaporates a thin protective film remains.

Although varnish films assist in sealing the cavity and reducing acid sensitivity, they are too thin to be effective in reducing thermal conductivity encountered with metallic restorations.

Cavity varnish cannot be used under composite resins or glass ionomer restorations.

Mixing systems

Cavity varnish does not require mixing.

Procedures and setting times

For this procedure you will need:

- cavity varnish;
- cotton pellets; and
- college tweezers.

Procedure

- Open the bottle of varnish and place a clean cotton pellet, held in clean tweezers (not having previously been used in the patient's mouth), into the liquid (but try not to touch the varnish or the bottle with the tweezers).
- Recap the bottle to prevent the liquid from evaporating and then thickening.
- Pass the pellet in the tweezers to the operator.
- If a repeat application is required, it might be wise to use a micro-brush to prevent cross-contamination.
- Repeat these steps if further layers of varnish are required.
- Wipe the tweezers with varnish thinner immediately after use to prevent varnish build-up on the instrument.

Safety issues

If the varnish container is not tightly stoppered, evaporation of the solvent causes the varnish to become thick. Before it can be used, it must either be carefully thinned with the correct solvent or discarded.

Calcium hydroxide (CaOH)

Properties

The original form of this material was a non-setting paste consisting of calcium hydroxide mixed with distilled water. It was used to cover exposed pulps in an attempt to promote secondary dentine formation and this form is still available.

Later formulations were produced as pastes that set to a hard mass and were designed to act as a barrier to the acid present in silicate cements.

Clinical uses

Calcium hydroxide has advantages in all cavity situations due to its effectiveness in promoting the formation of secondary dentine. It has also come into more general use under direct filling resins.

Mixing systems

Calcium hydroxide is available as two pastes (base and catalyst) or in powder and liquid form.

Procedures and setting times

For this procedure you will need:

- calcium hydroxide (tubes of base and catalyst paste, or powder and liquid);
- a small-tipped spatula and suitable greaseproof paper mixing pad (some mixing pads have a coating on them which is not suitable for CaOH); and
- a CaOH applicator (also commonly called a dycal applicator).

The procedure is outlined below.

- Put very small, equal quantities of the two pastes (catalyst and base), or one drop liquid and one scoop of powder, on a paper pad.
- Place one paste on top of the other or carry the powder into the liquid.
- Mix quickly for about 15 seconds.
- Mound into a small pile near the edge of the mixing pad.
- Hand the paste and applicator to the operator and wipe the spatula clean.
- Throw away the used top sheet of the paper pad after use.

Safety issues

Ensure that the mixing pad is not contaminated by either mixed material or dirty hands.

Zinc oxide-eugenol (ZOE)

Properties

When zinc oxide is mixed with eugenol (oil of cloves) it forms a weak cement that can be strengthened by the addition of resin or ortho-ethoxybenzoic acid (EBA).

Clinical uses

Zinc oxide-eugenol is regarded as an obtundent (pain reliever) and it is used as a sedative lining for most restorative materials or as a temporary filling material. It can also be used for impression taking (see later in this chapter).

Mixing systems

This material consists of a base and the catalyst is eugenol (oil of cloves) that are supplied in two separate tubes.

Procedures and setting times

The required amount of powder and oil is mixed on a mixing pad with a spatula. When a uniform mix is obtained, the dentist places it into the cavity, either as a liner under amalgam or as a temporary sedative dressing.

Safety issues

Care must be taken if used under composite resins because any free eugenol reacts with, and may inhibit the setting of, the resin. Coating the lips lightly with petroleum jelly will prevent the paste from sticking when ZOE is used for impression taking.

Zinc oxide-eugenol cements cannot be used under GIC restorations.

Intermediary Restorative Material (IRM)

Intermediary Restorative Material (IRM) is a reinforced ZOE temporary dressing material developed during the Vietnam War. This filling material is stronger and can be left in the tooth for a number of months until a permanent restoration can be placed.

The procedure is the same as for ZOE. The powder and liquid must be dispensed in exact proportions with the measuring scoop and liquid dropper supplied. Spatulation is necessary until a firm, glossy mix is achieved.

Ledermix

Properties

Ledermix usually contains corticosteroids in small amounts to settle inflammation.

Clinical uses

This cement is water soluble and can be used as a treatment for pulpitis. The paste is used as an antibiotic and sedative dressing during root canal treatment.

Mixing systems

Ledermix comes as a paste or in powder and liquid form.

Procedures and setting times

Powder and liquid for cementation is mixed following manufacturer's instructions. Pastes can be dispensed onto a cotton pellet or micro-brush.

Dental cements

Dental cements set or harden by chemical reaction after mixing, and are used:

- as a material for cementing inlays, crowns, etc. (also called a **luting** agent); and
- sometimes as a lining or base material.

The term cement can sometimes be misleading since some cements can be used for either temporary or permanent filling, for example, ZOE, GIC. Cements may be used in most restorations as bases or liners, cementation materials, or temporary and permanent filling materials. The dentist will select the appropriate type of cement to use.

Zinc phosphate cement

Properties

Zinc phosphate cement is a luting cement and does not provide a glue-type adhesion.

■ **luting**: the sealing of the junction of two substances, such as a crown on the tooth, with a fine-grained cement, such as GIC or zinc phosphate.

Clinical uses

Zinc phosphate cement material is used to cement inlays, crowns and bridges permanently into place and sometimes for cementing orthodontic bands. It can also be used as a strong, hard base or lining under some restorative materials.

Zinc phosphate cement is available in a variety of colours and this is important in the cementing of translucent restorations such as porcelain jacket crowns. If possible, the cement should match the colour of the restoration. A dark-coloured cement may show through and affect the appearance of the crown.

Mixing systems

Zinc phosphate cement is available as a powder and liquid and in a pre-portioned, capsulated form. The manufacturer's instructions regarding the activation of the capsule and consequent mechanical mixing must be followed implicitly.

Procedures and setting times

For this procedure you will need:

- a cool, thick glass slab;
- zinc phosphate powder and liquid;
- a zinc phosphate dispenser and dropper; and
- a flexible stainless steel double-ended spatula.

The purpose of mixing is not only to combine the powder with the liquid, but also to produce a cement with the best possible smooth flow characteristics, enabling it to form a thin film. The thin film allows correct seating of the restoration and high strength, and ensures a lasting restoration.

Cleanliness and dryness of the slab and spatula is essential since particles of previously hardened cement incorporated into the mix can prevent proper seating of inlays or crowns.

The correct consistency for cementing crowns or inlays is reached when the mix is creamy and will 'follow' the spatula 25 mm before breaking in a thin thread. The mix will fall from the spatula in a viscous drop, hold its form for a moment and then spread on the slab.

The consistency when used as a base liner is correct when the cement hangs but does not drop from the spatula. The mix must have a putty-like consistency and will not follow the spatula when it is raised from the slab, but breaks away.

The liquid should be placed on the slab well clear of the powder and mixed as instructed in Procedure 23.1.

Procedure 23.1 Preparing and mixing zinc phosphate cement

- After dispensing the powder, it should be divided as shown. This is achieved by forming a square of the powder about 2 mm deep using the dry mixing spatula.

- The square is divided into quarters. One of the quarters is next divided into half and one of these portions is halved again. If the assistant is right-handed, make sure that the first small addition is on the right and closest to the front edge of the slab as shown in the figure. The reverse is, of course, necessary for a left-handed assistant.

- Hold the spatula blade firmly against the slab along the entire length of the blade and make the mix using linear 'stropping' motions.

- Use the dry end of the spatula to draw each increment of powder into the mix.

- Mix thoroughly over a large area of the slab.

- Several times, interrupt the mixing to gather the edges of the mix. The mix should be homogeneous before any subsequent portions are added.

- Follow the manufacturer's instructions carefully for different brands.

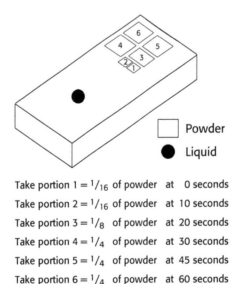

☐ Powder
● Liquid

Take portion 1 = $^1/_{16}$ of powder at 0 seconds
Take portion 2 = $^1/_{16}$ of powder at 10 seconds
Take portion 3 = $^1/_8$ of powder at 20 seconds
Take portion 4 = $^1/_4$ of powder at 30 seconds
Take portion 5 = $^1/_4$ of powder at 45 seconds
Take portion 6 = $^1/_4$ of powder at 60 seconds
Complete at 80 seconds

Factors affecting setting times

- Thicker mixes set faster.

- Within limits, fast addition of powder causes faster setting.

- Shorter mixing times cause faster setting.

- Higher slab temperatures cause fast setting. The ideal temperature for the slab is 20°C.

- Moisture gain causes fast setting and a weak cement. Moisture loss causes slow setting.

- Mix for the times shown in the illustration. The reaction caused by mixing the liquid and powder gives off heat. Thorough, slow mixing allows the cement to cool before the addition of the next lot of powder, and this slows the setting time of the cement. It is also important as it allows a smooth creamy mix to be achieved. Mixing over a larger area also slows the setting time.

- A hot or warm slab must not be used since heat causes the reaction to speed up, reducing the setting time and, most importantly, the amount of powder that can be incorporated into the liquid to produce the correct consistency. The slab should therefore be cooled but never below the dew point (i.e. the temperature below which water from the atmosphere will form as a mist of droplets on the slab).

- To prevent the material sticking to the dental placement instrument, a small amount of alcohol may be placed in a **dappen dish** for the dentist. The spatula used for mixing should be wiped immediately or placed into a small container with water until it can be cleaned.

Safety issues

When used as a base or hard lining under other restorative materials, a protective sub-base, such as zinc oxide-eugenol or calcium hydroxide, is often placed beneath the cement to protect the pulp from the effects of the phosphoric acid. This acid in deep cavities can cause severe irritation and in extreme cases can cause the death of the pulp.

When cementing inlays, crowns and bridges, you may be expected to apply the cement evenly and thinly to the cavity side of the inlay or crown while the dentist is applying cement to the tooth. Care must be exercised not to trap air.

Polycarboxylate cement

Properties

Polycarboxylate is a cement that is adherent to dental enamel and to a lesser extent to dentine. This cement is particularly bland to the pulp, has low solubility in normal mouth fluids and can produce a thin film.

Clinical uses

Because of its chemical nature and bland effect on the pulp, polycarboxylate cement is effectively used as a base, particularly under composite resins, and as a cementing agent in crown and bridge dentistry.

Mixing systems

The polycarboxylate cements are powder–liquid combinations. The liquid is a watery solution of poly-acrylic acid, while the powder is similar in composition to that used for zinc phosphate cements, being principally zinc oxide with some magnesium oxide and other salts to control the setting time. The powder and liquid are mixed together and the mix hardens into a cement consisting of the un-dissolved portions of the zinc oxide particles in a matrix of zinc polycarboxylate.

Procedures and setting times

For this procedure you will need:

- polycarboxylate powder and liquid;
- polycarboxylate dispenser and dropper;
- a glass slab or plastic pad; and
- a large, wide-bladed spatula.

The liquid is quite viscous and, in the past, some manufacturers produced liquids with different viscosities for lining and cementing purposes. However, most manufacturers now use a single viscosity liquid and vary the amount of powder to be added.

The mix should be made on a surface that will not absorb liquid and either a glass slab or the mixing pads supplied with the cement are suitable. The pad or slab should be cooled to just above the dew point, since a cool mixing surface slows down the reaction somewhat and provides a longer working time.

- Dispense the powder onto the pad, divide it into halves and recap the bottle.

- Dispense the required number of drops of liquid clear of the powder and recap the bottle.

- Draw half of the powder into the liquid and spatulate vigorously for about 10 seconds.

- Wipe the spatula clean on the pad and draw the remaining portion of powder into the liquid and complete the mix by about 30 seconds.

The mix should be similar to that described for zinc phosphate cements (putty-like for a base, creamy and flowing for cementation) and be glossy. The end of the working time of these materials is indicated when the cement loses its lustre and becomes stringy. It must never be used after this point.

■ **dappen dish:** a small glass or disposable plastic bowl, used for holding liquid dental materials during a procedure.

Safety issues

The disadvantages of polycarboxylate cements are lower strength than zinc phosphate cement and a high solubility in lactic acid. This high solubility can be very serious in mouths that develop considerable amounts of dental plaque.

Glass ionomer cement (GIC)

Properties

Glass ionomer cements are also known as glass polyalkenoate cements. They are probably the most commonly used cements. The cement is adhesive to both enamel and dentine and is tooth coloured.

The major advantage of glass ionomer cements is that they release fluoride.

Clinical uses

Glass ionomer cements are of particular importance in the cementation of some types of anterior crowns. They are considerably stronger than zinc phosphate cement, non-irritant to the pulp and are suitable for many forms of cementation and lining. They are also used for cementing orthodontic bands.

Some glass ionomer materials are suitable for restoring lost tooth substance such as occurs at the necks of teeth in older persons where incorrect use of the toothbrush can cause abrasion of cementum and dentine. As the material is adhesive, minimal cavity preparation is required, and true adhesion can be obtained to freshly cleaned tooth substance. Glass ionomer restorations can be used in place of composite cements in the anterior teeth.

Mixing systems

Glass ionomer cement is most commonly used in pre-packaged capsule form and is available as normal set and fast set. Glass ionomer cements are either self-curing or light cured.

Procedures and setting times

For this procedure you will need:

- glass ionomer powder and liquid;
- glass ionomer dispenser and dropper;
- paper mixing pad or glass slab; and
- a plastic or agate spatula.

Liquids based on polyacrylic acid are quite viscous, while the water-based liquids are considerably less so.

Because of the varying formulations of this material, it is not possible to give a powder–liquid ratio, but the manufacturer's instructions should be followed closely.

The mix should be made on a non-absorbent surface — either a glass slab or the disposable paper pad supplied with the material is suitable. The aluminous silicate powder particles are extremely hard and will abrade metals such as stainless steel. The incorporation of abraded metal particles will discolour the mix. For this reason, a stellite or agate spatula should be used.

- Dispense both powder and liquid onto the mixing surface according to the manufacturer's directions.
- Mix the increments as directed for the designated time, usually between 30 and 45 seconds.

The correct mix is similar in consistency to that of zinc phosphate cement and will be glossy but it is important that the mixed material be immediately conveyed to the cavity or preparation because some types of this material have a limited working time.

When used as a restoration, some carving and shaping can be done after about six minutes, and then the material should be protected from moisture contamination until completely set. Final shaping and finishing is best left until at least 24 hours after placement. Residue on mixing instruments may easily be removed by placing in water.

Safety issues

Do not use the cement after the working time has elapsed. The end of the working time is indicated by the material becoming rubbery. Any material, such as an exposed cement line, must be protected from moisture contamination, preferably for 24 hours, in order to allow the cement to achieve its highest resistance to solution in the mouth. Protection is gained by using the varnish supplied with most materials, or a coating of silicone grease.

Dental amalgam

Properties

Dental amalgam has been in use for over 100 years, although modifications are still being made to the basic alloy to improve its properties. It is affordable, strong and safe and used mostly for molar and premolar restorations. Amalgam is made by mixing mercury with an alloy.

Clinical uses

Dental amalgam is probably the oldest, most commonly used material for direct filling of cavities in posterior teeth.

Mixing systems

The alloy

Amalgam alloy is mixed with mercury to form the amalgam that is packed into the cavity. (An alloy is a mixture of metals.) Amalgam alloy is supplied to the dentist in numerous forms as follows.

- Lathe cut — these are needle-like particles usually produced by cutting a cast bar or ingot of the alloy in a lathe or milling machine.
- Spherical — the molten alloy is atomised or solidified in the form of fine spherical particles.
- Mixture — some brands of amalgam alloy use a mixture of spherical and lathe cut particles.

The shape of the particles affects the **trituration** of the amalgam and the ways in which it can be worked.

As well as these different forms of particles, the alloy may be supplied in various forms.

- Bulk powder — the particles are received as a bottle of loose powder either in 20g, 100g, or 1kg sizes.
- Tablets — the alloy is sometimes compressed into tablets by the use of pressure and heat.
- Pre-proportioned capsules are the most commonly used amalgams. Both alloy and mercury are supplied in a single-use capsule, accurately proportioned and suitable for mechanical mixing.

Mercury

The other component of the amalgam, mercury, is a metal that is liquid at ordinary temperatures. Liquid mercury, especially if finely divided into small droplets, gives off a poisonous vapour at room temperature. Mercury must never be splashed around, handled unnecessarily or squeezed onto the floor. Mercury is safe to use if good mercury hygiene is practised. Mercury must never be heated for any reason as this increases the production of poisonous vapour. If mercury is inadvertently spilt on the floor as much as possible should be picked up and the floor treated with a commercial preparation for the elimination of the hazard.

The amalgam alloy

The alloy is made up mostly of silver but may also contain smaller amounts of tin, zinc and copper. Both alloy and mercury are required to produce an amalgam. These components are combined by mixing mechanically in a mixing capsule. The mixing process is called trituration.

Reusable capsules

Reusable capsules are not very common but are still used by some dentists who prefer not to use pre-proportioned capsules. If this type of capsule is used, it should have a close fitting top that does not allow mercury to escape. This may be checked by placing a strip of adhesive tape around the capsule junction, and after mixing has taken place, examining the removed tape.

Dispensers may be used to load the capsules with alloy and mercury. The proportioned capsules should be mixed in the amalgamator for the time that produces the particular consistency that the dentist requires. It is essential that under-mixing, and a consequently dry mix, be avoided.

Pre-proportioned capsules

Pre-proportioned capsules contain pre-portioned alloy and mercury, which are kept apart. Before mixing, the capsules require activating (i.e. allowing the mercury and alloy to come into contact with each other). The capsules are produced in a variety of forms with differing methods of activation and it is essential that the manufacturer's method of activation and mixing times be adhered to.

If this is carried out, a consistently correct mix will be achieved.

Procedures and setting times

The dentist will usually instruct you on how to present the mixed amalgam before condensation so that it fits into the dentist's particular technique of condensation.

Safety issues

The most important aspect of amalgamation is the mixing procedure. It must be carried out long enough to achieve sufficient reaction between the alloy particles and mercury to produce a suitable plastic amalgam. This may be checked by ensuring that plastic, not sloppy or dry mixes, are employed. Dry mixes are extremely dangerous because failure of the restoration is inevitable since each packed layer does not unite with the preceding one.

trituration: the method of reducing a substance to a fine state by grinding, rubbing or pounding. Also used to indicate the mixing of dental amalgam alloy with mercury and other capsulated materials.

However, over-trituration should also be avoided, as the effect of this is to cause a contraction in the amalgam, which can affect the marginal integrity of the restoration.

See Chapter 15 for information about precautions when using mercury and procedures in case of a mercury spill.

Resin-based restorative materials

Properties

Resin-based restorative materials were previously known as direct filling resins or composite resins, but are now more correctly called resin-based restorative materials.

Clinical uses

Resin-based restorative materials form a tooth-coloured material that can be contoured to the shape of the tooth and which bond well to the tooth surface.

Mixing systems

Resin-based restorative materials have the following basic formulation:

- Resin bonding agent — this is usually the product of bisphenol A and glycidyl methacrylate (Bis–GMA) or a modification of this formula. The resin requires a catalyst and accelerator for hardening to occur.

- Filler — a powdered ceramic, such as quartz, alumino–phospho–silicate or special glasses, treated with vinyl or other silane materials so that bonding with the resin is possible. These add strength to the restoration.

- Other additives — ultraviolet filters which aid colour stability as well as other stabilising additives are present in these formulations.

The components of restorative resins can take the following forms.

- Paste with liquid catalyst — this consists of the resin-binder made into a paste with the filler while the catalyst is in liquid form.

- Two pastes — both pastes contain resin plus filler. One paste contains the catalyst, the other the accelerator. When both are mixed together in approximately equal quantities, hardening takes place.

- Powder and liquid — the powder is basically filler and the liquid is Bis–GMA resin diluted with monomeric methyl methacrylate or similar diluting agent.

- Encapsulated — the capsule is divided into two parts, one containing the filler and the other the Bis–GMA resin. The capsule is activated by bursting the separating membrane between the two components and then mixing in a high-energy machine.

- Single paste — all the required components of the resin system are present in this paste and polymerisation is initiated by either intense ultraviolet or white light. The light causes changes in the special catalyst, which starts the chemical reaction and leads to rapid polymerisation. Since 1983, white-light activated materials have virtually replaced the ultraviolet activated type.

Procedures and setting times

Resin-based restorative materials may be placed into the tooth in increments and light-cured after each increment.

Acid etchants

Properties

The etching liquid used is almost always a solution of phosphoric acid in water and the concentrations used range from 35 to 60 per cent. Gel-type etchants are also available. These are preferable where exact placement of the etchant is required, such as where a calcium hydroxide base has been placed. Gels are handled and act in exactly the same way as liquid etchants.

Clinical uses

Many dentists use acid etching before placing resin restorations. This ensures a clean surface (via removal of the smear layer) to improve the bonding of the restoration material with the dentine.

The acid, when applied to clean enamel, dissolves the enamel prism cones in some areas and the interprism areas on others. The object of the etching is to increase the surface and to expose clean enamel that is more suitable for bonding.

The etch is left on the tooth for the recommended time and then washed off thoroughly with copious amounts of water.

Procedures for use

For this procedure you will need:

- etching material and applicator;
- timer;
- cotton rolls or a dental dam to isolate the tooth;
- high-velocity evacuator; and
- triplex syringe.

In this procedure the dentist will:

- isolate the tooth using cotton rolls or a dental dam;
- clean the enamel surface with an oil-free prophylaxis paste;
- dry the surface (but not over-dry it);
- apply the etching agent (either liquid or gel) for the required time;
- use copious amounts of water to wash the etched surface free of acid and reaction products;
- keep the enamel surface free from contamination with saliva or oil from the air-line after etching and drying, and before application of the bonding resin or sealant;
- apply the permanent filling resin.

Safety issues

The patient should be wearing protective glasses and drapes, as etch is particularly damaging to eye tissue and fabric.

Bonding agents

Properties

The bonding material flows around an etched surface to provide a strong mechanical bond.

Clinical uses

Bonding agents improve the bond between the restorative resin and the enamel or dentine. They are applied after etching.

Mixing systems

Bonding agents are often light cured.

Procedures and setting times

Bonding agents may be applied with single use applicators from the special mixing palettes supplied.

Dentine adhesives

Properties

Two layers of dentine adhesives are recommended before restoring the tooth with either chemically or light-activated composite resin.

Clinical uses

A number of dentine adhesive materials are used with composite resin fillings. Bonding a resin to dentine can be more difficult than to enamel because the dentine contains organic materials.

These products provide reasonable adhesion to dentine and can be used in addition to bonding agents on etched enamel.

Mixing systems

Each product is supplied as two or three liquids that are mixed together and left to air dry, or as a single liquid that is light cured.

Procedures and setting times

Follow manufacturer's instructions for dispensing.

Safety issues

The liquids from different products and manufacturers are *not* interchangeable.

Impression materials

An impression is an accurate negative likeness of the dentition of either the upper or lower jaw. There are numerous techniques for impression taking and the choice of the appropriate method depends on the condition of the patient's mouth.

Alginate impressions

Alginate materials are supplied as a fine powder that is mixed with water before use. The powder, which is made of seaweed, contains a mixture of substances that react together when dissolved in water and set to form an elastic gel.

Although weighing is most accurate, it is more convenient to measure the proportions of powder and water using the scoops provided by the manufacturer. However, the tin must always be shaken well to loosen the powder in order to obtain a consistent quantity and quality. The mixture must be spatulated vigorously against the side of a flexible bowl using a broad flat spatula for at least 30 seconds.

Because alginate will not adhere to a metal impression tray, some stock trays are provided with perforations or a rim-lock to give mechanical retention of the material. Other trays may be painted or sprayed with a suitable adhesive.

Alginates are supplied in pre-measured individual packages. After removal from the mouth, models poured from alginate impressions should be cast within 15 minutes. This is because distortions occur within the set material which, together with water evaporation from the mass, leads to inaccuracies. If it is not possible to cast immediately, the impression may be wrapped in a damp towel or stored in a suitable container providing maximum humidity. Alginate impressions may be disinfected in diluted hypochlorite for three minutes. However, it should not be placed in water for long periods of time as serious distortion may occur.

Alginates are adequate for study models, constructing mouthguards and temporary crowns, providing casts are poured immediately.

Zinc oxide-eugenol (ZOE) paste

This material is also used as a cavity liner and is described earlier in this chapter. It is often the material of choice when taking an impression for a denture reline.

Elastomeric materials

Elastomeric materials are primarily used for impressions for partial dentures, crowns and bridgework. They are sometimes used as a thin wash similar to zinc oxide-eugenol paste.

Elastomeric materials are accurate impression materials that may be stored for a short period without distortion. They are usually supplied as two tubes of material — a base and an accelerator that are mixed in equal lengths on a slab with a spatula. Correct proportions are obtained by using equal lengths even though the nozzles of the tubes may be of different diameters.

Reversible hydrocolloid

Reversible hydrocolloid requires a special impression tray for the bulk of material and a syringe to carry the hydrocolloid onto the prepared cavities. It is very accurate but it is not widely used because it

requires the use of specialised equipment. Gingival retraction is used and the impression must be cast immediately.

Polyethers

Polyethers are exceptionally accurate, dimensionally stable materials. Two pastes are mixed together on a disposable paper mixing pad and then loaded into an impression tray. The material sets much faster and is stiffer than other silicone products. A thinner is provided if a more elastic impression is required. It must not be stored in water or in a moist environment as this will affect the dimensional accuracy.

Addition cured silicones (polyvinylsiloxanes)

Addition cured silicones are an excellent impression material. They are accurate and dimensionally stable as well as highly elastic. They are supplied as two-paste automix syringe systems in low, medium and high viscosities.

The material can be affected by storage temperature. If it is stored in the refrigerator it will be very fluid and have a longer setting time.

There is cross reactivity with latex rubber gloves and dental dams. Gloves must be removed before handling these materials in putty form.

Impression compound

Impression compound materials are not as commonly used today as they used to be.

This is a thermoplastic material (i.e. softens on heating and hardens again on cooling), which is made from a mixture of resins, vegetable oils and French chalk. It is supplied in tablets or as pencil-like cylinders called tracing sticks. The compound is softened in water at 55°C to 60°C for two to three minutes, then kneaded to a uniform consistency and placed in an impression tray. It will adhere well to a warm metal tray but must not be overheated or it will become sticky and if too hot could cause injury to the patient's tissue. After removal from the mouth, it is chilled in cold water and may be trimmed with a sharp knife.

Tracing stick compound may also be used to make additions to an impression and is applied by heating in an open flame. A spirit-filled torch is useful for moulding compound impressions.

Dental plaster and dental stone

Dental plaster and dental stone materials are made from gypsum and are used for making casts from impressions, and moulds for denture processing and for mounting casts on **articulators**. Dental stone produces much harder casts than dental plaster. Each is mixed with water to a thick consistency and sets in five to ten minutes.

Other materials used in the surgery

Waxes

Various types of waxes are used in prosthodontics in both surgery and laboratory procedures.

Baseplate wax is almost universally used for the construction of occlusal rims (bite-blocks) and to form the base for trial dentures. It is supplied in pink-coloured sheets and is used by softening in a flame or melting with a hot wax knife.

Sticky wax or model cement is supplied in sticks and is used for joining models or wax trial bases together.

Bite wax (registration wax) is a softer wax supplied in red, aluminium, or copper-coloured wafers or cylinders and is used to record the impression of opposing teeth on a registration rim or the relationship between opposing registration rims.

Tray wax is a soft, slightly sticky wax supplied in sticks. It is used to build up impression trays in order to control some impression materials.

Indicator wax is an extremely soft wax that is flowed on to the impression surface of a denture where it is used to show the location of pressure areas under functional conditions.

Temporary base materials

Temporary base materials are harder and stronger than wax and are used to make special impression trays and also to form the base-plates for bite blocks and trial bases on which the teeth are set. They may also be used merely to strengthen wax base-plates.

There are two types of temporary base materials:

❶ thermo-plastic; and

❷ self-curing.

A thermo-plastic material is softened by heating. It can then be moulded to the desired shape and allowed to cool and maintain this new form. Shellac base-plates are a thermoplastic material. They are supplied as thin sheets in two shapes, one for upper the other for lower base-plates.

The self-curing materials are generally a type of acrylic resin and are used by mixing together a powder and liquid to form a dough which is then moulded into the desired shape before setting. The bases may then be trimmed with burs and stones, and polished.

Summary

The materials discussed in this chapter do not represent the full range of dental materials. You should refer to the chapters on specialist dentistry in Section 6 for information about materials specific to those specialities.

chapter twenty-four
restorations

Introduction

The following series of steps is common to restorative procedures.

- Preparation and setting up — all instruments, materials, equipment, records and radiographs are prepared. The dentist decides on the appropriate material or materials for the restoration. The appropriate method for keeping the field dry is selected. If an anaesthetic is required, it is administered. The dentist decides on the appropriate material or materials for the restoration.
- The appropriate method for keeping the field dry is selected. If dental dam is utilised, it is put in place.
- The cavity is prepared.
- The cavity is lined if required.
- If a matrix band is required, it is placed.
- The restoration material is inserted.
- The restoration is shaped, carved or burnished as required.
- Occlusion is checked.
- Post-procedure instruction is given to the patient.
- If required, the filling is polished no less than 25 hours later.

Preparation and setting up have been discussed in other chapters. The remaining steps in the procedure are discussed in this chapter. Each restorative procedure requires different materials, instruments and accessories. In order to set up trays for these procedures, you will need to know which particular burs, stones, instruments, and so forth are likely to be needed for each procedure. Additionally, all dentists have their own preferences so each set-up will need to meet those preferences.

Keeping the field dry

This is one of your most important roles during any procedure. It involves keeping the mouth clean of debris, blood, saliva and excess water from the triplex syringe. Information about keeping the field dry can be found in Chapter 17.

Cavity preparation

The aim of cavity preparation is to remove decay but preserve as much as possible of the healthy tooth while doing so.

The cavity will be prepared in a way that is appropriate to the restorative material to be used. For example, an amalgam cavity may require some undercuts or notches that will help the restoration stay in place. A composite or resin filling will require acid etching before the restorative material is inserted.

The cavity may also be lined in order to protect the pulp and help to retain the restoration. Lining materials were discussed in the previous chapter.

Matrix retainers and bands

A matrix is used to provide a wall against which a filling material can be packed, to allow restoration of the original shape and contour of the lost tooth structure with the filling material. If matrix bands are used more than once, they must be checked and discarded when there are signs of wear.

Matrix retainers

Matrix retainers have a fine screw thread that has to withstand considerable pressure when applied to the tooth. Many are made from stainless steel. If they are not stainless steel, they should be dried before autoclaving to prevent rust or deterioration. Posterior and anterior types of matrix retainers include automatrix system, 'Siqveland' and 'Tofflemire'.

Matrix bands

On types having fixed bands, the bands should be replaced if any irregularities in shape develop — do not wait for bands to break before replacing them. If they have dents or creases, placing them between teeth is difficult and dangerous.

On types with removable bands, the band *must* be removed before sterilisation and should be straightened before packaging into autoclave pouches. Badly bent or distorted bands should never be put back in the instrument cupboard. They should be replaced. Metal matrix bands are considered to be 'sharps' and must be carefully disposed of into the 'sharps' bin.

Matrix materials include stainless steel band material, copper bands, celluloid bands and celluloid strips. Other types of preformed bands are also available.

How to prepare a matrix band

This is a responsibility that many dentists encourage the chair-side assistant to perform. More information is available in Figures 24.1 and 24.2.

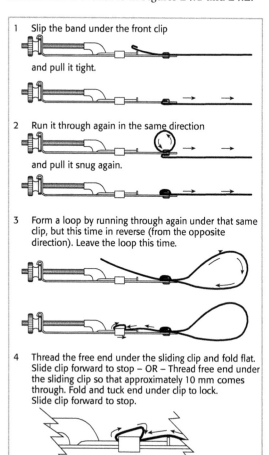

Figure 24.1 Threading Siqveland matrix retainer

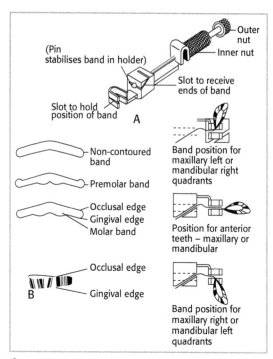

Figure 24.2 Threading Tofflemire matrix retainer

Wedges

Wedges are usually necessary when a matrix band is used and it is your responsibility to have a wide selection of cut wedges. The object of using a wedge is to prevent possible gingival overhangs developing if the filling material is forced out during packing. Wedges keep matrix bands in place and help to maintain a space between adjoining teeth.

Restoration of the tooth

Some dentists use hand-cutting instruments during the preparation of a cavity. See Chapter 19 for information about these instruments.

Amalgam restorations

See Table 24.1 for a description of the amalgam restoration procedure.

Condensation (filling of the cavity)

This term is given to the process of the dentist packing the amalgam into the prepared cavity. This process reduces the mercury content of the restoration and pushes the individual grains as close as possible to each other, leaving a minimum of matrix material.

Steps in the procedure	Equipment, instruments and materials required
1. Preparation and setting up for a composite filling. This is done by the DA.	Patient's records, relevant radiographs, gloves, masks and goggles for operator and assistant; anaesthetic syringe and required cartridge and needle, topical anaesthetic (if used); all required burs, triplex syringes, suction tips, saliva ejector (if used), composite/resin base instrument tray, matrix bands and wedges; cavity lining material, triturator (capsule mixer); articulating paper and holder, extra tweezers for retrieval of objects, tissues, cotton pellets and cotton rolls.
2. Cavity preparation. DA assists with lip and tongue retraction and aspirating. Adjusts operating light if required.	High speed and contra-angle handpieces, the dentist's preferred burs (diamond, tungsten carbide, steel), hand-cutting instruments if used.
3. Lining the cavity. DA mixes lining, loads it onto applicator and passes it to dentist.	The dentist's choice of lining material. Mixing pad and spatula for the assistant, a material applicator.
4. Placement of matrix band and wedge (if required) to form a wall replacing any lost tooth structure, against which the filling can be placed. Wedges placed to keep the matrix band patent (in position) and prevent overhangs.	The appropriate metal matrix band and retainer (e.g. Tofflemire or Siqveland) correctly threaded for the cavity being worked on. Wedges and cotton rolls. Saliva ejector if used.
5. Packing and condensing the amalgam into the cavity. The DA prepares amalgam, places into amalgamator and mixes for the required time, places into amalgam carrier (gun) and hands to dentist, alternating with amalgam packer/plugger.	Amalgamator (triturator) amalgam of choice, squeeze cloth, dental dam or rubber well and amalgam carrier. Dentist's choice of packer/plugger/condenser.
6. Carving and shaping the overfilled restoration to remove excess mercury and to reproduce as closely as possible the shape of the tooth. The DA retracts and aspirates.	Dentist's choice of carver (e.g. half Hollenbach, Walls discoid/cleoid, Wards carvers, or ball burnisher).
7. The occlusion is checked and adjusted as necessary. DA passes articulating paper.	Articulating paper and holder. Dentist's choice of carver.
8. Post-procedure instruction given to patient by dentist or DA regarding soft meals and care for at least eight hours.	Written instructions may be available.
9. Filling may be polished no less than 25 hours later.	Contra-angle handpiece and polishing burs or dentist's choice of handpiece and bur.

Table 24.1 Amalgam restorations

Multiple mixes should be used for large restorations so that setting of the amalgam has not progressed too far before the last portion of amalgam has been condensed. Successive mixes should be commenced early enough so that the condensation process is continuous.

Have various condensers available. The plugger used for condensation must consolidate the amalgam and not pass through it. This is particularly important with spherical alloys. A variety of condensers may be required.

The dentist will condense the amalgam with the greatest comfortable force. It is because of this condensation force that matrix bands must be used when proximal cavities are being restored.

The matrix band makes up the missing side of the cavity and must be well fitting and securely held by a wooden wedge at the gingival margin. This prevents amalgam from being forced out under the matrix band. If this occurs, an overhanging margin forms which can cause irritation to the gum.

As much mercury as possible is removed from the restoration during packing. The quality of the amalgam increases with a decrease in the amount of residual mercury. After packing each layer, the largest practicable plugger is used to bring the excess mercury to the surface. The dentist removes most of this mercury before adding the next increment of amalgam.

The dentist will over-fill restorations using perhaps twice as much material as necessary to just fill the cavity. The excess is then trimmed back to remove the mercury-rich layer from the top of the filling.

Amalgam restoration instruments

Amalgam gun

The amalgam gun (Figure 24.3) is used to carry the mixed amalgam into the prepared cavity. It is made of plastic or stainless steel. Each gun should be dismantled after every use and checked for fragments of set amalgam or excess mercury. Care should be taken when handling and disposing of excess mercury.

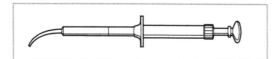

Figure 24.3 Amalgam gun

Amalgam plugger or condenser

The plugger (Figure 24.4) is used to pack or condense amalgam into the prepared cavity. The working end is referred to as the nib. Different types are available and are selected according to the size and shape of the cavity.

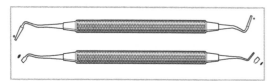

Figure 24.4 Amalgam plugger or condenser

Carver

Carvers are used to reproduce tooth anatomy in amalgam, wax, etc. All carvers have blades with sharp edges. A variety of carvers are used with amalgam restorations. See the example in (Figure 24.5).

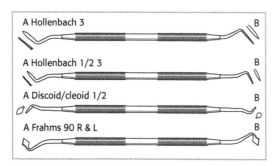

Figure 24.5 Amalgam carvers

Burnishers

These are designed to smooth and burnish amalgam and other restorative materials. All tips or blades are rounded (Figure 24.6).

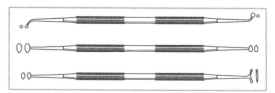

Figure 24.6 Amalgam burnisher

An amalgam tray set-up is shown in Figure 24.7.

Complaints about amalgams

Some time after a filling has been inserted, a patient might complain that a recently placed filling is painful. The first thing to do is determine what the patient means by painful. Is the tooth tender to bite on? If so, the new filling is possibly too high, and the patient should be brought back immediately to have this relieved, for a high filling is very uncomfortable.

Another complaint is that food collects behind a new filling. In this case the filling may possibly need replacement as the contact point may not be tight enough or has perhaps broken. An early, but not necessarily immediate, appointment is necessary.

The patient may experience electric shocks soon after the insertion of the amalgam. This is due to the new filling forming a part of an electric cell. As the filling completely sets, the 'electrical activity' normally ceases. The patient should be reassured, and told that this occasionally happens but only lasts for a short period.

When severe pain is experienced, this could be due to disturbance to the pulp of the tooth. These patients should be referred to the dentist for a decision on what is to be done. The patient should be given an immediate appointment.

Composite restorations

See Table 24.2 for a summary of the techniques involved in composite restoration placement.

Instruments and accessories

Many of the instruments used for amalgam restorations are also used when placing a composite resin restoration, including:

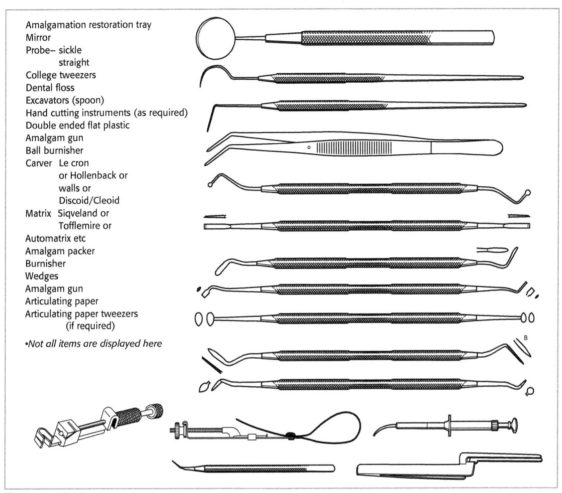

Amalgamation restoration tray
Mirror
Probe– sickle
           straight
College tweezers
Dental floss
Excavators (spoon)
Hand cutting instruments (as required)
Double ended flat plastic
Amalgam gun
Ball burnisher
Carver Le cron
           or Hollenback or
           walls or
           Discoid/Cleoid
Matrix Siqveland or
           Tofflemire or
Automatrix etc
Amalgam packer
Burnisher
Wedges
Amalgam gun
Articulating paper
Articulating paper tweezers
           (if required)

•*Not all items are displayed here*

Figure 24.7 Amalgam restoration tray set-up

- spoon excavator;
- lining applicator;
- flat plastic;
- wedge; and
- scaler.

In addition, there are instruments used specifically with the placement of composite resin restorations. These are generally made of teflon-coated plastic.

Composite placement instruments

Composite placement instruments are made of teflon, plastic or agate (Figure 24.8). This stops the resin from sticking to the instrument and prevents the resin becoming discoloured by contact with the metal of other instruments.

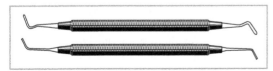

Figure 24.8 Composite placement instruments

Flat plastic instrument

Flat plastic instruments are used for the placement of thicker mixed materials, such as bases and composite resin, into the prepared cavity. Those designed for use with composite resin and GIC may be teflon-coated, nylon, or plastic. The flat plastic has a paddle blade (see Figure 24.9).

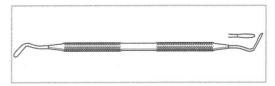

Figure 24.9 Flat plastic instrument

Celluloid matrix strip

This is used with composite resin restorations. A clear mylar strip, available in a variety of lengths, widths and contours, supports the restoration during the placement and curing. Because it is made of celluloid, it permits light transmission.

Steps in the procedure	Equipment, instruments and materials required
1. Preparation and setting up for a composite filling. This is done by the DA.	Patient's records, relevant radiographs, gloves, masks and goggles for operator and assistant; anaesthetic syringe and required cartridge and needle, topical anaesthetic (if used); all required burs, triplex syringes, suction tips, saliva ejector (if used), composite/resin base instrument tray, matrix bands and wedges; cavity lining material, triturator (capsule mixer); articulating paper and holder, extra tweezers for retrieval of objects, tissues, cotton pellets and cotton rolls.
2. Cavity preparation. DA assists with lip and tongue retraction and aspirating. Adjusts operating light if required.	High speed and contra-angle handpieces, the dentist's preferred burs (diamond, tungsten carbide, steel), hand-cutting instruments if used.
3. Lining the cavity. DA mixes lining, loads it onto applicator and passes it to dentist.	The dentist's choice of lining material. Mixing pad and spatula for the assistant, a material applicator.
4. Apply acid etchant and rinse with copious amounts of water.	Acid etchant and disposable brush.
5. Apply matrix and wedge.	Dentist's choice of matrix and wedge.
6. Apply bond and primer.	Dentist's choice of bond and primer, disposable brushes.
7. Apply composite or resin base. DA may be required to hold the curing light.	Dentist's choice of resin base. Composite placement instrument and curing light.
8. The occlusion is checked and adjusted as necessary. DA passes articulating paper.	Articulating paper and holder. Dentist's choice of handpiece and bur.
9. Polish restoration.	Contra-angle handpiece and polishing burs/discs or dentist's choice of handpiece and bur.
10. Post-procedure instruction given to patient by dentist or DA regarding avoiding heavily coloured foods (e.g. beetroot) for 25 hours.	Written instructions may be available.

Table 24. 2 Composite restorations

Spatulas

A range of spatulas is available to mix dental materials. A small stainless steel spatula is used to mix lining and base materials. Plastic, agate or teflon spatulas may be used to mix or transfer composite resin and GIC material.

Plastic instruments

These must be cleaned of all traces of cement and so forth before sterilising. Care must be taken to avoid scratching these instruments.

Dycal (or lining) applicator

These are used to place thin lining materials that will flow onto the prepared cavity floor. They are characterised by a small ball-shaped end on the tip. An example is shown in (Figure 24.10).

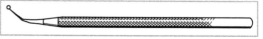

Figure 24.10 Dycal applicator

Moisture contamination

Composite restoration materials must be protected from moisture contamination until after hardening.

Acid etching

Many dentists use acid etching before placing resin restorations. This ensures a clean surface (via removal of the smear layer) to improve the bonding of the restoration material with the dentine. The smear layer is the very thin layer of debris and fluid that remains on the dentine after preparation of the cavity for the restoration. This layer closes off the ends of the dental tubules where they have been damaged by the cavity preparation.

Bonding

The bonding resin, when provided, is similar to the paste/paste restorative resin system but the pastes are less viscous and do not contain filler particles. The mixed resin is applied to the etched surface and bonds by forming tags which penetrate into the irregular enamel surface.

The bond can be affected by contamination of the surface by saliva, fluoride, oil or other organic material, and the etched surfaced readily absorbs or combines with these substances.

Contact points

Unlike amalgam, which must be packed to expand the matrix band and produce adequate contact points, placement of resin in some cavities requires special techniques and matrices. For Class II and Class IV cavities, specially designed metal matrices, which can be contoured, are very useful but adequate wedging is extremely important. The problem is less critical in Class III cavities. In all cases, burnishing of the matrix around all margins after placement of the restoration will ensure minimal

thickness of flash with consequent minimal finishing being required.

Finishing

Fine diamond burs can be used to remove gross excess and either fine plastic discs or wheels lubricated with silicone grease or special finishing discs can be used to produce the final smoothness.

Micro-filled resins are capable of taking a much smoother finish than those with coarser particle sizes. For this reason they are sometimes referred to as 'smooth surfaced resins'.

A sample composite restoration tray set-up is shown in Figure 24.11.

Summary

This chapter covers the basic restorative procedures carried out in general dental practice. To be able to assist efficiently and effectively it is essential that you become familiar with the instrumentation required so that you can anticipate the dentist's needs at each step of a procedure.

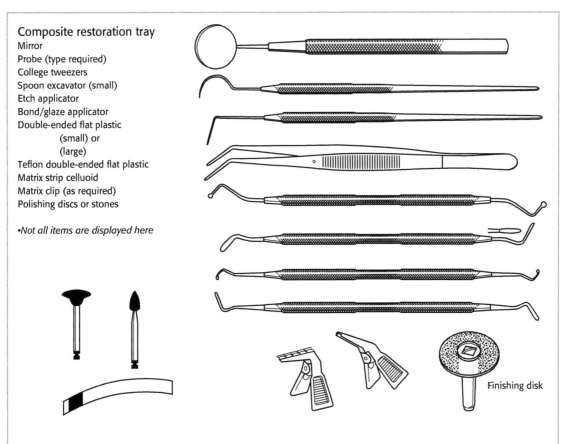

Composite restoration tray
Mirror
Probe (type required)
College tweezers
Spoon excavator (small)
Etch applicator
Bond/glaze applicator
Double-ended flat plastic
 (small) or
 (large)
Teflon double-ended flat plastic
Matrix strip celluoid
Matrix clip (as required)
Polishing discs or stones

•Not all items are displayed here

Finishing disk

Figure 24.11 Composite restoration tray

chapter twenty-five
fixed prosthodontics.

Introduction

Prosthodontics is the area of dentistry that specialises in restoring or replacing missing tooth structure. It aims to restore the physiologic health, function, form and appearance of the dentition. This type of restoration is required if there is tooth loss or tooth abnormality, such as after trauma or excessive tooth wear.

The speciality of prosthodontics includes:

■ removable prosthodontics;

■ fixed prosthodontics; and

■ implant prosthodontics.

Removable prosthodontics is the provision of dentures that patients can remove themselves. They are discussed in Chapter 30.

Fixed prosthodontics is the provision of a **prosthesis** that cannot be removed by the patient. These include inlays, onlays, veneers, crowns and bridges.

Implant prosthodontics is the provision of prostheses that are supported by implants instead of teeth. Implants may support individual crowns, bridges or dentures. There is a separate chapter on implants (Chapter 26).

This chapter will focus on *fixed* prosthodontics. Fixed prosthodontics includes:

■ crowns (cemented or bonded);

■ preliminary restorations for crowns (post and cores, direct or indirect);

■ bridges (cemented or bonded);

■ posterior inlay/onlays (cemented or bonded); and

■ anterior veneers (bonded).

These restorations are usually constructed indirectly i.e. outside the mouth. Teeth are prepared and the preparations recorded so that the restorations can be accurately made in the laboratory. They are then cemented or bonded onto the prepared teeth.

See Figure 25.1 for an example of a crown and bridge tray set-up.

Crowns

A crown is like a thimble, covering and supporting a single tooth. Tooth structure is removed circumferentially, leaving a peg-shaped crown preparation. An impression of the prepared tooth is recorded and then models and dies are prepared. The crown is made and then cemented or bonded into place.

Crowns may be used on teeth to:

■ restore the form of a badly broken down tooth;

■ improve the appearance of an unsightly tooth;

■ support a weak tooth; or

■ act as a retainer for bridgework.

Types of crowns

Porcelain jacket crowns

Traditional porcelain jacket crowns are made by mixing porcelain powders of various colours with water to form a paste. This mixture is carefully manipulated for colour and shape so that the finished crown will match the patient's other teeth. After the powders are shaped, the crown is dried, and placed in a furnace to fuse or bake the porcelain. After the porcelain crown is fired and finished it is tried in the mouth and, if it is satisfactory, it is cemented to the patient's tooth. The porcelain jacket crown is highly aesthetic but unfortunately prone to fracture. It has largely been superseded by porcelain fused to metal and all-ceramic crowns.

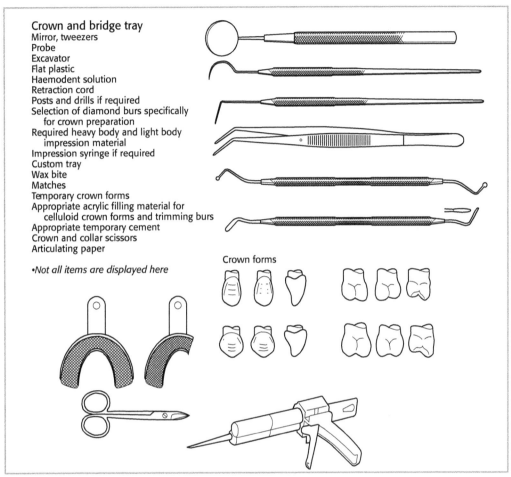

Crown and bridge tray
Mirror, tweezers
Probe
Excavator
Flat plastic
Haemodent solution
Retraction cord
Posts and drills if required
Selection of diamond burs specifically
    for crown preparation
Required heavy body and light body
    impression material
Impression syringe if required
Custom tray
Wax bite
Matches
Temporary crown forms
Appropriate acrylic filling material for
    celluloid crown forms and trimming burs
Appropriate temporary cement
Crown and collar scissors
Articulating paper

•*Not all items are displayed here*

Crown forms

Figure 25.1 Crown and bridge tray set-up

Porcelain fused to metal crowns

Porcelain fused to metal is the most common type of crown as it is both strong and aesthetic. A thin thimble of metal alloy is first cast and fitted to the die. The metal commonly used is gold alloy. Porcelain is then fused permanently over the metal casting to hide the visible metal and match the appearance of the patient's other teeth. The fused porcelain and metal casting then forms a single crown.

All-ceramic crowns

All-ceramic crowns are the most aesthetic crowns currently available. There are a number of different types. Depending upon the type, they may be cemented or bonded to the tooth. They are not as strong as the traditional porcelain fused to metal crowns and are generally used on anterior teeth.

All-ceramic crowns with a strong thimble of high-strength alumina or equivalent are strong and can be cemented or bonded to the tooth.

Some all-ceramic crowns do not have a strong internal thimble. These crowns are highly aesthetic but they require bonding to tooth structure for support.

Gold crown

The gold crown is made entirely from a gold alloy, and therefore its use is usually confined to posterior teeth, where it is less visible. It is a strong restoration that is especially useful if the patient has a heavy bite or if there is insufficient space for porcelain and gold alloy.

Acrylic resin crown

Acrylic resin crowns are easier and cheaper to make than porcelain and gold and are generally used as temporary crowns whilst the permanent crowns are made. Acrylic is not as aesthetic or strong as porcelain and tends to wear and stain. They can be made directly in the mouth or indirectly on a model.

Gold and acrylic crown

The gold and acrylic crown is seldom used in conventional crown and bridgework today. Greater strength and aesthetics can be gained with porcelain fused to metal. However, it is still utilised in implant dentistry.

Preliminary restoration before crowns

Most teeth requiring crowns are broken down. In order to prepare an ideal crown preparation it is necessary to rebuild the original tooth form. In a vital tooth this is called a core restoration and may be constructed of amalgam, composite resin or glass ionomer.

In a non-vital tooth, a lot of tooth structure has been lost. In order to retain the core restoration, part of the root canal space and pulp chamber is used for retention. This is called a post and core restoration. It may be made directly of either amalgam or composite resin and prefabricated post or it may be made indirectly and completely cast from gold.

In a direct post and core restoration a prefabricated post is selected and cemented into the canal space. Amalgam or composite resin is then packed around the tooth to restore it to normal form. The tooth is now ready for crown preparation.

An indirect post and core is made from an acrylic pattern or impression of the tooth. It is cast from gold at a laboratory. The cast gold post and core is later fitted and cemented. The tooth is now ready for crown preparation. A crown is then constructed and cemented on top of the core restoration.

Bridges

It is important to understand that the loss of teeth from the mouth can cause changes that create serious dental problems. Some of the problems created by tooth loss include:

- disruption to aesthetics and interference with speech;
- disruption of chewing efficiency; and
- remaining teeth becoming unstable. The teeth on either side of the spaces can 'tip' into the space. Teeth opposing a space can over erupt into the space. Tipped and over-erupted teeth can interfere with occlusion and function. Tipped teeth can create areas that are difficult to clean and render the region more prone to periodontal disease and decay.

For these reasons we generally try to restore spaces to protect individual teeth and maintain the stability of the remaining dentition.

Missing teeth can be replaced in three ways — with a denture, a bridge or implants. A denture is removable. The patient can take it out. A bridge or implant-supported crown is fixed and not removable.

A dental bridge is very similar to a bridge over a stream. It consists of a span supported at both ends (Figure 25.2). Teeth are required at both sides of a space for a bridge to be possible. Bridges may be used to restore small spaces caused by the loss of one or two teeth.

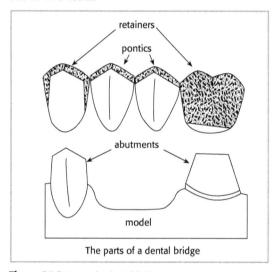

Figure 25.2 Parts of a dental bridge

There are two types of bridges. Conventional bridgework is usually made out of porcelain and gold alloy and is cemented on to prepared abutment teeth. Resin-bonded bridges are simpler in form. They may be made out of non-precious or gold alloy and porcelain. They are bonded to the abutment teeth.

The advantages of a fixed bridge are:

- The fixed bridge feels like the patient's own teeth. They can chew or laugh without fear of the appliance moving or dropping.
- The patients clean the bridge as if it were their own teeth.
- The fixed bridge does not interfere with speech, or encroach upon tongue space.
- The fixed bridge is aesthetic.

The disadvantages of a fixed bridge are:

- Adjacent teeth are committed to treatment — if these teeth would benefit from crown restoration then this is reasonable. If these teeth are sound teeth then it is biologically expensive to commit these teeth to bridgework.

- The patient must clean the area very carefully and have regular dental reviews. Teeth beneath bridges can still decay and develop periodontal disease resulting in failure of the bridge.

- Several lengthy appointments may be necessary. These must be coordinated to fit in with the complex laboratory procedures that are required.

- The fixed bridge is difficult to make, and therefore costly.

Pre-requisites for bridgework

Not all spaces caused by the loss of teeth can be restored by means of fixed bridgework. Some conditions preclude the possibility of bridgework, including:

- poor oral hygiene with active periodontal disease or decay processes;

- abutment teeth with poor prognosis such as traumatic history or excessive weakness from decay or previous fracture;

- no distal abutment tooth;

- a large number of missing teeth to be replaced; or

- the teeth adjacent to the space may be so tipped that they cannot be prepared to receive abutments parallel to one another without excessive cutting of tooth surfaces.

Where considerable spaces exist on both sides of the dental arch, a partial denture or implants may be more suitable.

Shade selection

For crowns and bridges (except gold crowns), the colours present in the patient's teeth must be closely matched in the restoration. A special shade guide is used to register and record the colour desired for the restorations. It is your job to ensure that this is recorded on the patient's file as it could be very useful, even years later.

A drawing of the outline of a tooth is often used additionally by the dentist to record areas of different colours or unusual markings on a tooth or teeth.

Shade selection is affected by the colour of the light falling on the teeth. Diffused daylight should be used. Coloured walls or curtains should be avoided. The colour of natural daylight varies with the time of day and with cloudy conditions, and so forth. Ideally, shade selection is easier and more accurate during the middle part of a clear day.

Anterior veneers and posterior inlays/onlays

Anterior veneers

A veneer is the restoration of a single tooth to correct irregularities in form and colour. It is more conservative of tooth structure than a crown but can only be used in specific situations where there is a lot of enamel tooth structure remaining and only minor shade correction required.

A veneer is like a false fingernail that is bonded to the front surface of a tooth. A thin layer of tooth enamel is removed to create space to place the veneer. A model is created from an impression of the prepared tooth and the veneer is made. Indirectly made veneers are usually porcelain. The veneer is then fitted and bonded into place with composite resin.

The veneer is fragile and only develops strength once it is bonded to tooth enamel. It must be handled very carefully or it will fracture.

Posterior inlays/onlays

Inlays

Inlays fit into the crown of the tooth. These are essentially the same as amalgam restorations but with modifications. The amalgam cavity has undercuts to retain the amalgam, but inlay cavities have walls flaring away from each other to allow withdrawal and insertion of the finished inlay.

Onlays

Onlays fit onto or around the crown of the tooth. They are used principally to protect remaining tooth structure and gain their retention from pinholes, grooves, slots or bonding.

Inlays and onlays are used when there has been extensive loss of tooth structure but a crown is not required. Cusps that are weakened can be reduced and protected with an onlay if they are subjected to heavy occlusal forces.

These restorations are usually made indirectly to enable control of restoration contour. Inlays and onlays can be used to restore ideal form where teeth are tipped or out of alignment.

Inlays are occasionally used as the supporting ends or retainers of a bridge. However, it is usually necessary to provide full occlusal coverage such as a crown-in-bridge retainer construction.

Types of inlays/onlays

Inlays/onlays can be:

- gold;
- non-precious metal alloy;
- ceramic or porcelain; or
- composite resin.

These restorations are all made indirectly. The tooth is prepared and an impression is recorded. A die is made from this impression and the restoration fabricated in the laboratory.

Gold

Gold inlays were once made from wax patterns carved directly in the mouth. It is now more common to take an impression of the tooth and create the wax pattern in the laboratory. The dentist takes an impression of the prepared and adjacent teeth. From this, a model or die of the teeth is made. The wax patterns can then be carved on the die and the restoration, when cast, can be fitted to the die and partly polished. When the patient comes in for the next appointment, the restorations are ready to cement into the cavities.

Non-precious alloys

These are used for bonded bridgework retainers.

Ceramic, porcelain and composite resin inlays

These are tooth coloured. Restorations are produced indirectly on models or may be computer milled out of ceramic blocks. Cavity preparations differ in that they are more rounded and tapered in form. These restorations are bonded in place with composite resin, not cemented.

Chair-side procedures for crown and bridge work

Infection control

It is important that best practice in infection control is maintained at all time, including when taking impressions and the transfer of all materials between the surgery and laboratory and vice versa.

The preparation of teeth for gold inlays, crowns or bridges requires you to be at the chair-side for most, if not all, of the time. Tray set-ups and their positions are important. Water-cooling sprays are always used, with air and water used alternately by the assistant to clear and cool the operating field. You will be responsible for water evacuation. Four-handed dentistry is essential.

Many procedures are precise and require excellent control of the field. The dental dam is essential for all bonded restorations such as porcelain veneers, inlays, onlays and bonded bridgework. It will also be utilised when preparing teeth or in procedures related to recording and cementing post and core restorations.

Control of gingival tissues

Margins of all restorations should be placed as far away from the gingival tissues as possible to ensure the long-term health of the periodontal tissues. Sometimes it is necessary to place the margins of crowns or inlays at or slightly below the crest of the free gingival margin. This may be because of:

- the appearance of an anterior crown where it is unsightly to show the margin;
- short clinical crown which has minimal retention; or
- a pre-existing restoration or caries that extends sub-gingivally.

In order to obtain a clear impression of the gingival margin of a crown or inlay preparation, the tissue must be retracted away from the tooth. Impression material can then be placed and will set without interference from the adjacent tissues. It is important that the gingival tissue is free from disease such as gingivitis before restorative procedures are commenced. Gingivitis can lead to excessive gingival bleeding, which can obscure the preparation, and hinder impression taking.

Retraction is usually accomplished by the use of retraction cord. The cord is available in a number of thicknesses. It is placed in the gingival crevice to displace the soft tissues away from the preparation.

Cord may be plain or impregnated with medicament to control bleeding. Various medicaments may be used including ferric sulphate and aluminium chloride. Bleeding must be controlled before the impression of the preparations is taken.

Electrosurgery is occasionally used as an adjunct to tissue retraction and haemorrhage control.

electrosurgery: surgery is performed with a special electric tip that can cut away excess tissue and control excessive bleeding.

Making wax patterns

Taking impressions

Taking impressions involves:

- setting up a special tray (if required);
- cavity preparation;
- gingival retraction;
- making a study model of opposing teeth or record of occlusion;
- bite registration;
- impression of the prepared teeth and other teeth of the jaw; and
- temporary restoration of the prepared tooth or teeth.

Assuming that the light-bodied and heavy-bodied materials are to be used, you must have the following items ready:

- special acrylic impression tray(s) and special adhesive;
- automix syringes of light body material;
- automix syringes of heavy body material;
- a special syringe for placing the light-bodied material around the tooth;
- gauze squares or tissues; and
- a clock or stopwatch for timing the mix.

Die materials

The dies or models on which the technician makes the wax patterns and restorations are made of one of either:

- die stone;
- electroplated copper; or
- epoxy resin.

These models are made in the laboratory and the technician occludes the model with the opposite jaw model by using a registration (bite) recorded by the dentist. This registration is usually made by placing soft wax, silicone or a quick-setting paste between upper and lower teeth and instructing the patient to close together. After the material has hardened, it is carefully removed and then later used by the technician.

Temporary inlays, crowns and bridges

After teeth have been cut and prepared to receive inlays, crowns or bridges, a temporary restoration is made for the patient. This is cemented to the teeth with a temporary cement and remains in place while the permanent restorations are being made in the laboratory.

Temporary restorations for small inlay cavities may be of gutta-percha, but for larger cavities (crowns, etc.) temporary restorations may be made of any of the following materials.

Anterior temporary restorations may be made from:

- crown forms, lined with acrylic resin; or
- acrylic or composite resin.

Posterior temporary restorations may be made from:

- crown forms, with acrylic resin inside;
- stainless steel; or
- acrylic resin, as for anterior teeth.

Temporary crowns are available to the dentist in a wide variety of tooth shapes, widths and lengths. They are essentially a thin hollow shell of material, shaped during manufacture to resemble a tooth crown. The dentist selects the particular tooth shape that best matches the patient's mouth and trims and shapes it at the chair-side to fit accurately to the tooth just prepared for a crown. This is then cemented to the tooth with a quick-setting temporary cement.

The temporary restoration performs the following functions:

- It protects the prepared tooth surfaces and the pulp from painful stimuli (hot or cold, sweet or sour).
- It maintains the tooth in its correct position in the mouth with respect to the adjacent and opposing teeth.
- It protects the fine margins of the prepared tooth from chipping or fracture during chewing.
- It protects the gum margin from becoming inflamed by food impaction, and preserves its correct contour.
- It temporarily restores the appearance of the teeth.

You should keep a list of times required for the various procedures, such as tooth preparation, impression-taking and cementation. In addition, you should have a list of the times that the laboratory technicians require to complete their work. This may vary according to individual dentist's requirements but will enable you to better arrange appointment schedules with patients.

Cementation

Cements used in the placement of crowns and bridges are discussed in Chapter 23. See the cementation tray set-up in Figure 25.3.

Patient instructions for care of crowns and bridges

After inlays, crowns or bridges have been inserted, the patient should be instructed to refrain from chewing at all, until the cement has hardened thoroughly. There are many types of cements and the dentist will instruct the patient depending upon the type of cement used. The forces exerted by chewing on the restoration before the cement has fully set may dislodge the restoration or may weaken the cement seal, leading to problems at a later date.

In the case of porcelain jacket crowns, the patient should be informed that they will withstand all normal chewing pressures but that sudden impact forces should be avoided. High impact forces can be caused by biting off threads, opening hairpins, cracking nuts, tapping the teeth with pencils, etc.

Inlays, crowns and bridges should receive thorough cleansing by the patient to prevent accumulation of plaque around them as it may lead to decay or gingival inflammation. The patient should be shown the use of dental floss, floss threaders or superfloss in cleaning around and under the pontics of a bridge.

Patients with complex dentistry, such as crowns, bridges and so forth, should be educated in the need for regular professional examination by the dentist as well as meticulous daily homecare. The dentist will specify the frequency of these.

Summary

By replacing missing teeth, the fixed prosthesis can prevent adjacent teeth from drifting, tipping or rotating into the space left by the missing tooth, and the consequent occlusal problems that can occur. It is an aesthetically satisfactory and functional method of replacing missing teeth.

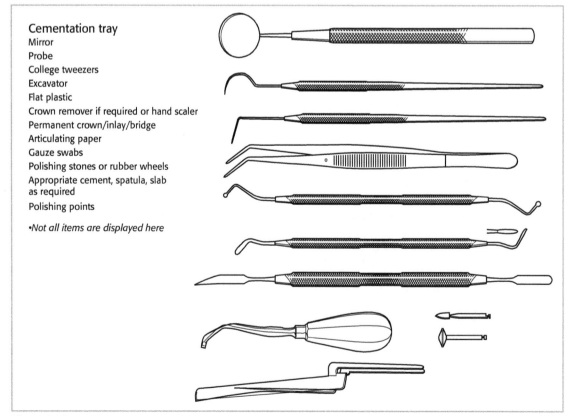

Cementation tray
Mirror
Probe
College tweezers
Excavator
Flat plastic
Crown remover if required or hand scaler
Permanent crown/inlay/bridge
Articulating paper
Gauze swabs
Polishing stones or rubber wheels
Appropriate cement, spatula, slab as required
Polishing points

•Not all items are displayed here

Figure 25.3 Cementation tray set-up

chapter twenty-six
implants

Introduction

Dental implantology is a speciality of dentistry in which an inert material (one that does not react with body tissue) is surgically placed into the jawbone so that it becomes accepted by the body. The implant becomes attached to the jawbone in such a way that the implant will be able to support teeth and satisfy both the requirements of function and aesthetics. That is, implants are the roots for natural looking replacements for a tooth (or teeth) that is anchored in bone.

The acceptance of the implant by the jawbone is a term called osseointegration. That is when the bone around the implant grows up to the implant and the bone cells actually grow into the small spaces and irregularities of the implant or fixture so that there is no space or membrane between the implant and the bone.

Implants today are made of titanium, either pure or an alloy. Many titanium implants are now coated in different ways to increase their surface area and bio-compatibility to bone cells. The coatings can be titanium plasma sprayed (TPS), hydroxyl apatite (HA) or TiUnite.

Successful implants can last over 20 years but their success depends on several factors. These include:

- the design and coating of the implant material;
- the bone quantity and quality of the patient;
- careful surgical technique; and
- the correct loading of the superstructures (i.e. crowns, bridges or dentures) onto the implant or implants.

Implants are used to replace missing teeth. They may be used to replace a single tooth or multiple teeth and may also be used to secure dentures which are either uncomfortable or unstable. Teeth may also be replaced by crown and bridge procedures; however, to do this entails cutting adjoining teeth to secure the missing tooth. Many patients prefer not to have this done and therefore implants are the closest thing to reproducing the patient's own natural teeth.

Implants are placed by general practitioners, prosthodontists, periodontists and oral surgeons.

Implant procedure

The implant procedure usually involves a series of appointments. At the first appointment there will be an examination of the patient, an assessment, x-rays taken and study casts made and a treatment plan will be formulated.

At the next appointment, the procedure, costs and possible complications that may occur, are explained to the patient. Patients are asked to sign a consent form before undertaking the surgical appointment.

The surgical appointment involves preparing the patient and the surgery to an almost theatre-like, sterile environment. The surgical placement of one or multiple implants in the jawbone is carried out carefully, usually under local anaesthetic. When the procedure is completed, the soft tissues are sutured and the mucosa completely covers the buried implants. This is followed by a healing period of three to six months to allow for bone maturation around the implants.

The second surgical appointment, some months later, is a less complex procedure, which is simply designed to expose the heads of the implants and connect attachments (healing abutments) that protrude through the soft tissue to allow the mucosa to heal around them. This allows subsequent appointments to be carried out a-traumatically and painlessly for the cosmetic reconstruction. A series of appointments may be necessary to complete the final prosthesis, which should be done very carefully, paying attention to load distribution and correct balanced occlusion. This is important to ensure long-term success.

Immediate tooth replacement

Alternatively, there are many practitioners now advocating immediate loading, especially in the edentulous mandible where three to six implants are placed in the anterior mandible and a temporary or permanent prosthesis is attached to these at the surgical appointment or within 24 hours.

It is now possible and often advisable to consider an implant before extracting a tooth. Once a tooth has been removed, the process of bone resorption begins. Therefore, whenever possible; consideration is now given to placing an implant immediately after extracting a tooth into the socket.

This procedure requires careful attention to certain protocols.

- The socket should be free from infection.
- The tooth must be removed very carefully (periotomes) so that there is no damage to the supporting bone.
- The implant should be placed past the position where the apex of the tooth was, into firm bone.
- The implant should ideally fill or obliterate the socket, therefore tapered implants are best suited for this procedure.
- Any gaps between implant and bone should ideally be filled with a bone-grafting material.
- Socket irrigation with saline and antibiotics prior to placement is advantageous.
- The implant should be very firm in the socket for it to be successful.

Immediate tooth replacement is an excellent way to replace a missing tooth and has many advantages when done correctly. The advantages include maintaining the gingival papilla and bone levels. The technique usually results in a more aesthetic emergence profile, which is the way the tooth appears to naturally erupt out of the gums into the mouth. Ideally, implant crowns should look like natural teeth. This is not always possible. However, the dentist will strive to achieve the best emergence profile in order to obtain the most aesthetic crown and gingival tissue appearance. See Figures 26.1 and 26.2 for examples.

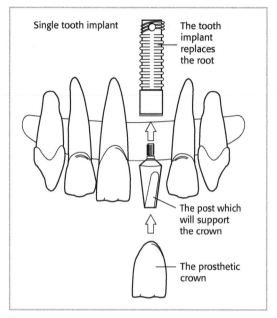

Figure 26.1 Single tooth implant

Preparation of the patient

Pre-operative preparation

- Check the patient's medical history (i.e. rheumatic fever, diabetes, etc.) as special precautions may be necessary.
- Check the patient has had only a light breakfast or lunch.
- Ensure that you have a contact number available if the patient decides they need an escort after the procedure.
- Ensure the patient is comfortable and at ease. Talk to your patient.
- Prior to surgery, any dentures are removed, cleaned and then soaked in a disinfecting solution.

Operating preparation

- The patient is informed before entering the surgery to expect gloves, masks, gowns and sterile drapes.
- All equipment should have been set up before the patient enters the surgery and everything checked for working order (e.g. handpieces).
- The operator gives the local anaesthetic before scrubbing for the operation. Have plenty of anaesthetic on hand and set up, ready to go. Check with the operator ahead of time as to the appropriate anaesthetic to be used.

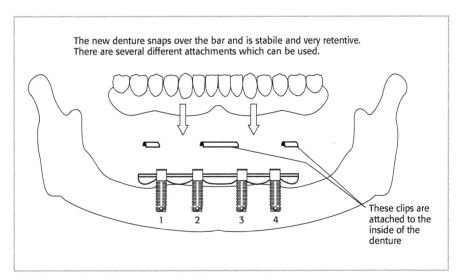

The new denture snaps over the bar and is stabile and very retentive. There are several different attachments which can be used.

1 2 3 4

These clips are attached to the inside of the denture

Figure 26.2 Bar overdenture

- The patient is then prepared (prepped). It is explained to the patient that it would be preferred if they didn't touch their face during and after the prepping procedure.

- The operator and assistants gown, scrub and glove. The patient is then draped while explaining what is being done. Ask the patient to keep their arms under the drapes, signalling if there are any problems.

- Suction and tubing may be connected to the drape on the patient's chest with a towel clip.

Operating procedures

Stage one

- An incision is made at the crest of the alveolus and may extend to the sulcus for reflection.

- In the case of an edentulous mandible, where implants are going to be placed near the mental nerve/foramina it is important that the mental nerve is located surgically and implants placed away from it. It is very important that if the operator asks you to retract a flap, you should retract exactly where the operator places it, to avoid any permanent damage to the nerve/patient.

- The bone is then drilled with varying burs and constantly irrigated. This drilling slowly enlarges the hole to the correct and final bur size to match the size of the implant to be used.

- Direction indicators may be used throughout the procedure to help with parallelism and direction. The operator may ask your opinion

on the direction of this indicator. It is important to be honest, so if you are unsure, say so.

- The fixture is then placed into the cavity with either a tension controlled handpiece at 45 rpm or manually with a torque tension wrench. It is most important that nothing touches the implant during the insertion stage as contamination may jeopardise compatibility.

- The operator may then remove the fixture mount to allow room to place the next fixture.

- Cover screws are then placed over the fixture.

- The gingiva is sutured back in place. Normally resorbable (e.g. Vicryl) sutures are used.

- The drapes are then removed (ensuring the overhead light is turned off).

- The patient is allowed to rest a while and then slowly sat up.

- Thorough post-operative instructions are given and post-operative appointments made for approximately two weeks time. This appointment is to check on the healing of the operation site and, if necessary, suture removal. Dentures are returned to the patient after being modified.

- It is most important to remember that titanium and stainless steel are un-like metals and, to prevent contamination of the titanium, should not be mixed. All titanium is handled as little as possible and titanium-tipped forceps should be used where possible.

- If you are unsure of the procedure check with someone who knows because a mistake could lead to a fixture being rejected in the patient's mouth, wasting a lot of money, time and effort and causing considerable distress to the patient.

Stage two

- Pre-operation preparation of the patient is the same as for stage one. The only difference is that handpieces are not usually required.

- The cover screws are located in the patient's mouth with the aid of a sickle probe. The cover screws may be visible as a grey area through the mucosa.

- There are two approaches the operator can use to expose the cover screws. An incision can be made along the alveolar ridge extending from mental foramen to mental foramen. Or separate cross incisions can be made just over the area of the fixture site; that is, if there are to be six fixtures, six incisions are made.

- A small screwdriver is then used to loosen and remove the cover screws placed at stage one.

- Once all cover screws are removed, the area is gently irrigated for better viewing.

- The operator checks around the fixture sites with a sharp instrument, such as a cumine scaler, to ensure if they are free from all tissue debris. To remove the debris that does not readily come away with the cumine scaler, the operator may use a scalpel blade or a small curette and Addison tissue forceps.

- The abutment is screwed in loosely and the operator checks again that no tissue is caught between the fixture and the abutment. An x-ray is usually taken to ensure the abutment is sitting exactly onto the implant before final tightening is carried out.

- If a long incision has been made the flap is closed by suturing.

- The drapes are then removed, ensuring that the overhead lights have been turned off.

- The patient is allowed to rest and then slowly sat up.

- Thorough post-operative instructions are given. Also inform the patient that if the dressing starts to fall off within a couple of days to phone and make an appointment to have a new dressing placed.

- An appointment is then arranged for a pack removal after one week.

If the patient has a denture which needs to be worn for aesthetic reasons, the denture is relieved and a soft lining (e.g. Viscogel) is placed to prevent undue pressure on implants during the healing period.

Decontamination of dirty instruments

- After completion of each case, all stainless steel instruments and stainless steel burs are placed in a large kidney bowl with a proteolytic solution for ten minutes. After ten minutes the instruments are rinsed with water and dried thoroughly. Do not leave instruments soaking any longer than ten minutes otherwise they will corrode.

- Titanium instruments are not immersed into the proteolytic solution but wiped with a disposable towel, dampened with neutral detergent, rinsed and dried.

- Wipe any blood off the handpiece with detergent.

- Line the sink with disposable towels so that small instruments are not lost down the drain. These instruments are extremely expensive, so great care must be taken.

- A clean towel is put on the side of the sink for the clean instruments to drain on.

- A toothbrush is used to scrub all the instruments clean with undiluted detergent placed into the bottom of a mouthwash cup.

- Scrub the instruments under cold running water, starting with the clean titanium instruments first, then the dirty titanium instruments and then going on to the stainless steel ones in the same order. Do not let the titanium and stainless steel get mixed together.

- Dry all instruments with gauze and distribute into beakers and test tubes for ultrasonic cleaning.

- Disconnect handpiece shank from head and spray with oil until it runs through clean. Wipe off excess oil with special methylated spirits and then place autoclavable pieces with all other instruments that need to be wrapped and autoclaved.

Summary

Dental implants are increasingly procedures of choice for replacing tooth loss. This form of treatment requires great precision and strict aseptic techniques, in which the dental assistant has an important role. Your knowledge of the procedure and the assistance required will make the dentist's job much easier, and the end result pleasing for the patient and the dental team alike.

Section 5

Preventive dentistry

A very large proportion of the world's population suffers from some form of dental disease. Since much of this disease is preventable, it is essential that the dental health team provide not only a treatment service but also a preventive program.

A healthy mouth contributes to the general health and quality of life of an individual. It is best obtained by the prevention of disease and the promotion of a healthy lifestyle.

Chapter 27 covers techniques used for the prevention of:

- dental caries;
- periodontal diseases;
- erosion, pathological attrition and abrasion;
- acquired orthodontic problems;
- traumatic injuries to the teeth and jaws; and
- oral malignancies.

It also discusses oral health promotion. Chapter 28 focuses on diet and nutrition.

chapter twenty-seven
preventive dentistry and oral health promotion

Introduction

Preventive dentistry is provided either at a community level (e.g. clean water, fluoridation of community water supplies) or by assessing risk factors in individuals and tailoring a preventive program to their specific needs. Dental examples of individual prevention based on risk assessment are topical fluoridation, use of fissure sealants, wearing of mouthguards and promoting good oral hygiene and dietary practices.

The three levels of prevention

Primary prevention

Primary prevention is the prevention of disease or injury. It is the goal that we try to achieve and, if successful, means that the patient has not suffered any injury whatsoever. Primary prevention is achieved through health education programs, specific preventive measures (e.g. sealants, immunisation, safe sex through use of condoms) or environmental modification (e.g. water fluoridation, clean air, radiation hygiene).

Secondary prevention

Secondary prevention means the early detection and prompt, minimally invasive treatment of disease. In this way, early clinical or preclinical conditions are identified by screening programs such as regular dental check-ups, glaucoma testing or mammography.

Much dental health care is devoted to secondary prevention. This includes check-ups, treatment of reversible gingivitis, remineralisation techniques, restoring early dental caries and the removal of calculus.

Tertiary prevention

Tertiary prevention means the limitation of any disability arising from disease, and rehabilitation of the patient. The object is to restore the person's function as much as possible, and to try to prevent recurrence of the disease or problem. Rehabilitation after a stroke is a common example. Dental examples include extensive periodontal treatment, complex restorative procedures and root canal therapy.

Unless otherwise stated, this chapter deals with the primary prevention of dental diseases, although dental practice obviously involves all three levels of prevention.

Preventive procedures

It is helpful to consider preventive strategies in terms of the *underlying disease process*. This consists of three events that must occur together.

❶ There must be a harmful agent e.g. micro-organisms, harmful chemicals, trauma.

❷ The agent must find a susceptible host, in this case the patient.

❸ The environment must be suitable for the development of disease.

On the following pages, these three factors are used to discuss the prevention of dental caries and periodontal disease.

Dental caries

For the formation of dental caries, the three events of the underlying disease process are as follows:

❶ The agent is the micro-organisms in the bacterial dental plaque.

❷ The host is the dentate patient, and the susceptible tooth surfaces, which may be affected by the caries process.

❸ The environment includes the level of exposure to fluoride, the quantity and quality of the patient's saliva, and dietary factors such as the frequency of exposure to refined carbohydrates, and sucrose in particular.

Prevention of dental caries

From the three events listed above we see that dental caries:

■ is a bacterial disease;
■ is influenced by the level of sucrose consumption;
■ is influenced by the frequency of meals;
■ is modified by fluoride; and
■ is influenced by the quality and quantity of saliva.

Recovery from acid attack is influenced by the thickness of the plaque. The thicker the plaque, the slower the return to normal pH levels.

A comprehensive approach to the *primary prevention* of dental caries includes:

■ Adequate exposure to fluoride over time — fluoridation of community water supplies at one part per million is a cost-effective method that makes no demands on the patient. Regular use of fluoride toothpaste is the next most useful strategy. Use of high concentration fluoride pastes and mouth-rinses, and various forms of topical application are used following individual risk assessment.

■ Dietary modification — the most effective method is to try to reduce the frequency of eating, in order to reduce the number of acid attacks to a level at which the repair processes can cope with any potential decalcification. Patients are counselled to reduce the frequency with which refined carbohydrates, particularly sucrose, are consumed. Advice is given to minimise consumption of cariogenic sweet sticky foods with a long **oral clearance time**. Dairy products have a protective effect against dental caries, and particularly hard cheeses which require vigorous chewing which stimulates saliva flow.

Artificial sweeteners can replace sugar, further modifying the diet to prevent caries.

■ Saliva stimulation, which promotes protective remineralisation — sugarless chewing gum can be recommended, including one that contains casein phosphopeptides. Chewing hard foods encourages the production of stimulated saliva, which has a high mineral content and high capacity to neutralise acids.

■ Effective oral hygiene has a role to play by reducing or removing concentrations of bacterial dental plaque. Although this method is important, it does place greater demands on the patient, and may be difficult to achieve with high-risk groups such as young children, elderly patients or the developmentally disabled. It is also difficult to maintain high levels of oral hygiene in substance abusers, and this problem is compounded by the fact that they often have drug-induced xerostomia. Toothbrushing will not remove plaque from deep pits or fissures or from proximal tooth surfaces.

■ Fissure sealants (particularly those which release fluoride) — used to prevent caries in pits and fissures, particularly in newly erupted teeth.

■ Combined mouth-rinsing programs using both Chlorhexidine gluconate and Stannous fluoride. These are sometimes used for very high-risk patients, or mothers who may infect their infants with cariogenic oral bacteria.

Secondary prevention of dental caries requires early diagnosis and recognition of reversible lesions, which are then treated by remineralisation, in addition to continuing primary preventive methods. Tertiary prevention includes all restorative procedures to limit the progress of individual lesions, protect the dental pulp, restore function and provide an environment in which primary prevention can be successful.

Periodontal disease

For the development of periodontal disease, the three events of the underlying disease process are as follows:

❶ The agent is the toxins produced by the micro-organisms in the subgingival dental plaque.

❷ The host is the periodontal supporting structures of the dentate patient.

❸ The environment includes predisposing or modifying factors such as the presence of calculus or other plaque-retentive factors, medication, smoking, environmental stress and diabetes and other hormonal conditions.

■ **oral clearance time**: the time taken for food to clear the mouth.

Prevention of periodontal disease

Periodontal diseases represent the effects of a host response to constant challenge from micro-organisms in **subgingival plaque**. That is, there is an inflammatory response to these micro-organisms as the host tries to overcome the bacterial challenge. This inflammatory response causes damage; that is, periodontal disease.

Neither the presence or absence of fluoride, or the buffering capacity of the saliva affect periodontal diseases. Except in certain extreme cases, periodontal diseases are not influenced by dietary frequency or quality. As we are currently unable to identify or modify host factors, mechanical plaque control remains the single effective preventive strategy available for the control of periodontal diseases.

Meticulous plaque control is the primary strategy for prevention of periodontal diseases. This requires a toothbrushing technique that will actually clean into the accessible gingival sulci, together with some form of interdental plaque control with floss or suitable interdental brushes or woodsticks. In some cases, antibacterial mouthwashes may be prescribed, usually for a limited period of time.

Environmental factors, which also require consideration, are assistance in quitting smoking by referring to an appropriate service, encouraging measures to limit environmental stress, control of diabetes and measures to relieve any xerostomia. Regular removal of calculus deposits is an essential form of secondary prevention. It is also important to improve the oral environment by removing plaque traps such as rough or overhanging margins of restorations.

Tertiary prevention involves periodontal treatment to arrest and limit the progress of any established disease.

Preventing attrition, abrasion and erosion

Pathological attrition occurs due to bruxism, and damage can be prevented by early recognition, appropriate stress management and counselling, and the construction of protective splints.

Abrasion can occur from aggressive use of a toothbrush and/or abrasive toothpaste.

It is also caused by certain habits such as chewing on hard objects like pipe stems or pens, or holding nails or needles in the teeth. Prevention is based on early recognition and appropriate advice.

The effects of erosion are prevented or minimised by early recognition and modification of risk factors such as gastric reflux or excessive consumption of acidic drinks. Advice should be given about the possible co-destructive effects of foods or drinks that can cause erosive softening of the tooth structure. For example, athletes who use acidic products such as 'sports drinks' for re-hydration should be counselled about the risk of enamel erosion. Patients suspected of bulimia or anorexia require sensitive counselling and referral.

Secondary prevention is based on recommending the use of various remineralisation techniques, in addition to dietary counselling.

Preventing acquired orthodontic problems

Many orthodontic problems are of a congenital aetiology, and are therefore not really preventable.

Some orthodontic conditions are due to prolonged childhood habits, or the early loss of arch space due to extensive caries, or early loss of the deciduous teeth.

Primary orthodontic prevention includes all efforts directed at maintaining healthy deciduous teeth, advice to parents on the effects of long-term use of comforters (dummies), and behaviour modification strategies for habits such as prolonged finger or thumb sucking.

Prevention of orofacial traumatic injuries

The use of professionally fitted custom-made mouthguards, and of protective headgear, is an efficient and effective method for preventing many dental injuries in both schoolchildren and adults.

Major maxillo-facial trauma can occur in motor vehicle accidents, and the routine wearing of seatbelts is essential.

Prevention of oral malignancies

Primary prevention is focused on advising patients of the role of smoking, and of alcohol consumption, in the aetiology of carcinoma of the oral cavity, coupled with careful investigation of any persistent, potentially premalignant lesions. Some cultural groups may require advice on the carcinogenic dangers of chewing betel nut or chewing tobacco.

■ **subgingival plaque:** plaque that forms in the gingival sulcus.

Specific preventive techniques

Specific preventive techniques include:

- toothbrushing, including plaque disclosing;
- using toothpastes and mouthwashes;
- interdental cleaning;
- care and cleaning of dentures;
- use of fluorides; and
- observing dietary considerations.

Toothbrushing

See Figure 27.1 for proper toothbrushing technique.

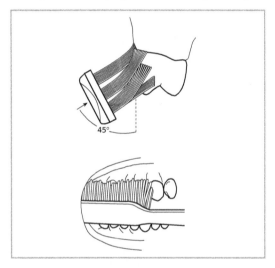

45°

Figure 27.1 Proper toothbrushing technique

The limitations of toothbrushing

Effective toothbrushing removes bacterial plaque from the accessible surfaces of the teeth, and provides a very simple and highly cost-effective vehicle for regular self-applications of low concentrations of fluoride. It does not contribute to gingival health by 'massaging the gums'.

Toothbrushing will also remove bacterial **substrate** from the oral cavity, although most damage to the hard surfaces is being done by acids produced within the plaque a short time after commencing to eat. What the toothbrush cannot do is remove plaque from deep pits and fissures, or from those surfaces of the teeth that are adjacent to and in contact with each another; that is, the mesial and distal surfaces.

In order to be effective, toothbrushing should be:

- regular;
- systematic;
- a-traumatic, without damaging either hard or soft tissue; and
- of adequate duration.

Choice of brush

Many commercially available toothbrushes are too large for most adult patients, and their bristles are potentially very abrasive.

Patients are advised to choose a brush with a compact multi-tufted head (child-sized for most brands), soft bristles and a comfortable ergonomically designed handle. Multidirectional bristle patterns have been shown to be as effective as flat trimmed bristles, and the choice of design is influenced by personal preference. If plaque control is seen to be adequate and a-traumatic then no change is indicated. Powered toothbrushes of the combined reciprocal and rotational type are equally as effective as hand-held brushes, and are particularly suitable for use by patients whose manual dexterity is compromised or whose oral hygiene is provided by carers.

Duration

Unsupervised patients tend to brush their teeth for one minute or less. The time required for adequate plaque removal is about three minutes for children and up to five minutes for adults. The use of an egg timer, or listening to a radio program of known duration, is a good way of ensuring that the time taken is adequate.

Frequency

For the majority of patients, twice a day is sufficient. High-risk patients may brush more frequently in order to increase their exposure to fluoride in toothpaste.

Last thing before retiring is a desirable time, again because it introduces fluoride into the environment before the nocturnal decline in saliva flow. After breakfast is also suitable, if time permits. However, if plaque removal is effective, then timing becomes less critical and can be left to the patient's discretion.

It is important to avoid toothbrushing immediately after consuming potentially erosive food or drink, such as acidic fruits or sports drinks, because the enamel will be in a temporarily softened state and highly susceptible to a combined abrasive/erosive

substrate: a substance containing particular enzymes.

effect. In these circumstances, patients can be advised to rise out with fluoridated water and delay toothbrushing for at least 30 minutes.

Toothbrush technique

The use of plaque-disclosing agents, both in the surgery and by the patient at home, is a very effective method for monitoring the effectiveness of toothbrushing. If plaque control is seen to be adequate, and there is no evidence of trauma, then the technique does not require modification. However, many patients instinctively use an ineffective and harmful method of horizontal scrubbing, and require additional advice.

Children should brush their teeth under supervision, and a series of overlapping small circular movements will be effective and manageable. For most adults, a modification of the Bass, or sulcular, brushing method is commonly accepted as being the most effective, in particular for patients at risk of periodontal disease. In this technique:

- the toothbrush bristles are directed horizontally and apically at an angle of 45 degrees to the long axis of the tooth;

- gentle force is used to introduce the bristles into the gingival sulcus and into the interdental spaces;

- a gentle vibratory motion consisting of short back and forth strokes is then applied, with approximately 10 strokes devoted to each small area (this is described as a jiggling motion);

- as the anterior areas of the mouth are approached, the head of the toothbrush is positioned more vertically, and the vibratory movement becomes more of an up and down stroke;

- after each cervical area is cleaned, the bristles can be rolled towards the occlusal surface to ensure that the whole tooth surface is cleaned; and

- the occlusal surfaces can be cleaned with a horizontal scrubbing action.

Toothpastes and mouthwashes

Toothpastes have two basic functions, cosmetic and therapeutic.

The cosmetic function includes a pleasant taste, foaming action, mild polishing and removal of stains. Although these make no direct contribution to the prevention of dental diseases, they make the procedure more pleasant and encourage people to clean their teeth longer and more frequently.

Toothpastes contain water, mild abrasive agents, humectants, flavouring, colouring, polishing agents, and foaming agents in the form of detergents. Detergents such as sodium lauryl sulphate and sodium-n-lauryl sulphate are contraindicated when patients have xerostomia, as they contribute to further dehydration of the oral tissues. Specially formulated fluoride toothpastes are available for these patients.

Most toothpastes also contain active ingredients for the prevention of dental disease.

Many of these are antibacterial additives that have only a limited short-term benefit, and make little significant additional contribution to the maintenance of oral health.

The most important therapeutic additive is fluoride, as repeated low dosage exposure to fluorides is the major post eruptive mechanism for primary prevention of caries and also secondary prevention by remineralising early pre-clinical lesions.

Another therapeutic ingredient in toothpaste may be some form of desensitising agent. It is however important to ensure that the product also contains fluoride.

Adult toothpastes contain 1000–1100 ppm of fluoride, while children's pastes contain 400–500 ppm. Adults at severe risk may be prescribed a higher concentration such as 5000 ppm.

Mouthwashes, like toothpastes, can be either cosmetic, therapeutic or both.

Most commercial mouthwashes are alcohol based, and will contribute to additional dehydration of the tissues in patients with xerostomia, particularly if they also contain astringents.

In general terms, mouthwashes only provide temporary superficial benefits. They will not penetrate very far into a periodontal pocket, so their action is mainly supragingival. They also lack substantivity, which means that their effect is not very long lasting.

Antibacterial mouthwashes based on chlorhexidine do have a role when used in the short term in the initial management of some periodontal diseases, or pre and post-operatively in oral surgery.

Neutral sodium fluoride mouthwashes are also used in the management of adults at identified high risk of dental caries. They are contraindicated in young children because of the risk of swallowing excess fluoride.

Interdental cleaning

The importance of cleaning the proximal tooth surfaces

Effective removal of the interproximal plaque is one strategy in the comprehensive approach to control of dental caries, although limited in its effectiveness. More significantly, periodontal diseases are predominantly interproximal diseases, which makes mechanical plaque removal from the proximal surfaces an indispensable preventive strategy.

Anatomical considerations

In a healthy person, the interdental papilla completely fills the interproximal space.

There is a normal crevice, the gingival sulcus, around the necks of the teeth at the margin of the free gingiva. This crevice ranges in depth from 0.5 mm to a maximum of 3 mm in a healthy periodontium.

The contact points between the teeth are relatively small, and are located above the interproximal space, close to the incisal edges or occlusal surfaces. Interproximal caries begin just beneath these contact points.

A toothbrush can only remove plaque from the occlusal surfaces (except of course from the depths of the fissures), and from the labial/buccal and lingual surfaces. Correct angulation of the brush will facilitate entry of the bristles into the gingival sulci of these surfaces.

The proximal tooth surfaces are not flat. They exhibit a substantial curvature in the bucco-lingual plane, which must be taken into account when attempting to clean these areas.

Interdental papillae are separated into buccal and lingual aspects by a depression called the col, which lies directly beneath the contact points between adjacent teeth.

Selection of aids for interproximal plaque control

The available materials and devices include:

■ dental floss, available in a bewildering variety of presentations including waxed, non-waxed, floss tape, teflon floss, flavoured and fluoride impregnated;

■ floss-holders, available in many designs for persons who have difficulty managing

conventional floss; some of these presentations are refillable (others, of which 'Flossettes' is a proprietary example, are used as disposables);

■ expanded dental floss, of which 'Superfloss' is a proprietary example;

■ interdental woodsticks; and

■ interdental brushes or interproximal brushes, of which the 'Proxabrush' (often miscalled a proxybrush) is one proprietary name of a large variety of products.

See the examples shown in Figures 27.2 and 27.3.

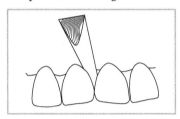

Figure 27.2 Interdental woodstick

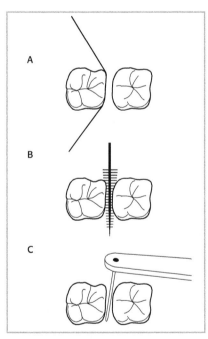

Figure 27.3 Floss, interdental brushes and interdental toothpick in holder

The decision on which of these devices to recommend to an individual is based on a variety of variables, of which the single most critically important one is the anatomy of the interdental space. If the interdental papilla completely fills the interdental space, then some form of floss is the only suitable material.

Where there has been slight recession (which means that a small interdental space exists) the choice may be either floss, or Superfloss, or a very small interdental brush, or woodsticks.

Larger interdental spaces are most efficiently cleaned by the larger interdental brushes, but if a patient is happily and successfully maintaining gingival health by using an alternative method, then the situation is best left alone.

Other variables which are important to take into consideration are:

- the manual dexterity of the individual patient. For example, children below the age range 8–10 years old lack the manual dexterity to use dental floss without damaging their tissues;
- cost;
- availability — if recommending any oral hygiene aid to a patient, ensure that you are able to direct them to an appropriate supplier; and
- convenience.

Which is the best product?

This is a frequently asked question. Numerous studies report small statistical differences in effectiveness between various types of products.

It is true that, in the correct location, interdental brushes are more effective than floss at removing plaque, and that woodsticks are statistically the least effective. However, these small statistical differences are of dubious clinical relevance.

Assuming that the choice has been based on sound anatomical principles, it appears that the most overwhelmingly significant variable is patient compliance, which will be largely determined by patient perceptions of ease and convenience of use, cost, comfort, apparent effectiveness and availability.

It is appropriate to be aware of the range of options available, in order to assist patients who report lack of success or specific difficulties.

Using dental floss

Floss is used to remove plaque from the adjoining proximal surfaces of the teeth, and from the proximal gingival sulci (Figure 27.4).

A strand of floss approximately 30–45 long is wrapped around the middle fingers, holding a 3 cm section tightly. The section to be used is held between the thumbs and the index fingers.

The floss is eased between the teeth at an angle of 45 degrees to their long axes. This greatly facilitates working the floss past the contact points without snapping it through and traumatising the gingiva.

The floss is curved around the tooth surface, and worked up and down. It is essential to work the floss under the free margin of the gingiva and into the gingival sulcus. This requires great care, as it is a common failing to attempt to take the floss too deeply. The adjoining tooth surface is then cleaned in the same way.

The floss is unwound and moved on during cleaning procedures so that a fresh segment is used in each space.

The distal surface of the last standing tooth is also cleaned.

If difficulty is encountered when removing the floss in an occlusal direction, it can be unwound from one finger and drawn out in a bucco-lingual direction.

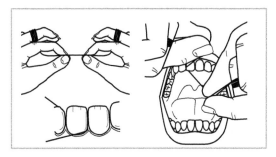

Figure 27.4 Using floss

Using interdental woodsticks

Note that these are not toothpicks. They are an entirely different shape, and are made from a different type of wood. Although they may have a secondary role as a toothpick, their primary function is the removal of bacterial dental plaque from the proximal surfaces of teeth where there is a sufficient degree of gingival recession for them to be used in an a-traumatic manner.

The woodstick should be moistened before use. No **dentifrice** is used.

Woodsticks have a triangular cross-section, designed to fit the triangular interdental space. The apex of the triangle always faces the occlusal surfaces or incisal edges; the flat base of the woodstick always faces the gingiva.

Insert the stick into the space, and move it backwards and forwards, whilst changing its angulation so that the sides actually contact the proximal surfaces of the teeth.

Although not the most efficient plaque removal method, sticks are relatively inexpensive, convenient to carry about, readily available and, most importantly, very easily manipulated by persons who lack the manual dexterity, motor skills or motivation to successfully use dental floss.

■ **dentifrice:** a paste, gel or similar material for cleaning teeth.

Using interdental brushes

It is essential to select a brush that is sufficiently small to fit the existing spaces. Too large a brush will contribute to additional gingival recession. Follow the guidelines set out below.

- Gross debris is first removed by conventional brushing.

- No dentifrice is used. The surfaces being cleaned are cementum, which are less mineralised than enamel or dentine, and therefore much more easily abraded.

- Short handled brushes, held between the thumb and forefinger, are significantly easier to use, particularly for persons with limited dexterity.

- Where possible, the brush is inserted into the space from both the lingual/palatal and the buccal aspects.

- Brushes should be rinsed and dried after use.

- In some situations, the brush may be dipped in an effective anti-bacterial agent such as chlorhexidine gluconate, before being applied to the tooth surfaces.

Care and cleaning of dentures

The surfaces of dentures provide extensive areas on which both plaque and calculus can accumulate.

Full denture wearers, particularly those who wear their dentures at night, are at high risk of developing 'denture sore mouth', which is a form of chronic monilial (thrush) infection. The problem is compounded if there is any degree of xerostomia.

Partial dentures have clasps, rests and connectors which can harbour plaque in protected sites contacting susceptible tooth surfaces. This contributes to the risk of dental caries and periodontal disease.

To minimise these possibilities, denture wearers are given specific advice on how to care for any remaining natural teeth as well as their dentures.

Full dentures

Dentures should be removed and cleaned after each meal where possible, and the mouth should be rinsed with water. The fitting surfaces should also be cleaned. Follow the guidelines set out below.

- Cleaning is best accomplished by using a soft brush and soap, such as liquid soap. Toothpastes and hard brushes can readily abrade the plastic of denture bases.

- To prevent breakage, dentures should be cleaned over a basin of water or over a wash cloth. It is not advisable to clean dentures under the shower.

- Because of reduced salivary flow, it is important that dentures be left out at night.

- Do not allow dentures to dry out. Soak full dentures at night in dilute (1/100) hypochlorite, which acts as a stain remover, deodoriser and antifungal agent. Remind the patient to rinse the denture with water before re-inserting.

- Never use harsh abrasives or scouring cloths on dentures. Persistent stains or calculus require professional removal.

Regular dental assessment of the fit and function of the dentures can prevent potential damage to the soft tissues.

Partial dentures

In general terms, the advice for partial denture wearers is the same as that for full denture wearers, but the following additional advice is also provided.

- Metal-based dentures should not be soaked in hypochlorite solution, as it may lead to corrosion of the metal. They may be soaked in plain water, or in a commercial denture cleansing soak.

- Particular attention should be given to cleaning any metal components which come into contact with the teeth or tissues.

- A small amount of fluoride toothpaste can be applied to metal components which contact the teeth.

- It is important to clean remaining teeth diligently.

- It is important to maintain regular check-ups of the dentures and the remaining natural teeth.

Dietary considerations

Dental caries is a disease that has certain distinct causes. The development of dental caries will be influenced by:

- the quantity and quality of the patient's saliva;

- exposure to both pre-eruptive and post-eruptive fluorides;

- the presence of bacterial dental plaque; and

- the frequency of exposure to cariogenic food and drink.

At the present state of knowledge, dietary factors do not appear to be directly related to the incidence or severity of periodontal diseases, except in rarely occurring extreme circumstances, such as scurvy or severe protein-calorie malnutrition.

Dental plaque bacteria metabolise carbohydrates (i.e. sugars and starches) and produce acids as a metabolic waste or by-product. Simple sugars break down more rapidly than the more complex carbohydrates, and sucrose (refined sugar) is regarded as the major dietary aetiological agent in the caries process. Many processed foods and convenience or 'junk' foods contain large amounts of sucrose, 'hidden sugars' as flavour enhancers and caramelising agents.

Carbohydrates that are retained in the mouth for long periods because of their sticky consistency are described as having a long oral clearance time, which means that their capacity to sustain prolonged acid production is very high. 'Health bars', 'energy bars' and 'breakfast bars' have very high levels of sugars, and are particularly sticky, which means an extended oral clearance time.

The most devastating dietary problem is 'bottle caries' or 'nursing caries', which occurs in young infants who receive comforter bottles containing sweetened liquids, acidic juices or expressed breast milk. A similar effect is produced when prolonged nursing at the breast is practised, as the lactose in breast milk is a fermentable carbohydrate. These sweetened liquids pool in the child's mouth, and during sleep the normal protective effect of the saliva is absent. Infants have had little time to develop adequate fluoride reservoirs, and deciduous teeth have relatively thin, and therefore susceptible, enamel.

Diet and nutrition are discussed in Chapter 28.

Fluorides

The use of appropriate fluoride treatments, including water fluoridation, is a cost-effective and minimally invasive way of both preventing and controlling dental caries.

Fluorides can benefit the dentition in two major ways.

❶ There is a pre-eruptive effect on the crowns of the developing teeth in children. In this case the fluoride is derived from drinking optimally fluoridated water, or consuming processed food or drink manufactured using fluoridated water. Some fluoride is also present in certain foods, and some may be derived if the child swallows any fluoride toothpaste. The greatest benefit of this pre-eruptive effect is to the deciduous teeth, and the pits and fissures of the developing permanent teeth.

Pre-eruptive fluoride is incorporated into the developing enamel of the teeth.

❷ There is now general agreement that the benefits of fluoride continue throughout life, and that the ongoing post-eruptive effects are far more significant than previously believed. The fluoride acts by interfering with the metabolic activity of plaque bacteria, and, more importantly, by establishing fluoride reservoirs on the tooth surface, and in plaque, pellicle and the soft tissues. When the tooth is subjected to acid attack, the fluoride in these reservoirs becomes mobilised, together with calcium from the tooth surface. These minerals then repair any damage which has been caused by acid attack.

Post-eruptive fluoride is derived from fluoridated drinking water, from the use of appropriate fluoride toothpastes, and from specifically targeted applications of topical fluoride varnishes, gels, solutions or mouthwashes. Maximum protection is given by repeated frequent exposure to low levels of fluoride to replenish the fluoride reservoirs.

Targeting high-risk sites in individuals

Specific surfaces and at-risk sites may be treated in the surgery in order to prevent dental caries (primary prevention) or to control or arrest existing lesions (secondary prevention). Newly erupted posterior teeth are often treated in this way.

Materials that are commonly used include fluoride varnishes, pastes and gels, or fluoride preparations such as stannous fluoride, which have an enhanced anti-microbial action.

Some restorative materials and fissure sealants, known as glass ionomer cements, contain fluorides which are gradually released in minute quantities, and contribute to caries prevention and control by maintaining levels of the fluoride reservoirs.

Water fluoridation

A major preventive strategy which is effective at the community level is the incorporation of fluoride into drinking water supplies, at a level of one part per million. In non-fluoridated areas, it may be appropriate to provide supplementation for children considered at risk, in order to gain the pre-eruptive effects. This is best done by dissolving a tablet containing the equivalent of one milligram of fluoride in a litre of water, and then using this water for drinking and cooking purposes.

Excessive fluoride consumption by children may produce white mottling, known as fluorosis. For this reason, supplements are prescribed on an individual basis, and young children are encouraged to rinse and spit after using fluoride toothpaste.

Fluoridated water provides substantial and lifelong post-eruptive benefits for both children and adults.

Fluoride toothpastes

Regular use of fluoride toothpaste is a valuable and important individual preventive strategy. The frequency of use is determined by individual risk. Twice a day is adequate for most individuals, and using fluoride toothpaste last thing at night before retiring will provide a top-up to the fluoride reservoirs at a time when protection from salivary minerals is reduced.

Adult fluoride toothpastes contain 1000–1100 ppm of fluoride. To gain maximum benefit, adults should spit out but not rinse after brushing. Small amounts of toothpaste may be applied to areas of early demineralisation, as a home-based topical application.

Children's fluoride toothpastes contain 400–500 ppm, and are used because of the risk of fluorosis from swallowing the more concentrated pastes. These junior formulations are used up to the age of six, after which a pea-sized amount of adult toothpaste may be used. Children should be supervised during brushing and, unlike adults, should rinse out and spit afterwards.

Concentrated pastes containing 5000 ppm are available for adult high-risk patients, and are particularly effective for older patients at risk of cemental (root) caries subsequent to gingival recession.

Fluoride mouth-rinses

Certain high-risk patients may be advised to supplement their primary preventive care by using fluoride mouth-rinses. Where repeated use is required, the use of neutral sodium fluoride products will avoid the risk of damage to porcelain surfaces or glass ionomer cement restorations, which may arise from using acidulated fluoride preparations.

Mouth-rinses are contraindicated in young children because of the dangers of swallowing.

Communicating oral health information

The primary prevention of dental disease requires commitment and compliance by patients. (The only exception is the significant anti-caries effect that is derived by the community from the fluoridation of the community water supplies.)

Patients frequently fail to comply with advice or guidelines about a healthy lifestyle. Educational programs about the risks of smoking, excessive exposure to sunlight, obesity, substance abuse or sexually transmitted diseases often fail in their objectives, and dental diseases are no exception.

The Becker Health Belief Model provides some explanation of what perceptions are necessary before patients will comply with a preventive message requiring them to implement a change in lifestyle. These perceptions are:

- The patient must believe that they are susceptible to the disease. A common attitude, particularly among younger people, is that 'this won't happen to me'.
- The patient must also perceive that the consequences of getting the disease are sufficiently severe to make them want to take preventive measures.
- The patient must be convinced that the preventive advice given is useful and practical.
- The benefits gained from the proposed action must be perceived to outweigh the costs of implementing the advice. Costs include not only time and money, but also the necessity to give up doing something enjoyable (such as eating lots of junk food), or the necessity to do something they consider unpleasant or difficult (having a mammogram, flossing their teeth).
- The patient must feel that the person who gives the preventive advice has credibility. This is essential.

Even if all these conditions are met, the patient may still not comply and make the necessary change in lifestyle.

What is necessary?

What is now required is a trigger or catalyst, something which finally motivates the patient to act on the preventive advice. This trigger is known as the 'cue to action'.

A cue to action may be either *intrinsic*, coming from the patients themselves, or it may be *extrinsic*, coming from another person or another source or medium.

Examples of intrinsic cues are experiencing symptoms ('I'm coughing a lot. I must give up smoking') or making lifestyle decisions ('I can't fit into any of my clothes. I must go on a diet').

Extrinsic clues may come from a concerned friend or relative ('It really worries me to see you smoking so much'), or from a television program, newspaper article, or perhaps the internet.

Giving oral health advice

When giving oral health advice to patients it is helpful to ensure that all the perceptions that have been listed in this model have been addressed.

■ The issues of susceptibility and the severity of the consequences are often well illustrated by showing patients areas of early changes in their own mouths (e.g. slight bleeding, early recession, subsurface decalcification or early abrasion and erosion lesions).

■ Try to describe the possible consequences in terms that the patients perceive to be relevant to themselves or their lifestyles. While the concepts of dental caries or periodontal disease may appear to be abstract to the patient, mention of the possibility of halitosis or of the teeth losing their lustre and becoming 'dull' may prove to be more meaningful because of their cosmetic implications.

■ Tailor the preventive program to the patients' specific needs, in order to minimise the costs to them both financially and in their time, or to minimise necessary alterations to their preferred lifestyle.

■ Explain the benefits from the point of view of oral health, but more importantly the social benefits, such as improved confidence, an attractive smile, fresh breath and the ability to enjoy all preferred foods without discomfort.

■ Your credibility as a 'prescriber' of preventive care will be based on the patients' perception of your non-critical acceptance of them as individuals, and your demonstrated empathy and willingness to listen and to assist. The oral health educator's role is one of a personal adviser, motivator or support person rather than that of a teacher or supervisor.

It is customary to describe the stages of oral health education as 'tell', 'show' and 'do', in that order.

Before telling the patient anything at all about their oral health, it is essential to listen to them and assess their perceptions of any problems, and also their expectations. This includes an assessment of their knowledge of oral health procedures. They may in fact be quite well informed and require encouragement and motivational support rather than new or additional specific rules or guidelines.

Showing the patient what to do should be preceded by observing what they are already doing. If it works, don't try to fix it. It may well be that all they require is a few modifications to an already suitable program. If demonstrating any procedures or making any recommendations, try to keep things as simple as possible, and do not overload the patient with excessive and possibly unnecessary information. Do make use of any suitable audio or visual aids, tapes, models, slides, illustrated atlases and tailored handouts. If providing pamphlets or brochures for home use, try to tailor the material to the patients' specific needs.

When dealing with families, and particularly with children, consider the possibilities of peer support by having family participation.

The final stage is providing the patient with an opportunity to *do* what is recommended, with the provision of support and guidance. Using disclosing solution and then allowing the patient to remove the stained plaque using a brush and floss is a useful opportunity to assist in refining their oral hygiene procedures.

As with any communication process, it is helpful to establish a non-threatening environment in which the oral health message can be communicated. One suggestion is for a dedicated room with a large mirror and a sink similar to that which would be found in the bathroom at home. It is more difficult for patients to practise procedures if they are lying down in the chair, or trying to juggle a hand mirror.

Summary

As most of the conditions listed above are diseases of lifestyle, they are largely preventable. However, lifestyle change is quite difficult to achieve, even for potentially fatal diseases. Oral health promotion requires excellent communication and motivational skills, as well sound, evidence-based clinical practices.

Be prepared for the fact that it takes time to implement behavioural change, and that the message will require frequent supportive reinforcement until the patient reaches an appropriate level of commitment and competence. This can only occur if the approach is supportive, accepting and non-judgmental.

chapter twenty-eight
diet and nutrition

Introduction

The human body requires food to develop and function. Food enables the body to grow and develop by providing:

- material for the building and repair of tissues;
- material for the production of energy;
- substances, which although present in small amounts only, are needed to keep the body in good working order; and
- water, needed to make up body losses from perspiration, breathing and excretion.

Although it is possible to survive as long as you receive sufficient energy from foods of any type, you will be much healthier if you receive your energy by eating a good combination of healthy foods.

Nutrients

A diet is all the food a person eats. However, it is the nutrients in the food that provide the continuous supply of chemical substances necessary for growth, energy and wellbeing. Nutrient requirements depend on a person's age, weight, activity level and gender, among other things. To be healthy a person must eat foods that provide sufficient nutrients. These nutrients may be divided into proteins, carbohydrates, fats, minerals and vitamins.

Although not usually classified as a nutrient, water must also be included in any discussion about nutrition. Water is essential for life. It is possible to exist for weeks without food but only for a few days without water in one form or another.

All these nutrients are available in a well-balanced diet. Many people take food supplements (e.g. vitamins and minerals) but these are generally not as satisfactory as a healthy diet.

Proteins

The basic material of every body cell is protein and the continual replacement of cells is necessary to maintain the body's tissues in good health. Proteins are the only nutrients that can build body tissues. Therefore, protein foods are necessary for everyone. Children from infancy to their teenage years, and women who are pregnant or nursing their babies, need a higher proportion of protein than other people.

If our intake of protein foods exceeds our requirements, or if there are no other energy sources (for example, in a low carbohydrate diet), the excess is converted into energy. If insufficient food is eaten, protein will be used by the body to provide energy at the expense of growth.

Proteins are made up of compounds called 'amino-acids', which are required in various combinations by the body tissues — bone, muscle, blood, skin, heart, liver and so forth — and also for internal secretions, such as enzymes and hormones. Proteins from animal sources, with the exception of gelatine, generally contain all the required amino-acids, though not necessarily in exactly the amounts needed by the body. The proteins in plants contain variable amounts of these amino-acids. A meal combination of animal and plant foods provides the body with the variety of amino-acids it requires for its various functions, including:

- growth of new tissue and repair;
- resistance to infection and disease; and
- recovery from injury and surgery.

Good sources of protein are:

- meat of all kinds, including poultry;
- fish;
- eggs;

- dairy foods (except butter);
- nuts;
- seeds;
- legumes, such as lima and soya beans; and
- wholegrain cereals.

Carbohydrates

Carbohydrates range in variety from simple sugars, such as glucose and sucrose (cane sugar), to more complex compounds, such as starch and cellulose. Most of the carbohydrates in food occur as starch, which is broken down in the body into glucose.

Carbohydrates are needed for:

- energy for all body processes, including growth, and for all activity; and
- proper metabolism of other foodstuffs, especially protein.

Sources of carbohydrates are:

- cereals such as wheat, corn, rice, oats, rye and products made from them;
- flour, bread, spaghetti, noodles, cakes, pastries and so forth;
- dried peas, beans and other legumes;
- dried dates, figs, prunes; and
- potatoes.

Complex carbohydrates

These are primarily found in vegetables, fruits and grains and they provide energy, minerals and vitamins. The structural parts of plants, the skins of fruit and the coverings of seeds, consist of complex carbohydrates (such as cellulose), which are not digested in the body and which are now referred to as fibre.

Refined carbohydrates

These are found in processed foods and often provide only energy but no fibre or nutrients. Examples are biscuits, cakes, sugar, soft drinks and some breads. Lollies, honey, jam and other sweet spreads have a high sugar content and are considered harmful to dental health.

Cariogenic foods

The process of the development of caries is discussed in Chapter 12. As a reminder, carbohydrates are broken down into the sugars that the body uses for energy. Plaque contains bacteria that uses these sugars for food, so a food that contains carbohydrates that can be used by the plaque in this way is called cariogenic food.

Complex carbohydrates are less cariogenic than refined carbohydrates. This is because they often clear the mouth before the breakdown into sugars begins. Refined carbohydrates often break down much faster and so are more cariogenic. If they are also sticky and stay in contact with the teeth, then they are very cariogenic. For example, a sticky lolly is more cariogenic than a soft drink.

Fats

Fats are a more concentrated fuel than carbohydrates, supplying 38 **kilojoules** per gram compared with 17 kilojoules per gram for carbohydrates.

Fats are needed for:

- energy and heat regulation;
- padding and filling for body organs;
- sources of vitamins A, D, E and K; and
- flavour and satisfaction.

Sources of fat are:

- cream, milk (and products of these such as butter and margarine) and cheese;
- vegetable oil such as corn oil, olive oil, peanut oil and sunflower oil;
- meat (especially pig meat such as bacon and ham);
- eggs; and
- foods such as avocados, chocolate and peanut butter.

Minerals and trace minerals

Large amounts of calcium and phosphorus help to make up the skeleton and teeth. Minute quantities of many other minerals and trace elements are necessary for the regulation of body processes. See Table 28.1 for more information about minerals.

■ **kilojoules:** formerly called calories, the unit to express the fuel or energy value of food.

Mineral	Function	Sources
Calcium, phosphorus and magnesium	Essential for healthy bones and teeth, muscle contraction, blood pressure regulation, healthy heart and nervous system and blood clotting. Magnesium is also essential for the production and transfer of energy, carbohydrate metabolism and transport of substances across cell membranes.	Milk, cheese, sardines, nuts, whole grains and green leafy vegetables. Supplements of calcium are not of proven value and should be combined with magnesium to be absorbed.
Iron	Essential for the oxygen transport and storage in the blood (haemoglobin in red blood cells) and muscles. Varies in importance throughout life. Menstruating women, growing children and pregnant mothers need more iron.	Liver, kidney, poultry, egg yolk, legumes, seeds, nuts, dried fruits and green leafy vegetables. Vitamin C improves iron absorption.
Fluoride	Has a proven strengthening effect on bones and teeth. It remineralises enamel and dentine.	Water (naturally in some mountainous regions and added to the water supply in others). Small amounts also found in tea, meat, fish, cereals and fruit.
Iodine	Essential for normal metabolism, growth and development because it is a component of thyroid hormones. Deficiency can lead to hypothyroidism and goitre.	Seafood of all sorts. Iodised salts. Is used to supply iodine to areas of soil deficiency. Vegetables grown in iodine rich soil, and milk, contain iodine.
Electrolytes, e.g. potassium, sodium chloride (table salt)	Electrolytes are vital for maintaining a normal balance of water between body cells and the surrounding fluids. Fluid exchange in the body. Digestion of food.	All animal foods (meat, butter, cheese, margarine, eggs, etc. Added to food directly. Used also to act as a preservative.

Other trace elements needed in minute quantities (usually found in multi-vitamin tablets) include: phosphorus, sulphur, boron, chromium, copper, manganese, molybdenum, selenium, vanadium, silicon, zinc.

Table 28.1 Minerals

Vitamins

Table 28.2 lists vitamins that are water soluble, which means they are rapidly excreted from the body. A constant daily supply of water soluble vitamins is required.

Table 28.3 lists vitamins that are fat soluble, which means they are stored in the body, and are therefore only required in small amounts.

Vitamin	Function	Sources
The 'B' Complex (Group)	Essential for the metabolism of carbohydrate, fats and proteins essential for growth, healthy hair, skin and the functioning of the nervous system.	Liver, kidney, whole grains, seeds, nuts, dairy products, eggs, wheatgerm, bran, brewer's yeast, green leafy vegetables, lentils, beans, peas, vegetable extracts.
Vitamin B_1 – Thiamine	Essential for releasing energy from food, converting excess energy to fat, for healthy skin, blood, muscles, the brain and nervous system. Alcohol metabolism.	As above. Supplements may be used to improve mental function in alcoholics and the elderly. To treat nerve problems and cardiovascular disease.
Vitamin B_2 – Riboflavin	Many of the above plus absorption of carbohydrates and proteins and many functions to do with general wellbeing. Normal growth and development and a healthy immune system. Vitamin B_2 deficiency causes lowered resistance to infection and loss of vitality.	All the above. Supplements may be used to treat anaemia, skin problems, migraine, stress and fatigue.
Vitamin B_3 – Niacin (Nicotinic Acid)	Energy control, healthy skin, blood cells, and function of the brain, nervous system and digestive system. Normal growth and development and hormone production.	Fish, liver, kidneys, yeast and vegetable extracts, nuts and cereals etc. Supplementation with nicotinic acid may be used to treat diabetes and some nerve disorders.
Vitamin B_6 – Pyridoxine	Needed to release the energy from food. For a healthy cardiovascular, nervous and immune system. For hormone production and protein metabolism.	As all other sources of B vitamins.

Other important vitamins in the B group are: **Folate (folic acid) B_{12}, Pantothenic acid and Biotin**.

Vitamin	Function	Sources
Vitamin C or Ascorbic Acid	Intercellular cementing in tissues (collagen) blood vessels, teeth, bones and cartilage development all depend on an adequate supply of Vitamin C. Acts as an anti-oxidant to help prevent disease. Severe deficiency leads to scurvy with symptoms of bleeding gums, joint pain, easy bruising and dry skin.	Fresh fruits and vegetables must be supplied adequately every day. Cooked vegetables are not good sources of Vitamin C.

Table 28.2 Water soluble vitamins

Vitamin	Functions	Sources
Vitamin A*	Growth and development of good vision (reduce the risk of developing cataracts) healthy skin (help in treating acne) and mucous membrane. Carotenoids act as powerful disease-fighting anti-oxidants.	Liver, butter, milk, cheese, egg yolk; occurs in red, yellow and orange fruit such as apricots, mangoes, apples, citrus and in vegetables such as carrots, tomatoes, spinach, broccoli, etc.
Vitamin D	Necessary for the normal growth and development of bones and teeth in children. Important in the prevention of osteoporosis in older people through the absorption and use of calcium and phosphorus in teeth and bones. It is also involved in muscle strength and the regulation of the heartbeat. Vitamin D is an important booster of immunity.	Food sources include oily fish, eggs, dairy products and margarine. Manufactured in the skin by ultraviolet light in sunlight. Exposure for 15 to 20 minutes three times per week is sufficient for the body's requirements.
Vitamin E	An anti-oxidant, it protects cells against free-radical damage, which is a known factor in the development of various cancers and cardiovascular disease. Development of red blood cells, muscle cells, and other cell tissue. High doses of Vitamin E may also have an anti-aging effect on skin and blood vessels, on the immune and central nervous system.	Vegetable oils, cereals, wheatgerm, seeds, nuts, brown rice, eggs, milk, soya beans and sweet potatoes. Also in dark green leaf vegetables.
Vitamin K	Essential for normal blood clotting, bone metabolism and kidney function. Thought to be helpful in relieving the discomfort of chillblains.	Manufactured by bacteria in the large intestine. Good food sources are dark green leafy vegetables, oils from green plants and some dairy products.

* (Carotenoids, including beta-carotene and lycopene in foodstuffs, is converted to vitamin A in the body).

Table 28.3 Fat soluble vitamins

A balanced diet

To ensure that your diet is balanced and contains the various nutrients in the correct quantities, the basic food guide should be followed daily (see Figure 28.1). Examples of one serving are listed below. If you eat a larger portion, it counts as more than one serving. For example, a dinner portion of pasta would count as two or three servings.

Milk and cheese

These are eaten for protein, calcium and vitamins. One serving is generally one cup of milk or yoghurt. Children, teenagers, and expectant and nursing mothers need about 600 ml per day. Use liquid milk, dried or evaporated milk or cheese. A 30 mm cube of cheese is equivalent to 1 cup of milk.

Meat, poultry, fish, dry beans, eggs and nuts

These are eaten for protein, vitamins and minerals. One serving equals about 60 to 100 g of cooked lean meat, poultry, or fish. Half a cup of cooked dry beans, one egg, or two tablespoons of peanut butter count as 30 g of lean meat.

Fruit and vegetables

Fruit and vegetables are eaten for vitamin C and other vitamins and minerals. Include one tomato or citrus fruit and some raw fruit each day. One serving equals one medium apple, banana, orange, $^1/_2$ cup of chopped, cooked, or canned fruit and $^3/_4$ cup of fruit juice. A serving of vegetables might be one cup of raw leafy vegetables, $^1/_2$ cup of other vegetables, cooked or chopped raw, $^3/_4$ cup of vegetable juice.

Bread, cereal, rice and pasta

Bread and cereals are eaten for energy, vitamins, minerals and some protein. Include whole grain cereals and bread. These provide more B group vitamins than white bread and refined cereals. One serving equals one slice of bread, 30 grams of ready-to-eat cereal, $^1/_2$ cup of cooked cereal, rice, or pasta.

Fats, oils and sweets

Fats, oils and sweets provide flavour and can provide energy and vitamin A. They should be eaten sparingly.

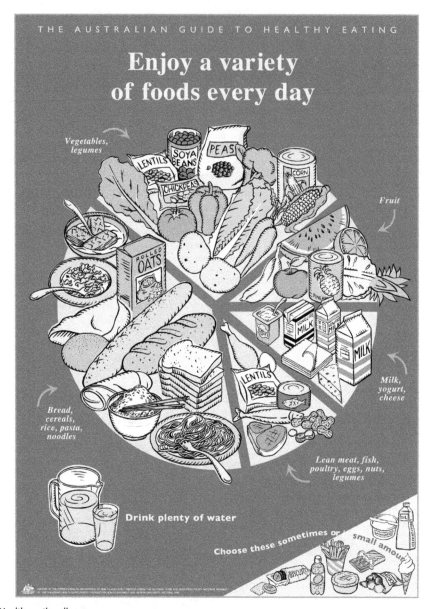

Figure 28.1 Healthy eating diagram
Source: *The Australian Guide to Healthy Eating*, The Children's Health Development Foundation, South Australia (1998).

Energy requirements of the individual

The principal uses of food are to supply energy to the living body and each of the three nutrients, carbohydrate, fat and protein, can provide this energy. The energy that is used even when the body is completely at rest is called the **Basal Metabolic Rate** (BMR) for that individual. When awake or active, people use increased amounts of energy.

The amount of energy food (that is, the number of kilojoules) needed every day is not a fixed figure. It varies according to age, sex, body build, physical condition and the amount of physical activity under-

taken. Because of their activity, the needs of children are greater than those of adults in proportion to their size.

If the body is provided with more energy than is needed for the day's activities, the excess will be stored in the tissues in the form of fat. If the food intake is too low, the reserves of fat are drawn upon for extra energy and the person loses weight. Weight loss can also be caused by physical or emotional factors that interfere with digestion.

■ **Basal Metabolic Rate (BMR):** the rate of energy utilisation during rest.

Diet and nutrition related to dental health

Having dealt with diet and nutrition in relation to general health and growth it is simple to relate it to dental health. The relationship is identical. The ideal diet for general health contains nothing more nor less than the ideal dental diet.

Development of a sound dentition requires the following.

Pre-natal nutrition

The diet of the mother must be well balanced and have adequate amounts of calcium, iron, iodine and vitamins A, B, C and D for her own health as well as that of the baby. It is an accepted fact that the baby will take all the nourishment it requires for growth and development so it is the mother who will suffer first where a deficient diet exists.

Post-natal nutrition

Breastfed children require the mother to have an excellent diet including high milk content — up to one litre per day — and adequate vitamin C. Liver is a good supply of required nutrients.

Nutrition in childhood

Generally, foods eaten by the young child are of great importance to long-term development. For sound health and development a balanced diet must be taken. Foods containing calcium, and vitamins A, C and D are essential for sound tooth formation.

It is also important for children to have fluoride, either in drinking water or as tablets.

Even at the age of 12, when the crowns of all the teeth have been formed and calcified, from a preventive point of view, the diet maintains its importance.

Many foods which contain sugar in a sticky consistency, or even in solution, play an active part in the formation of dental plaque and also contribute to disease of the soft tissue (gingivitis).

It is essential to note that these foods also add little or nothing to the maintenance of general health.

Temporary loss of appetite is common and usually easily explained. It can be caused by such things as teething and throat infections, or a decrease in growth rates at various ages, and by emotional upsets.

Nutrition in adulthood

Because of the cariogenic properties of food, adults also need to take care with what they eat. More information is provided in Chapter 27, under the heading 'Dietary considerations'.

Prevention of dental caries

To prevent dental caries it is necessary to change daily eating habits. Patients should reduce the frequency of eating, and in particular the frequency of eating (and drinking) things that have a high level of refined carbohydrates. What is crucial is not how much carbohydrate you eat, but how often you eat it, and how much of it is simple carbohydrate and refined carbohydrate such as sucrose (sugar).

Patients should try to avoid sweet sticky things that have a long oral clearance time.

Chewing hard foods or sugar-free chewing gum stimulates saliva, which has a high mineral content and promotes remineralisation.

Patients with a 'sweet tooth' should consider carbohydrate modified foods in moderation.

Saliva flow is minimal during sleep so it is important that patients avoid eating cariogenic foods either just before retiring or if they raid the fridge nocturnally.

Food intake diary

A poor nutritional state frequently produces a poor dental condition, affecting both teeth and gums.

In order to help a patient with poor diet, it is vital to first find out their normal eating habits. This can be done successfully through the use of a 'food intake diary' (Figure 28.2). If accurately compiled, it is easy to see where the patient has not eaten according to the five basic food groups, and therefore has not fed the body its required nutrients. The diary should be kept for five consecutive days, including a weekend or holiday.

With the information collected, the patient can be told how the diet may best be modified to eliminate the carbohydrates that are most caries-active, and replaced with fibrous, cleansing foods. Since the caries-active foods are usually the least nutritious, the patient's state of nutrition and therefore general health should be improved by modifications of this kind.

Name			Age	
Weight	**Height**	**Day**	**Date**	
	Food	**Drink**	**Extras**	
Breakfast				
Mid-morning				
Lunch				
Mid-afternoon				
Dinner				
After dinner				

1. Record foods in the order in which they are eaten.
2. Record every type of food consumed, solid or liquid, at meal time, between meals, while watching television etc. Also record chocolates, sweets, chewing gum, cough drops or syrups etc.
3. For each meal, list the food, preparation (fried, boiled etc.) and amount in household measures.
4. For fruits and vegetables, record whether raw, fresh, frozen or canned.
5. State amount of sugar or sugar products and cream or milk added to cereal, beverages or other foods.
6. Particular information on extras is most important. Do not leave out the slightest detail.
7. Record when teeth cleaned; brushed (TB) and/or rinsed (R).

Figure 28.2 Food intake diary

The completed diary can be used as a basis for discussion with the patient on the relationship between nutrition and dental health. Dentally harmful foods should be underlined and these should be discussed with the patient who can be encouraged to suggest alternatives that he/she is prepared to eat.

Food labelling

Understanding how to read food labels can assist with healthy eating. See Table 28.4 for information about food labelling.

Additives	These are used to improve either the appearance of the product or its lifetime. They can be shown by their name or a number. If there is a potential allergen in the food (e.g. peanuts) this is usually shown here, too.
Carbohydrate	Shown as total carbohydrate and sugars. Total carbohydrate includes starch, dietary fibre and sugars. Sugars include sucrose, fructose, lactose and glucose.
Cholesterol free or no cholesterol	May not contain cholesterol if from a plant source but this does not mean that the food is not high in fat!
Dietary fibre	This is an estimate of the total fibre. High fibre products are preferable.
Energy	This is the number of kilojoules (kJ). Usually shown per serve and per 100 g.
Fat	Shown as fat per serve and per 100 g.
Fat-free	Must not contain more than 0.15 g total fat per 100 g of food.
High fibre	The food must contain more than 3 g of dietary fibre per serving.
Ingredients	These are the main components of the products, listed in descending order by weight. For example, the component listed first is present in the product in the greatest quantity.
Lite or light	May be used to describe the taste, texture, energy or fat content. Check the nutrition panel for more information.
Low fat	The food should not contain more than 3 g of fat per 100 g.
Low joule or diet	These are usually low fat and artificially sweetened.
Net weight	The weight of the food without the packaging. This is important in determining the serving size.
No added sugar	No added sugars but the product may contain natural sugars.
Reduced fat or salt	25 per cent less fat or salt than the regular product. This does not mean low fat.
Sodium	The level of salt in the product. Low sodium products are preferable.
Storage instructions	Recommendations on how to store the product (for example, whether it needs to be refrigerated).
Use-by date	Shows the recommended date by which the product should be used, if it is stored as recommended.

Table 28.4 Food labelling

Appropriate dietary advice

- Eat three regular balanced meals a day. Follow the principles of sound nutrition.

- Reduce the frequency of eating, and particularly the frequency of sucrose consumption. Be aware of 'hidden sugars'. Use appropriate substitute sweeteners.

- Drink fluoridated water.

- Avoid sticky sweet foods that are retained in the mouth for long periods of time.

- Breastfeeding of infants is encouraged for the first six months, but not as a comforter for prolonged periods of time.

- If babies are bottle fed, introduce feeding from a cup between the ages of 6–12 months.

- Avoid sweetened water or sweetened formulas when bottle-feeding infants. Agents to avoid include sucrose, glucose, honey, molasses, expressed breast milk and sweetened vitamin supplements. If sweetened liquids have been started, progressively dilute the amount of sweetening agent as early as possible. The longer the infant has had to become accustomed to the sweetened formula or liquid, the more difficult it will be to break the habit.

- Avoid snacking at night after the teeth have been cleaned.

- Dairy foods have a protective effect due to their casein component.

- Chewing sugar-free chewing gum after meals encourages production of protective stimulated saliva.

- Foods which require vigorous chewing encourage the production of stimulated saliva which has a high potential for remineralisation.

While all these approaches will be useful when directed at the appropriate risk group, reducing the frequency of eating, and particularly reducing the frequency with which sucrose is consumed, are more attainable goals than attempting to impose very unrealistic restrictions, such as the complete avoidance of all sweets.

Acidic drinks

The acidity of a solution is described as its pH level. The lower the pH, the more acidic the solution. A pH of 7 is neutral.

The normal pH of saliva in a healthy mouth is very slightly acidic, just below 7.0. Below a pH of approximately 5.5, decalcification of enamel will commence. If plaque is present, it only takes between two to five minutes for the pH to fall below 5.5 after rinsing with a 10 per cent glucose solution. It then takes between one and two hours to return to normal resting pH levels.

Tooth enamel dissolves in acid, so frequent consumption of acidic (low pH) drinks will damage enamel. This damage can be seen as erosion (chemical 'wear') and increased caries (decay).

Table 28.5 compares the acidity of various drinks as tested in a laboratory, and as listed by the manufacturer.

When reading these results, please remember that tooth enamel begins to dissolve at pH 5.5, and that even enamel that has a high fluoride reservoir will begin to dissolve if the pH falls to 4.5 or below. For comparison, stomach acid has a pH of 3.2, which is the same as that of wine, and vinegar a pH of 3.0, similar to that of 'sports' drinks.

It is not only the pH of a drink that needs to be considered, but also the sugar content and the frequency with which it is taken. The mouth needs time to recover from the acid attack, and if a further acid drink is taken before it has had time to recover, the attack on the teeth continues uninterrupted. In other words, it is far better to drink the whole drink in a short period of time, rather than to sip it slowly over many minutes or hours.

Summary

Many patients do not clearly understand the link between diet, nutrition and oral health. You may be required to assist patients by providing them with clear and correct information on nutrition and dental health. To do this you will need a good understanding of how dental caries develops (e.g. the relationship between dental caries, the amount of sucrose that is eaten and the frequency of eating), as described in Chapter 12.

You will also be able to:

- encourage parents to be effective role models in improving their children's eating habits;

- assist patients in developing an appropriate food intake diary; and

- assist them in reading food labels for nutritional information.

Beverage	Measured pH	Manufacturer's pH
Fruitopia	2.8	Coca Cola 3.4
Powerade (Orange)	2.9	Coca Cola 3.4
Dura Fuel Isotonic Energy Drink	2.9	Aussie Bodies 3.0
Gatorade Lemon Chill	2.9	Pepsi Cola 2.9 – 3.4
Lemon Energizer Sport Drink	2.9	AWD (not supplied)
Coca Cola regular	3.0	Coca Cola 3.0 – 3.5
Iso Sport, Citrus fruits	3.0	Berrivale 2.9 – 3.3
Iso Sport Lite, Lemon-lime	3.0	Berrivale 2.9 – 3.3
Diet Coke	3.2	Coca Cola 3.0 – 3.5
Cordial (Berri raspberry diluted with water)	3.2	Berrivale 3.6 – 3.8
Schweppes Sports Plus	3.2	Schweppes 3.0
Stanley Cask Wine (Moselle)	3.2	Leasingham 3.2
Stanley Cask Wine (Riesling)	3.2	Leasingham 3.2
Stanley Wines (Claret)	3.2	Leasingham 3.2
Minchinbury White Wine	3.2	Penfolds 3.2
Lucozade Lemon	3.4	Smith Kline 3.2
Eagle Blue Ice Beer	3.4	SA Brewing Co 3.9 – 4.3
Fosters Lite Ice Beer	4.0	Carlton & United 4.2
West End Draught Beer	4.0	SA Brewing Co 3.9 – 4.3
Victoria Bitter Beer	4.2	Carlton & United 4.2
Mt Franklin Spring Water	4.8	Coca Cola 6.5 – 7.5
Gastrolyte Natural Flavour	5.0	Rhône-Poulenc 4.8
Milk (whole milk)	6.6	Dairy Vale 6.6
Adelaide tap water	6.8	SA Water 7.2

Table 28.5 Acidity of some common beverages

Section 6

Specialist areas of dentistry

Some of the specialist techniques described in this section are techniques that you will assist with in normal practice. For example, it is not uncommon for the dentist to be required to raise a flap in the course of an extraction or to perform root canal therapy. However, for complex or difficult cases, a dentist will refer a patient to a specialist oral surgeon or periodontist. These specialisations are discussed briefly. If working in a specialist area you will require specific on-the-job training.

chapter twenty-nine
patients with special needs

Introduction

Quite frequently, dentists are required to perform dental treatment on patients who have special needs. These patients may have some form of intellectual or physical disability, or a systemic disease. Often these patients require special care and consideration by both the dentist and dental staff.

You will be particularly responsible for allaying the fears of these patients by gentle handling and attention, by making the patient comfortable, and by reducing anxiety. The patient should *never* be left alone in the surgery.

If a patient has any of the conditions that are discussed below, it should become apparent from the medical history taken before the appointment. It cannot be stressed too much that you need to check the patient's medical history to ensure that the patient has completed every section and understands the questions, and you need to check that medical histories are regularly updated.

Medically compromised patients

Cardiovascular and blood conditions

Bacterial endocarditis

Patients who have congenital heart disease, who have an artificial heart valve or who have suffered rheumatic fever earlier in life often have damaged heart valves that can become infected by micro-organisms released into the blood stream during dental treatment (e.g. extraction, scaling).

Such patients are nearly always given prophylactic antibiotic therapy before, during and after dental treatment. Previously penicillin was always used, but as the mouth micro-organisms have now developed a high resistance to penicillin (up to 70 per cent of patients have mouth organisms resistant to penicillin), ampicillin, cephalosporins, amoxycillin or erythromycin are often used instead. These drugs should be given not more than one to one-and-a-half hours before dental treatment, and must be continued for three days after treatment. Patients at greatest risk should always be given these drugs by injection.

Heart disease

It is essential that the dentist know the nature of the patient's condition, the medications the patient is taking and other forms of management of the condition. For example, patients with heart disease may be taking drugs to prevent the blood from clotting, and this drug may have to be stopped for a few days if it is necessary to extract a tooth or carry out any surgery or deep scaling. Generally though, the patient should continue taking all medication before treatment, unless instructed to do otherwise by the dentist.

In some cases, the dentist may wish to discuss the patient's condition with the patient's cardiologist before beginning treatment. At the discretion of the dentist, the patient might be given supplemental oxygen throughout the procedure or sublingual nitroglycerin immediately before the procedure. Patients receiving some form of pre-treatment should be advised not to drive themselves to the surgery or drive home after the treatment.

Patients with heart disease often also have periodontal disease and should be advised of methods to improve that condition.

Blood disorders

Blood disorders have different causes and take different forms. Patients with these disorders are susceptible to bacterial infection.

Haemophilia is one form of clotting disorder. This is due to the absence from the blood of one of the clotting factors (Factor VIII). Von Willebrand's disease and Christmas disease are also due to missing clotting factors. Bleeding can also occur if the platelets in the blood are deficient (thrombocytopaenia). In all of these conditions there is a great risk of fatal bleeding if an injection is given, a tooth extracted or surgery or scaling carried out without the patient's clotting defect being medically corrected beforehand. A haematologist will replace the missing blood elements in the correct quantity to prevent prolonged bleeding. This has to be continued for several days until healing is established.

Concentrated, blood replacement products make it possible for some patients who have been trained (or whose parents have been trained) to give their own replacement factor intravenously at home, and then an hour later go to their own local dentist for routine treatment. The dentist is then able to safely use a local anaesthetic for restorations, but extractions or surgery must still be carried out in a hospital, with the patient admitted usually for several days.

Other blood disorders include anaemia and leukaemia.

HIV and AIDS

HIV (Human Immunodeficiency Virus) is a virus that attacks and can destroy the immune system by invading white blood cells. It is highly infectious. In the early stages of infection, the patient may have no symptoms. In fact, some patients are not aware that they have HIV and oral lesions are the earliest sign of the infection.

As the white blood cell count decreases, the condition progresses to AIDS (Acquired Immune-Deficiency Syndrome). Patients with AIDS are prone to oral infections. For example, ANUG is common in AIDS patients and, if untreated, results in tooth loss.

As a result, these patients need to institute excellent oral hygiene behaviours and may require education to allow this. They also need information that allows them to undertake oral self-examination to alert them to decreases in their immune responses.

Some AIDS medications can cause vomiting and that may result in tooth erosion. Some patients will also experience changes in taste and swollen or bleeding tongue and gums. Xerostomia can be a result of medications and artificial salivas are often recommended, as are fluoride mouthwashes.

Patients should declare their HIV status on their medical histories as their medications and the status of their immune system is vital information for the dentist. A note guaranteeing absolute confidentiality should be included on the medical history form.

Pulmonary disorders

Pulmonary disorders are disorders of the lungs and affect the patient's ability to breathe.

Exposure to stress or particular stimuli can cause the bronchial airways to contract and the patient may have what is called an asthma attack. This can also be caused by bronchial infection.

Asthmatic patients or those who suffer from multiple allergies are often treated with cortisone. Stressful dental treatment, especially oral surgery, or if general anaesthesia is used, may result in the patient collapsing. To prevent this, extra cortisone is given before, during and after such treatment. In some cases, the patient's physician may insist on hospitalisation for treatment, especially if general anaesthesia is to be used.

In chronic bronchitis, the bronchial airways are narrowed.

In emphysema, the air becomes trapped in the lungs and the lungs become over-inflated.

Active tuberculosis cases are not likely to be encountered in the dental surgery except when emergency dental treatment is required. Transmission-based precautions, as described in Chapter 14, must be adhered to if treating patients with active tuberculosis.

These conditions make patients more susceptible to bacterial infection of the lungs.

Appointments should be kept as stress-free as possible. They should be short, and if necessary, the dentist will choose appropriate sedation. Some patients benefit from increased oxygen. Nitrous oxide should not be used.

Kidney disease

Patients with kidney disease sometimes cannot absorb calcium properly and this can cause loss of bone from the jaws. As a result, teeth can become loose. Also, the tissues in the mouth and the salivary glands may become inflamed.

Patients may also present with bad breath because the kidneys cannot remove urea from the blood and this breaks down to form ammonia.

If patients are having dialysis, dental treatment should be within the following 24 hours. Patients with shunts may be at risk of bacterial endocarditis and should take antibiotics before dental treatment.

The dentist will probably consult with the patient's doctor before beginning treatment.

Head and neck malignancies

Radiation therapy is a common treatment modality for head and neck cancer. It may be used alone, or in combination with surgery and/or chemotherapy.

For effective treatment, tumouricidal doses of radiation must be administered, with their attendant adverse sequelae upon oro-facial structures. The severity and extent of these radiation side effects vary according to dosage, volume, shielding and type of beam used. Many of the sequelae can be averted or minimised by careful pre-radiation dental screening and post-radiation follow-up and management.

Radiotherapy of the head and neck region results in changes to the hard and soft tissues. These include radiation dermatitis, delayed skin and sub-cutaneous damage, as well as intra-oral changes such as acute mucositis and delayed soft tissue necrosis. Of relevance to dentistry are the changes that occur to mucous membranes, salivary glands, and bone and muscles of the face. These manifest as:

- radiation mucositis;
- xerostomia;
- taste loss;
- nutritional deficit;
- oral infections;
- 'radiation caries';
- trismus; and
- osteoradionecrosis.

Radiation mucositis

Mucosal cells of the oral cavity, pharynx and larynx have high turn over rates and low radiation resistance. As a result, radiation mucositis may appear by the beginning of the second week of a conventional irradiation protocol. Patients may experience difficulties with speech and symptoms of a sore throat in addition to pain, burning and discomfort, and dysphagia if the pharyngeal mucosa is in the treatment zone. The severity of the symptoms may be such that treatment may need to be suspended and the patient hospitalised for fluid and nutritional support. Suspension or cessation of treatment, or reduction of treatment dose, may compromise the patient's prognosis.

Xerostomia

Salivary glands are susceptible to the effects of ionising radiation, and radiation-induced xerostomia is a common and significant consequence of head and neck radiotherapy.

It is rapid in onset, progressive, persistent and largely irreversible at higher doses of radiation. Given the importance of saliva in the maintenance of oral health and the markedly increased proportions of streptococcus mutans and lactobacilli in xerostomic individuals, it is not surprising to find that a reduction in salivation may lead to a rapid, debilitating deterioration of oral health, and subsequent reduction of quality of life.

Management of xerostomia

Management of xerostomia is aimed at symptomatic relief, prevention or correction of the results of salivary dysfunction and treatment of any underlying disease. Treatments include increased hydration by way of frequent, small sips of water. Patients are encouraged to carry water in plastic water bottles or small aerosol bottles. Increased humidity using either cool or hot mist vaporisers at bedside may help with the disruption of sleep often experienced by xerostomic patients. Moisturisers and emollients applied to the lips are essential. Lanolin and creams containing vitamin E are well tolerated.

Efforts to improve salivary output range from simple techniques such as vigorous chewing of low caloric foods or sugarless chewing gum to acupuncture.

For the majority of patients the use of sugarless chewing gum is the most cost-effective means of stimulating salivary flow. However, it should not be used as a substitute for meticulous oral hygiene measures.

Chewing hard cheese elicits a rapid rise in plaque pH following a sucrose rinse. Cheese chewing also raises plaque calcium and phosphate levels, and facilitates enamel rehardening.

Taste loss

Taste loss is a common consequence of head and neck radiotherapy. This is to be expected given the role of saliva as a mediator of taste. Taste sensation is partially restored within 60 days and is almost always completely restored by four months post-radiation, although some patients are left with residual loss of taste sensation.

Nutritional deficit

After enduring radiation-induced xerostomia, mucositis, loss of taste and possible prior surgery, it is little wonder that many head and neck radiation patients become nutritional casualties, often losing any interest in food. The very act of eating becomes a painful and a less pleasurable prospect. Patients are restricted to soft, bland, often nutritionally deficient foods. Those patients who have undergone additional chemotherapy may also experience nausea and vomiting. Mastication and swallowing are often so difficult that **parenteral feeding** may be required to prevent dehydration and malnutrition. Hospitalisation not only increases the cost of treatment, but increases the risk of **nosocomial infections**.

Oral infections

Immunosuppressed patients are at increased risk of bacterial, fungal and viral infections. Most infections are caused by fungi, as irradiation causes shifts in the oral microflora creating favourable conditions for the emergence of candida albicans.

Candidiasis may develop well after the cessation of treatment, particularly with persistent xerostomia. Chronic forms of candidiasis present most commonly in the corners of the mouth and under dentures. This may be present even in the absence of radiotherapy. Continued smoking and alcohol consumption are also contributory factors.

Radiation caries

Xerostomia associated with radiotherapy reduces both the quantity and quality of saliva. As the plaque thickness increases, there is a simultaneous increase in the types of bacteria. Buffering capacity is reduced when salivary flow rates are low.

Radiation caries is often seen on smooth surfaces, notably incisal or occlusal, and around the neck of the tooth. Enamel appears desiccated (dried out) and is weakened, leading to progressive tooth wear and incisal chipping.

Trismus

Trismus is a common complication when the temporo-mandibular joint and masticatory muscles fall within the radiation fields, although the severity and extent is unpredictable. In severe cases, opening of the mouth is so restricted that existing dentures cannot be inserted, new prostheses cannot be constructed, and nutritional status and oral hygiene may suffer.

Osteoradionecrosis

Osteoradionecrosis (ORN) represents one of the most serious complications of head and neck irradiation. It involves death of bone cells due to radiation damage, with an ensuing chronic infection of bone (osteomyelitis). There is an ongoing **sequestration** of dead and infected bone.

The most commonly affected site is the mandible. Cases affecting the maxilla are rare. Advanced cases may lead to chronic pain, **sloughing** of soft tissues (gingiva), pathologic fracture, bad breath and pussy discharge.

Dental extractions are considered a risk factor for ORN. Most studies agree that while patients requiring pre-radiotherapy extractions are at higher risk of developing ORN than patients who did not require extractions, post-treatment extraction of teeth in the radiation fields is considered a significant risk factor.

Management of stomatotoxic consequences of radiotherapy

The above-named complications can drastically reduce a patient's quality of life. Some of these complications are unavoidable but transitory. Others vary in their severity depending on radiation fields, volume, dose and duration of treatment. Steps should be taken to minimise the harmful effects of these complications.

The first step in minimising the impact of the anticipated complications of head and neck radiotherapy is a comprehensive pre-treatment assessment.

Tooth removal accounts for the vast majority of trauma-related ORN. Therefore, all teeth located within the primary beam of the radiation portal should be closely examined and an assessment should be made regarding the prognosis of these teeth.

A high degree of patient awareness and motivation is essential to minimise the serious dental complications imposed by radiotherapy. Unmotivated patients are to be seriously considered for a regimen of aggressive pre-treatment extractions.

■ **parenteral feeding:** nutrients administered by infusion or injection, not through the alimentary canal. ■ **sequestration:** separation or splintering of a part of bone. ■ **nosocomial infection:** hospital-based infection. ■ **sloughing:** dead tissue separating from live tissue. ■ **immunosuppressed:** weakened resistance to infection possibly as a result of disease (e.g. HIV) or medication (e.g. chemotherapy).

Oral hygiene measures

Given the hostile oral environment produced by radiotherapy to the head and neck, it is hardly surprising to find meticulous oral hygiene featuring so prominently in pre- and post-irradiation protocols. Oral hygiene involves brushing, rinsing and flossing, and these elements are to be rigorously observed throughout the patient's life if dental disaster is to be averted.

Regular rinsing with saline, hydrogen peroxide, or sodium bicarbonate solutions (in various concentrations) has long been advocated. Sodium bicarbonate rinses are used extensively to elevate salivary pH and buffering capacity. They also suppress the overgrowth of acid-producing micro-organisms, especially mutans streptococci, and improve taste function in xerostomic individuals. Vigorous rinsing with one teaspoon of baking soda in a glass of water several times a day is encouraged. Fresh mouthwash should be prepared at least daily, and care should be taken not to ingest the solution.

Endocrine disorders

Diabetes

Diabetic patients may be stabilised medically on insulin (Type I diabetes) and with controlled diet, or often with diet alone (Type II). Patients with diabetes often have swollen and painful gingiva, may suffer from xerostomia, acetone breath and toothache. They are often slow healing. At the dentist's discretion, the patient may be given antibiotics to minimise infection after oral surgery.

Diabetics are also more likely to develop oral infections and periodontal disease. These can be severe and rapidly progressing. Diabetics also often experience xerostomia, oral candidiasis (thrush), and burning mouth and/or tongue.

Artificial saliva and fluoride rinses are often suggested for diabetics.

Appointments should be made for soon after meal times to prevent the patient having an insulin reaction due to a drop in blood sugar as a result of even slight emotional stress from dental treatment. Patients should be asked to have a normal meal before their appointment.

Techniques should be used to relax the patient and this can include soothing music and hypnosis, as well as oral sedatives.

Hypothyroid

Adults with this condition may have an enlarged tongue, delayed tooth eruption, periodontal disease and may be slow to heal.

In children, the condition may cause malocclusion, a protruding tongue, swollen gums, and an increased risk of gum disease and tooth decay. The teeth may not be properly shaped.

This condition occurs when the thyroid gland does not produce sufficient hormones. Most people diagnosed with this condition take medication to alleviate it. However, if the condition is not under control, they may have complications if treated with some sedatives and analgesics. The dentist will usually consult with the patient's doctor before beginning treatment.

Hyperthyroid

This condition is caused by an overactive thyroid gland. People with hyperthyroidism may experience severe gum disease. They are susceptible to potentially fatal hyperthyroid crises if they experience stress, pain or infection.

The dentist will consult with the patient's doctor before beginning treatment. People with hyperthyroidism can have severe cardiac problems and are very sensitive to some anaesthetics.

Neurological conditions

Neurological conditions are disorders of the nervous system. Patients will present with many different neurological conditions. Often these patients will be taking medication that can result in xerostomia and the associated oral health complications it causes. Mouthwashes, artificial saliva and manual floss holders are often recommended for these patients.

Where patients have a condition that impairs their ability to communicate, it may be advisable to request a carer to attend with them, or to schedule a slightly longer appointment that allows for clarification of information.

Patients with neurological conditions should be encouraged to have dental examinations at least twice a year, especially to manage caries and periodontal disease, and to correct defective bridges or dentures.

Many patients and their carers benefit from dental health education and a home care regime, especially in relation to the clients specific condition. This regime should be clearly explained and demostrated.

Patients who do not use electric toothbrushes may benefit from using them. In the advanced stages of the condition, if patients lose dexterity with their hands, a carer should take responsibility for their oral health care. The carer also requires education on best methods to use and should be advised on basic infection control procedures.

Epilepsy

Epileptic patients usually receive medication to control fits or seizures. These seizures can take the form of *petit mal seizures* which are brief (usually less than 30 seconds) and which may be barely noticeable. The patient may shake slightly or blink rapidly or stare into space.

Grand mal seizures are more significant and can be followed by loss of consciousness.

Patients with managed epilepsy usually only require routine dental treatment and should continue with their normal medication.

The drug most commonly used, Dilantin (phenytoin sodium), causes enlargement of the gums, which in extreme cases may cover the teeth. The use of chlorhexidine gluconate gel brushed on the gums will improve oral hygiene and remove inflammation, thus reducing the gum overgrowth by up to 50 per cent. Some patients can have their seizures controlled by newer drugs that do not cause gum enlargement.

Epileptic patients undergoing general anaesthesia must take their medication at the prescribed time, even during pre-anaesthetic fasting, to avoid the danger of fitting during or when recovering from the anaesthetic.

Stroke

Strokes can cause weakness, paralysis and speech difficulties as well as many other health complications. Patients present with a wide range of different symptoms of varying severity.

The dentist may wish to consult with the patient's doctor before beginning treatment.

Multiple sclerosis

This condition causes degeneration of the central nervous system. It can progress rapidly or slowly but is extremely debilitating and eventually causes paralysis.

As the muscles weaken or suffer from loss of control, good oral hygiene can be difficult to maintain. Additionally, paralysis may occur in facial or neck muscles. Selection of a good toothbrush may assist in better teeth cleaning.

Patients who wear dentures may have difficulties with their size and fit as the disease progresses.

Some patients experience spasms and may benefit from mild sedation. The dentist will consult with the patient's doctor if necessary. If they are wheelchair-bound, some patients will prefer to be treated in their wheelchair. Some patients will find it difficult to hold their mouths open for extended periods or to control their swallowing or the movement of their tongue.

Parkinson's disease

This disorder causes degeneration of nerves in the brain. This results in loss of muscle strength and tremors. As with many other neurological conditions, the common medications cause xerostomia. Because of decreased ability to brush teeth, many of these patients also have increased dental cavities and dental plaque, gum inflammation and periodontal disease, tooth mobility and pain.

Patients with dentures also find that the dentures do not fit properly over time.

Alzheimer's disease

In this disease, patients suffer from dementia, which develops over a period of time. Some patients have rapid deterioration of mental function (including loss of memory, increased confusion, depression and sometimes behavioural change) while in others it can occur over many years.

Often these patients have xerostomia caused by their medication. This has an impact on oral health, which may already be deteriorating because of reduced dental hygiene practices.

Appointments can sometimes be eased if they are scheduled during the patient's 'best time of the day' and if a carer remains with the patient. More information can be found in Chapter 36.

Cerebral palsy

People with cerebral palsy often have malocclusion. They might be grinding their teeth and often have difficulty with swallowing. Many will also have difficulty chewing. Additionally, some seizure medications cause gum overgrowth.

Patients may need to be treated in their wheelchair and may need assistance holding their mouths open for extended periods of time. Severe cases may need to be treated under general anaesthesia.

Musculoskeletal disorders

These are disorders of the bones, joints and muscles.

Arthritis

Patients with arthritis suffer from painful, inflamed and stiff joints. Some take aspirin and corticosteroids for relief of symptoms. Many will find sitting for extended periods to be quite painful.

Muscular dystrophy

Muscular dystrophy is a genetic condition that progressively causes weakness of the muscles. This affects the patient's ability to maintain good oral hygiene as they have trouble brushing and flossing. In the early stages of the condition, good selection of brushes and other oral health care needs can relieve some of this problem.

Some patients will need to be treated in a wheelchair and many will find sitting in the dentist's chair very uncomfortable.

In the later stages of the condition, many patients will have difficulty holding their mouths open or controlling their tongue movements. Additionally, the wastage of muscles will make breathing difficult and many patients lose their ability to cough.

Sedation and general anaesthesia should be avoided.

Osteoporosis

Osteoporosis is sometimes linked with bones of the oral cavity. This can cause loss of teeth and residual ridge resorption, which may result in difficulty in wearing dentures. It can also affect dental implant stability.

Women with osteoporosis are also at risk of developing periodontal disease and losing their teeth.

Patients with intellectual disabilities

As with any patient, patients with intellectual disabilities may be apprehensive about dental treatment. However, handicapped patients, especially children, have more limited resources for dealing with a stressful situation and require even more care and consideration. Patients who are too agitated may require sedation or anaesthesia. For this reason, it is important to practise prevention, and not crisis care.

Visits to the dentist should occur every three to four months. Carers may need special oral health education to give them the knowledge and skills they need to help the patient maintain good oral health. An electric toothbrush properly used by the patient, family member or carer can prevent plaque build-up.

Chlorhexidine gluconate brushing gel (or mouth rinse) can reduce plaque accumulation that leads to caries and periodontal disease. This can be used by the patient or applied by parents or carers by brush or special chewing brush applicator. Sodium fluoride gel (or mouth rinse) can also be used at home and helps to reduce the incidence of dental caries. Often, patients with intellectual disabilities cannot use a mouth-rinse efficiently, and the toothbrush applied gel is more suitable.

Routine conservative dental procedures should be undertaken as soon as caries is detected. The dentist may refer a child patient to a specialist paediatric dentist or hospital for more extensive treatment under pre-medication, relative analgesia, intravenous sedation, or general anaesthesia, as these patients are 'at greater risk' than the normal patient. With the healthy but older child or adult with a disability, it is possible for the general dental practitioner to carry out routine care in the surgery.

You can help both the patient and dentist a great deal by your understanding and by competent, sympathetic handling of the patient. If a parent or carer accompanies the patient, they should usually remain in the dental surgery in front of the patient, to assist with communication and comfort.

A detailed medical history is essential. This will be recorded by the dentist, you should familiarise yourself with the medical condition and its treatment. You should know how to help the dentist in the event of the patient's collapse, and where the resuscitation drugs and equipment are kept.

Behavioural, psychological and social disorders

As with the neurological disorders, these disorders are often treated with medications that can cause xerostomia. Additionally, some of the disorders, such as depression and schizophrenia, can result in inadequate dental hygiene. Treatment may need to be undertaken with the knowledge that dental hygiene will not improve until the condition is controlled.

Anorexia

Anorexia is a psychological condition, predominantly among young people, where the patient obsessively fasts. The consequence of this is that they do not get the nutrients required to maintain a healthy oral cavity.

Bulimia

Bulimia is a condition in which the patient induces vomiting after eating in order to reduce their calorie intake.

This vomiting can cause swelling of the salivary glands, chronic sore throat and small haemorrhages under the skin of the palate. It can erode the tooth enamel, especially on the lingual side of the upper front teeth. It can also lead to malocclusion if the back teeth are severely eroded. Malnourishment can also increase periodontal disease.

Patients who do not have their bulimia under control should be encouraged to brush their teeth and rinse their mouth with water after vomiting. Artificial salivas and fluoride mouthwashes might also be recommended. Some patients have an appliance made to cover their teeth and protect them from stomach acids.

Substance abuse related disorders

These may be related to legal substances (e.g. cigarettes, alcohol, tranquillisers and sedatives) or illegal substances (e.g. narcotics, amphetamines, etc). In many cases, substance abuse is accompanied by poor oral hygiene caused by neglect. However, with methadone (used as a heroin substitute under medical supervision), problems can be caused by the high sugar content as well as neglect.

It is important that the dentist be aware of a patient's substance abuse so that there are no complications caused by it. If you suspect that the patient may have an addiction or dependence, you should alert the dentist.

Pregnant patients

Good oral hygiene is essential during pregnancy and the patient might benefit from additional oral health education. Increases in oestrogen and progesterone during pregnancy may result in increased plaque, which can cause gingivitis. This can lead to periodontal disease. There is also an increased risk of 'pregnancy tumours', which are growths that develop on irritated swollen gums. These are normally left untreated.

It is safe to see the dentist while pregnant but anaesthetics should be avoided. Dental radiography is safe during pregnancy. Most patients see their dentists in the first or second trimester. Third trimester visits may cause discomfort if the patient needs to remain in the chair for extended periods.

Summary

It is important that all members of the dental health team pay particular attention to the emotional wellbeing of patients with systemic or chronic illness, or with intellectual or physical disabilities. Many of these patients have an added difficulty with communication and may find their anxiety difficult to express and control. Some patients may become aggressive if frustrated or scared.

Because of the complexity of treating patients with these conditions, there are specialist clinics available for patients with physical, developmental and psychological disabilities.

Your role, as you assist the dentist, may change for patients with special needs. There may be specialised techniques or equipment you will need to be familiar with. If you are unsure about these techniques or equipment, and the patient senses this, it may cause them to be more nervous, uncomfortable and unsettled during treatment.

You may also be responsible for providing information to the patient or the patient's family. You may be required to assist the family with a dental health program for the patient.

Procedures in the case of medical emergency are considered in Chapter 22 and should be regularly revised. Delay in action can be fatal and it is imperative that you be completely familiar with and practise the emergency routine to be carried out.

chapter thirty
removable prosthodontics

Introduction

Prosthodontics (also called dental prosthetics) deals with the replacement of missing teeth and tissues of the mouth with an appliance called a prosthesis.

Mention should also be made of maxillo-facial prosthetics. This is a branch of removable prosthodontics dealing with the restoration of appearance and, where possible, the function of tissues and/or teeth following their loss. This loss may be the result of disturbances of development, accident, surgery when treating malignant disease, or other causes. An example of an extra-oral maxillo-facial prosthesis is illustrated later in this chapter.

The use of implants is becoming increasingly important in both full and partial denture construction. They are considered in Chapter 26.

Considerations in removable prosthesis construction

Many factors must be taken into account when constructing an appliance or appliances for a patient regardless of whether the appliance is a partial or full **denture**. A variety of both extra- and intra-oral considerations must include such things as:

- patient motivation;
- ability to adapt to a prosthesis both mentally and physically;
- the age of the patient;
- economic factors;
- dietary habits;
- the amount of residual alveolar ridge(s);
- the condition of the oral mucosa and associated tissues;
- the status of any residual teeth.

Role of the dental assistant

There are five important aspects of assisting in prosthodontics.

❶ Appointment making. Appointments are usually arranged in advance. You should be informed of the treatment plan to allow adequate time for return of laboratory work that must be carried out between appointments. Remember that weekends and holidays are excluded from laboratory working time.

❷ Card entry making and recording. As instructed by the dentist, details must be entered on both treatment charts and laboratory instruction cards.

❸ Care of equipment and materials. All items must be cleaned and sterilised or appropriately decontaminated and set out as required. Materials require careful handling and storage.

❹ Assisting with treatment as part of the team.

❺ Assisting with the patient.

Complete dentures

See an example of a complete denture in Figure 30.1.

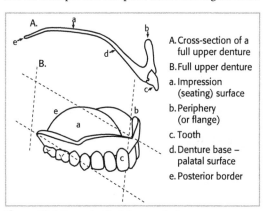

A. Cross-section of a full upper denture

B. Full upper denture

a. Impression (seating) surface

b. Periphery (or flange)

c. Tooth

d. Denture base – palatal surface

e. Posterior border

Figure 30.1 The parts of a full upper denture

■ **denture:** a set of artificial teeth that replaces all or some of the patient's real teeth.

The effects of total tooth loss

- There is loss of lower face height because of the decrease in the vertical dimension that results from loss of the teeth.

- There can also be harmful effects to the temporomandibular joint. Degenerative changes and re-modelling of the articulating surfaces can occur if vertical dimension is not restored by prostheses.

- Because of loss of alveolar ridge height, muscle attachments appear to reduce the depth of the vestibular sulcus.

Materials used in the construction of dentures

Materials that are used in denture construction but also in other forms of dentistry (impression materials, for example) are discussed in Chapter 23.

Denture base materials

Acrylic resin (polymethyl methacrylate)

Acrylic resin has been the most commonly used denture base material for many years. It has the following properties:

- a colourless, transparent plastic;
- light, clean and odourless;
- stable in temperatures below 75°C;
- relatively strong but may break on impact;
- may be dissolved (crazed) in some liquids (e.g. alcohol);
- supplied as a powder (polymer) and a liquid (monomer) — these are mixed to form a dough, which is then packed into a mould and processed.

Pigments are usually added to give colour to the gum tissues. This pigmentation may be varied in specific areas to 'characterise' the denture. In some cases the palate of the denture may be clear.

It is possible to have an allergy to acrylic resin or the colouring matter used, but this is rare.

Gold alloys

Gold alloy denture base materials contain gold together with platinum, palladium, silver and copper. These alloys are rarely used instead of acrylic resin for full dentures but have the following advantages:

- very high strength;
- may be cast to fit very accurately; and
- resist wear and abrasion.

A disadvantage is that it is difficult to modify the tissue fitting surface to compensate for changes that occur in the denture supporting tissues over a period of time.

Chromium-cobalt alloys

Chromium-cobalt alloys have great strength, even in thin sections. Both chromium-cobalt and, less commonly, gold alloys are used in partial dentures.

Patients with a powerful bite who have a history of fracturing dentures may require some kind of mesh metal framework to support the acrylic resin of a full denture.

Vulcanite

Vulcanite was a material almost universally used before acrylic resin became available, and as such is of historic interest only. It was a rubber material that came in 'gum' pink and base colours, pieces of which moulded together and formed the denture when processed (vulcanised) under heat and pressure. You are unlikely to see a vulcanite denture these days.

Additional materials for partial dentures

For partial dentures the method of impression-taking is different from full denture impression-taking because it is necessary to obtain an accurate **impression** of many teeth that are irregular in shape and inclination. For this reason, the material used must be tough and elastic so that it will pull out from the teeth and then return to its original shape. Three such materials are alginate, elastomeric materials (both discussed in Chapter 23) and agar.

Agar, or reversible hydrocolloid, is an extremely accurate material. It is a reversible material that softens on heating and returns to an elastic gel on cooling. This material is supplied in a plastic envelope and must be prepared by boiling for ten minutes, after which it may be stored at 80°C for any period before use. Just before being used, it is placed in a water-cooled tray and 'tempered' in a bath at 45°C for three minutes. Like alginate, it will not adhere to metal, so all water-cooled trays are perforated to retain the material. It should also be cast immediately after removal from the mouth, but may be left for a short period in a moist atmosphere.

impression: a negative likeness obtained by using an impression material. Dental impressions are taken of the teeth and supporting tissues, and models are cast from them.

Tissue conditioning materials

In addition to bony resorption, there is some flattening or distortion of the underlying soft tissues after complete dentures have been worn for a few years The tissues will recover after resting. So that impressions for new dentures are not taken with the tissue in this state of distortion, a material has been devised that is applied to the under-surface of the old dentures and kept in place for a few days to allow for tissue recovery. Under some circumstances, tissue conditioning materials may also be used for making impressions.

Soft lining materials

A number of different products are used as soft lining materials; for example vinyl resins, vinyl-acrylic resins and silicone rubbers. They are sometimes used when a patient is unable, because of tissue soreness, to adapt to the normal hard acrylic tissue fitting surface of the denture. In general, the heat-processed materials usually adhere better and the silicone types retain their softness much longer than the other kinds of liners.

The use of soft linings can only be regarded as a temporary measure, and inspection and replacement is generally required at regular intervals. Some soft lining materials may be damaged by soaking in overnight denture cleaning solutions.

Grinding and polishing materials

Grinding and polishing operations are used frequently during denture construction. Examples are:

- trimming impression trays and base-plates;
- grinding porcelain or acrylic teeth; and
- adjusting and polishing dentures.

An assortment of burs, trimmers and stones are required.

The chief polishing agents used for acrylic resin are pumice and tin oxide paste. These are applied when the denture is polished by means of cloth wheels on a dental lathe.

Infection control procedures in relation to denture adjustments are described in Chapter 14.

Instruments

Although varied by individual preferences, a standard set-up for prosthodontic treatment consists of:

- mouth mirror;
- dressing forceps;
- pair of calipers and/or a Willis gauge (see Figure 30.2);
- denture bowl;
- gauze squares;
- gentian violet or indelible pencil; and
- millimetre scale.

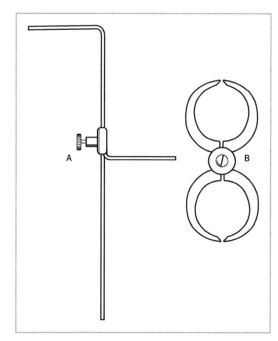

Figure 30.2 A: Willis gauge B: figure-of-eight calipers

The Willis gauge is a simple measuring device used to measure the proportions of the face and determine the vertical dimension which is the distance between the upper and lower jaws. Various forms of calipers or dividers may be required for measurements according to the dentist's preference.

The following instruments are typical requirements to be added to the basic prosthodontic treatment set-up listed above, as is appropriate for the procedure being carried out. Such requirements are usually specified by the individual dentist.

Burs

Large metal or tungsten carbide burs (either pear-shaped or round) in slow speed, straight handpieces are used for gross trimming of base-plates or denture adjustments. Small round burs (numbers 3 to 8) may be used for final adjustments to denture bases or cutting grooves in **models** or **casts**. Flat fissure burs of suitable size may also be used for cutting acrylic.

■ **model** or **cast**: a model of the impression of the jaws or other structures, usually poured in a type of artificial plaster or stone.

Trimmers

Large pear-shaped carborundum or alumina trimmers are used for grinding down acrylic bases or adjusting the thickness of the denture periphery. These may be used either with a dental engine and straight handpiece or a dental lathe.

Stones

Small mounted stones, either round or tapering, are used for making adjustments to the denture base. Wheel stones may be used during the try-in visit to grind porcelain or acrylic teeth in order to modify their shape or arrangement. Such stones are also used after the dentures have been processed for perfecting the occlusion.

With porcelain teeth, diamond stones of various shapes are often employed. After grinding, the teeth must always be polished. Rubber impregnated wheels and cones are useful for repolishing porcelain teeth.

For impressions

- Impression trays
- Rubber bowl and mixing spatula
- Compound knife (sharp) if compound is being used, or other impression materials
- Tray adhesive.

For registration and tooth selection

- Models and **occlusal rims** from laboratory
- Wax knife and wax spatula
- Le Cron carver
- Mould guide — shade guide
- Modelling wax and bite wax
- Face-bow
- Occlusal plane guide
- Some form of gas burner.

For try-ins

- Articulated models with teeth set-up in wax
- Wax spatula
- Le Cron carver
- Modelling wax
- Bite wax
- Some form of gas burner
- A large viewing mirror.

For insertion of dentures and adjustments

- Completed dentures — decontaminated and stored in water or sealed plastic bag
- Articulating paper
- Acrylic burs and artificial stones
- Disclosing wax
- Modelling wax (bite wax) and a wax knife
- A large viewing mirror.

All materials that have been in the mouth (such as impressions, occlusal records, bite rims, try-ins, dentures, and so forth) must be appropriately decontaminated before being handled in the laboratory, and again on their return from the laboratory.

In Table 30.1, the series of stages in complete denture construction, including both surgery and laboratory steps, is set out. Although these are generally accepted basic procedures, there are many variations in the procedural steps used. Each of the procedures is discussed in more detail under the following headings.

Steps in denture construction

1. Consultation

Consultation involves taking a medical history including what medications, if any, are being taken, a thorough oral examination including any necessary radiographs, such as a panoramic film (OPG), and any necessary photographs. The medical history could reveal, for example, a condition such as diabetes that could influence the ability of tissues to tolerate a denture. Similarly, medications could influence saliva flow and cause a dry mouth, and this may cause problems in the retention and comfort of the prosthesis.

It is necessary to discuss fully with the patient the proposed treatment plan, results to be achieved, and possible difficulties that may be encountered. In addition, the estimated fees may also be a part of this appointment. All details of the treatment plan should be recorded on the patient's record.

Following this consultation any procedures that are necessary before denture construction is commenced are completed. These could be surgical; for example, retained teeth or roots, soft tissue correction, removal of bony prominences or implant insertion. Operative procedures may be involved if an **overdenture** is prescribed. The use of soft tissue conditioners could be indicated.

Clinical procedures	Laboratory procedures
1. Consultation, history and examination. Discussion of treatment plan and estimated fees.	
2. Taking of primary impressions, in compound or alginate, using stock impression trays. Decontamination of impression before they go to the laboratory.	
3.	Pouring study casts. Constructing special trays in shellac or acrylic.
4. Taking final accurate impressions using special tray. Decontamination of impression before they go to the laboratory.	
5.	Pouring final casts. Constructing temporary base plates and occlusal rims (bite blocks).
6. Record taking. Determining the tooth positions using the occlusal rims. Registering jaw relationship. Taking face bow record. Selecting the teeth.	
7.	Positioning the casts in their relation to each other on an articulator. Setting up teeth in wax.
8. Positioning the casts in their relation to each other on an articulator. Setting up teeth in wax.	
9.	Making any necessary modifications to the set-up (clinical and laboratory).
10. Final try-in and check of occlusion. Decontamination of impression before they go to the laboratory.	
11.	Dentures processed and polished.
12. Insertion of dentures.	
13. Making post-insertion adjustments and occlusal check record. Decontamination of impressions before they go to the laboratory.	
14.	Remounting dentures on articulator for occlusal grinding.
15. Dentures reinserted.	

Table 30.1 Procedures for making a complete denture

2. Impressions

Primary impressions may be taken at the initial appointment or at a subsequent visit. Alginate is usually the material of choice for these impressions. Impression trays for the edentulous mouth are easily distinguished by the rounded form of the body, unlike the trays used when teeth are present. These have a square section to provide additional space for material around the teeth. Impression trays are usually of metal construction and may or may not be perforated. Disposable plastic trays are also available for use.

Lower trays differ from uppers in that space is provided to allow the tongue to remain uncovered when taking the impression (see Figure 30.3).

For impression taking, ensure that there is adequate protection for the patient's clothing and be unobtrusively ready to supply additional napkins in case of excessive salivation. At such times the dentist may prefer to use the aspirator. Mixing the impression material is part of the assistant's duties. The dentist may also require you to load the impression tray.

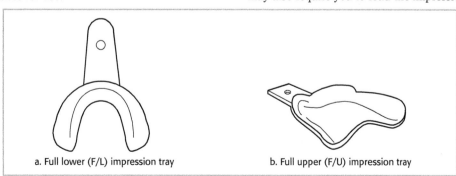

a. Full lower (F/L) impression tray   b. Full upper (F/U) impression tray

Figure 30.3 Impression trays

3. Study casts/special trays

The impressions are decontaminated and taken to the laboratory as soon as possible after they are taken and the study models poured in plaster or artificial stone. You may be required to pour these models if you have been trained to do so. In the laboratory they are then used to construct individual trays for secondary impressions as prescribed by the dentist.

If there is any unavoidable delay in pouring these models, the impressions must be kept in a moist and temperate environment to avoid distortion.

4. Final (secondary) impressions

Final impressions are taken using the impression material of the clinician's choice; usually ZOE or polyvinyl, and using a special tray.

5. Final models

After decontamination, the final impressions are taken to the laboratory and the final models are poured. Base-plates and occlusal rims are constructed on these models to the clinicians requirements.

6. Record taking

Record taking includes contouring the occlusal rims to the desired shape for aesthetics and function, determining and recording the **centric relation** and taking the **face-bow** readings.

The occlusal plane guide (Figure 30.4) is a flat metal template that some clinicians may use to indicate the inclination of the occlusal surface of the upper occlusal rim when placed in the patient's mouth.

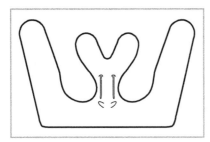

Figure 30.4 An occlusal plane guide

The face-bow (Figure 30.5) is an instrument used to locate the relationship of the upper arch to the temporo-mandibular joints (joints of the jaw). These joints are located just in front of the ears. The face-bow registration is then used to place the upper case in its correct position on the **articulator**.

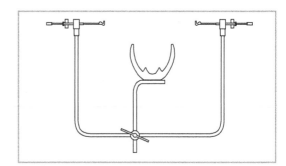

Figure 30.5 A face-bow

The artificial teeth to be used are also selected at this stage. The factors to be considered when selecting these are discussed later in this chapter.

7. Mounting models on the articulator

After registration of the jaw relationship, taking of other records and decontamination, the master casts are mounted with dental plaster upon an instrument called an articulator (Figure 30.6). This preserves the positioning of the casts. Some articulators are designed to simulate the movement of the lower jaw and thereby assist the technician in the accurate arrangement of the teeth. These articulators are termed adjustable or anatomical articulators. Those that are not adjustable are called plain line articulators.

The teeth selected are then set up (positioned) in wax.

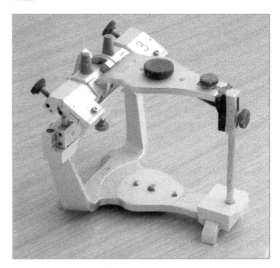

Figure 30.6 An adjustable articulator

8. First try-in

The appearance, speech, occlusal stability and retention of the dentures are checked at this stage, often with the patient in both the sitting and standing positions. Also, the patient is able to view the trial dentures and is invited to discuss their appearance. You may also be asked to comment.

If the registration of jaw relations must be changed, this may be done by taking a wax check-bite (i.e. by closing the teeth into soft wax). Naturally, if the registration of the jaw relations is changed, one of the casts (the lower) must be removed from the articulator and re-attached with fresh plaster in the new relationship.

In some instances it may be desirable to have a family member present at the try-in stage to ensure patient acceptance of the appearance of the finished denture(s).

9. Try-in modifications

When necessary, try-in modifications may be a combination of clinical and laboratory procedures. These may be carried out to adjust the occlusion, or alterations for aesthetic reasons.

10. Final try-in

Should major changes be necessary it is advisable to have a final try-in for another check of appearance, occlusion, speech, retention and stability, and to check for any further adjustments that might be required.

11. Processing and polishing

After necessary decontamination has been carried out the dentures are processed and polished. If some form of denture identification (and hence patient identification) is required, it is incorporated at this stage. A variety of methods may be used to achieve this. A metal tag or other insert within the denture plastic, inscribed with the appropriate information, is one method of denture identification.

12. Denture insertion

Dentures are inserted and again checked for appearance, stability, retention and speech.

13. Post-insertion adjustment

Any indicated minor adjustments are carried out. A new occlusal record is taken and the dentures are remounted on the articulator for occlusal adjustment.

14. Occlusal adjustment

Occlusal adjustment involves some additional adjustment of the tooth surfaces by grinding, and is advisable to ensure perfect harmony of tooth contacts during function. Any necessary grinding and polishing is usually carried out in the laboratory.

15. Denture reinsertion

The dentures are finally checked and inserted. Particular instructions in care, cleaning and use of the dentures are given. An appointment is usually made for a subsequent visit during which any further necessary adjustments may be carried out.

There is of course a great deal of variation in the above procedures according to the approach to denture construction used by the individual dentist.

Partial dentures

In general, the clinical and laboratory procedures followed in partial denture construction are similar to those in full denture construction. A partial denture (see Figure 30.7) is made up of:

- the artificial teeth, either made of porcelain or acrylic;
- clasps or attachments by which the denture is supported (occlusal rests) and retained by the remaining natural teeth (rarely you may see a denture designed without any attachments or clasps);
- a connecting frame that joins the components together — this may be constructed of acrylic resin, or metal (usually cobalt-chromium alloy, gold alloy, or stainless steel) or a combination of both acrylic and metal.

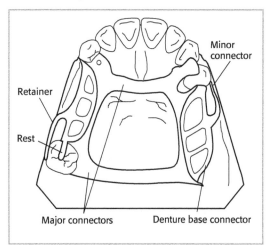

Figure 30.7 A partial denture

Nearly all partial dentures, however designed, contain some acrylic resin connecting the teeth to the base. When a cast gold or cobalt-chrome framework is used, it is frequently made in a single casting incorporating the clasps and attachments, and is termed a one-piece casting.

Another method is to construct the clasps of stainless steel or gold wire, which are then processed into an acrylic base together with the teeth. Frequently in partial dentures, a porcelain or plastic tooth would not be strong enough to withstand the force of the opposing teeth alone, and thus it must be provided with a suitable metal backing.

Procedures for making partial dentures

The clinical and laboratory procedures used in partial denture construction are similar to those used, and previously explained, in full denture construction. See Table 30.2 for a description.

Assistance during partial denture treatment

A standard prosthodontic tray for partial dentures would contain:

- mouth mirror;
- probe;
- dressing forceps;
- periodontal probe; and
- denture bowl.

To this should be added instruments and materials that are appropriate for the particular procedure, including:

- charts for history taking;
- x-ray film;
- scalers and rubber cups;
- primary impression trays (perforated or rim-lock) — impression trays for partial dentures differ in their form from those used for full dentures (the shape used depends on the presence or absence of standing posterior teeth, see Figure 30.8);
- tray adhesive;
- alginate impression materials (nearly always used for impressions for study models);
- wax knife;
- Le Cron carver;
- final impressions;
- individually constructed trays and tray adhesive;
- prepared agar, alginate or elastomeric impression materials;
- study models;
- stones or burs for tooth adjustment;
- final casts and occlusal rims if required;
- shade guides;

Clinical procedures	Laboratory procedures
1. Consultation and history. Examination and prophylaxis. Impressions for study models. Decontamination of impression before they go to the laboratory.	
2.	Cast study models.
3. Complete any necessary restorations, implant insertion and other treatment as required.	
4.	Construct individual impression trays and bite rims.
5. Design denture, perform any necessary tooth preparation for occlusal rests, etc.	
6. Final impressions. Decontamination of impression before they go to the lab.	
7.	Cast master models, duplicate them and cast working models. Construct occlusal rim(s) ('bite blocks') or construct attachments and set up teeth.
8. Registration and tooth selection. Try in cast metal framework if one is being used. Decontamination of impressions before they go to the laboratory.	
9. Try-in denture, check occlusion, make any necessary adjustments. Decontamination of impressions before they go to the laboratory.	
10.	Final wax-up and process denture(s).
11. Insertion of denture(s), check and adjust occlusion and retention.	
12. Post-insertion follow-up visit(s).	

Table 30.2 Procedures for making partial dentures

- metal casting(s) to be tried in;
- try-in;
- articulated models with trial denture(s);
- completed denture(s);
- articulating paper;
- registration wax;
- disclosing wax; and
- stones and burs for any necessary adjustments.

Immediate dentures

If a denture has been constructed before the extraction of the teeth and is inserted immediately afterwards, it is called an immediate denture. This type of denture may be either complete or partial. Sometimes these dentures are intended to be discarded after a few weeks or months and new dentures are then constructed. It is important for patients to understand the advantages and limitations of immediate dentures, and you should be able to give this information when required if trained to do so.

All immediate dentures require considerable adjustment because of changes that occur in the mouth with, and after, healing. If the correction required to the impression surface ('seating surface') of the denture is small, the denture may be relined by the addition of a thin layer of material to that surface.

If more than minimal correction is required, it is common practice to re-base an immediate denture. To correct for the changes described above during the re-basing procedure, that portion of the base of the denture in contact with the tissue is replaced and the teeth themselves are brought back into harmony with the teeth of the opposing arch.

The stages of construction for an immediate full denture are similar to the procedures described for complete dentures. However, some variations occur in the choice of impression materials and at the try-in stage.

It is not possible to try-in the dentures when the natural teeth are present. However, the patient can be assured of a natural appearance of the denture because, if desired, the arrangement of their real teeth may be copied accurately. Some patients may wish to change their appearance to one they consider more desirable.

Advantages of immediate full dentures

- There is no waiting period without a denture.
- Duplication of natural teeth is simpler since the existing appearance can be copied.
- There is quick adaptation of muscle function to the dentures.

Limitations of immediate full dentures

- Loss of retention of the denture during the first six weeks, due to mouth changes resulting from healing.
- Limitation in masticatory function (particularly on anterior teeth) as with full dentures. Necessity for relining after three months or sooner if required.

When a denture, either full or partial, is to be inserted immediately after the extraction of teeth, some special procedures are followed. Before insertion the denture is disinfected in an appropriate solution for the recommended time, as are the burs and stones that may be required for adjustment.

The patient needs to return to the practice/clinic 24 hours after initial insertion, and, until that time, the dentures should not be removed. At this visit, the denture is taken out, a prepared irrigation is used (such as warm saline) and any necessary adjustments made and the denture reinserted. Following this visit the patient is instructed to remove the denture after each meal, rinse the mouth with warm saline solution and brush the denture thoroughly.

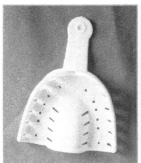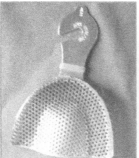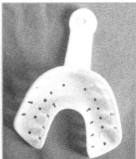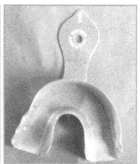

Figure 30.8 Partial upper and lower impression trays

Factors in tooth selection

Denture teeth are made of either porcelain or acrylic resin (Table 30.3). Large ranges of moulds (shapes) and shades are provided by various manufacturers. Anterior teeth are obtained in sets of six, while posterior teeth are in sets of eight for a single denture or 16 for a full denture. The sets are mounted on cards stamped with the trade name and two groups of numbers; one indicating the mould and the other the shade, e.g. Preceptor, Mould 3P, Shade R2 or Lumin Vacuum, Mould 637, Shade B2. Artificial teeth made from materials similar to the microfilled resin restorative materials are also available. These are more resistant to wear than acrylic resin teeth and do not fracture as easily as porcelain teeth if inadvertently dropped. However early types of such teeth appeared to be susceptible to staining.

The type of anterior tooth selected is influenced by:

- the shape, form, size, features and profile of the face;
- facial proportions;
- complexion and colour;
- inter-canine (between the canines) and facial width;
- smile line (lip length);
- sexual differences; and
- phonetics.

Old photographs of the patient when they had their own teeth are invaluable. Their old full dentures are also useful if the patient was happy with their appearance.

The selection of posterior teeth will be influenced by:

- the available space between the jaws;
- anterior crown height;
- mesio-distal space available;
- bucco-lingual/palatal space available;
- occlusal form — type of cusp indicated — this may be anatomic or non-anatomic (also known as flat cusp, zero degree or rational) occlusal form; and
- type of tooth selected (porcelain or acrylic).

Care of dentures

Complete dentures

- It is advisable to clean dentures thoroughly after meals, with a brush and soap, or denture cream, over a hand basin of water or a wash cloth. A scrubbing action should be avoided as it will cause abrasion. Avoid solvents and some antiseptics, as these will cause crazing of the denture. Dentures must be kept in water if not in use.

- Heavy calculus and food debris build-up may be removed by soaking the denture in undiluted white vinegar overnight and then cleaning the denture with a soft brush.

- To clean off stains and deodorise a denture it can be soaked in diluted bleach for an hour and then thoroughly rinsed.

- If completely comfortable, new dentures may be kept in place at night as an aid to muscle education. However, it is usual and beneficial to the tissues to remove dentures for a resting period. In mastication, commence slowly with non-sticky foods, and avoid the use of the incisors for biting until more accustomed to their use.

- If any tissue soreness arises the patient should return as soon as possible to have this corrected.

Partial dentures

In addition to the above, patients with partial dentures should be instructed that:

- Special care must be given to the cleaning of all natural teeth and the gingivae which are covered by the denture. Special instructions should be given in the particular methods required in each case.

Acrylic	Porcelain
Soft	Hard
Not wear resistant	Wear resistant
Can withstand impact	Break on heavy impact
Natural appearance	Natural appearance
Burn on heating in flame	Will not burn
Direct bond (chemical attachment to denture base acrylic)	Pins or undercuts are necessary for attachment to the base acrylic

Table 30.3 Comparison of the properties of acrylic and porcelain teeth

- The denture must be removed after each time food is taken and at least rinsed to remove debris. It must be brushed twice per day as shown.

- The denture must be left out of the mouth at night, unless otherwise instructed.

- The patient must return for examination at six-monthly intervals so that any changes in gingival tissues due to the wearing of the denture may be noted, and corrections made to prevent any periodontal problems becoming established.

Repairs and additions

Acrylic dentures may be repaired by a laboratory process in which a plaster model or key is made around the denture so that the broken parts may be prepared and replaced. The repair material may be of either the same acrylic base material as the broken denture, or a cold-curing acrylic resin that hardens quickly at room temperature. Broken parts of dentures and missing teeth may be replaced, although it is sometimes necessary to first take a small impression in compound or in alginate.

The dentist will decide the necessary procedure to be followed to repair the denture before it is taken to the laboratory. For example, it may not be possible to satisfactorily repair some dentures and others may require an impression. It is also important to find out the reason for the breakage, as this may influence the treatment. All repaired dentures should be checked and re-inserted by the clinician.

Patients should be instructed never to attempt to repair their denture themselves using superglue, for example. Such efforts can complicate and make a proper repair very difficult.

Maxillo-facial prosthetics

Maxillo-facial prosthetics is a branch of prosthodontics dealing with the restoration of appearance and function following extra- or intra-oral loss of tissues. Such loss may be the result of disturbances of development, accident, malignant disease and surgery, or other causes.

Every attempt is made to restore the appearance of the patient, and this is done once healing and any skin grafting is satisfactory. Prostheses are usually made of tinted acrylic resin or medical grade Silastic, although other materials may be used.

As can be seen from Figures 30.9 and 30.10, quite a natural look can be achieved.

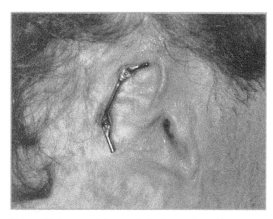

Figure 30.9 Tissue defect ready for impression taking

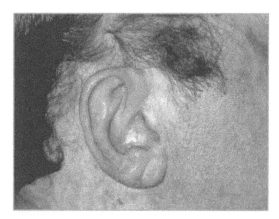

Figure 30.10 Prosthesis in place

Special adhesives and some minor utilisation of tissue undercuts are used to retain the prosthesis. Implants similar to those used to retain dentures are also employed, although radiotherapy treatment may contraindicate such a technique being used.

Summary

Although there is an increasing use of implants to replace missing teeth, dentures are still chosen by some patients. This may be for financial or other reasons. Dentures may also be used as an interim replacement for missing teeth before the placement of an implant.

In older patients, dentures are still common. The life of a denture depends on the type of materials used, patient maintenance, accidental damage and naturally occurring changes in the patient's mouth. The life of a denture may be as little as two years.

For these reasons it is likely that you will be required to assist in the construction, repair or maintenance of dentures. You must be familiar with the techniques and materials used.

chapter thirty-one

periodontics

Introduction

The two most prevalent dental diseases are dental caries and periodontal disease. Periodontics is the branch of dentistry concerned with periodontal disease.

This chapter will discuss the structure of periodontal tissues and what can go wrong with them in the common forms of periodontal disease. Treatment of periodontal diseases will also be discussed.

Some of the diseases discussed in this chapter are also referred to in Chapters 9, 11 and 27. You should refer to those chapters for additional information.

Some instruments used in periodontics are described at the end of this chapter.

Structure of the periodontium

If you look in your mouth you will notice a definite line separating the light pink gingival tissue from the darker red tissue (alveolar mucosa) lining the inside of the lips and cheeks. The mucogingival junction can be seen as a scalloped line marking the junction of the attached gingiva with the alveolar mucosa. The free gingiva is the unattached portion of the gingiva and forms the wall of the gingival crevice (gingival sulcus) (see Figures 31.1 and 31.2).

Periodontal disease

The two most common forms of periodontal disease are gingivitis and periodontitis. Gingivitis is inflammation of the gingiva. Periodontitis is inflammation of the deeper supporting tissue of the teeth. This inflammation can lead to loss of alveolar bone and periodontal ligament.

These conditions are **mixed infections** that are associated with a specific bacteria group usually found in the mouth. Whether a patient develops periodontal disease and how quickly the disease develops is dependent on the body's ability to control the bacterial infection.

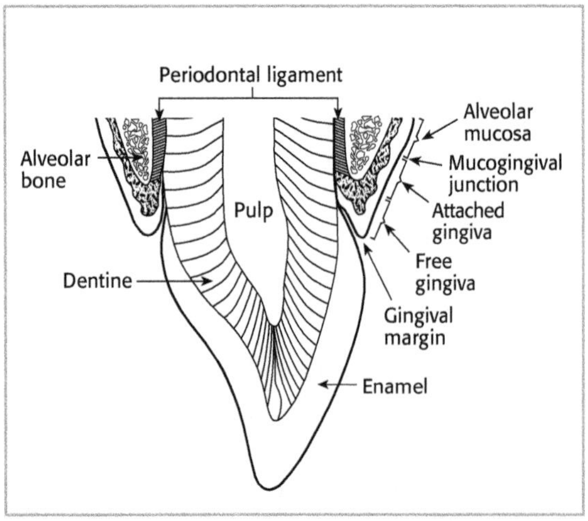

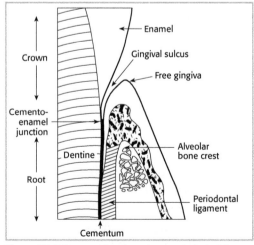

Figure 31.1 Periodontal structures viewed from proximal in longitudinal section

Figure 31.2 Cross-section through normal gingival tissues

■ **mixed infection**: an infection caused by a variety of organisms.

Development of periodontal disease

If bacterial plaque remains on the tooth near the gingival margin for a period of time, the gingiva adjacent to the plaque becomes inflamed. This inflamed gingiva appears slightly swollen, a deeper red colour, softer and less well **adapted** to the tooth than healthy gingiva. These are the classical signs of gingivitis that the dentist looks for when examining the periodontium. The signs become more obvious as the gingivitis becomes chronic. The earliest symptom of gingivitis is usually bleeding gums.

When this form of periodontal disease persists at the gingival margin for a prolonged time, the inflammation can begin to destroy the connective tissue and the alveolar bone beneath the gingiva. A periodontal pocket develops. The loss of the supporting alveolar bone leads to a loosening of teeth and the front teeth may drift from their position (see Figure 31.3).

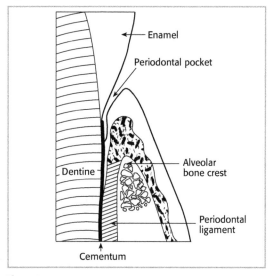

Figure 31.3 Pocket formation

Gingivitis

Gingivitis can be the result of poor oral hygiene but there are also systemic conditions that can cause symptoms. These conditions cause pathological changes, bacterial infections or hormonal changes that allow periodontal diseases to develop. Some of these conditions include leukaemia, haemophilia, Down syndrome, diabetes mellitus, HIV and pregnancy. Similar symptoms can also be caused by puberty, steroid therapy, and seizure or hypertension medications.

Development of gingivitis often accompanies stress, malnutrition and immunosuppression, especially when these are combined with poor oral hygiene. There may be a genetic predisposition to periodontal diseases. Smoking is a risk factor. The severity of the condition is proportional to the frequency and duration of smoking.

Diagnosis of periodontal disease

The signs of periodontitis may be similar to those of gingivitis or there may be few or none at all. Bleeding gingiva, unpleasant tastes, bad breath and, finally, loosening or wandering teeth are symptoms that patients with periodontitis might notice.

As the disease progresses and deep pockets are formed, much of the bleeding and redness may disappear because the site of the inflammation has become deep and hidden. In other words, there may be substantial loss of bone and yet the gingiva may appear healthy. So periodontal disease cannot be diagnosed from the patient's signs and symptoms alone.

Usually the dentist will diagnose the severity of the periodontal disease by measuring the depth of the periodontal pockets around the teeth. A periodontal probe is used to measure pocket depth. Its prime function is to determine how much bony support has been lost from around each tooth. For example, if the gingival margin is located at the cemento-enamel junction, a pocket of 6 mm means that 6 mm of support for that tooth has been lost at that point.

The dentist will also take into account the patient's medical history, occlusal problems and radiographs to determine the amount of alveolar bone loss.

The most common types of periodontal disease are:

- gingivitis, or inflammation of the gingiva;

- pregnancy gingivitis, thought to be caused by hormonal changes in the pregnant woman;

- pre-pubertal or early onset periodontitis, which is sometimes found in children at the time of the eruption of their permanent dentition;

- pubertal gingivitis, which is, as the name suggests, gingivitis that becomes more severe during puberty;

- juvenile periodontitis, found in adolescents who are otherwise healthy;

- adult periodontitis, also called adult onset periodontitis;

- periodontitis associated with systemic disease;

- acute necrotising ulcerative gingivitis (ANUG); and

- refractory periodontitis (that is, periodontitis that resists treatment).

The prevention of periodontal diseases

Prevention is wholly dependent on meticulous plaque control, particularly at the gingival margin and interproximally.

The environment is improved by the dentist or hygienist, who will eliminate plaque traps and remove all supragingival and subgingival calculus. This is essential to permit effective home care.

Patients are assisted with effective oral hygiene using toothbrushes, electric toothbrushes in some cases, and interdental aids such as dental floss, superfloss, woodsticks or interdental brushes.

Quit smoking programs are recommended.

Antibacterial mouthwashes may be prescribed in some cases. Disclosing solutions are particularly helpful in assisting patients to locate plaque deposits and monitor their own progress in controlling its formation.

Periodontal disease can be prevented by good dental hygiene. These methods are discussed in Chapter 27.

Treatment of periodontal disease

Gingivitis is a disease that can be reversed through effective treatment. This treatment eliminates or reduces inflammation and that allows the gingiva to heal. Treatment for periodontitis aims to stop the damage to supporting structures and, if possible, to repair some of the damage.

The treatment of existing periodontal disease is divided into surgical methods and non-surgical methods.

Non-surgical treatment — scaling, root planing and curettage

This is the first stage of periodontal treatment regardless of whether the patient has gingivitis or advanced periodontitis.

Once gingivitis has developed, there will usually be deposits of calculus above (supragingival) and beneath (subgingival) the gingiva. The dentist will use ultrasonic and hand instruments to remove or 'scale' these deposits. Additionally, any rough edges or overhanging margins on restorations that extend beneath the gingival margins will be smoothed off. This process is referred to as 'root planing'. It results in a smooth, clean root surface which will resist new calculus formation and enable the patient to keep the area clean.

Some patients may require gingival curettage in addition to scaling and root planing. This involves scraping the gingival lining of a periodontal pocket to remove any remaining necrotic tissue from the pocket wall.

When periodontal pockets are shallow (3–4 mm deep) these will usually disappear and the gingiva will often be restored to health by removing all subgingival calculus and rough edges on fillings, and establishing effective oral hygiene practices. Occasionally the dentist may prescribe an antibiotic if there is a risk of an infection. Mouth rinses are also effective as home treatments.

Although patients who have more advanced periodontal disease will benefit considerably from this treatment, additional treatment in the form of periodontal surgery may be necessary to prevent further periodontal breakdown. Regular periodic checks on plaque control is essential to maintain gingival health following treatment.

Surgical treatment

The most common reasons for a dentist to perform periodontal surgery are:

- to eliminate periodontal pockets;
- to gain a clear view of the roots of the teeth so the subgingival calculus can be completely removed; and
- to reshape the gingiva to make tooth cleaning easier for the patient.

The operator may treat advanced periodontal problems either with a **gingivectomy** or a flap procedure. The flap procedure, or gingivoplasty, is more commonly used because, unlike the gingivectomy, it exposes the bone around the roots of the teeth. The exposed bone can be reshaped to remove defects caused by uneven bone destruction. Any calculus remaining on the teeth is also visible for removal. After the alveolar bone is reshaped and the calculus removed, the flaps are sutured back to cover the bone. The techniques of flap surgery are discussed in Chapter 32.

Periodontal packs

These act as a protection for the gums and promote healing after surgery.

Eugenol-based packs may be used after surgery or for displacement of tissues in order to provide

gingivectomy: the surgical removal of the gingival tissue that is no longer attached to the teeth.

access. They consist of a powder and a liquid. The powder is mainly zinc oxide, resin and a **haemostatic agent**. The liquid is mostly eugenol. When mixed and applied to the gums, the paste sets to a relatively hard and sometimes brittle mass.

Non-eugenol based packs are only used after surgery. They are made from synthetic substances supplied in two tubes. When mixed together the paste sets to a relatively hard and non-brittle mass. Antiseptics are also present. These packs are less irritating to gums than eugenol packs.

Other disease affecting the soft tissues (gingiva)

Many other diseases are discussed in Chapter 12. You should refer to that chapter for more information.

Acute necrotising ulcerative gingivitis (ANUG)

This is a painful condition in which ulcers form between teeth. It used to be seen in young (male) adults who were 'run down' and often under emotional stress. It is now mostly seen in immunosuppressed organ transplant patients, people in the acute stage of drug withdrawal and those with HIV/AIDS.

It is not contagious and is probably an acute 'flare up' of what would have been simple chronic gingivitis in a healthier patient.

This condition may respond to removal of all irritants (calculus, etc.) from the teeth and mouth washes. Sometimes antibiotics (e.g. Flagyl) are used as part of the treatment. Patients should be discouraged from smoking. Patients should be instructed in effective home care.

Gingival hyperplasia

In this condition, the gingivae increases to abnormal size. Sometimes they can even cover the teeth. It can be caused as a side-affect to some drugs but it can also have a genetic component. Gingival hyperplasia is most common in people under the age of 20 and may be caused by hormonal imbalances, especially during puberty. (It also occurs during pregnancy.)

Acute herpetic gingivostomatitis

This virus infection results in blister formation and ulceration of the gums, the tongue and the insides of the cheeks and lips. The disease is very contagious. It usually affects young children and commonly spreads through a whole family.

Patients with the virus are quite ill and will refuse food because their mouths are painful. There is no specific treatment but patients can be given aspirin to relieve the pain. Patients' mouths should be kept clean by gently swabbing with a weak salt solution on cotton wool and they should be encouraged to take frequent drinks. Bed rest is advisable.

Gingivitis during pregnancy

During pregnancy the gingiva react to irritation in an exaggerated form. They tend to become more swollen and purplish-red in colour. Careful and complete scaling and removal of rough edges from fillings together with careful home care results in very rapid healing.

Periodontal abscess

Occasionally patients with deep pockets will develop abscesses due to a blockage occurring in the pockets so that pus cannot escape. This produces a moderately painful swelling of the gum over the tooth. Periodontal abscesses are treated by lancing the tissues to allow the pus to escape, and then surgically eliminating the pocket after the acute inflammation has subsided.

Gingival recession

Some people use very hard toothbrushes with and incorrect action and/or too much force. This damages the gum margins and allows micro-organisms to grow on the tooth at the edge of the gum. The result is loss of gum tissue so that the teeth appear longer. The exposed root surfaces may become sensitive. Treatment involves developing a more careful, more thorough, but less brutal, brushing method using a softer brush. Before this treatment is commenced, a desensitising paste may have to be brushed on to any sensitive root surfaces to prevent pain being felt when these surfaces are brushed.

■ **haemostatic agent:** chemical substances (medicaments) that prevent or reduce bleeding.

309

Pericoronitis

Occasionally patients present with a sore gum around an erupting tooth. This inflammation is caused by infection in the pocket of gingival tissue that covers the partially erupted tooth. Treatment may vary depending on the severity of the complaint and the tooth in question, but antiseptic mouthwashes, antibiotics, excision of the tissue flap, and removal of the tooth are all possible solutions.

Pericoronitis is most commonly seen around impacted third molars, and in severe cases may be accompanied by tenderness of the lymph glands draining the area and possibly some degree of trismus.

Instruments used in periodontics

Curettes

Curettes are types of scalers designed for the treatment of a periodontal pocket with sub-gingival curettage and the removal of calculus deposits from the root surface. These instruments should be checked regularly and sharpened when blunt. Some curettes are designed for specific tooth surfaces in particular areas of the mouth. See Figure 31.4 for examples.

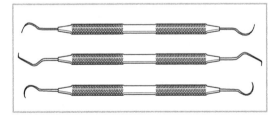

Figure 31.4 Curettes

Sharpening hand instruments

A sharpening stone (Figure 31.5) is used with oil to sharpen all hand-cutting instruments. A plastic test stick is used to check the sharpness of the instruments. The dentist will normally do the sharpening of instruments. If instrument sharpening is one of your duties, make sure you receive appropriate training beforehand.

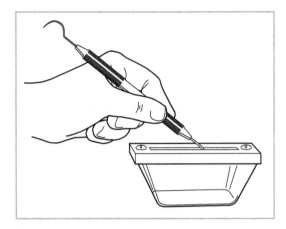

Figure 31.5 Sharpening hand instruments

Summary

Periodontal disease is primarily caused by the bacteria in dental plaque that cause inflammation in the periodontium. Periodontal disease is the most common cause of tooth loss in adults. However, it can be prevented and can also be controlled with proper treatment, even when quite advanced.

As well as assisting the dentist in procedures to treat periodontal disease you may, with the permission of the dentist, be responsible for educating the patient on the cause of the disease and its prevention. You will require a thorough understanding of the anatomical structures involved and the progress of the disease if this is your responsibility.

chapter thirty-two
oral surgery

Introduction

The quantity and type of oral surgery in general practice varies considerably. In some practices no oral surgery is performed, while in others, much oral surgery is performed.

The most common oral surgery procedures performed in general practice include:

- surgical removal of teeth and roots;
- removal of impacted teeth;
- apicectomies;
- implants; and
- periodontal surgery.

It is not within the scope of this chapter to give detailed nursing instructions for the various operative procedures, but rather to give some basic principles that govern all operative procedures.

Every operation may be divided into three basic phases:

❶ pre-operative phase;

❷ operative phase; and

❸ post-operative phase.

Instruments used in oral surgery are discussed at the end of this chapter.

The dental assistant's role in oral surgery

While assisting in oral surgery, you will be required to:

- comfort and calm the patient — most patients will be, at the very least, apprehensive, although many will deny this;
- use suction to keep the operative field clear of blood, saliva and debris;

- assist without obstructing the dentist's line of vision;
- adjust the dental light as required;
- retract tissues gently to optimise the surgical site;
- have all equipment readily available so there is no disruption of the procedure while searching for the correct instrument; and
- periodically reassure the patient.

Pre-operative phase

It is important that the dentist has an accurate medical history as this may have a direct bearing on the patient's treatment plan and the dentist's method of operating.

Many patients, particularly female patients, are reluctant to discuss their medical history with the dentist but will occasionally pass on information to the assistant. If this is the case you must pass on to the dentist any information you are given so that its significance in relation to the treatment can be assessed.

You should also impress upon patients the need for truthful answers to questions and try to make them understand that the history is not being taken with the idea of prying into their private lives, but for their own safety in relation to treatment and drugs that may be used. Some dentists prefer to give patients a written questionnaire to fill in and follow up any particular point with further questions later.

Translation of the medical history forms into various languages can be of considerable value in obtaining the necessary information from persons who do not read or speak English, or for whom English is not a first language. You will also require the patient to complete a medical history (as shown in Figure 32.1) and sign an informed consent form.

Patient/Parent's name:		Phone No:
Home address:		Post code:
Your Medical Practitioner:		Phone No:

Please answer YES or No.

Have you ever had a general anaesthetic (operation while asleep in hospital)? Yes _____ No _____

If yes, did you have any problems? (please specify) _____

When was the last time you had a general anaesthetic? _____

If no, have any family members had problems with anaesthetic? _____

Have you ever had or do you suffer from:	Yes	No
Rheumatic fever or infective endocarditis?		
Heart disease, angina or had a heart attack, heart murmur or an artificial heart valve?		
Chest pain in exercise, swollen ankles or palpitations?		
Kidney disease?		
Lung disease (bronchitis, asthma, etc.)?		
Prolonged bleeding after injury or surgery or spontaneous bleeding? Do you take Warfarin or other anticoagulants?		
Any longstanding illnesses (diabetes mellitus, epilepsy, goitre, etc.)?		
Indigestion?		
Allergies (including hay fever)?		
Complications with local analgesia or general anaesthesia?		
High blood pressure (hypertension)?		
Have you had jaundice or hepatitis?		
Porphyria, scoline apnoea or hiatus hernia? (please circle)		
A prosthetic joint (e.g. a hip replacement)?		

Are you at present, or have you recently:	Yes	No
Taken corticosteriods (within the last two years)?		
Been receiving medical treatment?		
Taking medicines, tablets or capsules for any reason? Please list them below.		
Possibly pregnant?		
Had deep ray therapy?		
Any serious operation, medical illness or stay in hospital longer than one month?		
Had an infectious disease (including colds)?		
Do you drink and/or smoke?		

Please list any medications here and any other information that you think may be relevant. _____

Figure 32.1 Sample medical history form for oral surgery patients

Premedication

The majority of patients who present for oral surgery are apprehensive. A word of encouragement and reassurance from you can be of great benefit and can go a long way towards allaying their fears. To those of us familiar with surgery, these fears may seem trivial but to the patient they are very real. In some patients the fear of surgery presents such an insurmountable psychological barrier that a sedative may have to be given prior to the operation.

The types of drugs used for premedication will vary according to the wishes and techniques used by the dentist. The most common groups include anti-anxiety agents such as diazepam or temazepam, and some antihistamines such as phenergan. The drugs may be administered orally before the scheduled appointment or, in some cases, they are given by injection at the surgery immediately before treatment.

Patients who require premedication *must* arrange for a responsible adult to bring them to the surgery and to accompany them home post-operatively. Premedication drugs frequently leave the patient drowsy and slow the reflexes so that judgment is affected. Patients should not drive or sign legally binding documents and should not be left alone for the remainder of the day.

Preparation of the surgery

It is essential that all equipment used in procedures is sterilised and *best practice* in infection control is maintained at all times.

In many surgeries the operator may find it convenient to keep prepared trays ready and sterilised for a particular procedure; for instance, for surgical removal of a fractured tooth root or **apicectomy**.

If prepared trays are not used, the sterilised instruments must remain in their pouches and should be

apicectomy: removing the apex of a tooth to enable retrograde (reverse) root filling.

placed on a sterile towel on a trolley or bracket table, covered by a further sterile towel until required for use. All instruments and towels should be handled only with sterile cheatles lifters. If this procedure is not carried out the chain of asepsis is broken and the advantages of adequate sterilisation are lost.

The sequence of events in the pre-operative phase is as follows:

- Place radiographs on the viewing screen.
- Prepare basic set-up for administration of local anaesthetic.
- Set up surgical instruments on a sterile bracket table; or place the prepared trays of instruments for a specific procedure. The number of instruments should be kept to the minimum, otherwise a tray becomes cluttered. Any additional instruments that might be needed can be kept in their sterilised pouches or wraps in a covered area at the assistant's side until the operator decides whether or not they are required.
- The patient should be comfortably seated with the head rest correctly adjusted, so that the head, neck and trunk are in a straight line. For the female patient, paper tissues should be provided to remove lipstick and excess make-up.
- Place protective goggles on the patient.
- Place drapes consisting of sterile towels or sheets over the patient to prevent contamination and to protect clothing.
- Some operators like to cleanse the patient's skin to reduce the risk of introducing foreign bacteria into the mouth. The skin may be wiped over with an antiseptic solution such as chlorhexidine.
- The patient may also be given an antiseptic mouth rinse.

The operative phase

Exodontia

Sterility in **exodontia** is as crucial as it is in other forms of surgery. Every attempt should be made to avoid the introduction of pathogenic micro-organisms.

You may occasionally be asked to support the patient's head during a tooth extraction. This will help prevent the patient's head from being moved when pressure is applied to the extraction forceps by the dentist.

Raising of flaps

In order to gain access to the deeper tissues it is necessary to raise a muco-periosteal flap. In other words, a portion of the periosteum together with the overlying mucosa is lifted from the bone as one layer. The size of the flap is carefully considered before the incisions are made. The quantity of bone that is to be removed to gain access is planned and the flap is designed so that the edges can be replaced over bone. This means extending the flap so there is good visibility. Having been raised, the flap is then held back out of the way with a retractor. This must be done gently to prevent trauma to the tissue of the flap itself.

Removal of bone

Once the flap has been retracted it may be necessary to remove the bone overlying a buried tooth, tooth root, cyst or other pathology being sought. The bone may be removed with a surgical steel bur. A sterile water or normal saline (salt) spray is essential to keep bone cool while a surgical bur is used. If bone becomes overheated it may cause a delay in healing. This water spray will also prevent the bur from clogging.

Impacted teeth

To facilitate removal of impacted teeth, it may be necessary to divide a tooth. This may be accomplished by the use of burs, or the use of burs together with an elevator. In the latter, a slot is cut and an elevator is placed and twisted. The tooth will then fracture, allowing elevation of the fragments to occur.

Special tungsten carbide oral surgery burs are available that cut bone more efficiently than normal dental burs. Teeth may be cut with ordinary small round or steel fissured burs but they become blunt more quickly.

Removal of debris

When the removal of the bone and the sectioning of tooth substance is completed, any rough edges of bone are filed and smoothed. Following this, all bone and tooth debris must be removed from the wound area. This is usually performed with a syringe filled with a sterile solution, either saline or water. The whole area is thoroughly irrigated and the slurry carefully removed with high velocity, low volume, fine bore suction. Any debris left behind can be considered as dead organic matter. This is ideal material on which micro-organisms can feed and multiply. Debris left behind may result in an infected wound, with resultant breakdown in the healing process. This cleansing of a wound is often referred to as **debridement**.

■ **exodontia:** tooth extraction.
■ **debridement:** removal of any foreign matter from tissue (e.g. root canal).

Replacing the flap

After cleansing away all debris, the tissues themselves must be repaired. Thus, the wound edges are brought together accurately and held in place by sutures, enabling healing to take place more readily.

If there is no possibility of replacing the wound edges on a firm bony base, particularly where there is a large defect beneath, the operator may pack the wound open with a material such as iodoform gauze, allowing the wound to heal by granulation. The healing in the first instance is slow and the filling in of the bony cavity takes longer.

Suturing the wound

The suturing of the wound edges may be made with two types of surgical suturing materials. The most commonly used materials are set out below.

Resorbable/soluble materials

- Plain catgut, which provides for faster healing of the mucous membrane.
- Chromic catgut which slows healing, allowing internal tissues to heal first.
- Soluble synthetic material, such as Vicryl.

Non-resorbable materials

- Black silk.
- Nylon.
- Polyester fibre.

These materials provide strength and some elasticity, but need to be removed five to seven days after surgery.

Surgical silks are plaited and treated with a silicone material to prevent any capillary action and also to prevent cells of the healing wound growing into the material which would make it difficult to remove later on. Sutures should be tied only just tightly enough to bring the wound edges together.

For patient comfort it is preferable to use a resorbable suture. This is especially important in certain groups who make visiting the dentist difficult or traumatic (e.g. small children, patients with disabilities), and patients who are travelling to an area in which there is no medical assistance.

As an approximate guide, plain gut will take some 10 to 12 days to absorb and chromic gut will take 17 to 21 days before absorption. Both silk and gut are obtainable in a variety of sizes, usually varying between 2/0 and 5/0, the 2/0 being relatively heavy material and the 5/0 being a very fine material. The most widely used size is 3/0.

You will be responsible for locking the suture needle, already threaded, into the holder and then passing it to the dentist. While the dentist is placing the suture, you will retract the cheek or the tongue. The dentist will probably cut the suture material a few millimetres from the knot, but you may be asked to do it. When the suturing is finished, the dentist will pass the materials back to you. You may also be required to mark the number of sutures on the patient's record.

Abnormal bleeding

Before suturing, the operator should ensure that bleeding has ceased and that the wound is filled with an adequate clot. In most cases, bleeding will cease spontaneously within three to five minutes but occasionally the patient will continue to bleed and action has to be taken to overcome this problem.

First, the operator will need to determine exactly where the bleeding is coming from and you can help by ensuring there is good light and suction. Once the bleeding point has been established, pressure should be applied over the area using a gauze swab or dab. Pressure is maintained for at least 10 to 15 minutes. Care should be taken to remove the gauze gently, as rough handling may cause bleeding to recommence by dislodging the formed clot, or damaging the end of a vessel wall. It should be remembered that pressure alone, if applied in the correct place for a sufficient length of time, will almost always stop haemorrhage unless that patient has a general blood abnormality. Haemorrhage can also be controlled by packing with haemostatic agents, such as oxidised cellulose. Vessels in soft tissues may need to be tied off if pressure alone fails to arrest bleeding.

In surgical procedures, a vessel within the bone may be severed and it is sometimes difficult to apply pressure to it. In these cases surgical bone wax may be pressed into the cavity in the bone, using a periosteal elevator or similar instrument, to seal it off. All excess bone wax should be removed as it tends to act as a foreign body if left in the bone cavity. Alternatively, bone overlying the bleeding point can be crushed with an instrument to enable pressure to be applied.

Post-operative stage

After all operative procedures, patients should be given clear and concise instructions to assist in promoting a rapid and trouble-free recovery period. It is desirable that they should also be given these instructions in writing to refer to when they get home (see the example in Figure 32.2). Most patients are not very receptive following a surgical procedure and will have forgotten spoken instructions almost before leaving the surgery.

Post-operative instructions

- Apply ice packs to the cheek over the area (outside the mouth).
- For the first eight hours, do not rinse out your mouth. The blood clot in the socket needs to stabilise and rinsing may dislodge it.
- Do not interfere with the surgical site. Exploring the wound with your tongue, or sucking around the wound may dislodge the blood clot. Your fingers carry disease-causing bacteria that can infect an open wound.
- You may eat or drink warm foods and drink immediately. Do not consume hot food or drink or you may burn yourself. Your mouth may still be numb from the local anaesthetic.
- After eight hours, start hot salt mouthwashes – just a pinch of salt in a tumbler of hot water, hourly for the first day and then four times daily (preferably after meals) for a week.
- Some patients may like to rub Vicks Vapourub onto the cheek skin, OUTSIDE the mouth. This sometimes acts as a counter-irritant and may help deflect the pain.
- Avoid smoking, alcohol and vigorous exercise for at least four days.
- Clean your teeth normally as soon as possible.
- Use vaseline or a similar lubricant to prevent your lips from drying out.
- Swallow normally as saliva is continually produced. Do not spit out.
- If bleeding recurs, bite on a gauze pad (or a clean handkerchief) firmly, then leave undisturbed for one to two hours. Sit upright. Do not use tissues for this as they fragment and leave fibres in the wound.
- Sleep with an additional pillow to allow you to lie in a more upright position.
- Take medicines as directed.
- Ensure you have a post-operative appointment.
- If you have any concerns, call your dentist.

Medications and your operation

For pain control, ibuprofen (e.g. ACT-3, Actiprofen, Nurofen, Rafen, Triprofen) obtained from your chemist is usually effective, or others as advised/prescribed. Preparations containing codeine are alternatives.

To minimise the risk of post-operative infection, antibiotics may be given before surgery. Further antibiotic therapy is usually not required.

Figure 32.2 Post-operative instructions

Specific instructions will vary according to the operation performed. The use of ice packs following surgery will help to minimise post-operative swelling. Two or three cubes of ice should be crushed, placed in a polythene bag and applied to the skin overlying the operative field. The application of cold contracts the capillaries in the region and prevents an excessive exudation of fluid into the tissues.

To be effective, the ice should be applied for a period of four to five hours post-operatively, with occasional removal of the ice bag to prevent acute discomfort when the anaesthetic wears off.

The dentist may prescribe an analgesic to be taken before the anaesthetic has worn off which may be taken as per manufacturer's instructions if necessary for relief of pain.

Mouthwashes

Most operators like their patients to commence hot saline mouthwashes once the blood clot has stabilised, at least eight hours after the operation. These consist of no more than a pinch of salt in a tumbler full of water, as hot as the patient can reasonably stand, hourly for the first day and then four times daily (preferably after meals) for a week.

The salt has a cleansing effect, helping to remove mucus and allowing debris to be washed away. In addition, the heat increases the blood flow to the region, increasing the presence of cells involved in the inflammatory response.

Patients should be given a further appointment before they leave the surgery for a post-operative check-up to see that they are healing normally. The precise time for this visit will vary from one practice to another, depending upon the wishes of the dentist; usually seven days following the procedure. All patients should be followed up until the dentist is certain that healing is adequate and no post-operative problems are present.

Post-operative sequelae

Post-operative **sequelae** are possible problems that might arise after surgery. They will vary with the area in which surgery has taken place and patients should be warned what to expect before leaving the surgery. For example, following third molar removal a patient may expect some swelling at the angle of the jaw, trismus and pain when the anaesthetic first wears off.

Most sequelae are quite normal and soon disappear but others, such as post-operative infection, may require treatment with antibiotics.

Dry socket

One sequel which will cause the patient intense pain is the so-called dry socket in which, for various reasons, the blood clot breaks down, giving the patient a foul taste in the mouth and leaving bare, bony walls to the tooth socket. On contact with

■ **sequelae**: events or circumstances after a procedure or event.

saliva and oral bacteria, a localised **osteitis** or inflammation of the bony lining of the socket is produced, which is accompanied by intense pain one or two days after surgery, which may even extend to four days. It can be treated by careful irrigation with warm saline followed by insertion into the socket of a suitable antiseptic and sedative dressing. A visit to the dentist/oral surgeon is essential.

Oro-antral fistula

A fistula is a tract joining a body cavity with the external or skin surfaces and is usually lined with epithelium.

Sometimes when a tooth in the upper molar region is extracted, the roots, which may protrude into the antral cavity, may cause the thin antral floor to be removed with the tooth, thus tearing the antral lining. This produces a hole from the mouth through to the antrum. Under normal circumstances the socket will fill with blood which will clot and go through the process of repair. Should the clot be lost through infection, or by the patient blowing their nose hard, there will be an empty socket across which the skin cannot grow. Instead the epithelial cells will creep across the bone. In so doing the cells will cover the socket walls, will meet and unite with the epithelial cells of the antral lining. This will then give an epithelialised tract joining a body cavity (the antrum) with the skin surface inside the mouth. This is called an oro-antral fistula. It may require surgical intervention.

Surgical instruments

Some examples of surgical instruments and tray set-ups are shown in Figures 32.3 to 32.8.

Scalpels

Non-disposable handles must be protected during sterilisation by bagging. The tendency now is to use pre-sterilised disposable blades and handles. The blades are available in various shapes. The most popular are #11 and #15.

Bone removing instruments

These include chisels, burs, files and rongeurs. It is most important that these instruments be kept sharp.

Rongeurs (Figure 32.3) are similar in shape to forceps but they have cutting edges. They are used to trim alveolar bone.

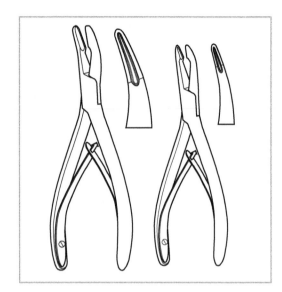

Figure 32.3 Rongeur or bone nibblers

Sutures

Be sure an adequate supply of needles for sutures is available, sterile, stored for use in sterile envelopes and ready for threading. There are different types of thread and these are discussed earlier in this chapter. Sutures are supplied by the manufacturer in sterile pouches. Ensure that the item has not expired and that the pouches have been stored to maintain sterility.

Root canal instruments

These instruments are discussed in detail in the Chapter 33, Endodontics.

Forceps

Remove all debris and blood from forceps before sterilisation. Particularly inspect the inside of the beaks where debris is harder to remove. Hinge joints are very prone to rusting and you should oil them regularly and manipulate them each day until they are moving freely. Clean the oil off the forceps before autoclaving. See Figure 32.4.

Elevators

As depicted in Figure 32.5, elevators come in various shapes and sizes. They may be used during tooth extraction to achieve leverage by loosening the tooth from the periodontal ligament. They may also be utilised to remove any residual root fragments and for lifting teeth that have been sectioned (cut vertically) with surgical burs.

osteitis: bone inflammation.

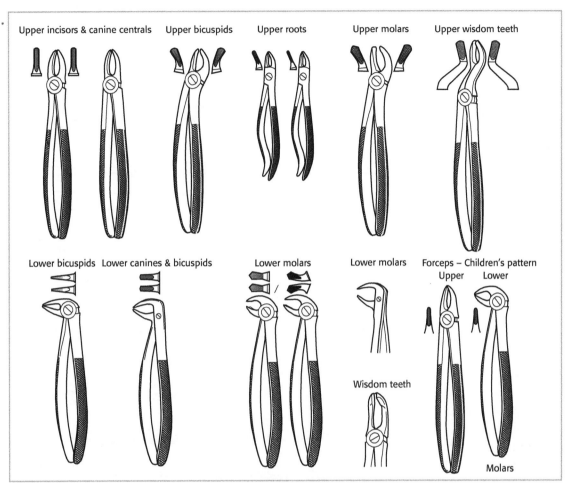

Figure 32.4 Forceps

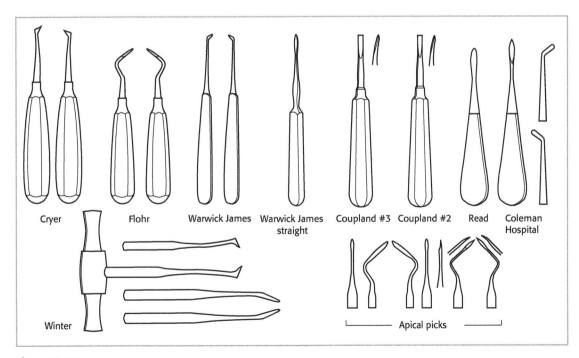

Figure 32.5 Elevators

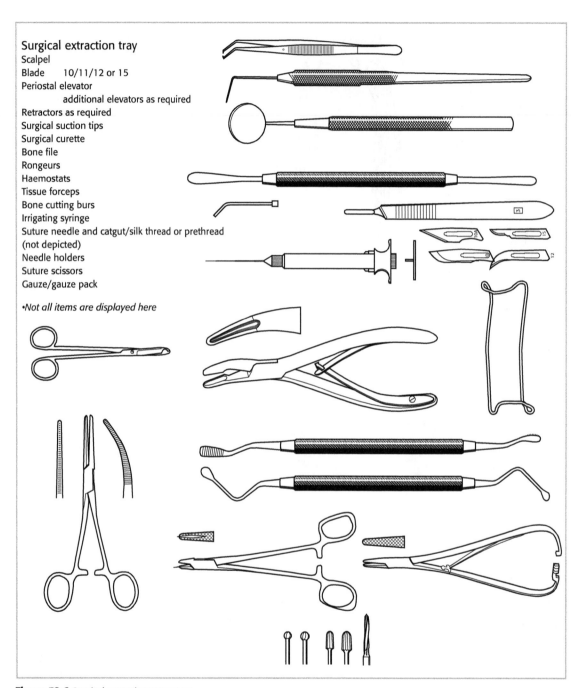

Surgical extraction tray

Scalpel
Blade   10/11/12 or 15
Periostal elevator
        additional elevators as required
Retractors as required
Surgical suction tips
Surgical curette
Bone file
Rongeurs
Haemostats
Tissue forceps
Bone cutting burs
Irrigating syringe
Suture needle and catgut/silk thread or prethread
(not depicted)
Needle holders
Suture scissors
Gauze/gauze pack

•*Not all items are displayed here*

Figure 32.6 Surgical extraction tray set-up

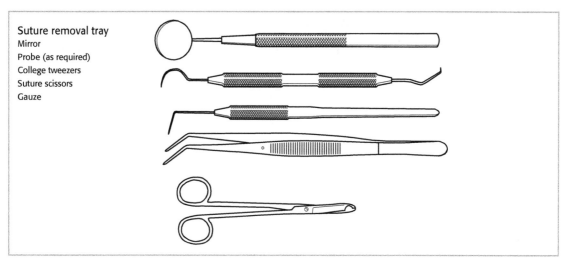

Figure 32.7 Suture tray set-up

Suture removal tray
Mirror
Probe (as required)
College tweezers
Suture scissors
Gauze

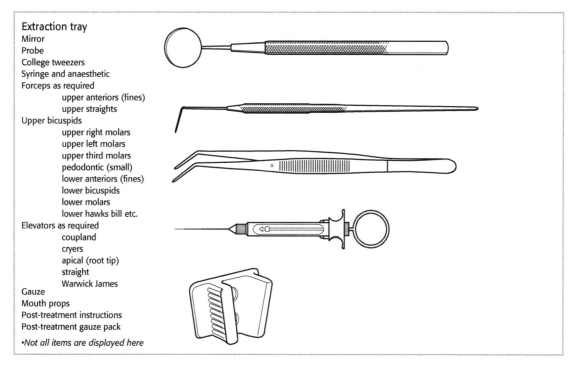

Figure 32.8 Extraction tray set-up

Extraction tray
Mirror
Probe
College tweezers
Syringe and anaesthetic
Forceps as required
    upper anteriors (fines)
    upper straights
Upper bicuspids
    upper right molars
    upper left molars
    upper third molars
    pedodontic (small)
    lower anteriors (fines)
    lower bicuspids
    lower molars
    lower hawks bill etc.
Elevators as required
    coupland
    cryers
    apical (root tip)
    straight
    Warwick James
Gauze
Mouth props
Post-treatment instructions
Post-treatment gauze pack

•Not all items are displayed here

Summary

As you will be assisting in the operative field, it is important that you understand the necessity for gentle handling of tissues and careful use of instruments during an operation, for much of the post-operative comfort of the patient will depend upon your care. The less the tissues are traumatised, the better the wound will heal.

Best practice in infection control is also essential.

chapter thirty-three
endodontics

Introduction

Endodontics is the branch of dentistry concerned with the diagnosis and treatment of diseases of the dental pulp and periapical tissues.

It is advisable to treat a diseased pulp as soon as it is recognised (usually an infection of the pulp via caries) because it is likely to become a source of secondary infection in the jaw, which in turn may flare up at any time. The alternative is extraction of the diseased tooth, which may be unavoidable if:

- the abscess is too advanced;

- endodontic treatment cannot reverse the situation; or

- an earlier endodontic treatment has failed.

Endodontic treatment consists of:

- removing the pulp or **necrotic** tissue from within the tooth;

- cleansing, enlarging and shaping the pulp canal; and

- completely sealing the canal with a filling material.

Conservative endodontic treatments are also possible and are discussed in more detail later in this chapter.

Pulp

The pulp of the tooth, contained in the pulp canal of the root and pulp chamber of the crown, is one of the two sources of nutrition of the tooth. The pulp depends for its survival on blood and nerve supply entering via the **apex**. The other source of nutrition is the numerous blood vessels coming from the surrounding tissues that sustain the periodontal ligament attachment. A critical component of this

is the cementum that covers the root surface, which after root canal therapy (RCT) becomes the more important means of keeping the tooth healthy. Therefore, a tooth with the pulp removed is not a dead tooth but rather a 'pulpless tooth', or 'non-vital'. So long as harmful bacteria do not occupy the space where pulp previously existed, the periodontal ligament which is attached to the tooth will continue to nourish the tooth. If it remains internally infection-free, the tooth is capable of staying in the jaw for the rest of the patient's life.

By contrast, if a tooth was avulsed (knocked out) and not put back immediately, the periodontal structures would not permanently reattach no matter what is done in the **root canal** to help. Then the tooth becomes a 'dead tooth'.

It was once common practice to remove a tooth with a diseased pulp, since it is easier to extract than to treat such a tooth. However, it is now recognised that it is not always easy to replace a tooth with a satisfactory artificial substitute. Bridges and implants are now commonplace but these sorts of non-denture replacements require a great deal of time and expense and efficient oral hygiene compared to saving the tooth.

Today, fortunately, many dental patients prefer to retain their own teeth wherever possible, not only for cosmetic reasons. Most patients wish to maintain a well-functioning dentition. No degree of dental skill will ever construct the perfect replacement for an extracted tooth. Retaining a tooth with endodontic treatment can often mean the difference between having to wear a fixed bridge, implant or removable denture. However, it is important to realise that not all teeth can be treated endodontically.

Occasionally, shortly after a blow or an accident, a tooth may discolour, due to bleeding within the pulp. Apart from this, pulpless teeth do not necessarily discolour and do not turn black. The discoloration that used to be associated with endodontically treated teeth (ETT) was due to old-fashioned drugs used inside the tooth. These are generally no longer used. Nevertheless, pulpless teeth may still develop or already have some variation in shade. In many cases it is possible to either bleach the tooth back to its original colour, or cover it with a direct composite, laminate or porcelain veneer. Teeth too broken down for these methods of help can be crowned, often with a metal post placed into the endodontically treated tooth's root to anchor a **coronal** core.

Pulpless teeth do not endanger the patient's health. Once they have been treated and all infection eliminated, pulpless teeth cannot cause trouble anywhere else in the body. In order to make sure that a root-treated tooth becomes and remains free from infection, a patient should be recalled periodically to ensure that periapical healing has taken place and is maintained. This means checking, by means of a radiograph, to observe that originally missing bone has returned, or a normal bone picture has been kept.

Pulp preservation and protection

It is the aim of the dentist to protect and preserve the vitality of the dental pulp whenever this is possible. The benefit is that RCT therapy can be avoided if the pulp is still alive and can respond favourably to conservative measures.

Protection of the pulp is provided:

- by adequate water-cooling of dentine during high-speed bur cavity preparation and by the avoidance of excessive dehydration and irritating chemicals;

- by the use of a lining material that will protect the pulp from chemical, thermal and micro-leakage irritation; and

- in very deep cavities, by the use of calcium hydroxide, glass ionomer or zinc oxide/eugenol cements so that secondary dentine may be stimulated.

Diagnosis of pulpal and periapical disease

Correct treatment planning is dependent upon the dentist's ability to diagnose diseases of the teeth and their supporting tissues. Diagnosis of pulpal and periapical pathology requires:

- a knowledge of the patient's dental history and symptoms;

- clinical signs of pathology;

- vitality tests; and

- radiographic examination.

Dental history and symptoms

The presence of pain is often due to the build up of pressure somewhere, which in turn usually indicates inflammation. Frequent pain indicates severe, possibly irreversible (acute), inflammation of the pulp, which is called pulpitis. This pain can be extreme, sometimes described by patients as more painful than childbirth.

Once acute inflammation has become established beyond the intercanal pulp space, its presence is usually indicated by soreness of the tooth to biting or tapping.

Clinical signs

The clinical signs include:

- crown discoloration due to pulp death (mainly in anterior teeth);

- exposure of the pulp from caries that has invaded too deeply or during cavity preparation;

- faulty restorations that cause pulpal irritation;

- apical soft tissue swellings due to periapical inflammation — where swelling is localised it is often referred to as an abscess; where it extends more widely into the surrounding tissues it is called **cellulitis** and can become very serious); and

- presence of a sinus or 'gum boil' from a draining abscess — this is found on the jaw surface, not necessarily immediately adjacent to the root/tooth responsible.

In some cases of chronic infection there may be no clinical signs or symptoms (e.g. no pain) and the diagnosis will depend on vitality tests alone (see below), usually with a radiograph providing confirmation.

Vitality/sensitivity tests

With these tests, a stimulus is applied to a tooth to intentionally create a painful response. If a tooth does not respond to any of these tests, it is non-vital, meaning the pulp tissue has been destroyed or otherwise broken down. This is called pulp necrosis. This situation will generally require endodontic treatment, unless the tooth has already received RCT. One or more of the following stimuli may be applied to the tooth as a vitality test.

- Heated gutta-percha, using a white rod of what is called temporary stopping. A flame is needed to provide the heat source.

- A cotton pellet saturated with a refrigerant spray (from a can) or a dry ice pencil (carbon dioxide, or CO_2, stick). The CO_2 stick is much more powerful and often the only way of getting a response from a tooth with a porcelain jacket crown.

- Electric current via a battery device (e.g. digilog or analytical technology pulp tester). These have a numerical scale to show the intensity of the current. The level reached may need to be recorded. To guarantee that the electrical stimulus is conducted through the enamel or dentine to reach the pulp, a conductive agent needs to be applied to the tooth surface (unless there is metal-to-metal contact). Traditionally, this has been a blob of toothpaste, but a spot of etchant gel will be more certain of performing this task. It needs to be wiped off the enamel surface immediately after it has served its purpose.

Reasons for pulp treatment

There are four main reasons why pulps are treated.

1. Vital carious exposure

As decay progresses into a tooth, the previously healthy pulp may become exposed. That is, the caries has carried through to the pulp's previously protected territory. An exposed pulp could become infected by its contact with the caries. It has to be removed and endodontic therapy may be needed.

2. Necrosis of the pulp

After decay has reached the pulp, death of the entire pulp will ultimately result.

The pulp may also die if a tooth receives a heavy blow or accident without actually becoming exposed. In this case the blood vessels that enter the apex (**apical foramen**) are broken by the severity of the **trauma**, are incapable of reconnecting through such a tiny opening, and the pulp cannot recover. Even though bacteria do not enter at the time of the traumatic event, they somehow get in

and take over the internal 'dead space' after the pulp tissue disintegrates from loss of blood supply. A tooth that has been avulsed is in this category, except sometimes for very young children.

In all cases where the pulp has become partially or totally necrotic, it is necessary to carry out endodontic therapy.

3. Vital accidental exposure of a normal pulp (mechanical or traumatic exposure)

Both an injury that causes a tooth to fracture or the careless use of a cutting instrument may result in the exposure of a normal vital pulp. Such an uninflamed pulp may be able to repair itself if a suitable cement or medicament is placed over the exposure immediately. If the exposed pulp has been left open to the oral environment for more than a couple of hours, or if it is becomes contaminated, the need for endodontic treatment is almost inevitable.

4. Elective removal of pulps (pulpectomy)

When teeth that are badly broken down coronally need to be rebuilt, sometimes it is necessary to use part of the root canal to accommodate a post to hold the restoration or artificial crown in place. In this case, normal pulp is removed and replaced with a canal filling in the apical half of the root (**pulpectomy**). The cervical half is used to secure the post, or if done in gold, the post/core.

Endodontic techniques

Endodontic techniques may be classified into conservative and radical. Conservative endodontics is performed on teeth that have vital pulps. The aim in these cases is to maintain pulpal vitality (pulp survival) in the treated tooth. Radical treatments involve removing all the pulp from the tooth.

Conservative treatments include:

- indirect **pulp capping**;
- direct pulp capping;
- vital **pulpotomy** (which can be partial or complete); and
- mummification.

Radical endodontic techniques include:

- **apexification**;
- root canal therapy (RCT); and
- **apicectomy**.

apical foramen: small hole in root apex for the entry and exit of pulpal vessels and nerves. ■ **trauma**: a knock, blow or injury. ■ **pulpectomy**: total removal of a vital pulp. ■ **pulp capping**: protective covering placed over a pulp exposure. ■ **pulpotomy**: opening into and partial removal of pulp. ■ **apexification**: stimulation of the root-end formation following death of pulp in immature teeth. ■ **apicectomy**: (also apicoectomy) endodontic surgery involving cutting of the root apex.

Other endodontic therapy includes the treatment of abscesses and cellulitis and the use of bleaches to whiten teeth.

Conservative endodontic techniques

Indirect pulp capping

This treatment is indicated when the pulp is vital but is likely to become exposed if the deepest remnants of caries or softened dentine are removed from the cavity.

Treatment includes the following steps.

- The tooth is isolated to exclude saliva. A dental dam is best for this if the situation is suitable for its placement.

- Caries is removed, except for a small layer left over the pulp. This remaining carious dentine is covered with a calcium hydroxide lining. This will destroy remaining bacteria and stimulate the formation of secondary dentine.

- The tooth is then temporarily restored with a fortified cement (e.g. GIC) or an amalgam restoration.

- After a few months, the temporary filling is removed to allow removal of the remaining caries.

- If treatment was successful, the permanent restoration is then put into a caries-free tooth.

- If treatment was not successful and removal of the remaining soft caries leads to a pulp exposure, RCT is needed.

Direct pulp capping

Accidental exposure of the pulp during cavity preparation allows the use of a direct capping technique provided the exposure is small, uncontaminated and the pulp is vital. No pulp tissue is removed as it is expected to be normal, or very close to normal. Basically, the dentist is dealing with a wound and applying a dressing to it. Calcium hydroxide in various paste forms, GIC or ledermix cement, may be flowed over the exposure site (as long as there isn't a bleeding point there). It is important that the capping agent contacts the exposed pulpal tissue and that the capping is immediately sealed with a base material and then permanent restoration.

The vitality of the tooth should be checked after a six-week period, and whenever the patient returns for recall examination. Later removal and replace-

ment of the restoration is not part of this procedure because all caries is removed before the pulp cap is placed.

Pulpotomy

This is an operation usually performed on a tooth with an open apex (i.e. the apical foramen is large in a young patient) where caries has reached the pulp or where the pulp has been exposed by an accident. In either scenario, part of the pulp in the coronal pulp chamber is removed with a sharp instrument (a spoon excavator or a bur in a handpiece). Calcium hydroxide is placed over the pulp stump of a mature tooth. A zinc oxide/eugenol cement is placed over the partial amputation site of a pulp in an apically immature root. A strong cement base follows this and then the final restoration. Long-term review for this procedure is also important because it is difficult to determine the normality of the un-amputated pulp tissue. See Figure 33.1.

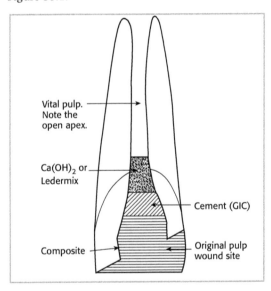

Vital pulp. Note the open apex.

Ca(OH)$_2$ or Ledermix

Cement (GIC)

Composite

Original pulp wound site

Figure 33.1 Tooth in which pulpotomy has been carried out

Mummification pulpotomy

This is used for deciduous teeth and occasionally for permanent posterior teeth, where a carious exposure exists but some vital pulp tissue also exists. After amputation of the infected portion of the pulp, formocresol is applied to the stump on a cotton wool pellet. Formocresol liquid:

- renders the remaining pulpal tissues 'non-vital' (it mummifies and preserves the pulp until the tooth exfoliates); and

- destroys remaining bacteria.

Apexification

If a tooth dies as a result of trauma before the apex has fully developed, conventional endodontic therapy cannot be carried out because the apex is wide open. This usually happens through traumatic injury to children's permanent incisors when there is no apical foramen closure yet, just a large funnel-shaped opening at the end of the developing root.

Any attempt at root filling would result in sealer and gutta-percha points being forced out into the **periapical** region. In this situation, treatment is carried out in two stages. The first stage consists of biomechanical debridement, followed by filling the canal with a calcium hydroxide paste.

This is usually carried to the apex by a lentulo spiral. The canal is sealed with a semi-permanent restoration and growth of the apex is monitored by radiographs taken periodically.

Such growth may take six to 24 months. When this is complete, the second stage of treatment is carried out. This consists of removal of the calcium hydroxide and its replacement by a conventional root filling.

Abscess and cellulitis

Acute abscess

An acute alveolar abscess is a localised collection of pus in the bone at the root of a tooth in which the pulp has become necrotic. It results from infection passing through the apex of the tooth into the nearby bone tissue. There is usually severe, throbbing pain locally, and sometimes swelling of the cheek tissues, or the roof or the floor of the mouth near the tooth. Tenderness of the tooth when biting is common and sometimes the abscess breaks through the mucosal surface near the apex of the tooth to form what is frequently called a 'gum boil'. This pimple-like formation may burst of its own accord or if disturbed or incised (lanced).

Treatment consists of establishing drainage immediately to allow the pus to escape. The best and most straightforward pathway for the release of pressure is via the root canal. This is usually done by drilling through the tooth to the pulp chamber.

Another method is to incise the gum over the tooth using a scalpel. This is usually done when a local-ised swelling is present. It is usually a secondary measure if canal drainage is not feasible for some reason, or if drainage is attempted but nothing emerges from the canal. The incision is then kept open by means of a wick made from dental dam. These wicks are cut in the shape of an 'I' or 'T' and are frequently sutured into the incision to prevent them from being dislodged.

The situation will take 24 hours or so to settle down and it is then treated like any other necrotic pulp tooth. If RCT is then not begun, the flare-up is likely to return.

Cellulitis

Where the swelling is not localised but extends over a larger area it is known as cellulitis. In this case the infection is controlled by systemic antibiotics combined with treating the source of infection (by cleaning the canal of the offending tooth). Once the cellulitis has subsided, endodontic therapy can be completed, usually over two extra appointments.

Chronic abscess

A chronic abscess is a longstanding moderate infection of the jaw surrounding the apex of the tooth. It is a progressive development following death of the pulp with extension of the infection out of the canal space and into the bone. Sometimes an untreated acute abscess, or one that has settled as a result of antibiotics only, can convert to the chronic form. Periapical abscesses will never resolve without either RCT or extraction. Antibiotics can only help in the short term.

A chronic abscess is usually symptomless, has minimal swelling and is often detected only by x-ray examination, or occasionally by the presence of an opening, known as a sinus, through the surface tissues. The pathway between that outlet and the root-tip of the offending tooth is called a fistular tract. It can usually be painlessly traced by a gutta-percha point to show on a radiograph which tooth is responsible. Diagnosis is often aided by the fact that the patient may remember a severe pain that went away abruptly and left the tooth feeling quite comfortable.

Treatment of a chronic abscess consists of sterilisation and filling of the root canal. This allows the bone in the chronic abscess area to heal.

■ **periapical:** referring to the area around the root apex.

Radical endodontic techniques

Root canal therapy (RCT) — the procedure

The general principles for root canal therapy are the same for all teeth, regardless of the disease status of their pulp. Root canal therapy begins with the removal of infected pulp tissue (known as exterpation) whether necrotic or vital. Indications for RCT are:

- the pulp is in an irreversibly inflamed state;
- the pulp is necrotic;
- an alveolar abscess is present; or
- the tooth has been replanted following avulsion.

The stages of the treatment are:

- isolation and asepsis;
- removal of pulp or pulpal remains and measuring the length of canals;
- biomechanical shaping and enlargement of the canal;
- sterilising the canal's dentine walls; and
- filling the canal close to the apex (**obturation**).

Asepsis

Since the aim of treatment is to kill or otherwise eliminate all bacteria in the root canal before filling, steps must be taken to prevent other bacteria being introduced from the mouth, from instruments or from the dental surgery environment (often transferred by hands).

Length of canal

The length of the canal must be determined first and is necessary to know before the mechanical shaping and enlarging can proceed (Figure 33.2).

The operator inserts a metal instrument of known length (usually a small, smooth broach) into the canal and then takes a radiograph. It may be your responsibility to record the length of the instrument on the patient's chart. The dentist will dictate the correct measurements (length and gauge) to be recorded.

You then process the exposed film. An inspection of the radiograph by the operator enables the correct working length of the canal to be determined and this is also recorded on the patient's chart.

If it is a multi-rooted tooth being treated, there will probably be different lengths for each root, and it is often likely for each canal to utilise a different cusp as its reference point.

In more recent years, electronic apex locators have been available as a means of determining correct length. This can by-pass the need for x-rays to provide this information. However, electronic apex locators are not 100 per cent reliable for all canals.

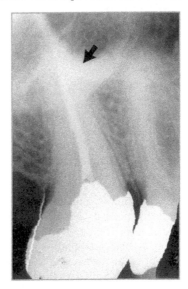

Figure 33.2 Determining the length of the canal

- You can then set all instruments to be used for the canal to this length. To do this, small pieces of rubber (e.g. cut from a rubber band) or small coloured plastic discs especially made for the purpose are used. They can be different shapes and can be slid along the non-cutting portion of the file shaft. They vary from 1, $1^1/_2$ to 2 mm in thickness. Most manufacturers put these on their files. Where they have to be independently applied, ensure that they are correctly positioned and sterile techniques are used.

Biomechanical cleansing

When the dental dam is in place, the pulp or necrotic tissue is removed with suitable instruments. The dentist aims to create a continuous conical form in the pulp canal while leaving the apical foramen undisturbed or as small as possible and in its original position.

The biomechanical cleansing of the tooth is then carried out. This is perhaps the most important aspect of endodontic treatment and usually takes the most time. The cleansing process is carried out just short of the tip of the apex of the tooth, and

- **obturation:** sealing of the root apex.

definitely not beyond it. An apical stop to close the apex is created inside the apical foramen and this is where the tip of the final root filling will be located.

The canal is flooded with a sterilising solution by means of a hypodermic syringe. A 1 per cent hypochlorite solution is the most popular. Some operators use other solutions (e.g. normal saline or other sterile solution) in addition to hypochlorite. Both you and the dentist must guard against any of the hypochlorite solution dripping onto the patient's clothing as it is a powerful bleaching agent.

The canal is then cleansed and its wall smoothed using reamers and files.

The dentist will ensure that a used instrument visibly carrying gross debris is superficially cleansed (e.g. on a piece of gauze or cotton roll) before being reintroduced to the canal. If two types of files are being used on the same canal, keep them in separate spaces within the work area.

When canal cleansing is completed, or no further progress can be made at that appointment, absorbent and size specific paper points are used to dry the canal. A medicated paste is then inserted into the empty canal space using a lentulo spiral filler. Following this, a pledget of cotton wool is inserted near the canal orifice to condense the paste into the canal and to stop occlusal temporary filling from getting into the canal space. The canal is then sealed with a temporary cement, usually of the zinc oxide-eugenol type, Cavit or GIC.

Sterilising the canal

The process of biomechanical preparation contributes to sterilising the canal. In addition, drugs (dressings) are used to assist in sterilising the canal. These include antibiotic mixtures, pastes of calcium hydroxide (non-setting) and iodoform, all of which can be rinsed or easily filed out of the canal at the next visit. This sterilisation takes place between visits and it can take from a few days up to one week. The patient should be advised to contact the surgery if pain persists or the temporary dressing is dislodged.

It is essential that the occlusal access opening is tightly sealed between visits to exclude fresh bacteria. A lost seal means that the canal is re-contaminated and treatment is delayed or compromised.

Obturation (filling the root canal)

The root canal is ready to be filled and sealed when:

- the tooth is comfortable and free from any soreness to percussion (tapping);
- any periapical exudate has been controlled; and
- any sinus that was present is now closed.

Once the root canal is suitable for filling, it will be sealed with a non-irritant filling. A root filling using the lateral condensation technique consists of three parts:

❶ master point (prime cone) gutta-percha;

❷ root canal sealer; and

❸ accessory points.

Master point (prime point) gutta-percha

This is a tapered piece of gutta-percha that is manufactured to correspond with the sizes of the reamers and files. The dentist chooses a point the same size as the last reamer or file used. This should fit tightly at the apical end of the canal. The point may have to be trimmed or the end may have to be softened by momentarily dipping its apical end in chloroform or eucalyptol. The point should reach within 1–2 mm of the apex, but not beyond it and this is checked with a radiograph.

The master point is then pressed against the root canal walls by passing a spreader into the canal and compressing the root filling laterally.

Root canal sealer

This point is sealed into place using an adherent root canal sealer. The sealer may be placed into the dry root canal by using a lentulo spiral filler, a hand reamer or fine plugger.

Accessory points

To ensure that the canal is properly sealed, a number of smaller sized accessory gutta-percha points should be inserted between the master point and the canal walls.

These are fine points that are inserted into the space obtained by lateral condensation of the master point. There is only one master gutta-percha point per canal but there may be as many as ten accessories, so you need to ensure they are available and set them out in a suitable way. This technique is called lateral condensation (Figure 33.3).

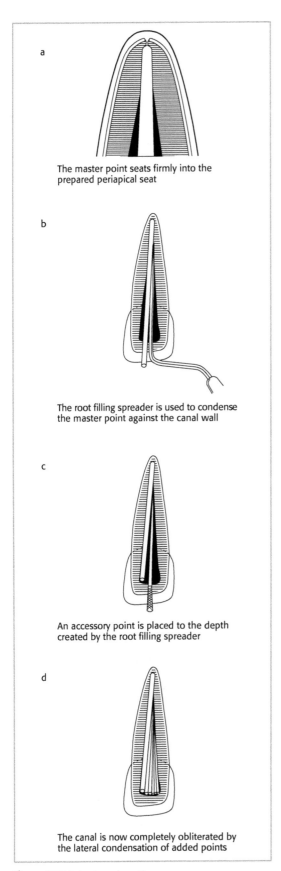

a

The master point seats firmly into the prepared periapical seat

b

The root filling spreader is used to condense the master point against the canal wall

c

An accessory point is placed to the depth created by the root filling spreader

d

The canal is now completely obliterated by the lateral condensation of added points

Figure 33.3 Lateral condensation

To prevent discolouration of the crown, all excess gutta-percha and paste is removed using a heated spoon-shaped excavator (endo-spoon) and the pulp chamber is cleaned with a solvent such as chloroform. A final radiograph should be taken to check the adequacy of the root filling. The tooth is then restored (Figure 33.4).

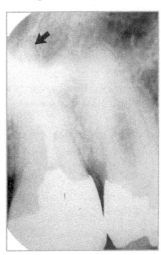

Figure 33.4 Root filling space

Another, simpler technique is as follows. The root canal space may also be filled by warming gutta-percha and packing this material into the canal. The master cone is warmed and placed in the root canal after this has been coated with sealant. The gutta-percha is then packed vertically with a plugger smaller in diameter than the root canal. It may be your role to select the gutta-percha points required by the dentist, to mix the root canal sealer and to coat the master point with sealer prior to passing it to the dentist.

Apicectomy (periradicular surgery)

Indications

In some cases, normal endodontic therapy must be supplemented with apical surgery. Where the apex cannot be reached by the usual means (i.e. through the root canal) surgery is needed in order to gain access to the apex. There are other cases where persisting diseased tissues surrounding the apex in the alveolar bone have to be cleaned out. This is termed 'periapical curettage'. Other situations exist which do not come under these headings; for example, surgically sealing a perforation (hole) half-way along a canal. For this reason, the term 'peri-radicular surgery' (i.e. surgery around the root) is to be preferred to the commonly used term of api-cectomy (which strictly means cutting off the apex).

Some of the indications for periradicular surgery are:

- Inability to reach the apical region of a tooth.

- Perforation of the canal where its location is accessible. Perforation is a hole extending from inside the tooth (root canal) to the root surface. This may be traumatic in origin, or caused by internal resorption.

- Lack of time — this is rare and fairly extreme. For example, the patient may live in a war zone or a great distance away. Immediate canal preparation and root filling is carried out in conjunction with periapical curettage.

Inability to reach the apical region of a tooth

This may be caused by:

- the presence of an unremovable post-crown on the affected tooth;

- fracture of the apical region that is causing complications;

- inadequate bone repair — this may occur when a good quality root canal filling has been placed, but periapical bone repair has not occurred or the lesion has become even worse;

- a broken instrument is wedged in the canal and cannot be bypassed;

- abnormal curvature of the root that standard files, etc. cannot negotiate; and

- calcified or impenetrable canals.

Procedure

This is a full surgical procedure (Figure 33.5). It involves:

- raising a flap in the soft tissue adjacent to the tooth;

- drilling through the alveolar bone to gain access to the root;

- removing about 2 mm of the apex of the root to open a space back into the root; and

- placing a suitable sealing filling close to the canal.

This is called a retrofill and the procedure is termed **retrograde cavity preparation**.

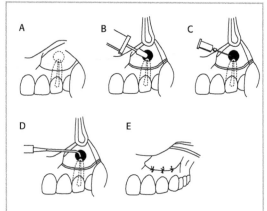

The patient is draped with sterile towels.
(A) To gain access to the apex of the tooth, a flap is raised.
(B) The position of the apex is determined and the buccal bone is removed with a sterile bur and water coolant. The apex is completely exposed.
(C) Additional local anaesthetic may be required, applied into the bone and round the lesion.
(D) The area is cleaned using fine curettes. The root tip is amputated and a retrograde seal or restoration is placed.
(E) The soft tissue flap is sutured in position.

Figure 33.5 The operation

Bleaching

Root canal therapy can also be elective, carried out on teeth with discoloured crowns. These may often be restored to their original colour by bleaching. This can only be attempted after an adequate root filling has been placed. The crown is filled with a paste consisting of sodium perborate and hydrogen peroxide followed by a seal of temporary cement or zinc oxide-eugenol. This is left in place for one to two weeks and may have to be repeated. When bleaching has taken place, the paste is removed and the crown is filled with a light translucent filling, such as a restorative resin.

Maintaining asepsis in endodontic therapy

Dental dam

When the pulp of a tooth is to be treated, the tooth is isolated using a dental dam. More information about dental dams can be found in Chapter 17.

Sterile trays and instruments

Endodontic instruments are classed as critical items and must be sterile at the point of use.

There are many ways in which sterile endodontic instruments may be arranged and sorted and all dentists have their own preferences. Two arrangements are as follows.

■ The sterile towel kit. This consists of two sterile towels, into which are placed all the long-handled instruments such as mirror, probe, tweezers, excavator, plastic instruments, etc. A stainless steel ruler, cotton wool pellets (pre-packed in a paper bag or metal container) and a syringe for irrigation are also required. This towel kit is then bagged and sterilised in the autoclave. When needed, the towels are spread over the bracket table, and this provides a sterile surface on which to work.

■ Metal boxes. These boxes, usually made of aluminium, have compartments of varying sizes to be used for storage of instruments such as tiles, reamers, barbed broaches, silver and paper points, and files sorted according to size. Special purpose boxes, for example, are for root filling. This box could contain a spreader, plugger, spatula and mixing slab. For apicectomy, surgical instruments can also be set out in boxes. All of these boxes can be sterilised by autoclave at 134°C for the prescribed time or in a dry-heat oven at 120°C for two hours. The type of box is important. A perforated box must be used in an autoclave and requires wrapping for storage. A non-perforated box can be used for dry heat sterilisers. As with all instruments, they must be perfectly dry and cooled upon removal from the autoclave.

Methods of sterilisation

Apart from the autoclave, which is essential and which follows ultrasonic and other cleaning, a glass bead or salt chair-side steriliser may be used for emergency re-sterilisation. This consists of a chamber filled with thousands of 2–3 mm glass beads or salt that is electrically heated to a temperature of 220–250°C. Previously autoclaved instruments are inserted into the beads for ten seconds with just their plastic handles protruding. These are not the primary steriliser of the file but a secondary, chair-side aid only. See Chapter 14 for more information on sterilisation. The extreme heat can damage small instruments.

The small instruments specifically made for endodontic therapy are not the only ones that require cleansing and sorting. The long-handled instruments must be cleaned of all cement and debris before sterilisation. Irrigating syringes and needles should be single use only. An irrigating syringe must never be used for the injection of local anaesthetic.

Post-operation

Obviously there is blood and debris on many of the instruments, most of which are sharp. Cleaning them afterwards, as well as the immediate environment of the room, bracket table and so forth, requires great care and thoroughness.

Suction tubing must be thoroughly flushed through with cold water.

Soaking all blood-soiled instruments in an enzymatic solution before cleaning and ultrasonication is recommended because the danger of blood-borne transmission of a pathogen in this type of work is higher than for more routine duties.

Instruments required

The general surgical tray is likely to include:

■ mouth mirror;
■ probe;
■ tweezers;
■ scalpel (with disposable pre-sterilised blades);
■ periosteal elevator;
■ curettes (small and large);
■ sutures (pre-sterilised, threaded and packed in individual envelopes);
■ needle holder;
■ suture scissors;
■ sterile gauze squares;
■ fine aspirator tips; and
■ other instruments the dentist prefers and which may vary from one tooth to another.

Where bone has to be removed, sterile bone burs, or tooth burs (round and fissure) for the straight handpiece, and a bone file may be required.

Where a retrograde filling has to be placed into the apex of the tooth a good number of other instruments will be required.

The complexity of equipment and access difficulty often make this procedure sufficiently difficult to justify referral to a specialist. Sometimes an operating microscope is required.

Endodontic instruments

See Figure 33.6 for some examples of specific endodontic instruments.

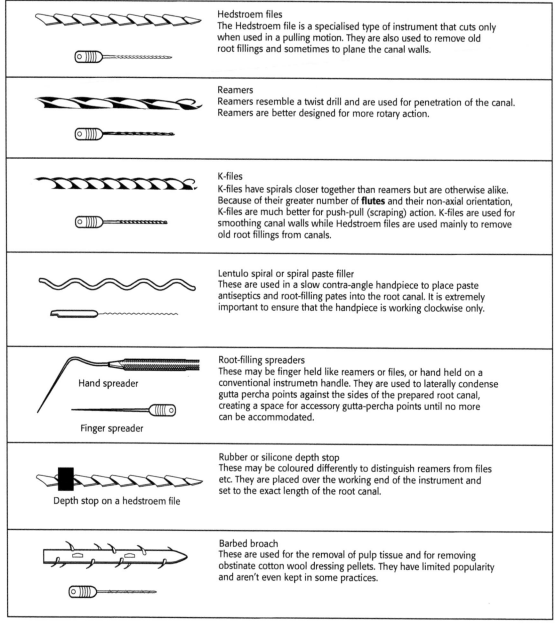

Hedstroem files
The Hedstroem file is a specialised type of instrument that cuts only when used in a pulling motion. They are also used to remove old root fillings and sometimes to plane the canal walls.

Reamers
Reamers resemble a twist drill and are used for penetration of the canal. Reamers are better designed for more rotary action.

K-files
K-files have spirals closer together than reamers but are otherwise alike. Because of their greater number of **flutes** and their non-axial orientation, K-files are much better for push-pull (scraping) action. K-files are used for smoothing canal walls while Hedstroem files are used mainly to remove old root fillings from canals.

Lentulo spiral or spiral paste filler
These are used in a slow contra-angle handpiece to place paste antiseptics and root-filling pates into the root canal. It is extremely important to ensure that the handpiece is working clockwise only.

Hand spreader

Finger spreader

Root-filling spreaders
These may be finger held like reamers or files, or hand held on a conventional instrumetn handle. They are used to laterally condense gutta percha points against the sides of the prepared root canal, creating a space for accessory gutta-percha points until no more can be accommodated.

Depth stop on a hedstroem file

Rubber or silicone depth stop
These may be coloured differently to distinguish reamers from files etc. They are placed over the working end of the instrument and set to the exact length of the root canal.

Barbed broach
These are used for the removal of pulp tissue and for removing obstinate cotton wool dressing pellets. They have limited popularity and aren't even kept in some practices.

Colour of handle	Instrument	Number	Diameter
Grey	08		
Purple	10		
White	15	45	90
Yellow	20	50	100
Red	25	55	110
Blue	30	60	120
Green	35	70	130
Black	40	80	140

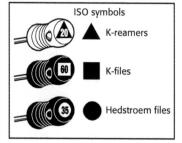

ISO symbols

K-reamers

K-files

Hedstroem files

Figure 33.6 Types of endodontic instruments

Size of instruments

In order to sort the root canal instruments into sizes, handles are made of coloured plastic. Each colour represents a standardised size. Root canal instruments are manufactured to standardised sizes (diameter) and a uniform taper. The standardised size expresses the diameter (or gauge) of the instrument in hundredths of a millimetre, measured 1 mm from its tip. This system allows the dentist to use instruments from different manufacturers, knowing that a certain size will always be the same width, regardless of the brand used.

The coloured handles of the small hand instruments have a hole punched through them. This enables a length of dental floss or thread to be tied to the instrument when a dental dam cannot be used (e.g. if there are badly broken down adjacent teeth). This is a safety measure to prevent losing the file in the patient's mouth. It may be your job to thread the files before giving them to the dentist to use.

Most modern instruments have their size stamped somewhere on the handle in a square (for the K-files), triangles (for reamers) or circle (for Hedstroem).

Sorting instruments

It is your task to sort and clean all instruments and to return them to their appropriate compartments. When doing this, the instruments must be carefully inspected and any bent, kinked or visibly damaged instruments should be discarded. If there is any evidence of strain, it will show up as an unwinding or 'concertinaing' of the spirals on the file.

Bent instruments should never be straightened as this could lead to breakage within the root canal the next time the instrument is used. A broken instrument within the root canal cannot usually be retrieved and this can frequently lead to the forced extraction of the tooth concerned.

A file that has been pre-curved by the manufacturer for use in a curved canal is not dangerously damaged by the pre-curvature put on it. There should be no attempt to straighten it.

Most small endodontic instruments that are used to file the canal/s are now recommended to be single-use instruments or, alternatively, individual patient file packs are sterilised in pouches, labelled and kept with the patient's records.

Summary

Endodontic treatment usually takes from two to four visits depending upon the complexity of the case. Surgical intervention may also be necessary in the management of some teeth but is always additional to whatever help is possible within the tooth first.

Due to the large number of pulpal and periapical diseases that may be associated with teeth, a range of endodontic techniques have been developed. New techniques are always being devised, usually to make the task easier or quicker. You will require specialised on-the-job training for specific techniques used in your surgery.

occlusion: the relation, when the jaws come together, of the upper and lower teeth. ■ malocclusion: a non-ideal relationship of the upper and lower teeth, the occlusion being the way in which the upper and lower teeth interdigitate (fit together) when the jaws come together. ■ morphology: the study of the form or structure of an organism or part of an organism.

chapter thirty-four
orthodontics

Introduction

Orthodontics is the branch of dentistry concerned with the supervision, guidance and correction of the growing and mature dental and facial structures. The most common type of orthodontia involves the movement of teeth, using braces, to correct the patient's **occlusion**.

Orthodontists deal with **malocclusions** that can be genetic or environmental. These malocclusions can be due to:

- crowding or spacing of the teeth (Figure 34.1);
- disharmony of the skeletal elements of the face;
- abnormal soft tissue **morphology**; or
- factors such as variation in size and number of teeth.

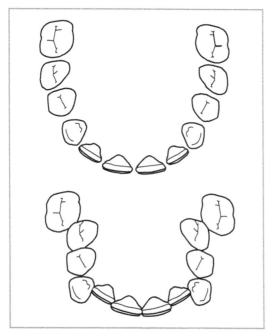

Figure 34.1 Crowding and spacing

This chapter includes discussion of:

- growth and development of the face;
- normal occlusion and malocclusion;
- management of orthodontic problems; and
- your role as an assistant to the orthodontist during orthodontic treatment.

Growth and development of the face

A knowledge of facial anatomy and growth is essential so you can discuss orthodontic procedures with patients. However, a detailed understanding of facial growth is not necessary and what follows is a discussion of growth and development of the face as it applies to orthodontics.

The cranial vault is influenced in its growth by the growth of the brain, which it protects. It provides a site of attachment for facial muscles.

The cranial base

The cranial base forms a base on which the brain rests. The anterior limb of the cranial base articulates with the upper facial skeleton and the posterior limb of the cranial base articulates with the mandible. There are two areas where cartilage provides growing sites and these are the spheno-occipital and spheno-ethmoidal synchondroses. Growth at these sites influences the length of the cranial base and so influences the relationship between the mandible and maxilla. See Figure 34.2.

The maxilla

In early life the prime growth centre for the maxilla is the nasal septum and this leads the maxilla to grow downwards and forwards. **Apposition** of bone occurs on the surface and in the sutural areas. The nasal septum has completed its function by seven years of age and at this stage the maxillary sinuses reach half their adult size. The palate descends downwards with the maxilla and there is surface apposition on the oral side and **resorption** on the nasal floor.

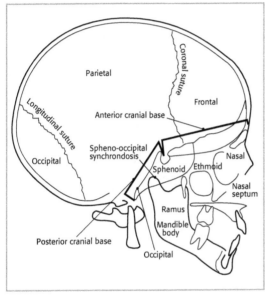

Figure 34.2 Sagittal section of the skull and facial bones

The mandible

The active growth site here is primarily in the cartilage of the condyle. The mandible, therefore, grows downwards and forwards from this site. There is also surface apposition on the bone and, in the ramus, resorption anteriorly and deposition of bone on the posterior aspect. This allows increase in dental arch length.

Proportional growth

The growth of the face and jaws will influence the eventual relationships of the teeth in the mature adult. Growth is increased in size in all directions; in depth, in height and in width. From the infant stage the following growth changes take place:

- After age one, the facial area grows more rapidly than the cranium.
- The upper face and the jaw grows up and forward. The lower face and jaw grows down and forward.
- As the small face becomes larger it appears to grow out from beneath the cranium and increases in height because of the divergent growth of the upper and lower jaws.
- The lower jaw grows more rapidly than the upper jaw.

In the majority of individuals there are changes in proportions in the parts of the face during this growing phase. Whereas the cranial vault is nearly seven-eighths of the bulk of the head at birth, in the adult it only forms half to two-thirds of the bulk of the head. See Figure 34.3.

Growth of the cranial vault is completed by six years of age, whereas the facial skeleton continues to grow until 16 to 18 years of age in females and 20 years of age in males. Most growth occurs at puberty.

These changes in facial characteristics result in a young child having relatively prominent teeth but this becomes less pronounced as the mandible continues to grow. The rounded profile of the child develops into the straighter profile of the adult.

Growth is not always predictable or uniform in amount or direction. The above considerations hold true in the majority of cases but there are always exceptions to the rule and sometimes paths

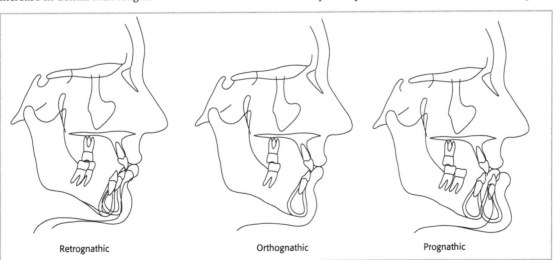

Retrognathic   Orthognathic   Prognathic

Figure 34.3 Facial types

■ **apposition:** cell growth onto existing layers of cell.
■ **resorption:** re-absorption of bone cells.

of development are followed that lead to dramatic changes in the developing occlusion. This is particularly seen in boys who have a tendency towards a prominent mandible and a Class III incisor relationship (see Table 34.2).

Growth of the dental arches

The jaws grow in width to accommodate the broader permanent anterior teeth. This change in width ceases after about the age of eight years. The arches grow in length as a result of the forward growth of the face and jaws. This provides space for the first, second and third molars. Growth in length ceases later than growth in width and finishes when all body growth ceases.

Dental alveolar growth and development

The alveolar bone fills in between the teeth in the maxilla and the mandible (which are known as the basal bones). Growth of the alveolus is by surface apposition and this must occur to accommodate the permanent teeth as the deciduous teeth are shed. The deciduous dentition is completed by $2^1/_2$–$3^1/_2$ years of age. There is no appreciable lateral growth in the arches during the period of 3–$5^1/_2$ years but during the eruption of the permanent incisors there is an increase of about 3 mm in the intercanine width. It is normal for space to occur between the upper central incisors. This is not related to the labial fraenum but rather to the anterior root crowding which is present. The roots of these teeth are compressed by pressure from the upper canine crowns, which are high in the alveolus at this stage of development. Ideally there should be some space between the deciduous incisor teeth, as it has been shown that 40 per cent of patients that do not have a space between their incisors have crowding in the permanent dentition. As the unerupted canines come into occlusion, the gap between the incisors generally closes up. Teeth may develop into areas where there is insufficient bone for their size and crowding or spacing may result. The eventual relationship of the teeth with each other, and to the dental base, will also be affected by the soft tissue environment.

The growth of the soft tissues of the face

As the teeth erupt, they come under the influence of muscular forces of the tongue, cheeks and lips and subsequently the teeth of the opposing arch.

The soft tissues of the face form a muscular envelope for the skeleton. The shape of the soft tissue varies during general body development from infancy to adult life. In the new-born infant the tongue is relatively large and often rests in contact with the lower lip between the gum pads. Later in development the tongue falls back to mould the dental arches. The facial musculature appears to become more tense with age and patients develop postures of their lips that may have the effect of restricting the size of the dental arches.

Occlusion

Normal occlusion

■ Centric relation is the relationship of the mandible to the maxilla when the mandible is in its most retruded position. This is the ideal occlusion of the teeth (Figure 34.4); that is, the ideal way in which the teeth come and fit together in centric relation. There is a smooth symmetrical curve to each arch and the arches coordinate or match each other in shape.

■ All the teeth contact on each of their mesial and distal sides (except for the last teeth).

■ There is precise interdigitation (or interlocking) of the upper and lower teeth.

■ Each upper posterior tooth is relatively distal to its lower counterpart.

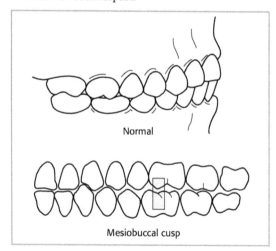

Figure 34.4 Ideal occlusion

Malocclusion

Any departure from ideal or normal occlusion is described as malocclusion. This may range from the malposition of a single tooth to major discrepancies of the jaws.

Malocclusion may involve:

- the relationship of the adjacent teeth to one another in the same arch;
- the relationship of upper teeth to lower teeth;
- the relationship of the upper jaw to the lower jaw; or
- any combination of the above.

Orthodontic classification

In order to communicate findings in examining the patient, the dentist and orthodontist use a universally accepted classification (see Tables 34.1 and 34.2 overleaf). Malocclusion is divided into three classes based on the relative positions of the upper and lower first permanent molars.

Other aspects of the classification overbite

Overbite is the amount by which the upper anterior teeth overlap the lower anterior teeth when the posterior teeth are in occlusion. The normal or ideal amount of overbite is about two millimetres. However, this can be affected by factors such as tooth size. Overbite (see Figure 34.5) may be incomplete — when the lower incisors are not in contact with the upper incisors or the palatal mucosa when the teeth are in occlusion — or complete, when the incisors are in contact with the upper incisors or palatal mucosa.

In severe cases the lower anterior teeth may be completely concealed or overlapped by the upper anterior teeth. This is called deep overbite.

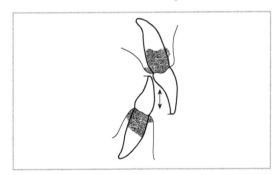

Figure 34.5 Overbite

Anterior open bite

Anterior open bite occurs when the posterior teeth are in contact but some of the upper and lower teeth are not in contact and there is an open bite

(see Figure 34.6). Thumb- or finger-sucking habits or tongue habits can cause this. It may also be associated with an increase in lower face height or with a tongue behaviour pattern that separates the anterior teeth.

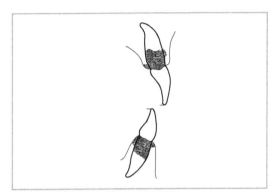

Figure 34.6 Anterior open bite

Overjet

Overjet (see Figure 34.7) is the amount that the upper incisors protrude beyond the lower incisors in a horizontal direction. This amount is normally measured in millimetres. Generally speaking, the ideal amount is about 2 mm.

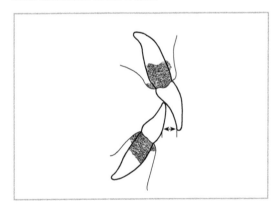

Figure 34.7 Overjet

Crossbite

Ideally, the buccal cusps of the lower posterior teeth occlude in the central fissures of the upper posterior teeth. In the anterior region, the incisal edges of the lower anterior teeth occlude lingual and gingival to the incisal edges of the upper anterior teeth. A crossbite (see Figure 34.8) may involve anterior or posterior teeth. When the upper teeth occlude lingual to the lower teeth the teeth are in a crossbite relationship. If a crossbite occurs on one side of the mouth it is unilateral while if it occurs on both sides it is bilateral. One or more teeth may be in a crossbite relationship.

Class I	In a Class I malocclusion, the mesiobuccal cusp of the upper first permanent molar occludes in the buccal groove of the lower first permanent molar and the maxilla is in an ideal relationship to the mandible. Class I malocclusions are the most common and include crowding, spacing, protruding teeth, space loss, extra or supernumerary teeth, crossbite and rotated teeth.
Class II	In Class II malocclusion, the lower first molar is distal to its ideal relationship to the upper first molar. The mandible is distal to its normal relationship to the maxilla. There are two divisions of Class II malocclusion depending on the degree of overjet and the inclination of the upper incisors.
Class II division 1	The upper anterior teeth protrude, giving an overjet greater than ideal. The molar relationship is Class II.
Class II division 2	The upper central incisors are often inclined lingually, a deep bite exists and the lower incisors may not be visible. The upper lateral incisors are often proclined. The molar positions are Class II.
Class III	In Class III malocclusion, the lower first molar is mesial to its ideal relationship with the upper first molar. The lower jaw may be mesial to the ideal relative position with the upper jaw giving the patient a prominent look to the lower jaw. There may be an anterior crossbite as a result.

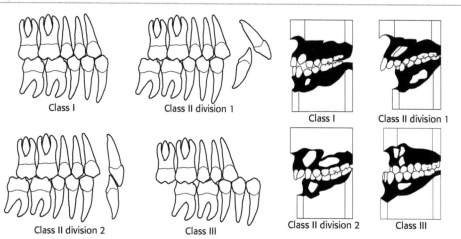

Table 34.1 Orthodontic classification

Class I	Class I lower incisors occlude with the middle third of the palatal surface of the upper incisors, there being an average overbite (3 mm) and an overjet.
Class II division 1	There is an increase in the degree of overjet present that is greater than 2 mm.
Class II division 2	Both the upper and lower incisors lean lingually to give an increased inter-incisal angle. There is an increase in incisor overbite and typically the upper lateral incisors protrude.
Class III	The lower incisors occlude anterior to the middle third of the palatal surface of the upper incisors and there may also be a reduced overjet and overbite. Edge-to-edge relationships and reverse overjet incisor relationships occur. This incisor relationship may be due to two teeth meeting edge-to-edge and subsequently the mandibular teeth gliding forwards into a displaced position characteristic of Class III incisor relationship.

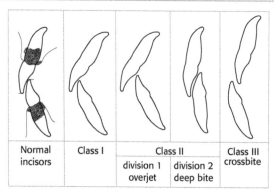

Table 34.2 Incisor classification

336

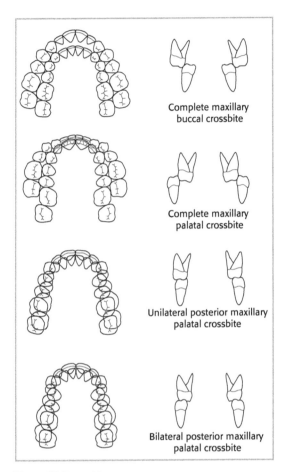

Complete maxillary
buccal crossbite

Complete maxillary
palatal crossbite

Unilateral posterior maxillary
palatal crossbite

Bilateral posterior maxillary
palatal crossbite

Figure 34.8 Crossbites

Mandibular displacement

Mandibular displacement is dislocation of the condyle in an anterior direction, past the articular eminence.

Skeletal pattern

Using either clinical estimation or **cephalometry**, the relative positions of the most anterior parts of the maxillary and mandibular dental bases relative to the bridge of the nose may be described as Class I, II or III.

Soft tissue patterns

When the mandible is in a relaxed position and the lips come together without effort, they are considered to be competent lips. When the lips are normally apart and the oral seal is only achieved by muscular effort, the lips are considered to be incompetent lips.

Speech

Sigmatism is the inability to produce the 'S' sound.

Causes of malocclusion

Hereditary and congenital causes

Hereditary malocclusions are those that are inherited through genetic causes. Children often have malocclusions similar to their parents.

Congenital malocclusions are those present at birth (e.g. cleft palate related malocclusions).

Developmental causes

Growth irregularities can also result in malocclusion, as follows:

- If the forward growth of the lower jaw is insufficient, a Class II malocclusion will result.
- If the growth in the lower jaw is excessive or if the forward growth of the upper jaw is insufficient a Class III malocclusion will result.
- If the growth in the length of the dental arch is not sufficient, posterior teeth may be crowded (e.g. third molars may become impacted).
- If growth in the width of the dental arch is not sufficient, permanent anterior teeth may be crowded.

Dental causes

- Premature loss of primary teeth — drifting of adjacent permanent teeth may occur and lead to space loss and associated malocclusion. Tooth decay that causes the loss of substantial amounts of tooth structure may cause space loss.
- Loss of permanent teeth — teeth adjacent to where teeth are lost may drift in all directions and lead to malocclusion.
- Prolonged retention of primary teeth — erupting permanent teeth may be deflected or delayed in their eruption due to the primary teeth being retained for too long.
- Missing and supernumerary teeth — upper lateral incisors, lower second premolars and third molars are commonly missing and this may give rise to undesirable drifting or spacing of teeth.
- Supernumerary or extra teeth may delay or deflect the eruption of adjacent teeth and take up space intended for other teeth.

- **cephalometry:** the measurements of the dimensions of the human head taken either directly or by means of x-ray.

- Abnormal fraenum attachments — often in the upper midline, the labial fraenum may contribute to spacing between the upper central incisors.

- Badly shaped restorations — under-contoured or over-contoured restorations may affect the relationships of adjacent teeth.

Habits

If thumb- and finger-sucking are prolonged and intensive, an open bite, proclined upper anterior teeth and lingually inclined lower incisors may result. This would mean an increase in the overjet. Crossbites affecting the posterior teeth may also result. Whether these changes occur depends on the intensity and the duration of the sucking and the position of the fingers (see Figure 34.9).

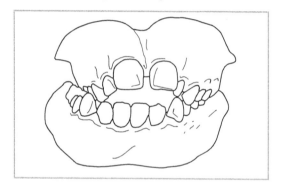

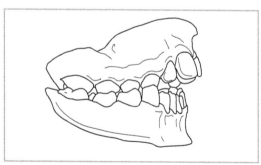

Figure 34.9 Effects of thumb-sucking

Other habits which can lead to malocclusion problems are:

- Dummy-sucking may cause a slight open bite but is not as serious a concern as digit sucking.

- Mouth-breathing may cause constriction of the upper arch leading to crossbite affecting the posterior teeth. The palatal vault may narrow as a result. The anterior teeth may procline and an anterior open bite may result due to the forward position of the tongue.

- Forward posturing of the tongue during swallowing and speech may produce an open bite and proclined anterior teeth.

Malocclusion and speech

Loss of anterior deciduous teeth may make articulation difficult and abnormal patterns of speech may develop. Malposition of individual teeth and adverse dental base relationships may make speech uncomfortable to perform and the child may speak in a manner that causes least discomfort. Orthodontic appliances may render speech temporarily defective due to the space they occupy in the mouth. The orthodontist and speech pathologist should consult with each other when a malocclusion is to be corrected and, at the same time, a speech irregularity is present.

Patient assessment

Management of the orthodontic problem can be divided into patient assessment, appliance therapy and retention.

Patient assessment involves:

- a clinical examination;

- taking records of the patient's present condition for analysis — such records include models, radiographs and photographs;

- making an analysis of the occlusion;

- formulating a treatment plan; and

- estimating the duration of treatment and indicating the prognosis to the patient.

Clinical examination

The clinical examination will assess:

- Reason for attendance — it is important to know why patients want orthodontic treatment, in order to motivate them satisfactorily and also to treat the problem for which they have sought advice. Medical and dental histories are often compiled by a questionnaire that you can help the parent to complete while the child is being examined. It is important to learn of any medical conditions that may conflict with orthodontic treatment.

- General morphology — the patient's general body size and development are assessed by taking height and weight measurements and comparing these with what is considered normal, and also by assessing the skeletal maturity level from hand and wrist radiographs and development of secondary sexual characteristics.

- General dental condition — this will include an assessment of caries incidence and periodontal condition. Patients may require general dental treatment before beginning their orthodontic treatment.

- Dental arch analysis — this will consider irregularities in arch form such as ovoid, square or tapering arches.

- Dental occlusion — this will include the incisor relationship, the molar relationship, overbite and overjet.

- The soft tissue pattern, which will include a description of tongue and lip activity, and their positions at rest.

- Cephalometric findings. These will indicate the linear and angular measurement of the dentist's choice to allow a geometric analysis of bony and soft tissue patterns.

Diagnostic records

To assist with the assessment of the patient's treatment needs and to assess the treatment progress, a number of diagnostic records are taken.

- Upper and lower study models indicate the way the teeth occlude at the beginning of treatment. The models are also useful to check arch form and general progress during treatment.

- Lateral cephalogram, OPG and periapical radiographs are commonly used to assess the patient prior to treatment, to assess tooth and jaw relationships and look for abnormalities of tooth and root form or the presence of pathology or other abnormal dental and bony features. Soft tissue form can also be analysed, particularly on the lateral cephalogram. A hand and wrist film may be taken if an assessment of the skeletal maturity of the patient is required.

- Full face, profile and intra-oral photographs are also useful records for soft tissue and dental assessment.

With the clinical and cephalometric assessment available and with record models and photographs also at hand, the dentist or orthodontist will be ready to analyse the case to determine the patient's growth pattern, the degree of crowding and spacing in the arches, the number of rotations present, whether or not there is mandibular displacement producing an eccentric occlusion and also to assess any skeletal disharmony and adverse soft tissue pattern. The position of any impacted or any unerupted teeth will be noted and at this stage the dentist will make an assessment as to the patient's

interest and that of the family in commencing orthodontic treatment.

Treatment planning

Orthodontic treatment should be considered as part of total dental care of the patient. It may be that the patient requires observation only for the time being, as the occlusion is not fully developed. Alternatively, interceptive procedures may produce a more favourable dentition during the developmental stages. This may or may not be followed by appliance therapy (generally between the ages of 11–14). Active orthodontic appliance therapy may be required. (Refer to separate heading below for a discussion of appliance therapy.) The extent and nature of tooth movement required to align teeth and establish a Class I incisor relationship should be noted. The dentist will decide whether these tooth movements, depending on the angulation of the teeth and other factors, will call for fixed or removable appliance therapy.

During appliance therapy the anchorage segments may need support by extra-oral appliances or inter-maxillary elastics.

The need for surgery in combination with orthodontic treatment will be considered. This may take the form of dento-alveolar surgery to remove supernumerary teeth or to expose un-erupted teeth or skeletal surgery aiming to correct gross disharmony of the basal bones. An orthodontist will decide which form of treatment will give the best result. Extractions may be required to relieve crowding as an interceptive measure, and this may be followed by appliance therapy later.

Preventive and interceptive orthodontics

Preventive orthodontics

These techniques aim to prevent the development of malocclusion. For example, the aim of the treatment may simply be to prevent premature loss of a tooth through decay. When teeth are lost prematurely, neighbouring teeth can crowd the space and that can mean there is insufficient room for erupting permanent teeth. If a tooth cannot be saved, a space **maintainer** may be required.

Preventive orthodontics also aim to correct habits that may be damaging. For example, preventive techniques may be required to teach a child not to suck their thumb.

■ **maintainer:** a device developed to fill a gap created by the loss of a tooth. A method to prevent malocclusion.

Interceptive orthodontics

These techniques involve intervention during the development of orthodontic malocclusions to lessen the severity of the case. Commonly, they involve the removal of teeth to prevent overcrowding, or the removal of deciduous teeth that are contributing to a malocclusion. Crossbites may also be corrected at this stage.

Appliance therapy

Appliance therapy involves the movement of teeth and/or the jaw using fixed or removable appliances or, commonly, a combination of the two. When the matter of orthodontic treatment is discussed with the family, photographs of orthodontic appliances should be available so that the orthodontist can illustrate the method of treatment with the patient.

As well as instruction at the insertion of the appliance, the family will require reassurance regarding certain features common to both fixed and removable appliances.

■ When the teeth initially move, they will become tender for several hours after the force is applied but this should resolve within the first three days. Analgesics may be prescribed in order to help the patient over this initial period of discomfort.

■ Speech may be temporarily distorted, especially where removable appliances are worn.

■ There may also be some irritation of the lips, cheeks and tongue during this initial period of adjustment to appliance wearing. If any severe irritation occurs, the patient should seek advice from the orthodontist, but minor irritation from fixed appliances may be overcome by applying soft medicated wax to any rough areas found on the appliance.

The patient should expect the teeth to move at the rate of 1 mm per month. During tooth movement some irregularities in the appearance may occur. This should not be a cause for any undue concern.

Removable appliances

Removable appliances may consist of:

■ a plastic base;

■ clasps that allow the appliance to be fixed to the teeth;

■ a labial bow, which can be used as a support or as an active component to align teeth;

■ the active component, which can either be resilient wire springs, a labial bow, or screw; and

■ bite-planes, or plates (see Figure 34.10), which may be incorporated in the plastic base in order to disengage the occlusion. They may be placed palatal to the upper anterior teeth, or capping the occlusal surface of the molar and bicuspid teeth.

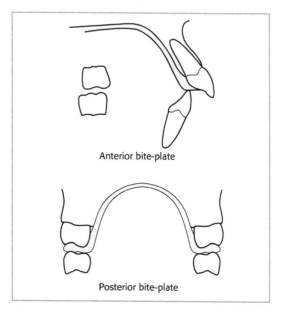

Anterior bite-plate

Posterior bite-plate

Figure 34.10 Bite-plates

There may also be additional hooks or spurs to maintain teeth in place or act as attachments for elastic traction or extra-oral traction. Removable appliances exert point pressure on teeth by means of springs or screws. Their mode of action is by tipping teeth into an improved position. Removable appliances usually have no facility for controlling root movement and they are also of little value in rotational movement of teeth.

Fixed appliances

Fixed appliances are orthodontic devices fixed to the teeth. Forces are applied by arch wires or auxiliaries via attachments welded to bands or brackets. This system allows precise control over tooth movement.

The type of tooth movement that can be achieved is increased in scope by use of fixed appliances. They are capable of more easily rotating and uprighting teeth than removable appliances. However, as in removable appliance treatment, the teeth must be moved to a position of muscular balance well supported by the alveolar bone. See Figure 34.11.

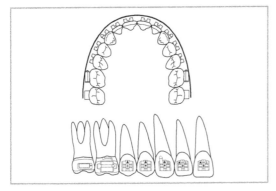

Figure 34.11 Straight wire appliance

Bands are preformed into various sizes to fit the teeth. They circle the tooth and are cemented to it and are most commonly used on the molars. Brackets, which are bonded directly to the tooth, are mostly used on anterior teeth and premolars. Bands (see Figure 34.12) and brackets are also called attachments. They allow controlled forces to be applied to the tooth. Before bands can be placed, the teeth must be separated to make a suitable space. Separators are placed for periods of time long enough to allow the separation to occur before the placement of bands (usually five to seven days before).

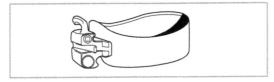

Figure 34.12 Orthodontic band

Arch wires may be round, or rectangular and may be formed in the contour of the dental arches. They are secured to the brackets or the bands by either soft wire ligatures, plastic rings or pins.

Auxiliary springs may be added to the arch wire or connected to the brackets to give additional force where required. Latex bands (Figures 34.13 a and b) are also used between groups of teeth to transmit forces from one group of teeth to another in the same arch or in opposing arches (intramaxillary or intermaxillary traction).

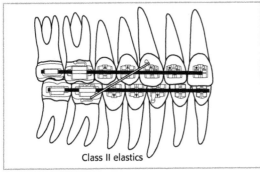
Class II elastics

Figure 34.13a Elastics

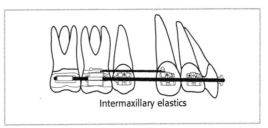
Intermaxillary elastics

Figure 34.13b Intermaxillary elastics

A great deal of patient cooperation is required if they are to wear fixed appliances satisfactorily. They must be careful not to damage the appliance by eating tough, fibrous or sticky food. It is imperative that the latex rubbers and extra-oral traction devices are worn as prescribed.

The management of orthodontic appliances retention

Following a course of orthodontic tooth movement, the teeth are held in position by retainers (Figure 34.14) that may be fixed or removable. Depending on the type of malocclusion that was corrected, the retainer may be worn full-time for part of the retention period and subsequently at night only.

It is important that the patient understands the necessity for wearing retainers during this phase of treatment, as failure to do so could lead to the occlusion returning to its previous state. The patient must realise that bone takes nine to 12 months to return to a stable pattern following orthodontic tooth movement and that retention may be necessary during completion of facial growth and of the dentition.

The period of retention will vary case by case. Some patients may need to wear retainers indefinitely to ensure stability for the treatment result.

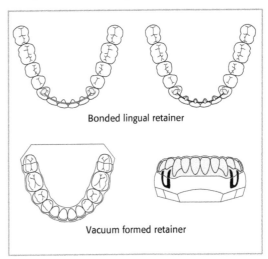
Bonded lingual retainer

Vacuum formed retainer

Figure 34.14 Retainers

Care of teeth and gums

Providing that the patient's plaque level is low and there is no chronic marginal gingivitis in the mouth, it is unlikely that the orthodontic appliance will damage the oral tissue. It is useful if a plaque scoring system is used to estimate the patient's standard of oral hygiene in order to avoid hyperplastic gingivitis and enamel decalcification during orthodontic treatment. It is essential that any patient about to undergo orthodontic treatment be instructed in toothbrushing and flossing technique and also about diet (and in particular about the level of intake of refined carbohydrates).

Care of removable appliances

Removable appliances should be inserted and worn as directed by the orthodontist and must be cleaned regularly, using toothbrush and toothpaste, following meals or snacks. The appliance should never come into contact with very hot water as this may distort the acrylic. At the same time the teeth and gums should be cleaned thoroughly. Screws and springs should be cared for as directed by the orthodontist. The patient should definitely be instructed not to play with the appliance or move it up and down with the tongue. The patient should be warned that there may be slight difficulty in eating and talking for the first 48 hours and the teeth may be painful to touch during the initial period.

Care of fixed appliances

Patients wearing fixed appliances should be advised to avoid eating sticky food and especially hard candies. They should also be advised not to eat raw carrots, celery or hard apples as biting these foods, particularly on the anterior teeth, will dislodge attachments. Should they become distorted or dislodged, the patient should contact the surgery immediately for an appointment. Should any wires become distorted the patient should likewise arrange an immediate appointment with the orthodontist so that adjustments can be made, otherwise unwanted tooth movements may occur.

The teeth and the appliance should be cleaned with particular care using a horizontal movement of the toothbrush across the brackets and arch wires, in order to avoid dislodgement of any wires or elastics that may be present. Toothbrushes that accommodate orthodontic brackets are available.

The dental assistant's role in orthodontic treatment

During orthodontic treatment, you have many duties, including:

- ensuring that the surgery is equipped and laid out to care for the dentist's and the patient's needs and that the necessary instruments and dental material are available for patient treatment when required;
- ensuring that infection control procedures are carefully followed;
- assisting the orthodontist at the chair-side, ensuring that all equipment and materials are ready and available for use, and assisting in the manipulation of these instruments and materials in the patient's mouth; and
- being available to help the patient and ensuring that the patient and the family are made comfortable in the dental surgery. You must also ensure that any questions that arise are answered by the orthodontist so that the patient is fully informed of the procedures intended and those that are being undertaken.

The instruments

The instruments required for orthodontic treatment vary with the type of work that is being undertaken.

When the orthodontist has completed the treatment procedure, you will be required to clean the bracket table and work surfaces with a surface decontaminant. You will need to scrub the instruments in a detergent solution to remove all traces of oral fluid and cement and then sterilise the instruments in an autoclave using a tray system. You will need to periodically check the sharpness of the cutting instruments and that the joints of all pliers are free moving.

Record taking

At initial examination for orthodontic treatment, the orthodontist will note clinical details and you should record these on an assessment form. You can also assist in taking a social and medical history that the orthodontist can use as a basis for discussion with the family. You may be asked to weigh and measure the patient to assess the level of maturity. The orthodontist will also make models of the mouth so you will need to prepare alginate and impression trays.

Radiographs and photographs

The orthodontist will require a full mouth radiographic survey. Usually an orthopantomogram (OPG) and lateral skull radiograph are taken as a bare minimum. Other radiographs may supplement this. Lateral skull radiographs will be required in order to analyse the patient's facial form. This is assessed by tracing anatomical landmarks that can then be related to each other.

You have a part to play in the tracing and measuring of these various points. It is important to have photographs of the patient before and after orthodontic treatment. Full face, right profile and intraoral views of the anterior teeth and the left and right buccal segments are necessary in order to give an assessment of the malocclusion. Mirror views of the upper and lower dental arches may also be required in certain circumstances. It should be possible for you to participate in the taking of these standard photographic views and the filing of them.

During treatment

When the stage is reached that bands are to be placed, the orthodontist will decide on the need to separate the teeth to allow band placement. A separate appointment seven days before banding will be required to allow placement of separators. These may be plastic modules, soft wire or spring wire types. A thorough prophylaxis of the teeth precedes band selection and when bands have been fitted and the appropriate attachments welded to them, the cementation can be undertaken.

For this phase of treatment, the mouth must be kept scrupulously dry. The aspirator, retractors and cotton rolls will aid in this. This procedure may last up to an hour and the patient must be adequately prepared for sitting in the chair for this lengthy period. In some instances, sedatives may be prescribed.

Bonding of brackets

In most circumstances it is preferable to bond brackets directly to the teeth rather than placing bands. There is also an advantage from an aesthetic point of view as the patients prefer bonded brackets to bands.

For a proper bond to form, the teeth must be etched first. The tooth surface must be cleaned with a prophylaxis paste. After the field is dried, an etching agent (35 per cent phosphoric acid) is applied so that the bonding resin may make superficial penetration into the enamel. It is important that you

ensure that a dry field can be maintained during this procedure. Make sure you know how to prepare and use the bonding material before commencing the procedure.

Placing arch wires

You may be required to assist the orthodontist by retracting oral tissues to allow adequate access to the mouth while arch wires are placed. You may also assist in attaching auxiliary elastic bands and extra-oral traction appliances. The patient has to learn to manage these at home.

Removing orthodontic bands

The orthodontist will require you to set out equipment so that the bands and arch wires may be removed from the teeth. This procedure produces some discomfort as there is considerable pressure placed on the teeth during band removal and the patient may require reassurance during this time.

Following band removal, cement removal and polishing of the teeth will be undertaken and you will need to set up an ultrasonic scaler, suitable polishing paste and either rubber cups or brushes in a contra-angle handpiece. You will assist during these procedures by having an aspirator ready to collect the fragments of cement and to generally remove debris from the mouth and ensure the patient's general comfort. After band removal, alginate impressions will be required to take study models needed to make retainers.

At the routine adjustment of appliances you should do your utmost to motivate the patient to wear the retainers as instructed and ensure that it is quite comfortable and provides no problems. Should any problems arise, bring these to the attention of the orthodontist. The patient is often motivated by showing their fitted appliances in a hand mirror.

Making appointments

You should know the length of time required for each of the procedures in orthodontics in order to set aside appropriate periods of time in the orthodontist's appointment book. Banding procedures will require varying amounts of time depending on the procedure being undertaken and you should acquaint yourself with the operator's requirements so that each patient is seen at the appointed time.

In conjunction with the orthodontist you may discuss with the family the progress of tooth movement that is being made. Use of study models and photographs will give encouragement to the patient during the treatment period, which may extend over 18 months to two years.

If you know that the patient is nervous about future treatment, you should tell the orthodontist. You should also keep the orthodontist informed of changing social and financial circumstances in the family if they come to your notice.

You are a vital part of the team treating orthodontic patients and your *calm and positive approach* can favourably turn the balance when patients are nervous or embarrassed by meeting friends or speaking for the first time with a new appliance in place. You should take an informed and intelligent interest in the management of the orthodontic treatment.

Orthodontic emergencies

Problems that arise in removable appliance orthodontic treatment usually consist of the acrylic or wire abrading the mucosa. Where removable appliances have broken, the assistance of the dental technician will be required and the technician should be warned before the patient attends. In situations where the patient has been unable to wear the appliance, it may now be a poor fit and a new appliance may be required. Liaison with the dental technician is necessary for construction of a new appliance.

Where fixed appliances are being worn, the most frequent problems that arise are bands or brackets that have become dislodged, ligatures and elastics that have become displaced and arch wires that have become distorted or broken. In many instances, where the band has become dislodged, a new band or modification of the existing band will be required and you should therefore set out the appropriate instruments, both for band selection and seating, and for arch adjustment.

When patients telephone for an appointment because of a broken appliance, whether it is removable, fixed or of the extra-oral type, you should endeavour to make arrangements for the patient to be seen within 24 hours. Further delay could cause unwanted tooth movement and seriously disturb the progress of the treatment.

Summary

The aim of orthodontic treatment is to align the teeth in a new and stable position. This treatment is not simply cosmetic, although it will often improve the appearance of the teeth and face. It will also reduce the likelihood of caries and periodontal disease because it will allow better plaque removal. Treatment can often make chewing more efficient and can sometimes improve the formation of some speech sounds.

Additionally, irregularities in the occlusion can sometimes cause pain and dysfunction of the temporomandibular joint and related musculature. Jaw misplacement can cause swallowing diffiulties. Correcting the occlusion will often relieve these symptoms.

chapter thirty-five
paedodontics

Introduction

Paediatric dentistry is a recognised dental specialty in Australia and many other countries of the world. It encompasses the comprehensive dental care of children including those needing:

- preventive therapy;
- restorative treatment;
- behaviour management techniques;
- trauma management;
- treatment of oral pathology;
- minor orthodontic treatment; and
- minor surgical treatment.

Although all children can be seen in specialist paediatric dental practice, the specialty focuses on those who have complex dental treatment needs, behavioural difficulties, medical compromises and special needs, orofacial and dental developmental anomalies and trauma.

A good understanding of child development is essential for all members of the dental team who are involved in dentistry for children. In order to effectively manage children of all ages, with their differing psychological development in addition to their wide range of dental needs, the dental team must have a practical knowledge of child development. Children's psychological, **somatic** and dental development can all progress at different rates for their chronological age. In addition, male and female development can be quite different at particular stages. The dental team should use their knowledge of child development to communicate effectively and have appropriate expectations of each individual child patient.

In addition to the stages of child development each child has a unique personality. An assessment and understanding of a child's personality type is important for the child's effective dental management. While some children have an easygoing nature and can easily handle changes in plans, others need to be given more time to adjust to new situations.

General stages of pre-school child development

The two-year old

Two-year-olds are usually very active and curious. They have a short attention span and explore their surroundings using all of their five senses: touch, taste, sight, smell and sound. As the mouth is a very sensitive part of the body they often explore unfamiliar objects by mouthing them to see how they feel and taste.

The two-year old is developing both gross and fine motor skills rapidly but at this age often shows clumsy movements and finds it difficult to handle small objects. There is usually a very close bond with the mother or primary care giver and these children are reluctant to be separated from them for any length of time.

Language is only just beginning to develop and is often limited to single words or short phrases. However, the level of understanding (receptive language) is usually far greater than the child's own language (expressive language). Explanations and instructions should be kept simple and short, and statements rather than open questions should be used. For example, it is more effective to say, 'Come and have a ride on our magic chair,' than, 'Would you like to ride on our magic chair?'. The latter allows the child to give the familiar two-year-old response of, 'No!'

■ **somatic**: of the body (as opposed to of the mind).

345

During this age, feelings of frustration are often shown by temper tantrums due to the lack of expressive language skills. Distraction is an effective method of management of two-year-olds as their attention is often easily diverted by something else of interest.

The three-year old

Three-year-olds have developed greater skill in observing their surroundings using sight, sound and smell, and rarely explore objects by placing them in their mouths. Their gross motor skills have developed sufficiently to be able to move around confidently and with ease. The fine motor skills continue to develop enabling them to handle smaller objects and begin to draw and colour-in purposefully.

Expressive language is quite variable at this age with some children still limited to short phrases whilst others have the ability to carry out extensive conversations. Receptive language has also developed to the point where more detailed explanations and instructions can be used.

Three-year-olds often show better self-control and increased language skills so temper tantrums are less common. They like to please adults and receive praise for compliant behaviour but their independence often leads to resisting adult assistance. Whilst distraction can be useful for three-year-olds the adult needs to be more resourceful in the distraction technique. Other methods of management that are useful for three-year-olds are 'tell-show-do', playful humour and positive reinforcement.

The four-year old

Four-year-olds often show much greater independence now that their skills in observation, gross motor and fine motor are becoming much more developed. Their expressive language is usually quite understandable and four-year-olds are usually able to take part in everyday conversations.

Individual personalities can become quite identifiable at this age so there will be a wide range of personalities, from shy to bossy, or cheeky. Receptive language is now well developed and the four-year old will be able to comprehend most adult conversation. For this reason it is very important to be mindful of conversations directed to the parents/carers and not assume that the child is either not listening or not comprehending what has been said. It is also important to choose dental terminology carefully while in the child's presence. Consider how the words 'gross' and 'acute' (a cute) may be interpreted by a child of this age.

Despite four-year-olds' newly gained independence, they often still hold a very strong maternal (or primary carer) attachment so it is still most often desirable to avoid separating the child and parent during the dental visit.

Four-year-olds' attention span, whilst improving, is still limited and they may find it difficult to lie still for an extended period of time. Try keeping appointments short and where that is not possible, give children a chance to rest or 'wriggle' during appropriate times throughout longer procedures.

The five-year old

Five-year-olds have become skilful in both gross and fine motor control, being capable of unaided dressing and feeding and showing greatly improved dexterity. Expressive language is catching up to receptive language, enabling this age group to participate in involved conversations.

The commencement of formal schooling brings greater socialisation and the importance of rules. This can be used to great advantage in the dental setting where ground rules for behaviour in the dental surgery can be set and the child can be encouraged to follow them. It is still beneficial to keep appointment as short as possible and give the five-year old suitable breaks.

Childhood habits

Thumb/finger/dummy-sucking is a common habit during the preschool years. Babies have a natural sucking reflex that begins before birth and is often carried into childhood as a soothing habit. Prolonged thumb/finger/dummy-sucking into the permanent dentition can cause proclination of the upper incisors, retroclination of the lower incisors, a constricted maxillary arch and formation of an anterior open bite. Management of thumb/finger/dummy-sucking usually involves a programme of self-control, use of removable or fixed appliances and/or orthodontic correction of the resultant malocclusion.

Bruxism is common in children, especially during times of eruption of new teeth. In the primary dentition bruxism can cause severe wear of primary tooth structure, even causing pulp exposure in extreme cases. Stress and life changes can initiate or exacerbate episodes of bruxism so management may need to involve counselling.

The clinical environment

The dental practice

A child's dental experience begins long before they sit in the dental chair or even arrive at the dental practice. They may enter the practice without hesitation, having had no prior dental experience, or they may come with a series of past memories or transmitted emotions from parents, siblings or others. For this reason it is essential that a child is taken care of from the moment they enter the dental practice.

The reception area/waiting room

On entering a dental practice a child patient should be made to feel comfortable and welcome. The reception area should cater for child patients by offering appropriate seating, books and toys. These items should be sturdy and easy to clean. They should be assessed for potential safety hazards. A special children's play pit or corner is ideal.

Young children should not be left alone in the reception area/waiting room if the parent is receiving treatment. You may be able to use this opportunity to begin talking with the child and perhaps introducing the child to the dental environment in a spare surgery.

Wherever possible, children should not be kept waiting excessively, as long delays can have a negative impact on timid and nervous children. The dentist or dental assistant should greet the child in the waiting room (without wearing a mask) and accompany them into the dental surgery. This is a good opportunity to begin a conversation with the child. This helps to distract them from the unfamiliar environment they are entering. By having a friendly and sympathetic nature and by engaging the child in appropriate conversation (i.e. favourite TV shows, best friends, school etc.) you and the dentist will show that you are genuinely interested in the child. Remembering these things at subsequent appointments will help begin new conversations and will make a child feel particularly special, and may put them at ease more quickly.

An interview room or non-surgical environment is often useful for new patients who are apprehensive about the dental treatment.

The general design and décor of the dental surgery should be appealing to all patients, including children. This can be achieved with the use of soothing colours and a clean, uncluttered layout. Any dental equipment not required during the appointment should be out of view wherever possible.

The surgery

Most often, it is desirable to have the parent or carer accompany the child into the dental surgery to support the child during the dental visit. However, if parents or carers are unable or unwilling to provide such support, then it may be more appropriate that they remain in the waiting room.

The dental surgery should be prepared in such a way that all potentially threatening objects, such as dental instruments, dental handpieces and so forth, are kept out of sight until the child is seated and settled, ready for the treatment to begin. At this time instruments can be passed from dental assistant to dentist behind the child's line of sight. The dental chair should be adaptable to a small child, and where necessary, a cushion can be used to improve comfort during lengthy appointments.

It is especially important that children are introduced to the dental environment at a pace that suits their stage of development and their personality. While some children will enter the surgery freely and sit in the chair without prompting, others may need a little time and some explanation before they feel at ease.

The staff

Whilst in the dental surgery the dentist and dental assistant should take a primary role in communicating with the child. Parents or carers can be politely encouraged to take a secondary role whilst still offering support to the child. This is best achieved when the parent or carer is seated in proximity or direct contact (i.e. holding the child's hand or leg) but without interrupting the flow of conversation between the dentist/dental assistant and child.

Role of the dental assistant in paediatric dentistry

General dental practitioners play a vital role in the dental care of children so it is essential for all dental assistants to have a good understanding of children and their dental care. Often the dental assistant will be the first person that a child patient interacts with on visiting the dental surgery. It is important that this relationship begins well so that the child has an opportunity to gain confidence within the dental environment and accept dental care.

Appointment scheduling and types of treatment

Each child will react and feel differently when entering the surgery because children are individuals and have different personalities and past experiences. Some will be relaxed, whilst others may be unsure, anxious or frightened. Children who are familiar with you and the dentist and have had pleasant experiences in the past, will often come into the surgery freely and without any anxiety. However, if there has been a previous negative experience a child may be apprehensive and reluctant to enter the surgery. Worse still is the reaction of a child who has previously been threatened or lied to by his parents/carers or the dentist/dental assistant.

It is important to realise that children show fear in many ways. Some are shy or quiet while others behave negatively to keep away from the source of their fear. A child with negative behaviour (screaming, kicking and biting) may be masking a severe anxiety towards dental treatment. It is difficult to overcome such fear and anxiety but showing empathy and being patient and understanding often works to gain the child's confidence. The child should be made to feel safe and given time to adjust to the sometimes overwhelming environment of the dental surgery.

Remember, with children:

- speak quietly and with a friendly tone;
- do not encroach on the child's personal space any more than necessary;
- give the child time to move toward you and become friendly rather than moving too quickly towards them;
- do not talk too much but engage the child in a conversation that you think will interest the child; and
- use appropriate language for the child's stage of development.

First appointment

Ideally the first visit to the practice for a child will be an appointment for another family member or carer. This will allow the child to experience the dental environment and observe a routine dental appointment. This kind of familiarisation avoids children being expected to 'perform' in an unknown environment and allows them to gradually become used to the dental setting.

The Australasian Academy of Paediatric Dentistry recommends that children be brought for their first dental visit following the eruption of their first tooth and no later than the age of one. This visit will ideally result in the child experiencing the dental environment by observing a parent/carer or sibling, having a ride in the dental chair and possibly being introduced to basic dental instruments and equipment (mouth mirror, triplex, evacuator). The benefits of having an early visit are that the dentist can discuss dietary and oral hygiene practices with the parent/carer and hopefully avoid any bad habits from starting. Also at this time, if any potential or existing problems are detected they can be managed early. Most importantly, though, it will start the child on a path of regular dental care that can carry through into adulthood.

Emergency examination

A planned first dental appointment contrasts a situation where a child attends for the first time, in oral pain and discomfort and requiring examination and/or treatment immediately. Under these circumstances there is less opportunity for gradual familiarisation and where there are extensive treatment requirements it may result in a child having the treatment carried out under general anaesthesia.

When an emergency examination is required for a young child in acute pain or following a traumatic incident, the 'knee-to-knee' examination is often the most successful. Using this technique the parent/carer and dentist sit facing each other on normal chairs. The child sits facing the parent/carer on their knee and is then laid back into the dentist's lap. The parent/carer can then apply mild restraint to control the child's arm and leg movements. The child's head is positioned on the dentist's knee where it can be supported by the inside of his/her wrists. This position gives the dentist good control of the child's head and allows an excellent view into the oral cavity for examination. If they are present and actively involved in the examination, the parent/carer is less likely to be disturbed if the child is uncooperative.

Subsequent appointments

Subsequent appointments may pass without any emotional tension or upset. Alternately, following a successful first visit the child may unexpectedly be hesitant, reluctant or completely uncontrollable. Some children do not show their apprehension of the dental environment at the first visit but on re-entering the dental surgery become overwhelmed.

For this reason it is important that the child's experience during subsequent appointments reinforces a sense of order, safety and control.

You play an important role in greeting the child and putting them at ease. By repeating the familiarisation process carried out at the first visit, the child will often settle and take comfort from the sense of routine. Some children will require extensive familiarisation (more than one appointment) in order to commence treatment.

While the child continues to improve and accept further treatment the process should be considered a success. If, however, the dentist is unable to progress past an initial examination then other management techniques or referral of the child may need to be considered.

Behaviour management techniques

The goals of behaviour management in paediatric dentistry are to allow successful dental treatment to be carried out and to instil a positive dental attitude. Behaviour management encompasses a whole range of techniques from the use of facial expressions and voice tone to carrying out dental treatment under general anaesthesia. The most common techniques used in paediatric dentistry are used every day and on every individual patient to a certain degree.

Some child patients require no more than a good explanation of proposed treatment and a calm and unhurried approach but others may find it difficult or impossible to tolerate dental treatment while conscious. Some of the following techniques can be carried out by general dentists while others are more commonly used following referral to a specialist paediatric dentist.

Familiarisation and behaviour modification

Familiarisation of child patients is used universally with both cooperative and uncooperative children. The techniques most often used are voice control, non-verbal communication, positive reinforcement, tell-show-do and distraction. These are variously used on their own or in combinations that are targeted to the individual patient and their unique stage of development, personality and level of anxiety.

Voice control is simply a controlled alteration of the voice volume, tone or pace to influence a patient's behaviour and gain attention and compliance. Voice control is extremely common and is most often used in combination with other behaviour management techniques.

In a similar way, non-verbal communication uses contact, posture and facial expressions to reinforce and guide behaviour.

Positive reinforcement seeks to encourage good behaviour using positive voice changes, facial expressions, praise and rewards. This is another method used almost universally by those treating children.

Tell-show-do is a method of behaviour shaping used by many professionals who work with children. Firstly, verbal explanations of procedures are made using language appropriate to the child's age and developmental level. Secondly, the procedure is demonstrated in some way for the child in a controlled and non-threatening setting. Most often this stage is carried out extra-orally so that the child can see the procedure and experience how it feels, sounds and smells. For example, a prophylaxis cup can be used on a child's fingernail to demonstrate the slow-speed handpiece. Finally, the procedure is attempted.

Distraction is a method quite different to tell-show-do, where the child's attention is diverted from a potentially unpleasant procedure. This technique is used commonly for procedures such as the administration of local anaesthesia, where it would be inappropriate to use tell-show-do.

Prophylaxis and oral hygiene

The traditional method of dental prophylaxis using a rubber cup or bristle brush with prophylaxis paste has been found to remove fluoride-rich enamel from the surfaces of teeth. For this reason, toothbrush prophylaxis has gained wider acceptance for use during initial and recall examination visits.

Toothbrush prophylaxis has many benefits during a child's dental visit. It instils a sense of importance for the child of this routine home-care procedure, it allows the dentist to correctly demonstrate the procedure for the parent/carer and the child and it conserves the fluoride-rich enamel surface while enhancing the uptake of fluoride.

However, dental prophylaxis using a rubber cup only is often an excellent introduction to dental treatment as it is painless and introduces the child to some basic dental equipment. You play an important supporting role during prophylaxis. This procedure offers the dentist a perfect opportunity to begin the 'tell-show-do' process (see the 'Behaviour management techniques' section above) with an inexperienced child.

Fissure sealants

With the introduction of fluoride into community water supplies and toothpastes, the rate of smooth surface caries has declined dramatically. In fluoridated communities today, caries almost always begins in pits and fissures and interproximal contact points; areas where the topical action of fluoride is least effective.

The most effective way to prevent pit and fissure caries is by fissure sealing. Fissure sealants should be placed on susceptible teeth as soon as possible after eruption and when adequate isolation can be obtained. The permanent first molar is the most susceptible to fissure caries as it is the first permanent molar tooth to erupt into the mouth. At the time of eruption, at six to seven years of age, the child's level of dexterity is limited and adequate plaque control is often not achieved. Furthermore, the fissure pattern of these teeth is extremely variable from individual to individual, and where the fissure pattern is extensive and deep the risk of developing caries is higher.

Composite resin is recommended over glass ionomer cement as the material of choice as it has superior retention over time. An ideal fissure sealant should be placed under dental dam isolation and be opaque for ease of detection at future examinations.

Home care — the role of parents/carers

Toothbrushing

Parents/carers should be advised to begin cleaning children's teeth when they first appear in the mouth, at 6–9 months of age. Initially, a soft cloth can be used to wipe over the teeth. Once the child has become familiar with the tooth-wiping routine a small soft bristled toothbrush can be introduced to gently brush away plaque. Ideally, a twice-daily toothbrushing routine should be developed as soon as possible to set up a good oral hygiene habit that will be carried through into adulthood.

The ideal toothbrush for a toddler has a small head and soft bristles to reach all areas of their small mouth. It is essential for an adult to supervise toothbrushing, helping to clean all the tooth surfaces and encouraging spitting rather than swallowing or eating the toothpaste.

Only a smear of fluoride toothpaste should be used. Specially designed fluoride toothpastes with low fluoride levels are available for children six years and under. It is ideal for parents/carers to continue to assist with toothbrushing until the child is around 6–7 years of age and has sufficient dexterity to remove plaque effectively.

Disclosing solutions and tablets can be an effective aid for children and their parents/carers. The periodic home use of disclosing solution/tablets to show areas being missed by oral hygiene methods should be encouraged.

Flossing

Flossing can be introduced in the late preschool years. At this time the interproximal surfaces of the primary molars become more at risk of caries. To begin, parents/carers should be encouraged to floss for their children but once children gain sufficient dexterity they can be taught to floss themselves. There are commercial floss holders on the market that can make flossing easier until such time as the child is able to floss effectively on their own.

Fluoride therapy

The caries-preventive effect of fluoride was first discovered in connection with fluoridated drinking water in the early 1900s and for many years it was thought that the formation of a more resistant surface layer in enamel during tooth development was the primary anti-caries role. However, in recent years the importance of incorporation of fluoride in the enamel has come to be questioned.

The topical effect of fluoride is now recognised to be the most important for caries prevention. Even at very low concentrations, such as 1 part per million found in community water supplies, fluoride acts to enhance remineralisation and prevent demineralisation of enamel.

The saliva surrounding teeth is supersaturated with calcium and phosphate and in the continuous presence of small amounts of fluoride, remineralisation of enamel is favoured. When remineralisation takes place in the presence of fluoride the rebuilt enamel is more caries resistant than the original structure. This fluoride-rich surface layer of enamel develops post-eruptively in the presence of fluoride from fluoridated water, toothpaste and professionally applied fluoride products.

Brushing with fluoride toothpaste is another very effective fluoride delivery system. Regular adult toothpastes contain between 1000–1500 parts per million fluoride and specially formulated children's pastes contain 400–500 parts per million. This level is significantly higher than that found in the water supply and acts to provide a mini-fluoride treatment to teeth when brushing twice-daily.

There is now very limited need for the use of fluoride supplements in the form of tablets and drops. Even in communities with non-fluoridated water supplies, individuals acquire fluoride from multiple sources — commercially prepared food and drinks, toothpaste and professional fluoride products (such as rinses, gels and varnishes). Therefore, recommendation of fluoride tablets/drops should only be made for individuals with a high caries risk who have limited other sources of fluoride exposure. When prescribing fluoride tablets/drops the most effective method of usage is for the fluoride supplement to be added to household drinking water at 1 part per million. Using this method the topical effect of the supplement will be maximised.

Whilst the caries reduction achieved by the use of fluoride has been a major public health achievement, there is a need to use fluorides responsibly in order to minimise the effect of fluorosis. Fluorosis is a defect of enamel caused when there is excess fluoride present during the development of tooth enamel. It is most commonly seen in its mildest form — producing white flecks on the enamel of permanent teeth.

As the permanent teeth begin forming from birth onwards, it is essential that fluoride over-exposure from eating or swallowing excessive amounts of toothpaste is prevented. This period coincides with a time when toddlers and preschoolers want to show their independence during everyday tasks such as toothbrushing, so it is important that parents/carers are aware of the dangers of fluoride over-exposure and are urged to supervise their children carefully.

Professional fluoride solutions such as rinses, gels and varnishes are extremely concentrated (1000–25,000 parts per million) and should never be left within the reach of children. Often the amount of fluoride contained in such products is sufficient to cause acute toxicity requiring medical treatment and/or hospitalisation of young children. When providing or prescribing such products for adult patients it is essential that they be advised to store the product out of the reach of children. Children under the age of six years are unable to spit out effectively and should not be prescribed mouth-rinses until after this time. Concentrated gels and varnishes should be used very sparingly during dental preventive treatment as they can also cause acute toxicity in small children.

Radiography with children

Dental caries in the primary dentition may begin very early but remain clinically undetected for quite some time. The primary molars have a very low contact point, making interproximal caries (especially on the distal surface of the first primary molar) very difficult to detect visually. Bitewing and periapical radiographs are often quite difficult in the very young child, even when small films are used. Whilst OPG radiographs do not give the same quality of information, they are usually more easily tolerated by an uncooperative child.

For cooperative children three years and older, small film bitewing radiographs are preferable for detection of caries. The use of a lead apron with a thyroid shield is essential for radiation hygiene.

The dental operators should not assist the child during the exposure. If assistance is required, a parent/carer wearing a lead apron is the best option. When required, the parent/carer can sit on the dental chair with the child on their lap and assist the child in remaining still and holding the radiographic film in place where necessary. This technique can also be used for periapical radiographs for the examination of trauma or dental anomalies.

Anaesthesia and sedation for children

Local anaesthesia

Once successfully achieved, local anaesthesia will provide the potential for painless dental treatment and the basis of a good attitude towards dentistry.

Special care must be taken when first introducing a child to local anaesthesia. Initially, the child should be prepared for the experience using an explanation of what he/she will experience in words that are age appropriate. With the use of a good topical anaesthetic agent and allowing adequate time for it to act, many children will not find the experience unpleasant.

Preparation of the needle, syringe and carpule is ideally done before the child enters the surgery or unobtrusively and out of sight of the child. The prepared local anaesthetic syringe can then be passed to the dentist below the line of sight of the child. You can play an important role in distracting the child, offering support by holding the child's hands and/or preventing the child from any sudden movements that may be dangerous during the process.

Sedation

The use of nitrous oxide/oxygen sedation for child dental patients is extremely common. This safe and effective behaviour management technique offers a rapid effect and complete and fast recovery. The nitrous oxide/oxygen is administered via a nasal mask and results in relaxation, loss of time perception and decreased gag reflex. It does not provide anaesthesia and is most commonly used in conjunction with local anaesthetic. For an anxious child, once the nasal mask is accepted, it allows an increased level of cooperation while still conscious.

Other forms of nasal and oral sedation and premedication of children can be undertaken by qualified practitioners who possess appropriate equipment and facilities. However, many of the agents used give unpredictable results when used for the first time in children. In most circumstances, children requiring oral or nasal sedation should be managed by a specialist paediatric dentist within an approved facility.

General anaesthesia

For some children, their age, level of cooperation or complexity of dental treatment may necessitate the use of general anaesthesia. The objective of general anaesthesia is to provide a safe environment under which quality dental care can be provided efficiently and effectively to those who are otherwise unable to tolerate treatment. The decision to use general anaesthesia must not be taken lightly and informed consent from the parent/guardian is essential.

General anaesthesia should only be administered by a qualified medical practitioner within an accredited anaesthetic facility.

Developmental considerations

Primary dentition

There are 20 primary teeth (four incisors, two canines and four molars in each arch). These begin erupting from about six months of age. The

formation, calcification and eruption sequence of the primary dentition is fully covered in Chapter 9. Discussed here are some problems that child patients may experience and which you may see in your surgery. Some of these conditions have also been mentioned in Chapter 8.

Teething

Teething can cause some localised pain and discomfort for babies, including red, swollen and sore gums. This can often make babies irritable and can cause excessive drooling, flushed cheeks and changes in eating patterns. Systemic effects that can be seen at the same time include raised temperature, changed bowel movements and nappy rash. It is not known whether these changes are directly linked to teething or result from another simultaneous minor viral/bacterial infection. However, signs of serious illness should not be attributed to teething and medical advice should be sought.

Babies often find that pressure relieves the discomfort of teething and so they often place their fingers or other objects into their mouths during teething times. A clean cold teething ring is recommended for this purpose. Foods and other small objects should be avoided for use as teethers due to the hazard of choking. Non-aspirin based teeth gels, available at pharmacies without prescription, can also be of value during teething.

Developmental anomalies

Disturbances of the number of teeth

Missing primary teeth are much less common than missing permanent teeth. Anodontia is a total lack of teeth. Hypodontia or oligodontia is missing one or more teeth.

Supernumerary teeth are extra teeth. They are most commonly found in the permanent dentition in the premaxillary region (mesiodens). They can be normal shape or conical.

Disturbances of the number of teeth can be found in some syndromes involving the head and neck (e.g. missing teeth are associated with ectodermal dysplasia, Down syndrome and clefting, supernumerary teeth with cleidocranial dysostosis).

Disturbances of the size and/or shape of teeth

Macrodontia are teeth larger than normal. Microdontia are teeth smaller than normal. Macrodontia and microdontia can be individual tooth or several teeth or complete dentition.

Double teeth are more common in the primary dentition than the permanent dentition. It can involve two teeth of the normal dentition (primary or permanent) or can involve a supernumerary tooth. Double teeth include:

- concrescence — two teeth joined by cementum;

- fusion — two teeth buds joined by dentine and pulp;

- germination — budding of a second tooth from a single tooth germ;

- dens invaginatus — a developmental disturbance where there is an invagination of enamel and dentine into the pulp chamber (most common in upper lateral incisors);

- dens evaginatus — a developmental disturbance where there is an enamel covered tubercule projecting from the occlusal surface of the tooth (most common in premolars);

- talon cusp — an accentuated projection of the **cingulum** of a maxillary incisor tooth; or

- taurodontism — tooth/teeth with enlarged pulp chamber/s.

Enamel defects

These defects can be acquired or inherited. Acquired defects include:

- Intrinsic discolouration — this is caused by incorporation of products during enamel formation (e.g. tetracycline staining).

- Hypomineralisation/opacities — a qualitative defect of enamel altering the translucency. Hypomineralisation of enamel produces porous white opacities that can become stained post-eruption (e.g. mild fluorosis, or mild trauma to developing tooth bud).

- Hypoplasia — a quantitative defect of enamel altering the surface continuity (e.g. severe fluorosis, severe trauma to developing tooth bud, and other developmental disturbances during enamel formation). Chronological hypoplasia describes a pattern of hypoplasia throughout the dentition at different levels on each crown depending on the stage of crown formation at the time the disturbance occurred.

Inherited defects include, for example, amelogenesis imperfecta, which affects both primary and permanent dentition of the individual. All teeth in both arches are affected. Amelogenesis imperfecta results from defective genes causing a disturbance during enamel formation causing hypoplastic and/or hypomineralised forms.

Disorders of dentine

Dentinogenesis imperfecta is an inherited disorder of dentine causing amber/grey/bluish discolouration of teeth, pulpal obliteration, short clinical crowns and narrow roots. The enamel often chips or flakes away post-eruption due to a defective cemento-enamel junction. This condition can occur alone or it may be associated with the systemic condition osteogenesis imperfecta.

Other disorders include dentinal dysplasia, vitamin-D resistant rickets, regional odontodyplasia and dentinal cysts.

Eruption disorders

Natal/neonatal teeth are teeth present at or soon after birth. These teeth can be the normal primary teeth or supernumerary teeth. They are usually extremely mobile as root development has not yet commenced.

Ankylosis is loss of the lamina dura of the root surface, which causes fusion of cementum and bone. Teeth appear to submerge as the alveolus and surrounding teeth continue to develop. It can occur in primary or permanent teeth. It is a common sequelae of replanted avulsed or intruded teeth.

Disturbance of root development

Root development can be delayed, altered or arrested by systemic illness. The most common cause is radiotherapy of the head/neck region (refer to Chapter 29).

Early childhood caries

Early childhood caries (ECC) is the name given to a pattern of tooth decay that can develop in infants and toddlers. It usually begins on the upper primary incisors and progresses to the molars as they erupt into the mouth. The lower incisor teeth are usually spared as the tongue lies over these teeth during suckling and because of the protective influence of the sublingual and submandibular salivary glands.

When infants and toddlers are allowed to suckle for prolonged or frequent periods during the day or night (longer than required for nutritional purposes), their teeth may be at risk of developing ECC. Any fluids in baby bottles other than water can cause ECC including formula, breast milk, cow's milk,

■ **cingulum:** lingual elevation within the cervical third of an anterior tooth.

flavoured milk, juice, cordial and soft drinks. The risk of ECC is increased in infants and toddlers who suckle during sleep times as the salivary production decreases during these times. Early childhood caries can also result from the frequent use of a dummy that has been dipped into a sweetener such as honey.

In order to prevent ECC, children should not be put to sleep with a bottle containing any fluid other than water. Continual night-time breastfeeding practices should also be modified to decrease the frequency of exposure of the teeth. During routine dental visits parents/carers should be counselled about the risks of placing fluids other than water, breast milk, formula or cow's milk into baby bottles at any time.

The introduction of a drinking cup should start as soon as the child is able (at around 12 months) and weaning from bottle-feeding should follow. Infants' teeth should be cleaned by parents/carers from the time of eruption to further reduce the risk of ECC.

Periodontal disease in children

Gingivitis is extremely common in children and is characterised by the presence of reversible gingival inflammation without any loss of bone or clinical attachment. The sole cause of gingivitis is plaque accumulation at the gingival margin of teeth. Other factors can further aggravate the response of the gingival tissues; such as, hormonal changes, drugs and inadequate margins of restorations. As plaque plays the major role in the initiation and development of gingivitis, plaque control is fundamental to achieving healthy gingival tissues. Brief descriptions of periodontal disease follow, but for a detailed discussion on periodontics refer to Chapter 31.

Puberty gingivitis

During puberty there is a more marked reaction of the gingival tissues to plaque accumulation caused by poor oral hygiene.

Periodontitis

Chronic and aggressive forms of periodontitis occur rarely in children in both localised and generalised forms. As in adults, periodontitis is a progressive form of periodontal disease resulting in loss of bone or clinical attachment.

Acute herpetic gingivostomatitis

This is caused by the first infection with the Herpes Simplex Virus. It results in systemic illness including fever, malaise, irritability and ulceration of the gingival and oral mucosal tissues.

Gingival overgrowth

Gingival overgrowth can be inherited (hereditary gingival fibromatosis) or drug-induced. It causes an overgrowth of the gingival tissues aggravated by plaque accumulation. When severe, it can cause delayed or **ectopic** eruption of teeth due to the bulk of fibrous tissue present.

Restorative dentistry for children

Restorative treatment

Restoration of primary teeth is significantly different from that of permanent teeth. The shape of the primary molars results in broad interproximal contact points that are closer to the gingival margin than in their permanent counterparts. The enamel layer of primary molars is proportionally thinner and the pulp chamber is proportionally larger than in permanent molars. Young permanent teeth also exhibit large pulp chambers that need to be taken into consideration during restoration.

Despite these differences, the principles of restoration of the primary and young permanent dentition remain the same as that of the mature permanent dentition. Caries should be removed and appropriate outline, resistance, retention and convenience form should be established dependent on the restorative material to be used.

The choice of material for restoration depends on several factors including:

- Age of the child and how long the restoration is required to last (time until exfoliation of primary teeth).
- Cooperation of the child — is the treatment being carried out with or without local anaesthesia and dental dam? Does the child require general anaesthesia or sedation, making repeated restoration more difficult?
- Caries risk — fluoride-releasing materials such as GIC's, composite resin strip crowns and stainless steel crowns providing full tooth coverage are considered.

Amalgam, glass ionomer cements and composite resins all have their place in the restoration of primary and young permanent teeth. Each child should have an individual treatment plan that takes into account the factors listed above. Two restorations that are extremely durable in the repair of primary teeth are composite resin strip crowns for anterior teeth and stainless steel crowns for molars. These full-coverage restorations have the advantages of good retention, low recurrent caries and ease of placement.

Composite resin strip crowns

Commercially produced crown forms for the primary dentition are used to place composite resin crowns on the primary anterior teeth following caries removal and protection of exposed dentine. These restorations provide excellent aesthetics, are easily placed and provide a durable restoration that is at low risk of recurrent caries.

Stainless steel crowns

Pre-formed stainless steel crowns are the most durable restoration available for primary molars. Although they are non-aesthetic, they provide a restoration that most often outlasts the lifetime of the tooth.

Pulp therapy in the primary dentition

The decision whether to restore or extract a pulpally involved primary tooth depends on several factors.

- Is the tooth restorable? Can the tooth be adequately restored following pulp therapy?
- Is the tooth close to exfoliation?
- Is there an odontogenic infection (an condition occurring during the development of the tooth)?
- Is the tooth mobile?
- Does the child have a medical history that contraindicates pulp therapy (congenital heart disease or immunosuppression for example)?
- Can the child tolerate the complex treatment required?

There are four recognised pulp therapy procedures.

❶ direct pulp capping;

❷ indirect pulp capping;

❸ pulpotomy; and

❹ pulpectomy.

These procedures are described at length in Chapter 33.

Direct and indirect pulp capping are rarely successful in cariously involved primary teeth where the pulp is already inflamed.

Pulpotomy involves the removal of vital pulpal tissue from the coronal chamber and placement of a medicament over the radicular pulp stumps to fix or stimulate repair of the remaining vital radicular pulp. This procedure can only be carried out where there is a vital pulp (reversible pulpitis) and therefore is not appropriate where there is an acute abscess, **furcation** involvement or mobility of the tooth.

There are several medicaments that can be used for a pulpotomy procedure. In Australia, formocresol is most commonly used. Following placement of the medicament, the pulp stumps are sealed and a restorative material is placed within the coronal pulp chamber. Ideally a full coverage restoration (anterior composite resin strip crown, posterior stainless steel crown) should then be placed in order to achieve a complete seal.

A pulpectomy involves the removal of pulpal tissue from the coronal pulp chamber and the root canals. It can be carried out where there is irreversible pulpitis or total pulpal necrosis. The canals are then obturated using a material that is resorbable during subsequent root resorption and exfoliation of the tooth. Materials commonly used for pulpectomy obturation in the primary dentition are zinc oxide eugenol, calcium hydroxide and iodoform paste. As with pulpotomy, the ideal restoration following pulpectomy is either a composite resin strip crown or a stainless steel crown.

Where pulp therapy is contraindicated for a particular patient or a particular tooth, extraction is the treatment of choice. Extraction of primary incisors and primary first molars have limited consequences for space loss. However in cases where extraction of primary canines and primary second molars are required, the placement of space maintainers is advantageous.

Traumatic injuries

Traumatic injuries are extremely common in children and may be the first presentation of a child to a dentist. Trauma in children is distressing for both the child and the parent/carer and so you and the dentist play a vital role in calming and reassuring the family.

Thirty per cent of children suffer trauma to the primary dentition and 22 per cent of 14-year-olds

■ **furcation:** junction where the roots of a multi-rooted tooth meet.

have experienced trauma of their permanent dentition. Twice as many boys as girls suffer dental injuries. Most injuries result from play accidents and falls, so the risk of injury is high in the six-month to three-year age group where toddlers are learning to walk, climb and play. Primary school children most often sustain injuries in the playground and from bicycles, and teenagers tend to sustain injuries from sports, fights or accidents.

Sadly, a small but significant percentage of oro-facial trauma results from child abuse. Injuries that do not match the given history should be investigated further and detailed notes should be made in the patient's dental records. All health professionals, including dentists, are required by law to report suspected child abuse injuries.

The type of injury suffered depends on several factors including velocity of impact, shape of object (blunt or sharp), resistance of the object (fixed or mobile) and angle of impact. Trauma to primary teeth most often results in tooth **luxations** and soft tissue injuries, and less frequently tooth fractures. This is due to the relative elasticity of the bone at this stage compared with the permanent dentition. Increased overjet is a major predisposing factor for dental injuries — where an overjet of 3–6 mm doubles the frequency of trauma to incisor teeth and an overjet of greater than 6 mm increases the risk of trauma threefold.

Traumatic injuries to the oro-facial region can be broadly grouped into four categories:

❶ soft tissue injuries;

❷ tooth fractures;

❸ luxation injuries; and

❹ major oro-facial trauma

Soft tissue injuries

Bruising is the simplest and most common type of soft tissue injury and usually does not require any treatment. It often occurs in combination with other soft tissue and dental injuries.

Lacerations can affect the skin, oral mucosa or a combination of both. When a laceration penetrates from the skin through the full thickness of tissue to oral mucosa it is called a *through-and-through laceration*. Most often lacerations require suturing back into position. Through-and-through lacerations require several layers of sutures to repair the skin, muscle and oral mucosal layers.

De-gloving is the term for a stripping of the gingival tissues off the bone. This injury is often overlooked as the flap of tissue may remain in its correct position during examination. All but very minor de-gloving injuries require suturing back into place.

Tooth fractures

Crown infraction is a crack in the enamel surface without loss of tooth structure. No treatment is required. See Figure 35.1 for classifications of fractures of teeth.

Crown and root fractures can be categorised into uncomplicated crown fractures and complicated crown fractures.

Uncomplicated crown fractures affect enamel only or enamel and dentine. These fractures are treated depending on how much tooth structure has been lost. Very small fractures (especially in the primary dentition) can be treated by smoothing or discing the rough surface and leaving it unrestored.

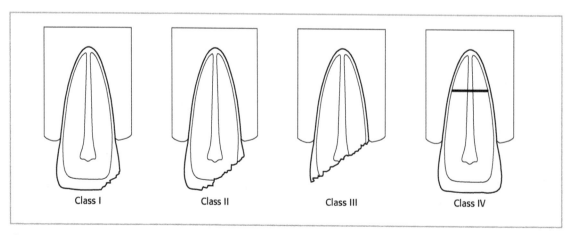

| Class I | Class II | Class III | Class IV |

Figure 35.1 Classification of fractures of teeth

luxation: loosening of a tooth from traumatic injury.

Significant fractures of enamel and enamel/dentine usually require composite resin restoration with protection of exposed dentine surfaces.

Complicated crown and crown/root fractures affect the pulp in addition to dental hard tissues. Complicated crown fractures require pulp therapy prior to restoration of the fracture. This may require a pulp capping, pulpotomy or pulpectomy procedure depending on the individual case. Crown/root fractures in the primary dentition are often non-restorable and may require extraction. Crown/root fractures of the permanent dentition pose difficult treatment challenges and complex procedures, with extraction often required.

Root fractures affect cementum, dentine and pulp. These can occur in the coronal, middle or apical third of the root. Treatment in the primary dentition involves review and monitoring. In the permanent dentition splinting of root-fractured teeth may be required depending on the degree of tooth mobility.

Luxation injuries

Luxation injuries involve displacement of the tooth within the alveolar bone. They can be categorised into:

- Concussion — injury resulting in no displacement or mobility of the tooth. No treatment apart from monitoring pulp vitality is required.

- Subluxation — injury resulting in mobility but no displacement of the tooth. No treatment apart from monitoring pulp vitality is required.

- Luxation — injury resulting in mobility and displacement of the tooth. This can be intrusive (back into the socket), extrusive (out of the socket) or lateral (buccal, lingual or lateral displacement). In the primary dentition teeth can often be gently guided back into position or left to reposition naturally by tongue and lip pressure. In the permanent dentition treatment is on an individual basis taking into consideration obstruction of occlusion, potential for re-eruption and mobility of the tooth. Permanent teeth often require splinting for some period of time following luxation injuries.

- Avulsion — complete extrusive luxation resulting in the tooth being lost from the tooth socket. Primary avulsed teeth should never be replanted due to the risk of damage to the underlying permanent successor. Permanent avulsed teeth should be replanted as soon as possible following the injury. The success rate of reimplantation is dependent on the extra-oral time period and degree of damage to the periodontal ligament and root surface. If teeth cannot be replanted immediately they should be stored in fresh milk ensuring that there is minimal handling of the root surface. Avulsed teeth almost always require flexible splinting and pulp extirpation should be carried out within 7–10 days. Reimplanted teeth have a variable long-term prognosis as the complications of root resorption and ankylosis are common. Instructions for dealing with avulsed teeth can be found in Chapter 33.

Major oro-facial trauma

This involves fractures of the alveolus, maxilla and/or mandible in combination with soft tissue and dental injuries. Treatment most often occurs in hospitals where there is a multi-disciplinary team approach.

In treating children and adults with trauma there are important stages to follow.

- Take a careful history (including immunisation status).

- Carry out a thorough examination.

- Take appropriate radiographs (intra-oral and/or extra-oral films).

- Assess pulp vitality of affected teeth (thermal and electric pulp testing, percussion and transillumination).

- Make detailed notes in the patient record.

- Carry out required treatment or refer the patient to a specialist paediatric dentist for management.

The prevention of trauma begins with education of parents/carers to ensure that children wear appropriate mouthguards for sports, helmets for bicycle riding and child restraints/seat belts in cars. Mouthguards should be worn during training sessions as well as games. Parents/carers should be aware of the emergency management for dental injuries (especially for avulsed permanent teeth).

Summary

The vast majority of Australian children receive their routine dental care in general dental practices and school dental health programs. It is vital for all dental health care practitioners to understand paediatric dentistry and child development and make appropriate decisions regarding the diagnosis and treatment of children. Where the scope of a child's needs falls beyond that of a particular general dental practice the child should be referred to a specialist paediatric dentist for comprehensive care.

chapter thirty-six
dentistry for the ageing

Introduction

Geriatrics is the medical study and treatment of the aged. Geriatric dentistry (also called geriodontology or geriodontics) is the study of ageing processes as they affect the tissues of the oral cavity and related structures.

Ageing is influenced by factors such as the mode of living, accidents, disease, stress and heredity. Scientific and medical advancements have resulted in large proportions of the population living to an advanced age. The over-65 sector is the fastest growing sector of the population.

People in the over-65 sector vary widely in their physical and mental condition. Many are physically well, requiring little or no medication for physical conditions. Others have complex health problems requiring substantial medical intervention. Many have fixed or removable prostheses.

Older Australians are now retaining more of their natural teeth and the dental problems faced by the dental profession are becoming increasingly complex. Indications are that in years to come more and more people over the age of 70 will retain most of their natural teeth.

For many of these people, physical wellbeing has an impact on their oral health. It is important that the dental health team be able to distinguish which of the patient's signs and symptoms are caused by disease, which are caused by ageing and which are side effects of medication.

Additionally, aged patients with oral health problems may have deteriorating general health and happiness because of their oral health problems. For example, problems with mastication may lead to decreased nutrition, and ill-fitting dentures may cause problems with self-esteem and communication.

Medical histories

Taking a patient's medical history is particularly crucial for the elderly patient who may be taking a number of medications or could have conditions that can complicate dental treatment, cause side-effects or drug interactions.

Elderly patients are usually health-conscious and may provide long and detailed medical and dental histories. These should be noted and given to the dentist for evaluation. The name, address and telephone number of the patient's present medical practitioner should be recorded.

Common dental problems in the elderly

Elderly patients often have problems that make mastication painful and inefficient. Some of these problems include those discussed below.

- Reduced salivary flow can produce a partial or complete dryness of the mouth (xerostomia). These patients may have thick, sticky saliva. It is often seen in patients following radiation therapy and is a common side effect of medications. The lack of saliva influences the retention of dentures and complicates the mastication and digestion of food.

- Loss, attrition, erosion and abrasion of natural teeth can cause pain that may affect the amount and nature of the diet.

- Abnormal taste and burning sensations may be related to xerostomia, hormonal disorders and vitamin B deficiencies. Inflammation of the tongue (glossitis) and corners of the lips (angular cheilitis) may deter patients from eating certain foods and may lead to dietary deficiencies that further complicate diagnosis and treatment.

- Periodontal disorders are common in elderly patients and may be exacerbated by slower healing.

- Unsatisfactory dentures often result from excessive bone resorption and hypersensitive soft tissues. Fungal infections may occur on the tongue and under ill-fitting dentures.

- Old, poor quality restorations may have persistent tooth decay around them.

Patients with dementia

An appreciable proportion of the population over the age of 65 has some form of dementia. Patients with dementia experience significantly higher incidence of all forms of oral disease, including oral mucosal lesions that are denture-related, increased plaque, gingival bleeding and caries (both root and coronal). The likelihood of oral disease in dementia patients increases if the patient has severe dementia, is institutionalised or has a primary carer who finds maintaining a good oral health care program to be difficult.

Many dementia patients stop wearing their dentures. This can lead to several complications. The first is dietary. Some patients suffer from nutritional deficiency because they cannot chew a wide range of foods.

Other complications can be caused by the loss of vertical height in the lower third of the face. That is, the upper lips fold over the lower ones. Saliva can seep or pool in the angle of the mouth and a fungal infection called 'candidiasis' forms. (Some people also develop candidiasis under their dentures.) Sometimes candidiasis forms over another type of inflammation, called 'angular cheilitis'.

Additionally, removing the dentures can also affect speech.

Appointments

Appointment times may need to be slightly longer for the elderly patient for a number of reasons. In particular, time must be allowed for detailed medical history taking. Appointment times should be written down and should be made for times suitable to an old person. For example, in the mornings when fatigue is minimum is preferable. Try to avoid peak hour traffic times.

Patients may be very talkative, particularly if they live alone. You should be prepared to speak clearly and listen carefully. By engaging the elderly patient in polite conversation before the dental appointment you may find invaluable information regarding the patient's life situation, including changes in medication, in social circumstances (e.g. death of spouse), their oral health status (e.g. pain on eating, comfort of denture, appearance of teeth) or new medical conditions the patient might forget to tell the dentist.

You should ensure that background noise is reduced to ensure the elderly patient can follow instructions easily.

People with dementia may require you to break down tasks to easily understood instructions. For example, 'Take a seat in the clinic' might be taken literally and the patient might attempt to pick up a seat and carry it into the clinic. Task break down would be: 'Step here, bend your knees, and sit in the chair'.

When the elderly patient is in the dental chair you will need to take care that there are no sudden movements of the dental chair as this may affect the patient's back, blood pressure or general medical condition. The position of the dental chair may need to be more upright than usual, particularly for patients with swallowing problems. Some elderly patients prefer to sit rather than to lie in the prone position.

Your role in settling the patient in the dental chair, addressing them directly and making them feel comfortable cannot be over emphasised.

Preventive dental care for the elderly

Your role in preventive dental care is very important for the elderly patient.

- Ensure regular recalls, three-monthly for professional dental hygiene care if required.

- Be available to give advice on preventive care devices, such as anti-microbial mouthwashes, fluoride rinses, salivary testing kits and suction toothbrushes.

- Assist the dentist in filling out patient care plans that are easily readable by the elderly patient for use at home.

- Geriatric patients often require additional advice on diet. With medical cooperation, a dentist may advise multivitamins and a higher protein intake. Usually the aged person has a lessened stimulus for eating and, combined with a limited budget, malnutrition may occur.

Where natural teeth exist, medicinal acids may aggravate exposed dentine and cementum. Patients can be advised to take acidic preparations through a straw or in capsules. Patients should try to consume citrus fruits by eating the whole fruit and brushing the teeth or rinsing soon afterwards, rather than consuming juices.

Summary

Dental assistants have a special role in recognising the normal signs of ageing and understanding the problems of elderly patients. For example, it is normal for most of these patients to have skin and hair changes, decreased elasticity of muscles, diminished eyesight and hearing, and slower healing processes.

Many patients in this age group have a strong cancer phobia and you should understand this and encourage the need for an early examination by the dentist should the elderly patient have any concerns.

chapter thirty-seven
forensic odontology.

Introduction

Forensic odontology (forensic dentistry) is a branch of dentistry that deals with the application of the knowledge of dentistry to legal problems. It is mainly concerned with identifying people by means of the teeth. This may involve:

- comparing dental records with the teeth of deceased persons, including those who have died in mass disasters or terrorist acts;

- identification from saliva by means of DNA comparison or bacterial flora; or

- identification or exclusion of individuals or animals as being the cause of bite marks.

Sometimes forensic odontologists become involved in complaints about malpractice or questions of fraud in dentistry, and in any other areas where dentistry and law come into contact. They may also work with archaeological specimens, and occasionally they may be required to visit archaeological sites. They tend to work closely with forensic pathologists and often also with forensic anthropologists. They frequently appear in courts as expert witnesses.

Forensic odontologists (or forensic dentists) are qualified dentists who have chosen to specialise in the forensic area. They most commonly practice in this field in an Institute of Forensic Medicine or Pathology, depending on the state or territory in which they work, and may appear in courts in whatever jurisdiction applies to a particular case. Because forensic odontology is not usually a full-time occupation, most forensic odontologists also work in general dental practice, or with a university or in the public sector. In the event of a mass disaster, forensic odontologists may travel to the disaster site. This may be within Australia or overseas.

The techniques used in forensic odontology are described on the next few pages. You will see that accurate record keeping in the dental surgery is crucial to effective forensic odontology. Your role in forensic odontology is described towards the end of this chapter.

Forensic identification of deceased persons

Identifying people

The civil recording of births, marriages and deaths was begun in 1837 in England and Wales and in 1855 in Scotland. In Australia, civil registration of births, marriages and deaths became compulsory at different times in different states: Queensland and New South Wales in 1856, Victoria in 1853, South Australia in 1842, Western Australia in 1841 and Tasmania in 1838.

As a result, when we come into the world, our legal existence begins with the issue of a birth certificate. In the same way, it is terminated with the issue of a death certificate. In some circumstances, this may be issued following the completion of a medical certificate of the cause of death by a medical practitioner. In other circumstances, the case lies within the jurisdiction of the Coroner and, in such cases, a death certificate cannot be issued until the Coroner is satisfied that the deceased person has been identified beyond doubt.

Until a death certificate is issued, the legal affairs of a person cannot be finalised. In some circumstances, financial affairs cannot be completed, insurance benefits may not be payable and the surviving spouse may not be free to marry again. The family cannot complete its grieving process.

While visual identification by family members or friends may be possible in some cases, where significant decomposition or trauma has occurred, it may not be desirable or possible for this to be undertaken. In such cases, more specialised forms of identification may be required, and these may include the services of a forensic odontologist.

The unique nature of the dentition

Dental identification is based upon the premise that each dentition is unique. While this may seem like commonsense, it has never been proved. (Similarly, the uniqueness of fingerprints has never been proved.) However, we generally accept that dentitions are unique in the same way that we accept that people are physically unique — two people may look similar but on close examination even 'identical' twins have differences.

By comparing the dentition of deceased persons with dental records, forensic odontologists attempt to identify those deceased persons.

Routine forensic identification of deceased persons

The forensic odontologist is most commonly called upon to perform routine identification services when identity needs to be established to the satisfaction of a Coroner. The identification may be problematic because of decomposition or trauma that renders the deceased beyond visual identification. Such cases commonly include motor vehicle accidents, incinerations, gunshot cases, suicides and cases discovered some time after death. Skeletonised material may also require identification.

The normal procedure is for police to investigate the circumstances of the death, and establish the likely identity of the deceased person. They will then attempt to find the dental practice(s) or clinic(s) that treated the suspected deceased and request dental records. These will be provided to the forensic odontologist who will attempt to compare them with the teeth of the deceased.

The outcomes of the process may be:

- that the deceased is identified beyond question;
- that the deceased is excluded as belonging to the individual to whom the records belong; or
- that the comparison is inconclusive and more records or a different method of identification is required.

Missing persons

Sometimes police may suspect that a deceased person may be a missing person. That is to say, their absence has been a matter of record for a period of time, and information about them is held by a missing persons department in a police jurisdiction. The police will investigate and attempt to find the practice(s) or clinic(s) that treated the suspected missing person, and request their records.

These will then be provided to the forensic odontologist who will compare the teeth of the deceased to the supplied records.

The outcomes of the process may be:

- that the deceased is identified beyond question;
- that the deceased is excluded as belonging to the individual to whom the records belong; or
- that the comparison is inconclusive and more records or a different method of identification is required.

Mass disasters, including terrorist attacks

Whittaker and MacDonald (1989) define a mass disaster as one 'in which the normally available forensic services would be stretched beyond acceptable limits and organised teamwork becomes a necessity'. In Australia, a working definition is that a mass disaster involves four or more deceased persons in a single incident and requires specialised identification procedures.

There are two distinct types of mass disaster: those in which the number and identities of the victims are likely to be known (for instance, a plane crash where a passenger manifest and a list of crew is available), and those in which the number and identities of the victims are not initially known (for instance, a terrorist bomb attack). These are called a 'closed disaster' and an 'open disaster' respectively. The identification procedures in each of these types of incident are different, and in both cases they differ from those used in routine identifications as well.

In a closed disaster police immediately begin the process of finding and retrieving dental records. As they arrive, they are transcribed onto special yellow Interpol forms in a standard way. Meanwhile, teams of dentists examine the deceased persons and transcribe their findings onto similar pink Interpol forms for comparison. The deceased persons are thoroughly documented with comprehensive radiography and photography undertaken. Subsequently, the ante-mortem records are compared with the post-mortem records and identities established wherever possible. Dentists work in pairs and this helps to reduce errors. Similar procedures are undertaken by other specialist groups, including DNA biologists, fingerprint teams, pathologists, and police comparing and tracing property found with each of the deceased. Subsequently, each group presents its findings to an identification board, and this is where final identification is certified. Ideally, the deceased are not released until all the identifications are completed.

In an open disaster the situation is different because a list of the deceased persons is not initially available. Indeed, the number of deceased may not become clear for some time. As reports of missing persons possibly associated with the incident begin to arrive, police investigate and begin to compile dental records. These are transcribed onto yellow Interpol forms as per a closed disaster. Teams of dentists begin the examination of deceased persons recovered from the disaster site. Other specialist groups (dealing with DNA, fingerprints, property and pathology) also examine the remains. When sufficient evidence is felt to be present to identify a deceased person, this is presented by representatives of each specialist group to an identification board. This board certifies the identity of the deceased if they believe the strength of the evidence is sufficient. Unlike a closed disaster, deceased persons are released as they are identified.

The role of the forensic odontologists in such disasters is a crucial one. Dentistry and DNA are the only identification methods felt to have sufficient strength of evidence that they can be used alone to identify a victim. Other methods have supplementary value, or make a case in the absence of DNA or dentistry only when several different methods agree. Wherever possible, several different methods are used simultaneously to triangulate and improve the strength of the conclusion.

Bite mark identification

Bite marks are being recognised more frequently as a method of identification as people's awareness is raised as to how common they are and what they look like. Bite marks may be found on people, either alive or dead, or they may be found in substances such as foodstuffs, for instance apples, cheese or chocolate or other substances.

Their analysis is a difficult and exacting occupation. Recently, digital techniques have made the analysis and presentation of bite mark evidence simpler.

In the event that a bite mark is recognised on a patient, it should first be reported to the senior dental officer or the practitioner in charge, who in turn would report it to police. The wound, if fresh, should be swabbed with a cotton swab for DNA before washing. The wound will then be photographed by a police photographer using rigid L-shaped measurement scales, and impressions may be taken if indentations are present. Photographic appointments may continue for several days to preserve different features of the injury over time.

Once the forensic odontologist has identified the wound as a human bite mark, an attempt is made to match individual features of a suspect's dentition to the features of the bite injury. (Investigation to determine the likely suspects is the responsibility of the police.) In general, if the wound is in an area that could be reached by the victim's own mouth, then the victim's teeth are also compared with the features of the injury.

There are three possible outcomes of the process. In order of likelihood these are:

❶ the suspect can be eliminated as a cause of the bite;

❷ there is insufficient basis for a reliable conclusion; and

❸ the suspect's teeth are likely to have caused the injury.

It is far easier, and usually more reliable, to exonerate an individual as a cause of a bite than it is to implicate them. If the evidence suggests that an individual cannot be exonerated as a cause, then the degree of confidence with which they can be said to be the cause will depend on the number of unique features present in the bite mark and the closeness of the match. In general, it is very difficult to state that a particular person is the only person who could have caused a particular injury, especially on something as resilient as human soft tissue. Where a likely match is found, the combination of the dental evidence combined with findings of a police investigation will contribute to the construction of a case against a suspect.

Bite mark evidence is usually circumstantial evidence. The fact that a bite mark belonging to a suspect in a murder case is identified on the deceased does not automatically indicate that the suspect murdered the victim.

Records required for forensic odontology

Written records

Written dental records are usually used for comparison with charting made from the dentition of a deceased person for identification. Written dental records should have been completed for every patient who has ever had a dental consultation. Sometimes they will contain a little useful information (for example a record of an emergency consultation resulting in a drug prescription), and at their best, they will constitute a complete written record of a patient's teeth and all of the dental work performed on them.

They must be accurate in order to be useful. For example, a patient with an upper left first molar tooth missing will not be correctly identified from written charts alone if the upper right first molar tooth is erroneously recorded as having been extracted.

Increasing patient mobility means that many patients see multiple dentists throughout their lifetime, and this can mean that the police investigation may need to find written records from multiple surgeries. Because not all records may be available or found, the forensic odontologist may have only a subset of the available information with which to work.

It is important to recognise that written records constitute only an often incomplete written description of a patient's dental state at a particular period in time. They are therefore not directly representative of a dentition in the same way that a radiograph or a photograph is. In addition, they are subject to recording errors. It is not uncommon to find that an incorrect tooth surface has been recorded as having been filled (for example, an MO rather than a DO), and this decreases the reliability of the comparison. It can even result in exclusion of a deceased as being a particular individual when they are one and the same person. For this reason, it is preferable not to rely on written records alone. In addition to written records, forensic odontologists prefer to have a direct image of the teeth, such as a radiograph or a photograph, with which to work, since images are not prone to the same kinds of recording errors that affect written records.

There is a strong argument to suggest that identity can never be established beyond question on the basis of written records alone, because irrespective of the number of concordant features, one is not directly comparing teeth with teeth; one is comparing writing with writing. Therefore, with written records forensic odontologists prefer to suggest that identification has a degree of probability in relation to the number of points used to assess it, rather than being definitely established.

Radiographs

Unlike written dental records, radiographs do constitute a direct record of an individual's teeth and therefore are not subject to the same kinds of recording error that may affect written records. Although there are many technical faults that can render radiographs less than ideal, most commonly they record an image of the teeth as they were at a particular point in time. This means they are an excellent medium for comparison, since as well as tooth crowns and the presence and shapes of restorations, they may record a wealth of additional information. This may include anatomical features of the teeth and roots and of the alveolar bone, the relative sizes and positions of structures, and the features, sizes and shapes of any pathological lesions that may be present.

Most commonly, bitewing and periapical radiographs tend to be available with dental records. Sometimes, OPGs, lateral skull, lateral oblique, postero-anterior or other radiographic views showing anatomical features of the teeth and skull are retrieved. Each of these may have something to offer the identification process. Because skull radiographs are often used for purposes other than dentistry, medical records should also be searched for radiographs.

When presented with **ante-mortem** dental radiographs in the dental records, the forensic odontologist will usually seek to take corresponding radiographs of the deceased, attempting to match them as closely as possible to those obtained from the dental or medical records. The two are then compared. The comparison may be documented in writing but radiographic comparison is most powerful as an exhibit in court if the two radiographs are superimposed to demonstrate the similarity.

Digital techniques may be used to analyse and demonstrate the similarity, and to provide an easy method of demonstrating the similarity to a lay audience or courtroom.

Bitewing and periapical radiographs are most commonly used for this purpose.

The major factors adversely affecting the use of ante-mortem radiographs in comparison work are:

- poor fixing and poor washing, leading to degradation of the radiograph in the time since it was taken;
- incorrect labelling; and
- incorrect orientation and mounting.

Bony sinus matching

On some skull radiographs the teeth may not be easily superimposed but other unique features may be visible. The classical features that are used in such cases include the frontal and, to a lesser extent, the maxillary sinuses. Frontal sinuses are especially useful since they are frequently and significantly asymmetrical, and appear quite distinctive. Frontal sinuses are often noted in postero–anterior skull radiographs.

Digital techniques

Techniques for digitally superimposing radiographs are useful at both the analysis and presentation stages. Using a commercial graphics program, separate radiographs can be stored in different picture layers and can then be assessed for the degree of correspondence between different features of superimposed images.

When two radiographs are overlayed digitally, one can be rendered as a negative and its opacity reduced so that the underlying radiograph becomes progressively more visible. As the corresponding positive and negative features of the two layers cancel each other out, any differences tend to stand out in sharp relief.

Other medical images

Other medical images including CAT scans, MRI scans and PET scans may also be useful in the comparison process, and they should be sought in the medical records wherever possible.

Photographs

Photographs are extremely useful in forensic odontology. While many people in a population are unlikely to have had recent dental radiography, very few have not recently had a photograph.

Photographs of individuals usually depict them smiling, and hence showing the only component of the skeleton that shows through the soft tissues in life: the teeth.

Once a photograph showing a smiling face has been obtained by police investigation, it is then fairly straightforward to assess the position and distance of the original camera from the subject when the photograph was taken. An experienced forensic or police photographer is invaluable in this phase. The teeth of the deceased are then photographed with the camera in a similar relationship, and the tooth images of the original life photograph and those of the deceased are superimposed.

If they belong to the same individual, an excellent match will be noted. This can be analysed and demonstrated in court using digital techniques in the same way as that which applies to radiographs.

Models

Dental models can be very useful for comparison with the teeth of a deceased. It is important not to rely on visual comparison alone, since this fails to be objective and can be a source of errors between superficially similar dentitions. It is better to photograph the model and the corresponding area of the dentition from similar distances and to superimpose them, examining the minute details to confirm the correspondence. One can also make a physical mould of the deceased dentition in rubberbase impression material and match it directly to the model, cutting the impression if necessary to show how it fits.

These objective tests allow a forensic odontologist to determine if the model belongs to the same dentition as the deceased, and to thus establish identity.

Mouthguards

The fit of a mouthguard directly on the teeth of the deceased can be assessed. Mouthguards can also be treated in some respects as negative dental models. Models can be poured from them and then analysed as discussed above. It should be recognised that the quality of the model that can be derived from a mouthguard will not approach the quality of a normal diagnostic cast but the technique can still be useful.

Dentures

Dentures can be useful in establishing identity, especially if they are marked in some way with an identifying label. Partial dentures are generally more useful than full dentures, because they can be demonstrated to fit a partially edentulous mouth. Cobalt-chrome partial dentures are better than acrylic dentures in that they have a more precise fit, and tend to be more easily marked for identification, but any denture that has an identifying label can be useful to corroborate other dental findings.

You can be helpful in terms of denture labelling by selling the idea to both the dentist and patient. It doesn't really matter what identifying mark is made, provided there is a record of it in the patient's chart. Many varieties of code have been suggested over the years but there is little that is superior to a patient's name. Patients can be advised not so much of the forensic implications of denture marking but rather the convenience of being able to identify their personal property in case of loss.

Denture marking is occurring in more and more nursing homes these days because it prevents mixing up of dentures that are cleaned in a central cleaning area, and also prevents remakes due to denture loss and later recovery, where the newly-found denture cannot then be identified.

Denture marking can be quick and easy. Several dental supply companies sell kits that can satisfactorily mark an acrylic denture in a few minutes with a mark that will survive for two or three years of normal use. Dentures can be marked more permanently at manufacture.

DNA

DNA from a previously living individual can be matched to DNA harvested from a deceased person. DNA can be recovered from tooth pulps quite some time after death. It has been successfully obtained after extensive decomposition and/or immersion months, or years, following the demise of the owner.

Common sources of DNA from someone presumed to be deceased include toothbrushes and other personal items. If DNA is not recoverable from such sources, it may be recovered from parents and/or siblings and comparison of that DNA with the DNA of the deceased may establish the likelihood that the deceased was related to the donor.

DNA matching is unlikely to take over from forensic odontology. At present it is still expensive, waiting lists are long and it can be invasive. However, even if it does become more affordable, rapid and routine, it will almost certainly still be used together with forensic odontology identification techniques to provide better reliability of results.

Patient identification implants

Patients in some countries and at different times have been fitted with identifying implants of one sort or another. Sometimes these have been in the form of tiny pieces of metal engraved with microscopic information that have been sealed into a small cavity on a molar tooth using distinctly coloured composite resin.

The signs that such a device is present are obvious and therefore such identifying **artefacts** in a corpse should be recovered and read by a forensic odontologist.

While none of these techniques has become universally popular, research continues into identifying artefacts, and surgical implantation of identifying items remains a real possibility.

Dental assistants and forensic odontology

Forensic odontology relies on the keeping of good quality records by dentists and dental assistants in public and private practices.

Recording of dental examination and procedures

The dental record is a legal document. As such, the operator who performs dental examinations and/or procedures assumes legal responsibility for its contents. In practice, and for infection control reasons, recording is most frequently performed by a dental assistant.

You should work carefully to ensure that errors in recording are kept to a minimum, since incorrect recording of an examination or a procedure can potentially result in the record excluding identity of a deceased person.

If possible, you should encourage the dentist to perform a full charting of each patient at the initial examination. It is worth noting that most dental boards mandate that full recording be done at the time of initial examination in their *Guidelines on Dental Records*. For instance, the Queensland Dental Board document typifies this approach: '3.2.1 On first attendance for examination the mouth should be fully charted both using an odontogram and text'.

If complete records are not kept, even notation that records which teeth are sound, decayed, missing and filled will provide a great deal of information to the forensic odontologist.

■ **artefact**: a substance, or structure, not naturally present in tissue, e.g. an implant.

In the morgue situation, it is not advisable for a forensic odontologist to both examine *and* record, for infection control reasons. There may be occasions in which a dental assistant may be able to assist a forensic odontologist in morgue examinations by performing recording of findings during examination of a body. Most commonly, however, this task would be carried out by a second forensic odontologist so that the examination of the first odontologist can be cross-checked by the second odontologist, as a quality assurance measure.

Labelling of items

You may be required to label radiographs, dental models, dental photographs or other materials relevant to a patient's dental history. Ensure that these are labelled correctly with the patient's name, the date, and any other details that are relevant to the item.

Incorrect labelling may lead to omissions in the record, or to extraneous and incorrectly labelled material appearing in the dental record. Either may be grossly detrimental to a forensic examination.

Radiograph processing and mounting

The processing and mounting of radiographs is of great forensic importance. Radiographs that are incorrectly processed may be difficult to read in future years. It is most important to ensure that radiographs are correctly washed for an adequate period to ensure that they remain in good condition for the life of the image, and do not discolour.

The correct orientation of x-ray film at the time of exposure is critical. If this is not done, then it may be extremely difficult later on to correctly orientate the radiograph. This is particularly true of bitewing and periapical radiographs.

Correct mounting and labelling of radiographs should be ensured. Incorrect mounting may be confusing, and incorrect labelling may cause the radiographs to be useless at best, and to exclude identity at worst.

Record retrieval

When asked for dental records to assist in a forensic investigation, you should carefully examine the dental chart to ascertain that all the records available for the patient in question have been included.

All radiographs in particular should accompany the written record. Other records such as dental models, mouthguards or dentures that have not yet been inserted, and photographs, are all useful. All records should all be retrieved. Failure to include records may prompt further requests to trace the missing items.

Retaining dental records

Most Australian dental boards recommend retaining dental records for at least seven years after the last entry, or in the case of children, at least seven years after they reach 18 years of age. The Dental Council of New Zealand recommends retaining dental records for ten years after the last entry. This does not constitute an instruction to destroy them as soon as this period has expired and most boards encourage dentists to retain their records for as long as possible.

For forensic purposes, it is preferable to retain dental records for as long as possible, even after the death of a patient has been communicated to the practice. Deceased persons may not be found until many years after death and it is tragic when records that could have been used to identify them are no longer available. Other deaths may later warrant police investigation, in which case records may then be required. All types of records should be retained, including radiographs, photographs and any other items.

What to do when dental records are requested

If you are asked to provide dental records to assist in a police investigation, the first thing to do is to ask for and record the name of the person requesting the records, along with the date and time. Records would normally be requested by a police officer who will come personally to collect them.

Retrieve the original dental records, including any radiographs, photographs and models and other items such as dentures or mouthguards that may be awaiting insertion. You should not add anything else to these records. You may wish to photocopy the original documents to keep in the practice.

If you can offer any other information such as recollections or a transcription of the records where handwriting may be difficult to interpret, then write these on separate sheets of paper and print your name and date on the sheets before signing them.

Place all of these items in a secure container, and label and seal the container.

When the police officer calls for the container, ensure that you are given a receipt for the property. This receipt must be retained, since it forms part of what is known as the 'chain of evidence' that may later be used in court to certify that the container has not been tampered with in any way.

The records will either be retained by the authorities until legal proceedings are complete, or may subsequently be returned to you, depending on the current procedures in your state or territory. If records are returned to you before legal proceedings, they should then be stored and kept, since they may be required in later actions. They will eventually be returned to you at the conclusion of any legal proceedings.

You should not provide copies of records to the police, since this will lead to a further request for the originals. You should not attempt to avoid supplying records. Police can issue a subpoena for them if you do not supply them.

Summary

It is very rare for dental assistants to be directly involved in the work of forensic odontologists. However, there is a possibility that the practice in which you are employed will be approached to provide records for use by a forensic odontologist. As this work relies on good quality records and radiographs, your work as the keeper of those records and developer of radiographs is crucial.

Reference

Whittaker, D.K. and MacDonald, D.G. (1989) *A colour atlas of forensic dentistry*. Wolfe Medical Publications, London, p. 100.

Section 7

Career options

As your career progresses you may find that your career priorities change. You might find, for example, that there are specialist fields you find particularly interesting. You might choose to extend your skill base by attending further education courses. You may simply decide to change employers for practical or personal reasons. Knowing the options that are available to you will assist you in making decisions of this kind.

chapter thirty-eight
employment opportunities

Introduction

The satisfaction you get from your career depends on having a clear vision of the career path that you want and finding the position that is right for you. Know yourself.

Make a list of your skills and abilities. Consider the range of tasks you undertake at your current place of work, skills and knowledge you have gained through training, and any interests or hobbies you have. For example, do you have skills with word processing or spreadsheets? Is there any way you can demonstrate you ability to work independently, or leadership or team skills?

You have a much better chance of gaining employment if you have a thorough understanding of your skills and abilities before you write an application or résumé, or attend an interview.

Employment prospects

There is currently a shortage of qualified and trainee dental assistants in every major city in Australia and in many overseas countries.

Dental assistants can be employed in:

- private and group dental practices;
- hospital clinics;
- health fund clinics;
- health departments;
- community dental health services;
- institutions presenting education and training;
- programs for dental auxiliary personnel; and
- the armed services (navy, army, air force).

There is ongoing and rapid change in technology and scientific understanding of disease and its prevention. Consequently, you should take every opportunity to update your skills and knowledge through study and attendance at conferences and workshops. Upgrading skills and knowledge not only improves practise as a dental assistant but also improves morale and enjoyment at work.

Finding employment

There is a wide range of ways of finding a position as a dental assistant in private or public practice. There is currently a shortage of qualified dental assistants so if you are genuinely interested in finding a position, you should be able to do so relatively quickly. The following headings provide suggestions for ways to find employment.

Newspapers

Newspapers are the most obvious starting point for finding a position. Do not limit your search to the health section of the employment pages as employers advertise in different locations; for example, the positions vacant section. Don't forget to look in different states' and national papers as well as local papers.

Many newspapers also have their employment sections available on the internet.

Web pages

There are websites that specialise in employment opportunities. Some of these have job vacancies and some allow you to enter your résumé so employers can contact you. Some do both. Some websites require a fee but others are free. Take the time to investigate these sites.

You may find overseas positions on the web.

Agencies

You might also want to contact public and private employment agencies. Look in the yellow pages phone book for their locations.

Professional organisations

Some professional organisations are listed in Chapter 1. There are considerable benefits in joining your local professional organisation. Apart from the advice and support these organisations provide, they sometimes also offer employment registers and can put you in touch with dentists looking for assistants.

Additionally, these organisations offer training opportunities and sometimes social events where you can meet other assistants. Through these meetings you might hear of positions that are available, or about to become available.

Door knocking

Door knocking involves visiting practices to ask if there are vacancies and to provide a brief statement with your name, contact details, dental assisting experience if any and a sentence about your interest in the field. Be prepared. Know what you want to say and have a paper and pencil ready to take notes. Make sure you have copies of your résumé and a cover letter ready to provide if requested. Dress as you would for a job interview.

Be systematic. Decide on the suburbs you can reach without lengthy travel times. Make a list of dental practices from the yellow pages phone book. Keep a record of all employers you contact, their response and any comments to remind you of the contact. Call them after two weeks. Keep doing this until a job comes along that you like.

Sending unsolicited résumés

Some people have success by sending their résumé with a cover letter to employers of interest. These letters and résumés (along with any that are left while door knocking) should be followed up a few weeks after they were sent/delivered. This follow-up can take the form of a thank you for the practice's time. This shows the employer that you are keen and reminds them to consider résumés they have forgotten in the interim.

Applying for advertised positions

Carefully analyse the advertisement for the position to discover exactly what you are expected to provide in your application. If there are specific criteria that you must meet, make sure that you address them in your application. If there are few or no criteria, ask for more information when you call about the position.

Look at the required experience, at the salary and duties. Make sure you know what will be expected of you in the position and decide whether this is the kind of position you want and can fill adequately.

Writing your résumé

Many people make the mistake of using the same résumé for all job interviews. You should ensure that the résumé and cover letter that you provide are tailored to the specific job you are applying for.

Make sure that your résumé is clear and concise. Have someone else read it and the cover letter to check that spelling and grammar are correct.

Take care with the layout. These documents should be printed on unlined white paper. The layout should be consistent. Don't use too many fonts. Make sure there is plenty of space around the text so that it is easy to read.

Your résumé and cover letter should make it clear that:

- you are keen to fill the position;
- you have good communication and social skills;
- you are practical and self-motivated; and
- you have suitable experience and training. Match your skills to those required by the employer and wherever possible, state experiences you have that demonstrate the abilities the employer asks you to demonstrate. If you do not have experience with particular tasks, demonstrate how you have taken steps to learn about the task or are willing to learn.

Ensure that your résumé includes:

- your name;
- contact details, including address, phone numbers, email addresses;
- your education, employment and training history; and
- names and contact details of at least two referees.

You might want to send details of personal and professional referees. Make sure that you contact these people and ask their permission before listing them.

You may want to include:

- interests and hobbies that demonstrate skills useful in the job (leadership, organisation, etc.);
- academic awards or achievements; and
- your professional goals

If you are required to fill in an application form, do so in pencil first, or make a draft copy, to enable you to fine-tune the final copy. Check that you answer all questions and have accurate spelling and grammar.

The cover letter

This should catch the employer's attention and highlight your strengths and enthusiasm. Your style should be clear and natural. It should match the style of the advertisement. A formal advertisement demands a formal response. A casual advertisement can have a casual response. An example of a fully blocked cover letter is provided in Figure 38.1. For further discussion, see the section titled 'letter styles' in Chapter 5.

Mary Osmond
42 Teeth Street
NICEVILLE NSW 2666
Ph: (02) 556 3927
19 May 2003

Dr P Relief
Dental Surgery
12 Upper Denture Street
EUPHORIA NSW 2034

Dear Dr Relief,

I am writing in response to your advertisement for a dental assistant in the *Sydney Morning Herald* (17 May 2003).

I am presently completing the Dental Assistant Certificate III Course with the NSW Dental Assistants' Association. This accredited course covered all the topics required for the endorsed National Competency Standards for dental assisting. I have two years experience in dental assisting.

[*You should focus on the things that seem most relevant to the particular job advertisement. For example, if they require a dental receptionist, then communication skills are the top priority.*]

I have been employed in my current position with Dr Smith for two years. During my employment I have gained extensive experience in …

I have developed my skills in …

[*You should try to add some specific details here, targeted at the job advertisement.*]

I enjoy working with people and feel that my natural empathy and enjoyment of hard work would fit in well at your dental surgery.

[*This part should focus on what you feel are your particular strengths or the specific requirements mentioned in the ad; for instance, sense of humour, ability to deal with stress, good phone manner and so forth.*]

I can be contacted on the phone number provided above and look forward to hearing from you.

Yours faithfully,

Mary Osmond
[*Your signature*]

Mary Osmond
[*Your name typed*]

Figure 38.1 Example of a fully blocked cover letter

Interviews

Be prepared. Be well presented. Practise possible answers before you attend the interview.

An interview can be one-on-one, by telephone or a group interview.

Before you go, learn as much as you can about the organisation. For example, if the practice specialises in orthodontics, know as much as you can about procedures before you go to the interview.

Anticipate questions you might be asked (especially about areas in which you are weak) and have some answers prepared. If you are asked a question that you do not understand, do not hesitate to ask for clarification.

Know what questions you want to ask the employer. You might like to ask about the composition of staff in the organisation, why the position is vacant, expectations of the position for the future, hours of work, possibilities for advancement, and so forth.

Asking for feedback

If you do not get the position you apply for, do not be discouraged. It is appropriate to ring the employer to ask for some feedback on the application and interview and ways in which you could improve your performance in future.

When offered the job

Once you have found a suitable position make sure the work conditions (roster, lunch breaks, etc.) are clearly explained. If asked to sign a contract, get advice from someone who knows about such contracts (for example, the state/territory dental assistants' association or union).

If there are conditions that are unfair that you would like to change or things that you would like to add, you are entitled to do so. You can ask for time to study the document.

Summary

Remember that the better prepared you are, the better chance you have of finding a position that meets your needs. Carefully consider your skills, abilities, knowledge and requirements before you start your job search. Take care with your presentation and applications that you present to potential employers. With care and persistence you will find the job that is right for you.

appendix

Contact information for useful organisations

Occupational Health and Safety Offices

New South Wales
WorkCover NSW
400 Kent Street
Sydney NSW 2000
Phone: (02) 9370 5000
Fax: (02) 9370 5999
Toll free: 1800 451 462
Website: *http://www.workcover.nsw.gov.au/*

Queensland
Workplace Health and Safety
Forbes House
30 Makerston Street
Brisbane QLD 4001
Phone: (07) 3247 4711
Fax: (07) 3220 0143
Toll free: 1800 177 717
Website: *http://www.dtir.qld.gov.au/*

National
WorkSafe Australia
Website: *http://www.worksafe.gov.au/*
NOHSC Switchboard:
Phone: +61 2 6279 1000
Fax: +61 2 6279 1199
Email: *info@nohsc.gov.au*

ACT
ACT Workcover
Level 3, FAI House
197 London Circuit
Civic ACT 2601
Phone: (02) 6205 0200
Fax: (02) 6205 0797

Northern Territory
Northern Territory Work Health Authority
Minerals House
66 The Esplanade
Darwin NT 0800
Phone: (08) 8999 5010
Fax: (08) 8999 6650
Website: *http://www.nt.gov.au/wha/*

Tasmania
Workplace Standards Authority
30 Gordons Hill Road
Rosny Park Tas 7018
Phone: (03) 6233 7657
Fax: (03) 6233 8338
Website: *http://www.wsa.tas.gov.au/*

Victoria
Victorian WorkCover Authority
World Trade Centre
Cnr Flinders & Spencer Streets
Melbourne Vic 3001
Phone: (03) 9628 8111
Fax: (03) 9628 8199
Website: *http://www.workcover.vic.gov.au/*

South Australia
WorkCover Corporation
100 Waymouth Street
Adelaide SA 5000
Phone: (08) 8233 2222
Fax: (08) 8233 2466
Toll free: (SA Country only) 1800 188 000
Website: *http://www.workcover.sa.gov.au/*

Western Australia
Worksafe Western Australia
1260 Hay Street
West Perth WA 6005
Phone: (08) 9327 8777
Fax: (08) 9321 8973
Website: *http://www.safetyline.wa.gov.au/*

Employer and union organisations

Australian Chamber of Commerce & Industry
Level 4, 55 Exhibition Street
Melbourne Vic 3000
Phone: (03) 9289 5289
Fax: (03) 9289 5250
Website: *http://www.acci.asn.au/*

Australian Council of Trade Unions
ACTU House
393-397 Swanston Street
Melbourne Vic 3000
Phone: (03) 9664 7310
Fax: (03) 9663 8220
Website:
http://www.actu.asn.au/

Other agencies

National Health and Medical Research Council Publications
The Publications Officer
ONHMRC (MDP 100)
GPO Box 9848
Canberra ACT 2601
Phone: +61 2 6289 9520
Toll free: 1800 020 103 (inside Australia only)
Fax: +61 2 6289 9197
Email: *nhmrc.publications@nhmrc.gov.au*

Australian Standards
http://www.standards.com.au/

CSIRO OHS Home Page
http://www.minerals.csiro.au/safety/saferes.htm

Manual Handling Centre
http://www.mhc.com.au/

Department of health

Australian Capital Territory Office
Ferntree House
8–10 Hobart Place
Canberra City ACT 2601
Phone: (02) 6274 5111
Freecall: 1800 020 102
TTY (02) 6274 5260
Fax: (02) 6274 5222

Northern Territory Office
Cascom Centre
13 Scaturchio Street
Casuarina NT 0800
Phone: (08) 8946 3444
Fax: (08) 8946 3400

South Australia State Office
55 Currie Street
Adelaide SA 5000
Phone: (08) 8237 8111
Freecall: 1800 188 098
Fax: (08) 8237 8000

Victoria State Office
Casselden Place
2 Lonsdale Street
Melbourne VIC 3000
Phone: (03) 9665 8888
Freecall: 1800 631 286
Fax: (03) 9665 8181
Central Office telephone: enquiries:
Phone: (02) 6289 1555
Freecall: 1800 020 103

New South Wales
73 Miller Street
North Sydney NSW 2060
Phone: (02) 9391 9000
Fax: (02) 93911 9101

Queensland State Office
Samuel Griffith Place
340 Adelaide Street
Brisbane QLD 4000
Phone: (07) 3360 2555
Freecall: 1800 177 099
Fax: (07) 3360 2999
North Queensland Office:
Phone: (07) 4727 2289
Freecall: 1800 019 030

Tasmania State Office
21 Kirksway Place
Battery Point TAS 7004
Phone: (03) 6221 1411
Freecall: 1800 005 119
Fax: (03) 6221 1412

Western Australia State Office
Central Park Reception
14th Floor 152-158
St George's Tce
Perth WA 6000
Phone: (08) 9346 5111
Freecall: 1800 198 008
Fax: (08) 9346 5222
Website:
http://www.health.gov.au/state.htm

terminology

Many dental and medical terms appear long and incomprehensible at first glance. However, almost all of them are made up of smaller parts joined together to make the whole word. If you use your commonsense, it is often possible to work out the meaning of the word.

The three parts that make up most medical/dental terms are:

❶ the prefix — this occurs at the beginning of a word to modify or add to its meaning; for example, hypo (too little, low);

❷ the suffix — this occurs at the end of a word to modify or add to its meaning; for example, ia (condition, state of); and

❸ the root word — this is the word base; for example, therm (relating to heat/temperature).

From these three parts, it is possible to work out the meaning of the word. The example here is hypothermia, which means the condition of having low temperature.

Prefixes

ana without; e.g. anaerobic, able to live without air or oxygen
a- or **an** absence of
aer, aero air, a prefix denoting relation to growth in air (e.g. aerobes)
bio denoting life
dens-, dent a tooth
dys painful, difficulty in
ecto situated on, without or on the outside
endo inside, within
exo outside, outward
gingiva gums
haema blood
hemi half
hydro water
hyper over, beyond the normal, excessive or above
hypo too little, low
intra into, within
mal bad, wrong
mega large
meso-, mesio middle
micro small
myo relating to muscle or muscles
odon-, odonto-, dent relating to a tooth or the teeth
ortho straight, correct
os a bone
oto ear
paedo/pedo children
para beyond, faulty or abnormal
per through, throughout
peri around, covering
poly many
post after
pre before
semi half
stomat/o mouth or oral cavity

Suffixes

-alg/algia pain
-aema/haema blood
-ectomy cutting out or excision
-ia condition, state
-itis inflammation
-ology science
-oma tumour, growth
-otomy incision, surgical cutting
-ostomy leaving an opening into
-phobia fear, dread
-pnoea breathing
-scope an instrument for examining
-therapy treatment

Root words

arthro joint
cardio heart
cerebro brain
derma skin
glyc sugar
hepato liver
neuro nerve
occlude come together, shut or close
oral mouth
os/osteo bone
oto ear
phagia swallowing
pneuma lung

Latin phrases in common use

in situ in the natural or normal place
in utero within the uterus
in vitro within glass; observable in a test tube
in vivo within the living body

Abbreviations — used in recording data in patient records

A/C	Account		NAD	Nothing abnormal detected
Adj	Adjustment		NP	New patient
AE comp	Acid etch composite		NV	Non-vital
AJC	Acrylic jacket crown		OHI	Oral hygiene instruction
Alg. imp	Alginate impression		OPG	Orthopantomogram
Am.R	Amalgam restoration		Ortho	Orthodontics
App.	Appointment		P/-	Partial upper denture
Ac/R	Account rendered		-/P	Partial lower denture
BA	Broken appointment		PA	Periapical radiograph
BP	Blood pressure		PDH	Previous dental history
BT	Broken tooth		Pedo	Pedodontics
Comp.R	Composite resin		Perio	Periodontics
Cr. Co	Chrome cobalt		Porc.	Porcelain
Endo	Endodontic		Post.	Posterior
Exo	Extraction		Pros.	Prosthodontics
F/-	Full upper denture		RA	Relative analgesia
-/F	Full lower denture		RCF	Root canal filling
#	Fracture		RCT	Root canal therapy
FTA	Failed to attend		Rest.	Restoration
GA	General anaesthetic		SnF 2	Symbol for stannous fluoride
GI	Gold inlay		T/A	Tooth ache
GIC	Glass ionomer cement		Temp. Rest	Temporary restoration
Imp.	Impression		TMJ	Temporo-mandibular joint
IRM	Intermediary restorative material		UE	Unerupted
LA	Local anaesthetic		UTA	Unable to attend
Mand.	Mandibular		V	Vital
Max.	Maxillary		VMK	Porcelain bonded to metal
M/guard	Mouthguard		Xbite	Crossbite
MMR	Maxillary mandibular relationship (bite)		ZOE	Zinc oxide eugenol

glossary

Abdomen The part of the body that contains the stomach, intestines and other organs. The abdomen is immediately below the chest but is separated from it by a sheet of muscle called the diaphragm.

Abrasion Abnormal wearing process due to friction. It may be caused by habits (chewing hard objects) or by poorly fitting retainers on removable appliances. The most common cause is the over-vigorous use of hard toothbrushes or abrasive toothpastes. Abrasion can also occur if the teeth are brushed immediately after contact with acidic drinks, when the enamel is still softened by the acid. Toothbrush abrasion lesions usually have very sharp edges, are often wedge shaped, and are located at the gingival margin (Class V). Occlusal abrasion is the normal wearing away of tooth substance under the stress of mastication.

Abscess A localised collection of pus within the tissues of the body.

Absorption Soaking up of a substance through the mass of another. For example, a stone cast, placed in water, will absorb the water.

Acute Of sudden onset. Having a short and relatively severe course.

Acute inflammation An immediate response to sudden or severe injury.

Adapted Well fitting. In the case of gingivitis, the gingiva is less well adapted to the tooth than healthy gingiva.

Aerobe Micro-organism that can only live in the presence of oxygen.

Aerosol Suspension of materials in vapour or gas. For example, fine spray created by the spinning of a high-speed handpiece and containing blood, saliva and micro-organisms.

Aetiology The causative factors which produce a disease.

Ala The fleshy parts on the outside edges of the nostrils.

Alignment The act of arranging in a line, the state of being arranged in a line.

Allergy Hypersensitivity to a substance.

Alloy Any mixture of metals. A silver/tin/copper/zinc alloy is used as a dental filling material when mixed with mercury.

Alveolar Relating to the alveolus (plural alveoli) or bone around teeth.

Alveolar process The portion of the maxilla or mandible that supports the teeth.

Alveolar ridge The residual ridge in which alveolar bone remains after loss of teeth.

Alveolectomy The operation of excising or cutting away any portion of the alveolar process.

Amalgam Any alloy in which one of the metals is mercury.

Anaemia Medical condition where there are too few red blood cells.

Anaerobe Micro-organism that can live in the absence of oxygen.

Anaesthesia General anaesthesia is a loss of consciousness produced by drugs. Local anaesthesia is loss of sensation of pain in a local area while the patient is still conscious.

Anaesthetic A drug that alters body function by acting on the central nervous system in producing loss of sensation, loss of consciousness, amnesia and loss of protective reflexes.

Analgesia Partial loss of feeling or sensation.

Analgesic Pain reliever. A drug that alters body function by acting on the central nervous system.

Anaphylactic shock An extreme form of allergic reaction associated with sudden swelling of the throat and oral cavity.

Anaphylaxis Sudden onset of allergic reaction which can include shock, cardiac and respiratory failure and which can be fatal.

Anatomy The study of the structures of the body.

Anginal pain A suffocating pain in the chest produced by an inadequate blood supply to the myocardial (heart) muscle.

Angle's classification A classification of the different forms of malocclusions set up by Edward Hartley Angle, an American orthodontist.

Ankylosis Fusion of a tooth to bone.

Anodontia The congenital absence of teeth. It may be partial (some teeth missing) or less commonly complete (all the teeth missing). Teeth most commonly missing are third molars, upper lateral incisors and lower second bicuspids. Complete anodontia occurs in some congenital syndromes, e.g. hereditary ectodermal dysplasia.

Anomaly Any marked deviation from that which is ordinary or normal.

Ante-mortem Before death.

Anterior Situated in front of. Used to denote the incisor and cuspid teeth or forward regions of the mouth.

Anterior teeth The four incisors and two cuspids of both jaws.

Anterograde amnesia Forgetting events that occurred after the anaesthetic was used.

Antibiotic A drug that alters the action of invading micro-organisms, either by destroying them (bacteriocidal action) or by interfering with their metabolism or reproduction (bacteriostatic action).

Antibody A substance produced in an animal (human) as a reaction to the presence of an antigen.

Anticariogenic Inhibiting or preventing the development of dental caries.

Antigen A substance that, under suitable conditions, stimulates an immunological response and reacts with antibodies.

Anti-inflammatory A drug that decreases the effect of inflammation on certain tissues of the body

Anti-pyretic Relieving or reducing fever.

Antiseptic A substance that inhibits the growth and development of micro-organisms without necessarily destroying them. Mostly used to clean skin.

Antrum An anatomical cavity within the bone, especially a sinus cavity.

ANUG Acute necrotising ulcerative gingivitis.

Apex (plural, apices) Tip or end of a tooth root. A general anatomic term for the top of the body, an organ or part, or the pointed end of a conical object.

Apexification Stimulation of the root-end formation following death of pulp in immature teeth.

APHG Acute primary herpetic gingivostomatitis.

Apical Relating to the apex of a tooth.

Apical foramen Small hole in root apex for the entry and exit of pulpal vessels.

Apicectomy Removal of the apex of a standing tooth.

Appliance A broad term commonly used to denote any dental prosthesis.

Apposition Cell growth into existing layers of cell.

Arches The arches formed by the teeth in the jaws. There are two arches; upper and lower, maxilla and mandible.

Artefact A substance, or structure not naturally present in tissue, e.g. an implant. On a radiograph, an artefact is any mark or image not related to the anatomy of the patient being examined. These may be fingerprints, earrings, scratches, etc.

Arterial pulse The heart contracts and beats approximately 70 times per minute but this varies from person to person and also in one person under different circumstances. The rate of the heart muscle contraction (or beat) can be felt as a wave of contraction along the arteries and is referred to as arterial pulse.

Arterioles Blood vessels smaller than arteries but larger than capillaries.

Articular cartilage Cartilage that covers and protects the joint surfaces of the bone.

Articular eminence The articular tubercle of the zygomatic process of the temporal bone, forming the anterior boundary of the mandibular fossa.

Articulating parts The parts that allow movement.

Articulating surfaces The surfaces between parts that allow movement.

Articulation Anatomical – a joint between bones, whether movable or not. Dental – the relationship of the upper teeth to the lower teeth, either natural, artificial or casts between the upper and lower teeth. Speech – the enunciation of words.

Articulator A mechanical device with movements simulating those of the temporo-mandibular joints, to which maxillary and mandibular models may be attached for the positioning of artificial teeth or of studying the manner in which the natural teeth meet.

Asepsis/aseptic Absence of infection, free from disease-causing micro-organisms.

Asphyxia Suffocation, lack of air/oxygen supply.

Aspiration The removal of fluids from a cavity by means of an aspirator.

Assault A wilful act without consent, an attack.

Atrophy The wasting away of tissue, organs or body parts from disease or defective nutrition.

Attrition Wearing away of tooth substance by friction from direct tooth-to-tooth contact. Some degree of attrition is considered physiological, due to normal chewing, and becomes more evident with age. Pathological attrition occurs in excessive tooth grinding (bruxism), and wear facets may be seen on the teeth. The process is accelerated when the enamel is worn away and the dentine exposed.

Autoclave A steriliser that utilises high-pressure steam and heat.

Autopsy Examination of a dead body to determine the cause of death.

Avulsed Knocked out.

Award Conditions of employment laid down by industrial legislation.

Axial surface Any surface of a tooth which is parallel to the long axis, such as the facial surface.

Axis An imaginary line through an object around which it might rotate.

Axon A threadlike extension from a nerve cell that transmits impulses outwards from the cell.

Bacillus (plural, bacilli) A rod-shaped micro-organism (bacterium).

Bacteria (singular, bacterium) Single-celled micro-organisms possessing no chlorophyll.

Bactericidal Able to destroy (kill) micro-organisms (bacteria).

Bacteriology The branch of medicine that deals with the study of bacteria.

Bacteriolysis The process of destroying bacteria by rupturing them.

Bacteriostatic Inhibiting the growth and reproduction of micro-organisms.

Band A thin strip of metal closely encircling the crown of a tooth horizontally (orthodontics).

Basal Metabolic Rate (BMR) The rate of energy utilisation during rest.

Bearing surface A load-supporting surface or point.

Benign Non-cancerous and generally not presenting a threat to health.

Bevel The slope or slant of a surface or edge (of an instrument).

Bicuspid A tooth with two cusps.

Bifurcation Division into two parts or branches, as any two roots of a tooth.

Bilateral Having two sides. Pertaining to both sides. Any partial denture having a major connector is said to be a bilateral appliance.

Bio-burden The types and numbers of micro-organisms on an item prior to sterilisation.

Biofilm A thin film of biological materials (including micro-organisms). Biofilms occur on many surfaces which are immersed in liquids, including instruments and parts of equipment. Bacterial dental plaque is a biofilm.

Biological indicator A system for testing the success or lack of success of the sterilising process.

Biology The science that deals with the structure and functions of living organisms.

Biopsy Diagnostic examination of a small piece of tissue removed from a living subject.

Bite A registration of the functional relationship between upper and lower arches (often in wax).

Bitewing A radiograph that includes only the crowns of the upper and lower teeth and is made by the patient biting on a right-angled projection from the centre of the film.

Blood dyscrasias A group of diseases involving the blood cells and the blood forming tissues.

Bone The material of the skeleton of most vertebrate animals.

Braces Metallic bands and appliances used to move teeth in the correction of the bite and tooth position. Known as orthodontic appliances.

Bracket A small metal attachment fixed to a band that serves as a means of fastening the arch wire to the band.

Bridgework The replacement of missing teeth with artificial teeth that are supported by the adjacent natural teeth. Bridges are usually fixed appliances.

Bronchioles Smaller branches of the bronchi which carry air to all parts of the lungs.

Bronchodilator A drug used by asthmatics to relax air passages to the lungs and make breathing easier.

Bruxism Grinding or gnashing movements of the teeth, especially during sleep.

Buccal Relating to the cheek or mouth, e.g. the buccal surface of a tooth is the surface next to the cheek.

Buccal frenum The stringlike mucous membrane which attaches the cheek to the alveolar ridge in the bicuspid region of each arch.

Buccal groove The groove which extends from the occlusal surface down into the buccal surface of a molar.

Buccal notch The v-shaped notch in the impression or denture by or for the buccal frenum.

Bur A rotary instrument used in a dental handpiece for cutting and smoothing tooth substance and dental appliances. Alternative spelling – burr.

Burnish To polish by friction; e.g. adapting the margins of a gold inlay to the tooth structure.

Calcification The process by which organic tissue becomes hardened by a deposit of calcium salts within its substance. The term 'calcification' is used in dentistry with a liberal interpretation to denote the disposition of any mineral salts which contribute toward the hardening and maturation of tooth tissue.

Calcified Become hard or stiff because of the deposit of calcium salts.

Calculus (tartar) Calcified material deposited on the teeth from the saliva composed chiefly of lime salts. A calcified mass found in a salivary gland or duct. Dark calculus found on the tooth surface under the gingival margin – sub-surface calculus.

Cancellous bone Mesh-like, or honeycomb bone as opposed to solid or cortical bone.

Cancer Any malignant new or abnormal growth or neoplasm.

Canine See cuspid.

Carbohydrates and sugars Chemical compounds that include starches.

Cardiac muscle Specialised heart muscle.

Cardiovascular system Another name for the circulatory system.

Caries Dissolution of the calcified tissues of the tooth by acid produced from ingested refined carbohydrates and micro-organisms in dental plaque. The process by which cavities are formed in teeth by gradual destruction of enamel and dentine.

Carrier A person who carries a pathogenic organism but who does not necessarily become sick. A person who has had a disease and recovered can be a carrier. Carriers can still pass the disease on to other people.

Cartilage Strong elastic tissue.

Cassette The metal 'plate' that holds an extra-oral x-ray film; e.g. an OPG film. Cassettes hold two intensifying screens.

Cast A reproduction of all or part of a dental arch in a material such as dental plaster or dental stone.

Cavity The excavation produced by decay in a tooth.

Cellulitis Inflammation of cellular tissues extension of acute infection into the soft tissues.

Cement A type of filling material used in dentistry.

Cementum A hard tissue that forms a protective layer over the root and to which the fibres of the periodontal membrane are attached.

Centric occlusion The relation of the occlusal surfaces of the teeth of one arch to those of the other when the jaws are closed and the teeth are said to be in the position of physical rest.

Cephalometry The measurements of the dimensions of the human head taken either directly or by means of x-ray.

Cervical Pertaining to the neck or to any cervix; i.e. that portion of the tooth near the junction of crown and root.

Cervix The neck of the tooth – a neck or constricted position.

Chemical indicator A dye that changes colour to show that a steriliser has reached the required temperature during the sterilisation process.

Chronic Long, continued, not acute.

Chronic inflammation A less dramatic but more prolonged response either due to slight irritation over a long period, or following incomplete resolution of an acute inflammation.

Ciliated mucous membrane A moist lining that secretes mucous and that is covered in tiny hairs (ciliated).

Cingulum A lingual elevation within the cervical third of an anterior tooth. A band-like enamel ridge rising crown-wise from the cervix.

Cleaning The process of reducing the bio-burden (any contamination that adheres to a surface).

Cleft palate A congenital fissure along the midline of the roof of the mouth, where the two bones of the hard palate have failed to meet during foetal development.

Closed bite A condition where the intermaxillary space is less than it should be.

Coccus (plural, cocci) A round-shaped micro-organism.

Collagen A protein found in connective tissue, skin and bone. It is fibrous.

Commensal A parasitic organism living on or within a host deriving benefit without harming the host.

Compound fracture A fracture in which there is an external wound leading to the break in the bone.

Concave Curving inward; dished in.

Condyle The rounded eminence of the mandible that fits into the socket (fossa) of the joint.

Congenital Occurring in the offspring before birth.

Congenital disease Any disease present at birth. A hereditary congenital disease is genetically transmitted to successive generations; e.g. haemophilia, Down syndrome. An acquired congenital disease develops in the foetus, often due to environmental influences such as maternal illness or lifestyle. Many of these are preventable e.g. rubella, effects of drugs, smoking. Some congenital diseases, such as cleft lip and cleft palate, occur due to incomplete development for unknown reasons.

Contact point The point at which adjoining teeth surfaces come together.

Contagious Communicable to other people, as a disease. Carrying or spreading a disease.

Contamination The condition of being soiled or impure as a result of contact or the addition of a foreign material or organism.

Contract An agreement between two or more parties. It can be verbal or written; e.g. making an appointment or an employment contract. The person entering a contract must be of legal age (18 years or over). A breach of contract is when part or all of a contract is broken.

Contractile Able to contract or tighten.

Contrast On a radiograph this is the difference in densities in adjacent areas of the film; e.g. dentine and enamel. Some areas are very dense, some are not dense.

Convex A surface which is curved outward toward the viewer; mounded.

Coronal Referring to the crown or visible part of the tooth.

Coronal plane An imaginary line that divides the body into front and back.

Corpuscle A cell in the blood or lymph.

CPR Cardiopulmonary resuscitation.

Cross-bite A condition in which maxillary teeth are in lingual version to mandibular teeth, bilateral, unilateral or involving only a pair of opposing teeth.

Cross-infection The indirect transfer of pathogenic organisms from one person to another.

Crown The part of the tooth that is covered with enamel (the part of the tooth usually visible in the mouth).

Culture medium Nutrient substance used to grow biological materials under controlled conditions.

Cusp An elevated, pointed portion of a crown of a tooth.

Cuspid A long, single rooted tooth, the crown of which consists mainly of one cusp.

Cutaneous Relating to the skin.

Cyanosis Blueness of the skin, especially the lips and nail beds, caused by insufficient oxygenation of the blood.

Cyst An epithelium-lined cavity that contains liquid or other materials, often present at the apex of a tooth.

Cytoplasm All of the parts of a cell apart from the nucleus.

Dappen dish A small glass or disposable plastic bowl, used for holding liquid dental materials during a procedure.

Debridement Removal of any foreign matter from tissue (e.g. root canal).

Decalcification Loss or removal of calcium salts from hard tooth substance.

Decay See caries.

Deciduous teeth Teeth of the primary dentition that are shed naturally.

Decontamination Removal of bio-burden from used articles or surfaces to make them clean.

Deglutition Swallowing.

Dehydrate To remove the moisture from a substance.

Dendrite An extension from a nerve cell that receives impulses from other nerve cells and transmits them to the centre of the cell.

Density On a radiograph this is the overall blackening or darkening of the radiograph when viewed by transmitted light such as from a viewing box.

Dental dam A thin sheet of rubber used to exclude moisture and maintain a sterile field during cavity preparation and endodontic procedures.

Dental dam clamp A spring clip that holds the dental dam around the neck of an isolated tooth.

Dental dam forceps Instruments used to place dental dam clamps on teeth.

Dental dam holder A metal or plastic frame or strap device used to hold the dental dam in position over the mouth, keeping the edges clear of the field of operation.

Dental dam punch An instrument used to punch holes of various tooth sizes in a dental dam.

Dental floss Waxed or unwaxed thread or tape used to clean in interproximal spaces of teeth as an oral hygiene homecare procedure.

Dental laboratory Manufacturer of dental prostheses; e.g. dentures.

Dentalgia Toothache.

Dentate Having natural teeth.

Dentifrice Tooth paste or powder.

Dentine The main mineralised substance of the tooth that surrounds the dental pulp and is covered by enamel on the crown and cementum on the root.

Dentistry The science that treats the dental apparatus, including its relation to the body as a whole.

Dentition The character, number and arrangement of the teeth. The process of eruption of a tooth.

Denture A set of artificial teeth which replaces some or all of the natural teeth.

Detergent A surface active cleaning agent, including soap, used for cleaning.

Diagnosis The determination of the character and kind of a medical or dental condition.

Diastema Naturally occurring spaces between teeth, and commonly between maxillary anterior teeth, particularly the central incisors.

Disease An illness or sickness. A disturbance in the function or structure of any part of the body.

Disinfection The destruction of pathogenic organisms and their products. The inactivation of non-sporing organisms by heat or chemical treatment.

Dislocation Displacement of any part from its normal position.

Distal Those surfaces farthest from the midline of the dental arch.

Distensible Able to expand.

DNA and **RNA** Deoxyribonucleic acid and ribonucleic acid. Chemicals that contain genetic information.

Downward displacement autoclave An autoclave in which steam gradually replaces any air in the autoclave.

Drill See bur.

Droplets Minute particles of moisture expelled by talking, sneezing or coughing and that may carry infectious micro-organisms.

Drug Chemical compounds, either naturally occurring or synthetic, administered to alter the function of the body or of an invading pathogen.

Drug Register A record of drugs kept, when drugs were used and to whom drugs were administered or given.

Dry socket Inflammation of a tooth socket following an extraction, due to loss of the blood clot from the socket, leading to inflammation of surrounding bone and delayed healing.

Dsyphagia Difficulty in swallowing.

Duct A passage or tube through which secretions and excretions can pass.

Ductless gland Because secretions go directly into the blood stream, endocrine glands are referred to as ductless glands.

Eccentric Off centre.

Ectopic Located away from the normal position.

Edentulous Without teeth.

Endoscopy Insertion of a tube into the body for diagnosis.

Electron microscope A very powerful, electronic magnifier.

Electrosurgery Surgery performed with a special electric tip that can cut away excess tissue and control excessive bleeding.

Elevator An instrument used as a lever to loosen and/or remove a tooth or tooth root.

Embolus May be a blood clot, bacteria or an air bubble that blocks a blood vessel. It may be carried to other parts of the body (e.g. the brain) by blood vessels.

Embryology The science of the development of structures during the early stages of life.

Eminence A projection or prominence; e.g. frontal.

Enamel The hardest tissue in the body. The mineralised tissue that covers the crown of a tooth.

Endodontic implant Metal post cemented to root canal and extending into jawbone to stabilise loose tooth.

Endodontics The branch of dental science that deals with the soft tissues within the teeth; i.e. pulp and root canal therapy. The treatment of the roots of non-vital teeth and the pathology associated with teeth.

Endotoxin Toxin or poison released on destruction and rupture of a pathogen.

Environmental wrapping Using plastic or foil barriers on equipment to minimise cross-infection.

Enzymes Proteins produced by cells and which start biochemical reactions.

Epiglottis A leaf-shaped flap at the entrance to the larynx. It assists in closing the airway when food is swallowed. It prevents food from 'going down the wrong way'.

Epilepsy A medical disorder that can result in loss of consciousness and convulsions or 'fits'.

Epithelium The skin and mucous membrane are types of covering tissue in which the first layer is epithelium. Epithelium is a thin layer of tissue that, as well as other things, lines the internal cavities.

Equilibrium A state in which the body's processes are in balance.

Erosion Loss of tooth substance due to chemical causes and not bacterial or frictional causes. A common cause is excessive consumption of acidic drinks, juices or sports drinks. It can also occur from acid regurgitated into the mouth in bulimia, anorexia and gastric reflux. In some cases erosion occurs for unknown reasons. This is known as idiopathic erosion.

Eruption The emergence of a tooth through the mucous membrane covering the jaws.

Erythema Redness of the skin due to widened blood vessels near the surface.

Erythrocytes Red blood cells.

Eustachian tube A tube that connects the middle ear to the back of the throat. The tube allows air pressure on both sides of the eardrum to equalise.

Excavator A hand instrument used for the removal of caries from a decayed tooth.

Exodontia That branch of dentistry that deals with the extraction of teeth.

Exotoxin Toxins produced and actively released by living pathogens.

Explorer or probe Also called a probe. An essential instrument on a basic examination tray. Used to detect carious cavities and marginal integrity of restorations.

Exposure The removal of the protecting enamel and dentine from the pulp of a tooth.

Extra-oral Outside the mouth.

Extrinsic Outside – (as opposed to inside or intrinsic).

Exudate Fluid rich in plasma proteins, cell materials and debris, usually present when there is inflammation.

Facebow A caliper like device used to record the relationship of the upper jaw to the temporo-mandibular (jaw) joint.

Facultative pathogens 'Good' micro-organisms that are capable of causing disease if they invade tissues and multiply.

Faecal-oral route Transfer of organisms from faeces to the mouth (usually because of lack of adequate hand-washing).

Filamentous Long strands of cells joined end to end.

Filling The procedure of inserting a material into a prepared tooth cavity. The material used in this procedure. A restoration.

Fissure A defect or crack in the enamel of the crown of a tooth.

Floss See dental floss.

Fluoridation The introduction of therapeutic quantities of fluorides into the water or the diet.

Fluoride A chemical compound SnF_2 that reacts with tooth enamel to make it more resistant to decay.

Fluorosis Hypoplasia and/or discoloration of teeth caused by excess concentrations of fluorides in the diet or water supply.

Flutes Cutting edges on endodontic instruments.

Foramen A naturally occurring hole in bone through which pass blood and lymph vessels and nerves.

Forceps Hand instruments with two beaks and handles, used to grasp and remove teeth. Fine instruments used to grasp flaps of tissue, blood vessels or pieces of bone or tooth.

Fossa A depression or pit; e.g. a depression on the surface of a tooth or bone.

Frenum (also fraenum) A membranous band of tissue; e.g. the mucous band that attaches the upper lip to the alveolar process above the incisor teeth, the fold that attaches the tongue to the floor of the mouth. Also called frenum, frenulum.

Full denture An appliance that replaces all the natural teeth of a dental arch.

Furcation Junction where the roots of a multi-rooted tooth meet.

Gag To retch without vomiting. A mouth gag is a device to prevent the closure of the teeth during dental procedures.

Gauge The diameter of the tube through which the solution passes into the tissues.

Gangrene The breakdown or necrosis of a part of the body (e.g. toe or foot) due to a lack of blood supply.

Gangrenous pulp An infected and dead pulp.

Germ Any micro-organism, especially pathogens.

Germicide An agent (usually a chemical) capable of killing some micro-organisms.

Gingiva (plural, gingivae) Gum tissue. It is a specialised form of oral mucosa quite distinct from mucous membrane.

Gingival margin trimmer Chisel used to bevel gingival enamel margins.

Gingival papillae The portion of the gingiva found between the teeth in the interproximal spaces below the contact areas. Also known as interdental papillae.

Gingivectomy The surgical removal of free gingival tissue at the level of the gingival attachment. This creates new marginal gingiva. Such a procedure may be indicated for a variety of reasons in the treatment of periodontal disease.

Gingivitis Inflammation of the gingivae.

Gland An organ of the endocrine system, a collection of cells that produce secretions.

Gnatho-dynamics The science of the movements of the jaw.

Gram-negative and gram-positive bacteria Bacteria can be classified by their reaction to a dye, called gram's stain. Micro-organisms are classified as gram positive (purple staining) or gram negative (pink staining).

Granuloma Collection of granulation tissue around the root apex following chronic untreated infection of the root canal.

Grinding surface The outer, biting (occlusal) surface of the posterior teeth used to crush food.

Gum See gingiva.

Gutta percha A rubber-like material used for filling root canals in endodontic therapy.

Haematoma (bruise) A haematoma is a localised collection of usually clotted blood in an organ, space or tissue.

Haematopoiesis The formation of blood cells.

Haemoglobin A substance in red blood cells that enables oxygen to be transported to the cells of the body.

Haemophilia A medical condition in which the blood clots more slowly than normally.

Haemorrhage Bleeding.

Haemostatic agent A substance that arrests bleeding.

Halitosis Unpleasant breath.

Handpiece or drill A mechanically operated instrument into which are placed burs, discs, stones and other cutting instruments used in cavity preparation and other cutting operations.

Hatchet A hand instrument used for trimming enamel margins.

Hemisection Cutting and removing one half of a tooth or jaw.

Heparin A substance present in the tissues and especially in the liver, which acts as an anticoagulant (anti-clotting).

Heredity Characteristics passed on from parents to children before birth.

Herpes A type of viral infection.

Herpetic keratoconjunctivitis A debilitating herpes infection of conjunctiva of the eye.

Herpetic paronychia A very painful infection of the nail beds.

Histamine A naturally occurring substance in body tissues that is released as a response to injury and allergy caused by animal stings, irritant chemicals and antibodies.

Histology The science that deals with the study of the microscopic structure of tissues.

Holding time The minimum time at which instruments in an autoclave must be held at a temperature that has been established to destroy all micro-organisms. See also penetration time and sterilisation time.

Homeostasis A state of equilibrium maintained by a cell or organism through biochemical processes.

Host Any living organism that parasites live on or within.

Hydrocolloid A type of dental impression material.

Hyperaemia Presence of excessive amounts of blood in tissue.

Hyperglycaemia A medical condition where the patient has too much sugar in the blood.

Hyperplasia Increase in the size of an area of tissue due to an increase in the production of the number of its cells.

Hypersensitivity A more than normal reaction to a stimulus.

Hypertensive Abnormally raised blood pressure.

Hypertrophy Increase in the size of an area of tissue due to an increase in the size of cells. Often due to an increased work demand of the existing cells.

Hypnotic A drug that alters body function by acting on the central nervous system. Hypnotics induce sleep.

Hypodermic needle A hollow needle used with a syringe for injection.

Hypoglycaemia A medical condition where the patient has too little blood sugar.

Hypoplastic enamel (**hypoplasia**) Under-development of enamel tissue.

Hypothalamus An area at the base of the brain which controls many of the body's automatic and hormone-related activities.

Hypoxia A state of reduced oxygen in the blood.

Iatrogenic Brought about by (dental or medical) treatment. Treatment-related condition.

Idiosyncrasy A tendency, individual peculiarity or characteristic.

Immediate denture A denture inserted immediately after the removal of the natural teeth.

Immunisation The process of rendering a person immune and protecting them against certain diseases.

Immunity Natural or acquired resistance to specific diseases or poisons. May be natural or acquired.

Immunosuppressed Weakened resistance to infection, possibly as a result of disease (e.g. HIV) or medication (e.g. chemotherapy).

Impacted tooth A tooth positioned in the jaw in a way that prevents it from erupting normally.

Impression A negative likeness obtained by using an impression material. Dental impressions are taken of the teeth and supporting tissues, and models are cast from them.

Impression tray A receptacle into which impression material is placed and is used to convey this material to the mouth. It then supports the impression material while it is setting.

Incisal Relating to the cutting edges of incisor teeth.

Incision A cut into body tissue.

Incisor teeth Term used to indicate the four anterior teeth of either jaw, which are the biting teeth.

Infection The successful invasion of the body tissues by pathogenic organisms. A person may have an infection but may not necessarily be contagious.

Infectious/contagious Causing or communicating infection.

Inferior Situated below.

Infiltration The introduction of a solution (usually an anaesthetic) into the tissues (e.g. those surrounding the teeth).

Inflammation The healing response of the body to disease or injury. The purpose is to: destroy and remove the cause of injury; limit and localise the extent and injury; and repair and replace the damaged tissue.

Informed consent When a patient makes an appointment for treatment it is implied that consent is given for treatment but this has no legal status. Before giving consent to proceed with treatment the patient is entitled to be fully informed of: the type of treatment; the alternatives (if any); the number of appointments needed; the cost of the treatment; any known side effects; and the prognosis. The parent or guardian must act (and sign) on behalf of a minor or a developmentally challenged person.

Injection The forcing, under pressure, of a liquid into some part or tissue of the body.

Inlay A type of restoration that is cast to fit a tooth cavity and cemented into position. Inlays are usually constructed from gold alloys, porcelain and composite.

Inorganic Chemically — a substance which contains no carbon. Biologically — pertaining to inanimate material (e.g. salt and sand).

Insertion The act of placing a finished denture or other appliance in the oral cavity.

Intensifying screens Sheets of semi-rigid plastic with fluorescent crystals rolled into them. The crystals fluoresce when x-rays strike them. This property is used to reduce exposure times, and thus patient radiation dose.

Intercusping The relation of the cusps of the premolars and molars of one jaw with those of the opposing jaw during any of the occlusal relations.

Interdigital spaces The spaces between the fingers.

Interproximal Between neighbouring (tooth) surfaces.

Intramuscular Within or into a muscle or muscles.

Intra-oral Within or into the oral cavity.

Intraosseous Within or into a bone.

Intravenous Within or into a vein.

Intrinsic Situated entirely within.

Investment Any mould material used in the processing or casting of dentures, crowns or inlays.

Irrigation The process of washing out a cavity using a liquid (usually a saline solution).

Ischaemic A localised lack of blood supply to a tissue causing it to look blanched.

Jaw The part of the skull concerned with mastication; i.e. the maxilla and/or mandible.

Junction (of hard and soft palate) The imaginary line at the beginning of movement of the palate; the boundary of the hard and soft palate.

Keratinised mucosa Mucous membranes that are becoming fibrous and hard.

Keratinising Able to produce keratin, which is a fibrous protein that is the basis of hair and nails. Keratinised epithelium has a tough, protective layer.

Kerato-conjunctivitis Inflammation of the cornea and the conjunctiva of the eye.

Kilojoules Formerly called calories, the unit used to express the fuel or energy value of food.

Labial Relating to the lip. The surface of the tooth that faces the lip.

Laboratory Manufacturer of dental prosthesis or working area where these are prepared in the surgery.

Lamina dura The layer of bone lining a tooth socket (literally hard layer).

Lateral Relating to the side.

Lesion An abnormality in structure, arrangements or functions of a part. Any hurt, wound or local degeneration.

Leucocytes White blood cells.

Leucopoenia A deficiency in the number of white cells in the blood. It may cause necrotic lesions in the mouth of a patient.

Leukaemia A condition caused by an excess of white cells in the blood.

Ligature A cord used for tying blood vessels.

Lingual Relating to the tongue. The surface of a tooth facing the tongue.

Litigation Legal action.

Lobe The part of tooth formed by any one of the separate points of the beginning of calcification A segment from which a natural tooth develops.

Local anaesthetic A drug that alters body function by acting on the central nervous system and producing loss of sensation in an area to be treated.

Long axis An imaginary line which might be drawn in a vertical plane through the centre of a tooth.

Lumen The bore or inner width of a tube.

Luting The sealing of the junction of two substances, such as a crown on a tooth, with a fine-grained cement, such as GIC or zinc phosphate.

Luxation Loosening of a tooth from traumatic injury.

Lymphadenopathy Swollen glands.

Macroscopic Large enough to be seen with the naked eye.

Maintainer A device developed to fill a gap created by the loss of a tooth. A method to prevent malocclusion.

Malaise Illness, feeling unwell.

Malignancy Tumour or neoplasm characterised by rapid growth, non-capsulated, invasive, destructive of the surrounding tissues, composed of uncharacteristic cells of the host tissue, capable of metastasis and usually fatal.

Malignant Cancerous; a tumour that invades surrounding tissue and can spread to other parts of the body.

Malleability The property of metal which permits it to be extended in all directions without breaking.

Malocclusion Abnormal occlusion of the teeth. An occlusion and positioning of the teeth that is not in accordance with the usual anatomical rule or form.

Mandible The lower jaw.

Mandibular fossa A fossa is a hollow or groove in a bone. The mandibular fossa is a hollow in the mandibular bone.

Mandrel A spindle or shaft used to hold cutting stones and polishing discs which is attached to a handpiece.

Marginal ridge The ridge at the outer margin of the occlusal surface of molar and bicuspid teeth.

Marrow Soft fatty tissues that fill the hollow cavities of bones.

Mastication The act of chewing.

Masticatory apparatus The first part of the digestive system contained in and around the oral cavity.

Matrix A framework. Basic material that binds together to form a mass or bulk.

Matrix band A thin band of metal or plastic used to provide a temporary tooth wall during the placement of a restoration.

Matrix retainer An appliance for holding a matrix band in position e.g. Tofflemire.

Maxilla The upper jaw.

Maxillary sinus A large cavity enclosed within the body of the maxilla below the orbit.

Medullary cavity The cavity in long bone which holds the bone marrow, where blood cells are formed.

Membrane A thin layer of tissue covering a part, or separating adjacent cavities.

Mesial That surface of a tooth facing towards the midline of the dental arch.

Mesiodens A supernumerary tooth is between the upper central incisors.

Metabolic activity Chemical interactions that provide the energy and nutrients needed to keep the organism alive.

Metabolism Chemical interactions that provide the energy and nutrients needed to keep an organism alive.

Metastasis Transfer of a malignant cell from one part of the body to another through blood or lymph vessels to form a secondary lesion.

Microbiology The study of micro-organisms.

Micro-organism Single cell form of plant or animal life visible only by means of a microscope.

Microscope An optical instrument for magnifying minute objects.

Midline A plane that divides the body into right and left equal halves.

Mineralisation The addition of minerals, such as calcium, to the body, which hardens certain tissues such as teeth and bone.

Mitosis The way a cell divides into two daughter cells that both have the same number of chromosomes as the original cell.

Mixed infection An infection caused by a variety of organisms.

Model or cast A model of the impression of the jaws or other structures, usually poured in a type of artificial plaster or stone.

Molar Grinding tooth. One of the multi-cusped teeth situated in the posterior part of the mouth.

Monitoring (the sterilising process) A programmed series of challenges and checks, repeated periodically and carried out according to documented protocols that demonstrate that the process being studied is both reliable and repeatable.

Morphology (tooth) The study or science of the form and structure of teeth.

Motile (mobile) Capable of independent movement.

Mucosa Moist epithelium and connective tissue. A moist lining that secretes mucous.

Mucous membrane Tissue containing mucous glands that lines the oral cavity and other internal cavities of the body.

Mutation The ability of viruses to change their genetic code so that they become resistant to current conditions and efforts to kill them.

Narcotic A drug that alters body function by acting on the central nervous system. Narcotics are the drugs of addiction. They relieve anxiety and pain, can induce sleep and a general feeling of wellbeing. Capable of causing loss of consciousness. May be addictive.

Necrosis Localised death of cells and tissue.

Necrotic Dead.

Negligence A careless act. Omitting to do something that a reasonable person, guided by the principles ordinary people live by, would do, or doing something that a prudent and responsible person would not do.

Neoplasm Abnormal swelling or lump in tissue. May be benign (walled off from surrounding tissue and only causing trouble due to size and interference with function) or malignant.

Neurones Nerve cells.

Non-vital tooth Tooth in which the pulp has died.

Nosocomial infection A localised or systemic condition that results from adverse reaction to the presence of an infectious agent or its toxin(s) and that was not present or incubating at the time of admission to hospital or other health care facility. That is, an infection developing in hospital or 14 days after leaving hospital.

Nucleus The central part of a cell vital to its functions, growth and reproduction.

Obtundent A pain-relieving agent.

Obturation Root filling.

Obturator (oral) A prosthetic appliance used to close an opening in the roof of the mouth. These openings are usually deformities patients are born with, (cleft palates) or the result of surgery for cancer.

Occlude To bring together, hence to bring the upper and lower teeth together.

Occlusal rims Equipment used to record the MMR (maxillo-mandibular relationship). That is the relationship of the upper to the lower jaw (the maxilla to the mandible). In the dentate individual this is established by the teeth in occlusion. In the edentulous person it is determined by the use of bite rims, also known as occlusal rims or bite blocks.

Occlusal surfaces (of teeth) The grinding surfaces of molars and premolars. Those surfaces of the teeth that come together when the jaws are closed.

Occlusal trauma Injury brought about by malocclusion.

Occlusion The natural closure and fitting together of upper and lower teeth. The relation of the mandibular and maxillary teeth when efficiency is obtained. When the teeth of the mandibular arch come into contact with the teeth of the maxillary arch in any functional relation, occlusion is established.

Odontalgia Toothache.

Odontoblasts Specialised cells surrounding living pulp, lining the inner dentine walls, responsible primarily for dentine formation.

Oedema Swelling produced by the accumulation of fluid in the tissues.

Oesophagus Long tube that passes through the neck (behind the trachea) and chest (behind the heart and lungs) and into the abdomen.

OHS Occupational Health and Safety.

Open bite More than the correct amount of jaw opening.

Operculum A structure like a lid or cover; e.g. a flap of gingival tissue over a partially erupted tooth.

Oral cavity The cavity forming the entrance to the alimentary canal; i.e. the mouth.

Oral clearance time The time taken for food to clear the mouth.

Oral hygiene The care of the teeth and the preservation of healthy tissues in the mouth.

Oral prophylaxis Preventive treatment for gingivitis and periodontal disease including the removal of calculus and other irritating material.

Oral surgery The type of dentistry dealing with extraction of teeth, soft tissue surgery, bone surgery and fracture repair and removal of pathology in the region of the mouth and face.

Organelles Specialised cell parts that are responsible for specific functions.

Organic matter Matter made of living things (cells, for example).

Organs Body parts. Each of these is a complete and independent part of an animal and has a specific function.

Orthodontic band A strip of metal formed so as to encompass the crown of the tooth on a horizontal plane. When employed in tooth movement procedures, the banding permits bodily movement of the teeth. A succession of welded orthodontic bands, when applied onto adjoining teeth with cementation, is useful for tooth stabilisation.

Orthodontics The specialty in dentistry concerned with the prevention and correction of abnormalities in tooth position and their relationship to the jaw.

Osseous tissue Bone.

Osteitis Inflammation of bone.

Osteoblast A cell from which bone develops.

Osteoclast A cell in bone that assists with the development of cavities and canals in the bone.

Osteogenic cells Bone-forming cells.

Osteomyelitis Inflammation of bone that includes the bone marrow.

Overbite That characteristic of the teeth in which the incisal ridges of the maxillary anterior teeth extend below the incisal edges of the mandibular anterior teeth when the teeth are placed in centric occlusal relation. The vertical overlap of the upper over the lower teeth.

Overdenture Also known as an overlay denture, this is a removable full or partial denture constructed over specially prepared natural teeth. It may involve the use of magnets to assist retention or the use of devices known as precision attachments that retain and stabilise the denture.

Overjet That characteristic of the teeth in which the incisal ridges or buccal cusp ridges of the maxillary teeth extend labially or buccally to the incisal ridges of buccal cusp ridges of the mandibular teeth when the teeth are in centric occlusal relation. The horizontal overlap of the upper teeth over the lower teeth.

Pack A dressing used on the gingiva and about the teeth during treatment of periodontal disease or after gingivectomy. A gauze and cotton wool pad placed over a tooth socket to prevent haemorrhage following tooth extraction.

Paedodontics (paediatric dentistry) The practice of dentistry restricted to children. The study and treatment of dental diseases and abnormalities in childhood.

Palatal Relating to, or facing the palate.

Palate Roof of the mouth.

Palliative effect Providing pain relief.

Papilla (plural, papillae) A small nipple-like protruberance.

Paraesthesia Partial loss of sensation.

Para-medical and para-dental auxiliaries Medical or dental staff member whose work supplements or supports medical or dental practitioners in their work. Dental auxiliary is sometimes used as a collective name for staff who work with, alongside or for dentists; i.e. dental assistants, dental receptionists, hygienists, dental therapists and technicians.

Parasite Any plant or animal (including micro-organisms) that derives its sustenance from another living organism.

Parenteral feeding Nutrients administered by infusion or injection into the tissues, not through the alimentary canal.

Parotid gland Parotid salivary glands lying below the ear on each side of the face. The largest of the salivary glands.

Partial denture A denture that replaces some of the natural teeth in one jaw.

Pathogen A micro-organism capable of causing disease.

Pathogenic Capable of initiating infection.

Pathogenic load The number of potentially disease causing micro-organisms on an item.

Pathology Structural and functional changes caused by disease or the study of those changes.

Pellicle Complex protein derived from saliva.

Penetration time The time required for every part of the load in an autoclave to reach the required temperature for sterilisation to take place. See also holding time and sterilisation time.

Periapical The region around the apex of the tooth root.

Pericoronal Around or in the region of a tooth crown.

Pericoronitis Inflammation of the soft tissues around the crown of an erupting or impacted tooth. A condition frequently associated with impacted or erupting third molars.

Periodontal ligament The ligament surrounding the root of the tooth and acting as a sling attaching the root to the alveolar bone (also called periodontal membrane).

Periodontics The type of dentistry that involves the treatment of soft supporting tissues (gums) of the teeth and surgical procedures for dental implants.

Periodontitis Inflammation of the periodontal ligament.

Periosteum The dense fibrous tissue closely adapted to the surface of a bone to which muscles attach.

Periphery The circumference or outer border of an object. The circumferential boundary.

Peristalsis Wave-like intestinal muscle contractions that move food and waste through the body.

pH hydrogen ion concentration. Neutral pH is 6.8 to 7.0. Anything lower is increasingly acid. Anything above is increasingly alkaline.

Phagocytosis The engulfing and destruction of invading pathogens by the phagocytes in white blood cells.

Pharmacology The study of drugs and their action.

Phonetics Pertains to the production of sounds in speech.

Physiology The science that deals with the normal functions of the body.

Pit A sharp pointed depression in the tooth enamel.

Plant Equipment including fixtures, e.g. dental unit.

Plaque Dental plaque is an organised colony of micro-organisms (i.e. bacteria) contained within an organic matrix and adhering to the tooth surface.

Plasma proteins There are two main types of protein present in plasma – albumin and globulin. These provide osmotic pressure to keep the fluid part of blood inside the vessels, to act as antibodies against infection and to help in the formation of blood clots, among other things.

Plaster A gypsum material used to make casts and investments for denture processing.

Plastics Materials used for filling cavities such as cements, gutta percha, acrylic resins and amalgam. Substances produced by chemical condensation used to make artificial teeth and dentures or to restore the size or shapes of a natural tooth.

Plugger A hand instrument used to condense dental amalgam into a tooth cavity.

Pocket formation An abnormal space developing between the tooth root and the gum.

Porcelain A material used in making denture teeth and ceramic crowns.

Positioner A resilient removable appliance covering the maxillary and mandibular teeth. Used to achieve limited repositioning of the teeth.

Posterior Behind, in the rear.

Potent Strong, powerful.

Potentiate Increase the effectiveness of a drug.

PPE Personal protective equipment.

Precision A specially machined male and female part used in some partial dentures for attachment of the teeth.

Premolar A bicuspid.

Prescription A written instruction for the preparation, composition and administration of drugs. A written instruction from a dentist to a dental technician for the construction of a prosthetic appliance.

Primary herpetic gingivostomatitis An inflammation caused by herpetic infection and involving more than the gingiva (i.e. oral and perioral mucosa, tongue, lips, cheeks, fauces, etc.). There are also major systemic symptoms.

Prion A protein capable of causing disease.

Probe A slender, sharp, flexible instrument used during an oral examination.

Process A part that grows on or sticks out on an organism. A slender projection of bone.

Prognosis An estimation of the probable course of a disease or condition.

Prophylaxis Measures taken for the prevention of dental or oral diseases and abnormalities. These include the removal of calculus and plaque from teeth.

Prosthesis An appliance to take the place of a natural part.

Prosthetics (dental) that branch of dental science that deals with the restoration of lost parts of the dental apparatus.

Prosthodontics The type of dentistry that involves full and partial replacement of fractured or lost teeth or other parts of the facial anatomy.

Protoplasm The liquid contents of a living cell.

Protrusion The condition of being thrust forward, such as the protrusion of the incisor teeth.

Protuberance Projecting part.

Proximal Next to, adjacent. Those surfaces of teeth that adjoin each other in the same dental arch.

Pulp The vascular connective tissue containing blood vessels and nerves within the pulp chamber and enclosed by dentine.

Pulp capping Protective cover over exposed pulp.

Pulpectomy Removal of the dental pulp from a tooth.

Pulpitis Inflammation of the pulp.

Pulpotomy Removal of part of the pulp of a tooth.

Pus Thick, yellow semi-liquid substance made up of a collection of dead tissue cells, micro-organisms and white blood cells resulting from an inflammatory response.

Putrefaction The decomposition of organic matter under the influence of micro-organisms and resulting in foul smelling discharge.

Quantity rate A rate some dental supply companies offer as a discount if you buy in bulk.

Quick cure resin Auto-polymerising acrylic resin.

Radicular Root part of the tooth.

Radiographs Often called x-rays. Exposed x-ray films.

Radiography Creating an image on film by passing x-rays through something.

Radiology The science of interpreting x-ray films (radiographs) in medical and dental practice.

Radiolucent Offering little resistance to the passage of x-rays, allowing them to travel through the area.

Radiopaque Resistant to the passage of x-rays.

Reamer A thin corkscrew-like instrument used for enlarging and cleaning root canals.

Recession The gradual shrinking back of the gums, leaving the tooth cervix, and part of the root, exposed.

Record(s) Files containing information about the registration and treatment of patients. Interocclusal record(s) relate upper and lower models during mounting on, and adjusting on, an articulator.

Red marrow Marrow that is rich in blood tissue. Produces blood cells.

Replantation Replacement of an avulsed tooth.

Resorption Physiological removal of tissue or body products, such as the roots of deciduous teeth, or of some of the alveolar process after the loss of the adult teeth.

Retractor A surgical instrument for drawing back the edges of a wound to allow access to deeper structures. Cheek and lip retractors used to improve access and visibility during a procedure.

Retrograde cavity preparation (also retrograde root filling) A filling placed surgically at the root apex.

RNA Ribonucleic acid. Chemicals that contain genetic information.

Root That part of the tooth that is enclosed in a socket of the alveolar bone. That part of the tooth covered by cementum.

Root canal The cavity in the long axis of the root of a tooth that contains the dental pulp.

Root planing Smoothing of root surfaces during scaling.

Rubber dam See dental dam.

Rugae Folds or ridges of tissue on the anterior part of the hard palate.

Sagittal An imaginary plane that divides the body into right and left sides.

Saliva The natural fluid of the oral cavity excreted by the salivary glands.

Saliva ejector A small bore apparatus (suction tube) used to suck saliva from the mouth during operative procedures.

Sanitising To reduce microbes to an acceptable level. A term normally used in the hotel or catering industry.

Saprophyte An organism that lives on decaying or dead matter.

Scaler An instrument used for the removal of calculus.

Scalpel A surgical knife.

Scavenger unit An exhaust system used to eliminate any stray fumes while using nitrous oxide.

Sedative Drug that alters body function by acting on the central nervous system. Sedatives relieve apprehension and anxiety.

Septicaemia Presence and multiplication of micro-organisms and their toxins in the blood. Blood poisoning.

Sequelae Events or circumstances after a procedure or event.

Sequestration Separation or splintering of a part of bone.

Sequestrum A piece of bone that has died due to lack of blood supply and separated from its original bone.

Serous A watery fluid.

Shell crown A metal cap designed to fit the prepared tooth and reproduce the crown. Usually made of gold plate.

Sinus Natural cavities in some bones of the skull; e.g. maxillary sinus or antrum. Drainage point, on a gingival surface, from a chronic abscess. A tract or channel through which pus is discharged.

Sloughing Dead tissue separating from live tissue.

Smear A small collection of material spread onto a glass slide for microscopic examination.

Smooth muscle Muscles responsible for the involuntary movements, such as transporting food in the alimentary canal.

Soil Visible dirt or debris that can allow micro-organisms to grow on an item.

Solder To join two metals with a third by means of heat.

Solvent A substance that is capable of dissolving another substance. For example, water is a solvent for salt.

Somatic Of the body, as opposed to of the mind.

Spacer An appliance used to prevent adjacent and opposing teeth from moving into a space.

Spatula A flexible blunt instrument used for mixing dental materials.

Spirochaete A wavy, spiral-shaped threadlike micro-organism.

Statute of limitations An Act of parliament that restricts the time after which legal proceedings can be brought. There is a time limit placed on people being able to sue for negligence or assault, etc.

Sterile Germ free, aseptic.

Sterilisation The complete destruction of all living organisms.

Sterilisation time The total time required for sterilisation to occur after the autoclave chamber has reached sterilising condition. It includes penetration time, holding time and a safety factor. See also holding time and penetration time.

Sterilised The state of being free from all forms of microbial life, including spores.

Steriliser An apparatus used for sterilisation.

Stimulus Anything that registers on our senses; e.g. light, pinprick, etc.

Stomatitis Widespread diffuse inflammation of the soft tissues of the oral cavity (gingiva, mucosa, lips, cheeks, tongue).

Stone A gypsum product used to make casts.

Striated muscle Muscles attached to the skeleton and capable of voluntary movement.

Subgingival plaque Plaque that forms in the gingival sulcus.

Subgingival scaling Scraping away of subgingival calculus.

Submandibular Below, under the mandible.

Substrate A substance containing particular enzymes.

Sulcus Groove or fissure, e.g. a groove on the surface of a tooth or the vestibule of the mouth.

Supernumerary teeth Extra teeth beyond the normal complement. They are often small, pointed and peg shaped. Fourth molars are not uncommon. The most common location for a supernumerary tooth is between the upper central incisors, when it is called a mesiodens. Some supernumeraries erupt normally, and others are detected during radiography.

Supplemental grooves A shallow linear groove in the enamel of a tooth. It differs from a developmental groove in that it does not mark the junction of lobes.

Suppuration Formation of pus.

Suture Natural junction of two bones. A fixed joint. A surgical thread for tying and sewing.

Symbiosis Two unlike organisms living together in which each benefits without having any effect on of the other.

Symphisis A junction of two bones separated by fibrocartilage. A fixed joint.

Synapse Junction between two neurones that transmit nerve impulses from one to the other.

Syncope Fainting. Temporary unconsciousness caused by cerebral anoxia.

Synovial membrane The innermost of the two layers of a synovial joint capsule. It is comprised of loose connective tissue that has a free smooth surface that lines the joint cavity and secretes a lubricant, the synovial fluid.

Syringe An instrument for injecting a liquid.

Systemic effect For example, nitroglycerine tablets placed under the tongue are absorbed through the mucosa and dilate the coronary arteries of the heart.

Tartar See calculus.

Tempering The procedure of imparting to a metal a desired degree of hardness, also called heat hardening. Not commonly used for dental alloys.

Temporo-mandibular joint The joint between the mandible and the base of the skull. The head of the condyle moves in the glenoid fossa.

Therapeutic Using pharmacological knowledge to prevent or treat disease, and for the relief of pain.

Therapeutics A branch of pharmacology: the art of using pharmacological knowledge in the prevention or treatment of disease and for the relief of pain.

Thermoplastic Materials that soften under heat and solidify when they are cooled with no chemical change taking place.

Thoracic Chest.

Thrush Candida albicans or monilia.

Tissue A group of cells in an organism. The four basic types of tissue are nerve, muscle, epithelial, and connective tissues.

Tissue retractor See retractor.

Torque A twisting force. A rotary force causing part of a structure to twist about an axis. In orthodontics, a rotation of a tooth on its long axis.

Toxin Poison. The product of metabolism in a pathogenic organism and which is poisonous to the host.

Toxoid A treated toxin, without its harmful properties, used to stimulate production of antibodies.

Tracing A line or lines or a pattern scribed by a pointed instrument or stylus on a tracing plate or tracing paper, used in orthodontics.

Tranquillisers A drug that relieves anxiety.

Trauma A physical injury.

Traumatic occlusion or bite An abnormal occlusal stress that is capable of producing, or has produced, injury to the tooth and/or its supporting structures.

Trigeminal nerve One of a pair of cranial nerves that supplies movement and sensation to the jaw, face and nasal cavity.

Trismus or lockjaw Spasm. Inability to open the jaws.

Trituration The art of reducing a substance to a fine state by grinding, rubbing or pounding. Also used to indicate the mixing of dental amalgam alloy with mercury and other capsulated materials.

Tubercle A small prominence or projection.

Ulcer An open sore in the soft tissues of the body. A break-down in the epithelial layer of skin and mucous membrane through its full layer, leaving underlying tissues exposed and raw.

Ultrasonic cleaning The cleaning off of debris by the use of ultrasonic waves passed through water containing detergent. This is done in preparation for heat sterilising.

Unerupted tooth A tooth that has not erupted into the mouth.

Uraemia Blood in the urine.

Utero (in utero) In the womb.

Validation The set of procedures used to obtain results, record them and interpret them to establish the efficacy of a procedure.

Vasoconstrictive Causing blood vessels to constrict (tighten) and reduce blood flow.

Vasoconstrictor A drug used in local anaesthetic solutions to prevent the anaesthetic agent from rapid systemic distribution by constricting the blood vessels near the injection site. By keeping the anaesthetic localised they prolong the analgesic effect of the solution and decrease bleeding in the treatment area and reduce the risk of any infection spreading from the treatment site.

Vector An organism, such as an insect, that carries disease from one sick person to another.

Vector transmission Transmission of a disease via a vector. For example, a mosquito or a tick can carry infected blood from one animal to another.

Vestibule Entrance. That part of the mouth between the cheeks and lips and the alveolar ridge.

Vicarious liability The employer is responsible for any negligent act of an employee if committed in the course of work.

Virucidal Capable of killing viruses.

Virulence The capacity of an organism to overcome the body's defences. An organism can have high or low virulence. Organisms capable of causing severe infection are said to be highly virulent and those producing only minor infections possess low virulence. A highly virulent disease is one that can overcome the body's defence mechanisms.

Virulent Extremely poisonous, infectious or damaging to organisms.

Viscosity A measure of a liquid's resistance to flow or its relative fluidity.

Vital Living.

Weld A process whereby metals are joined by the use of heat and pressure, or by the use of pressure alone, as with gold foil.

Xanthodont Person with yellow teeth.

Xerostomia Dry mouth due to lack of saliva production. May be caused by various medications and head and neck radiotherapy.

Yellow marrow Marrow that is rich in yellow fatty tissue where white blood cells are produced.

acknowledgments
for figures

Bath-Balogh, M and Ferenbach, MJ (1997) *Illustrated dental embryology, histology and anatomy.* WB Saunders, Sydney. Figures 8.4; 9.1; 9.8.

Bird, DL and Robinson DS (2002) *Torres and Ehrlich Modern Dental Assisting* (7th edn). Saunders, Philadelphia. Figures 8.10; 8.11; 8.15; 8.18; 17.1; 33.2; 33.4.

Children's Health Development Foundation (1998) *Australian Guide to Healthy Eating.* Children's Health Development Foundation, South Australia. Figure 28.1.

Cree, L and Rischmiller, S (2001) *Science in Nursing* (4th edn). Harcourt, Sydney. Figure 7.1.

Darby, ML and Walsh, MW (2003) *Dental hygiene theory and practice* (2nd edn). Saunders, Philadelphia. Figure 27.3 (adapted from p. 361).

Daskalogiannakis, J (2000) *Glossary of orthodontic terms.* Quintessence Publishing Co, Inc, Chicago. Figures 34.1 – 34.4; 34.8; 34.10; 34.11.

Kodak, Health Sciences Test (1989) *Radiodontic Pitfalls* (out of print). Figures 21.10 – 21.23.

Miles, DA, van Dis, ML, Jenson, CW and Ferretti, AB (1999) *Radiographic imaging for dental auxiliaries* (3rd edn). WB Saunders, Sydney. Figure 21.1 (adapted from p. 74); 21.4.

Robinson, DS and Bird DL (2001) *Ehrlich and Torres Essentials of Dental Assisting* (3rd edn). Saunders, Philadelphia. Figures 7.1; 7.3 (p. 28).

index

Lightning Source UK Ltd.
Milton Keynes UK
UKHW032018301219
356137UK00003B/17/P